THE DAY-BY-DAY
Pregnancy
BOOK

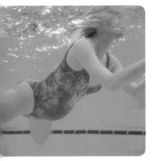
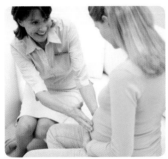
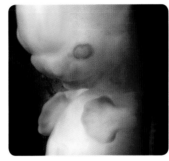
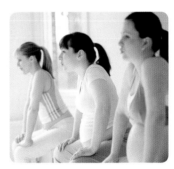
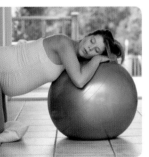
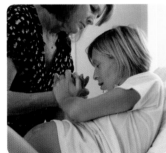
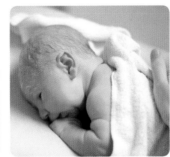
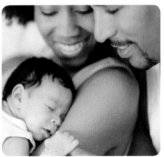

Editor-in-chief **Dr Maggie Blott**

Consultant Obstetrician

LONDON, NEW YORK, MUNICH, MELBOURNE, DELHI

Project Editors Dawn Bates, Claire Cross
Project Designers Emma Forge, Tom Forge, Peggy Sadler
Senior Editors Andrea Bagg, Anne Yelland, Emma Woolf
Senior Art Editors Sarah Ponder, Nicola Rodway, Liz Sephton
Production Editor Ben Marcus
Production Controller Alice Holloway
Creative Technical Support Sonia Charbonnier
Illustrators Debbie Maizels, Medi-Mation
Picture Researcher Sarah Smithies
Managing Editors Esther Ripley, Penny Warren
Managing Art Editors Glenda Fisher, Marianne Markham
Publisher Peggy Vance

UPDATED EDITION
Project Editor Martha Burley
Design Assistant Kate Fenton
Senior Pre-Production Producer Tony Phipps
Creative Publishing Manager Anna Davidson
Managing Art Editor Christine Keilty

Every effort has been made to ensure that the information
in this book is complete and accurate. However, neither the
publisher nor the author is engaged in rendering professional
advice or services to the individual reader. The ideas, procedures,
and suggestions contained in this book are not intended as
a substitute for consulting with your healthcare provider.
All matters regarding the health of you and your baby require
medical supervision. Neither the publishers nor the author shall
be liable or responsible for any loss or damage allegedly arising
from any information or suggestion in this book.

First published in Great Britain in 2009
by Dorling Kindersley Limited
80 Strand, London WC2R 0RL

This revised edition published in Great Britain in 2014
by Dorling Kindersley Limited

ISBN: 978-1-4093-4518-3

Printed and bound by South China Printing Co. Ltd
Reproduction by MDP, Bath

Discover more at **www.dk.com**

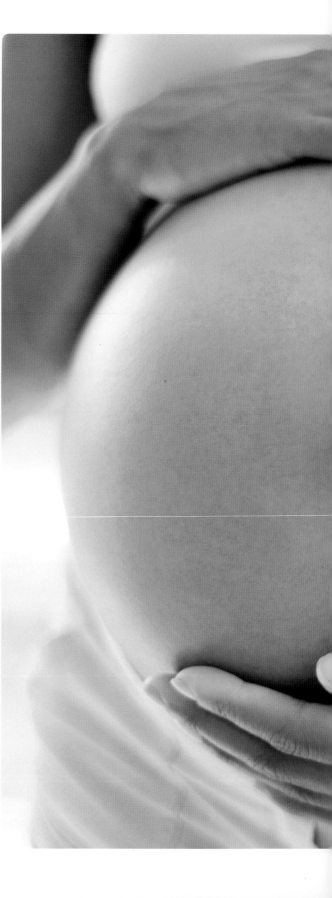

THE DAY-BY-DAY
Pregnancy
BOOK

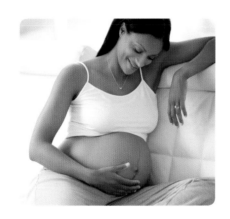

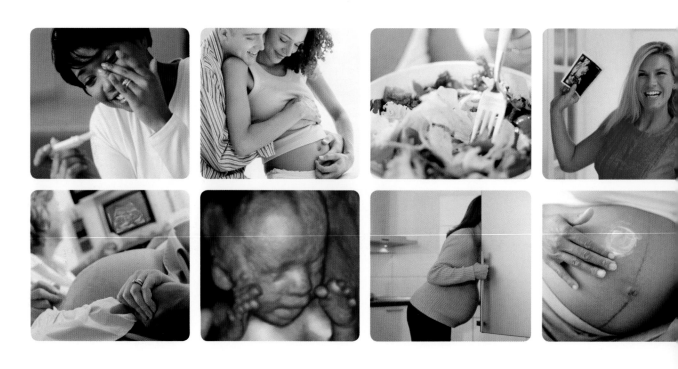

Comprehensive advice from a team of experts,
and stunning images for every single day

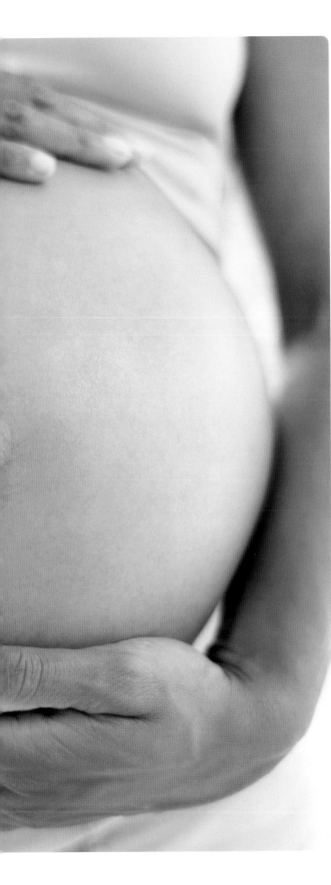

Editor-in-chief

Dr Maggie Blott MB BS, FRCOG

Dr Maggie Blott has worked for over 30 years in Obstetrics
and Gynaecology. Former Consultant Obstetrician at Kings
College Hospital and University College Hospital in London,
she was spokesperson for the Royal College of Obstetricians
and Gynaecologists and has also written a magazine column
for women with gynaecological problems. Dr Blott currently
works as an Consultant Obstetrician and Gynaecologist
in Abu Dhabi, where she is actively involved in antenatal
care and delivery.

Contributors

Dr Carol Cooper MA, MB, BChir (Cantab), MRCP General Practitioner,
London; Tutor at Imperial College School of Medicine, London

Ms Friedericke Eben FRCOG Consultant Obstetrician and
Gynaecologist, Whittington NHS Trust and Portland Hospitals, London

Dr Katrina Erskine MD, MRCP, MRCOG Consultant Obstetrician and
Gynaecologist, The Homerton Hospital, London

Dr Laura Goetzl MD, MPH Professor and Vice Chair for Research,
Department of Obstetrics and Gynecology, Division of Maternal
Fetal Medicine, Temple University, Philadelphia, Pennsylvania

Dr Belinda Green PhD Midwife, University College London Hospitals,
NHS Foundation Trust, London

Dr Deirdre Guerin MB BCh, BAO, LRCP and SI, FFA, or CSI Medical
Director of Resident Obstetric Services and Consultant Anaesthetist,
The Portland Hospital for Women and Children, London

Amanda Hutcherson DipHeMid, RM, PGCert Ed, MA Midwife
Practitioner, London

Dr Philippa Kaye MB BS Hons, MA Hons (Cantab), DCH, MRCGP,
DRCOG, DFSRH Works in general practice

Dr Su Laurent MRCP, FRCPCH Consultant Paediatrician, Barnet
Hospital, London

Mr Andrew Loughney PhD, MRCOG Consultant Obstetrician, The
Royal Victoria Infirmary, Newcastle upon Tyne

Dr Paul Moran MD, MRCOG Consultant Obstetrician, Head of Fetal
Medicine, Royal Victoria Infirmary, Newcastle Upon Tyne

Melinda Nicci BA (Psych), HDipEd Fitness and lifestyle coach and
founder of baby2body: pregnancy and post pregnancy health and fitness

Catharine Parker-Littler SRN, RSCN, SCM, DPSM (Advanced
midwifery), BScMid (Hons) Practising midwife; founder and former
midwifery director of midwivesonline.com, a website for midwives,
healthcare professionals, and parents-to-be

Dr Hope Ricciotti MD Associate Professor of Obstetrics, Gynecology,
and Reproductive Biology, Harvard Medical School, Beth Israel
Deaconess Medical Center, Boston, Massachussetts

Dr Vincent M. Reid PhD Lecturer in Developmental Psychology,
Durham University

Dr Mary Steen RGN, RM, BHSc PGCRM, PGDipHE, MCGI, PhD Professor
in Midwifery and Reproductive Health, University of Chester

Karen Sullivan ASET, VTCT, BSc Developmental Psychology; Childcare
expert and author

Sally Watkin Pregnancy and parenting author

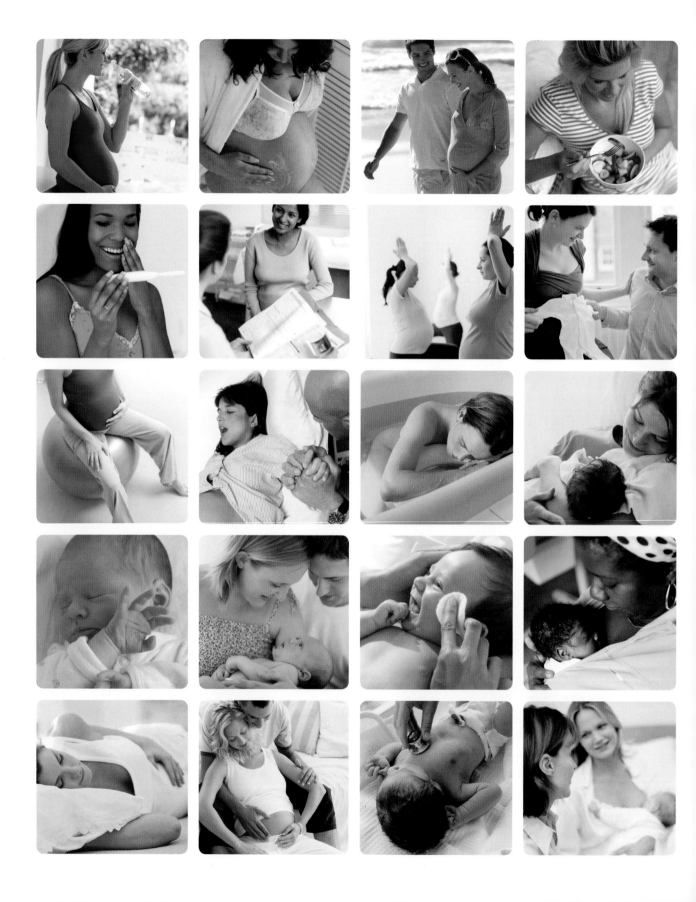

Contents

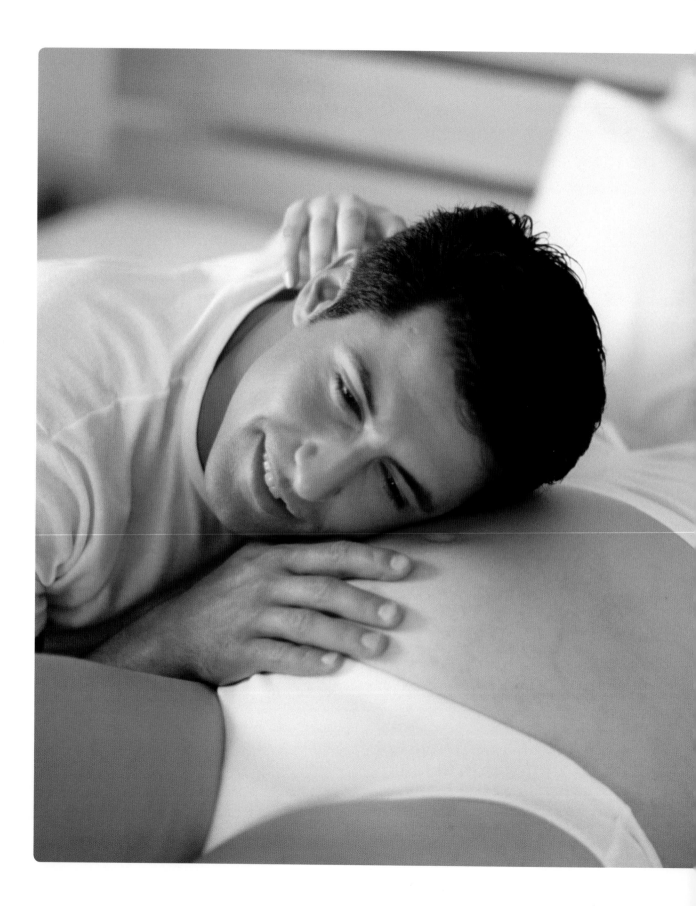

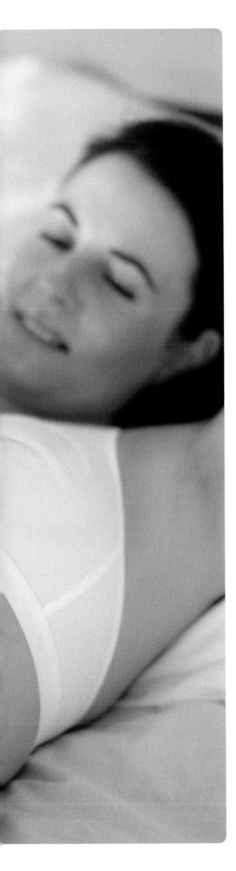

Introduction

Pregnancy is an exceptional time when women enter one of their most significant life stages and need to assimilate quickly knowledge and understanding of the process of pregnancy and birth. In the past, when women traditionally gave birth at home, cared for by midwives and female relatives, pregnancy and birth was a familiar event. Today, it's unusual to have such first-hand experience and a woman's knowledge of pregnancy and birth is often non-existent or limited to that which she gained in her first pregnancy. As a result, many, if not all, women contemplate pregnancy with a mixture of trepidation and curiosity. These feelings are often compounded by the recognition that their own lifestyle choices can have an enormous influence on their own and their baby's health. For all these reasons, there is a great need for women to be able to access information about pregnancy that is accurate, balanced, and accessible.

In *The Day-by-Day Pregnancy Book* information is gathered from a wide body of professionals, each with his or her own area of expertise. The midwives, doctors, obstetricians, and paediatricians who have contributed the core information in this book have between them cared for thousands of women at each stage of pregnancy and labour, delivered thousands of babies, and provided care and support for women and their babies after the birth. The exhaustive record of pregnancy, birth, and the postnatal period provided by their combined expertise is complemented by specialist knowledge on diet and exercise from a nutritionist and a lifestyle and exercise coach. The information presented – at once practical, detailed, and full of simple explanations and advice – will provide the vital tools women need to help them plan for pregnancy, negotiate the many changes they will experience, and develop a safe and appropriate birth plan.

Most pregnancy books are written for women. Today, many men also wish to follow closely the development of their unborn child, but have little information and often feel excluded. Within this book there are reassuring explanations for partners about the changes that occur during pregnancy as well as advice for women on how to include partners during pregnancy and the early days of parenthood.

Margaret J. Blott

Dr Maggie Blott

How this book is organized

This book starts with guidance on how to enjoy a healthy and safe pregnancy, with lifestyle advice that often applies to the preconceptual period, too. The core section of the book gives a day-by-day account of pregnancy with detailed explanations of the physical and emotional changes that take place in your body along with fascinating insights into how your baby develops within the uterus. A labour and birth chapter takes you through the delivery of your baby, followed by a summary of the first two weeks with your new baby. A final chapter deals with concerns and complications in the mother and baby in pregnancy, labour, and the postnatal period.

A healthy pregnancy

This chapter provides the information you need to make lifestyle choices that will maximize your own health throughout pregnancy and give your baby the best possible start in life. It includes guidelines for exercising safely, eating healthily, avoiding hazards, and dealing with illnesses. It also addresses concerns you may have about how the emotional and physical changes of pregnancy may impact on your relationships.

Pregnancy day by day

Here, the book takes you day by day through the extraordinary story of conception and pregnancy, counting down each of the 280 days until the onset of labour. Each day reveals how your baby is developing and the changes that are occurring in your body. The 280 days, or 40 weeks, of pregnancy are divided into three trimesters, each of which comprises around a third of the pregnancy. Apart from being a simple measure of time, each trimester represents a distinct phase in the development of the baby and in the pregnancy.

The first trimester The definition of the first trimester is given in this book as weeks 1–12, though you may also see weeks 13 and 14 included in other books. This trimester covers the time from the beginning of the menstrual period to the moment of conception, which is usually around two weeks. As the exact moment of conception is unknown, pregnancy is counted from the one definite date, the start of the menstrual cycle. Although technically your pregnancy may not begin until two weeks into your menstrual cycle, these two weeks are very important in helping your body to achieve a healthy pregnancy. Here, we explain day by day the changes that take place in your uterus to prepare it for conception and implantation of the early embryo, and offer dietary advice and recommendations from fertility experts to boost your chances of conceiving.

The first trimester is a period of extraordinary development, when all your baby's major organs form, and he or she will grow faster than at any other period in life. A day-by-day account is given of the changes that you and your baby undergo, and advice offered on how to cope with the exhausting changes that occur in early pregnancy. There's also an honest appraisal of the emotional feelings you're likely to experience, reassuring you that negative as well as positive emotions are normal. Practical information

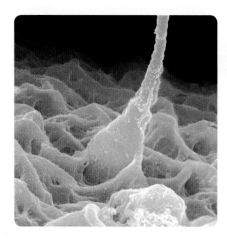
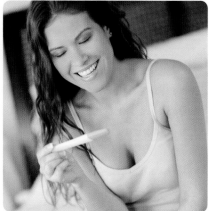
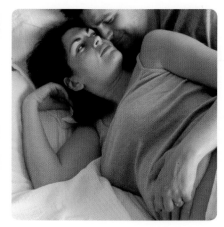

on accessing antenatal care and detailed explanations of the choices that are available help you begin to plan your pregnancy and think about your options for the birth.

The second trimester In the second trimester, which is designated as weeks 13–25, your baby's organs mature further and growth continues. This is an exciting time as your body starts to change shape to accommodate your growing baby and you feel your baby move for the first time. However, it is also a time when women can experience symptoms that are often due to quite normal pregnancy changes but that can occasionally indicate a problem. For example, abdominal pain can be due to ligaments being stretched or to constipation; however, it could also indicate a problem with the placenta. Symptoms such as these are discussed at the relevant point in pregnancy, with detailed explanations that will provide reassurance or alert you to the possibility of something more serious that should be brought to the attention of your midwife or doctor.

The third trimester In the third trimester, designated as weeks 26–40, your baby continues to grow and mature and, if born early, could survive life outside the uterus. During this time, your body starts to prepare itself for labour. We describe the changes taking place and explain why they occur, as well as providing pointers to what is normal and which symptoms need to be reported to your midwife or doctor. Women recount their experiences, and questions that are presented daily to doctors and midwives are reproduced to provide a bank of vital knowledge. Practical guidance on all matters, from maternity leave entitlement to reassurance that having sex won't harm the growing baby, helps you to navigate your way through the final weeks of pregnancy.

Labour and birth

One of the best ways to cope with labour is to understand its stages. In the labour and birth chapter, a team of professionals covers in detail the progress of labour, each providing their own expert insight. A midwife writes about normal births and discusses natural pain relief. An anaesthetist gives the options available for medical pain relief, including detailed descriptions of how epidurals are given and their pros and cons. While most women have a normal birth without complications, on average 25 per cent have a Caesarean section, and around 10 to 12 per cent have a ventouse or forceps delivery. An obstetrician writes about difficult births, describing complications and the medical interventions that may be required.

The first two weeks

Here, the early days as you adjust to life with your new baby are charted in the day-by-day format. A paediatrician addresses the practical issues of babycare, while a midwife focuses on the emotional and physical renewal you undergo as your body recovers from the birth and you step up to the new tasks of nurturing and feeding your baby.

Concerns and complications

This reference section is a concise guide to conditions in pregnancy and labour, and postnatal concerns in the mother and baby. Clear explanations enable you to digest medical information, understand which symptoms are not of concern, and feel reassured about how more serious conditions are managed in pregnancy, labour, and the postnatal period.

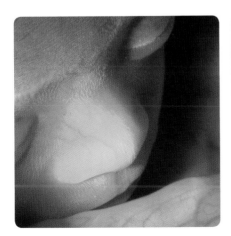
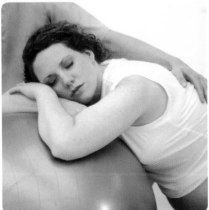
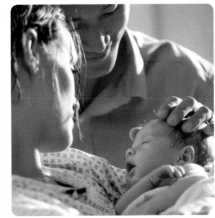

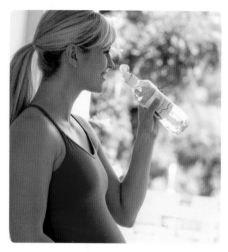 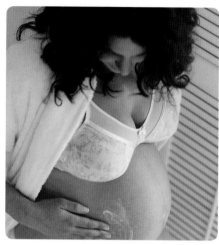 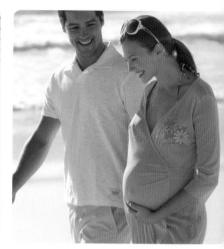

In pregnancy, feelings of awe and excitement are often mingled with concerns about your own and your baby's wellbeing. With an ever-growing body of knowledge on how a mother's behaviour in pregnancy impacts on her baby's short- and long-term health, women today have the opportunity to ensure that their lifestyle choices positively benefit their babies. Eating healthily, exercising regularly, and avoiding hazards will all help to give your baby the best possible start in life.

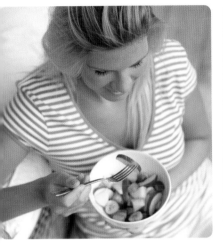 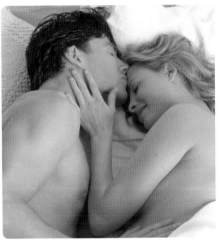 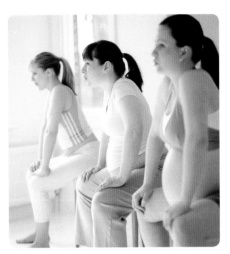

A healthy pregnancy

Your pregnancy diet

You can optimize your own health and your baby's future health by eating a nutritious, balanced diet throughout pregnancy.

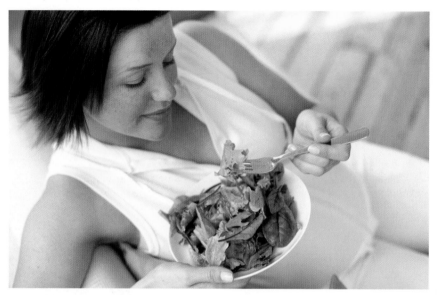

Eating regular nutritious meals and snacks throughout the day is vital during pregnancy to keep your energy levels up, and to provide your growing baby with all he needs to develop well.

In recent years, much has been learnt about what constitutes a healthy diet in pregnancy. The importance of folic acid (see p.16) in preventing birth defects is now well established and there is mounting evidence that many aspects of a person's future health may be influenced by the mother's diet in pregnancy. Current thinking is that good nutrition in pregnancy may reduce a baby's future risk of diseases such as obesity, diabetes, and heart disease.

As well as influencing your baby's health, good nutrition in pregnancy also optimizes your health, helping you to cope with the demands of pregnancy.

A healthy diet

Getting the right balance of protein, carbohydrates, and fats in pregnancy is simple, as the ratios are the same in pregnancy as at other times: 50–60 per cent of your calories should come from carbohydrates; 25–35 per cent from fats; and 20 per cent from protein. The components of these nutrients don't need to be in this exact ratio for each meal, or even every day, but you should aim to achieve this balance over the course of a week. A diet that includes plenty of vegetables, fruits, whole grains, and good proteins and fats will automatically contain the proper mix of nutrients.

Carbohydrates

Carbohydrates are an important source of fuel for you and for your baby as they are broken down into glucose, which passes easily across the placenta. Aim for four to six servings a day, a serving being equivalent to a slice of bread, 60g (2oz) of cereal, or 75g (2½oz) cooked pasta.

Carbohydrates are divided into two subgroups: refined and unrefined. In general, white is bad when it comes to carbohydrates, as refined foods such as white rice and white breads are rapidly broken down and enter the bloodstream in the form of a spike of glucose. It has been suggested that this spike may have health implications, such as a larger baby and risk of obesity later in life, but as yet there's no evidence to confirm this.

Unrefined carbohydrates are less processed, so they break down more slowly in the bloodstream and release glucose steadily. They are also a good source of fibre, which helps to prevent constipation. These are a healthier choice, and at least half, if not all, of your carbohydrates should come from unrefined sources. Examples include wholewheat or multigrain bread; brown rice; and wholewheat pasta and cereals.

Protein

Protein is essential for the growth of the baby and the placenta, as well as for your health. Pregnant women need around 60g (2oz) each day. Aim for two to three servings of protein-rich foods a day, a typical serving being 85g (3oz) red meat, or 150g (5oz) fish. As most adults get about 100g (3½oz) of protein daily, there is usually no need to increase your intake, especially if you have protein at each meal. If you're vegetarian, as well as protein at each meal, you should have a protein-containing snack. If you're having twins or more, you need around 80g (3oz) daily, and when breastfeeding, 70g (2½oz) daily.

Choose protein sources that contain less saturated fat, such as skinless chicken, lean beef and pork, tofu, low-fat cheese and yogurt, and skimmed milk. Fish, nuts, and seeds contain healthier unsaturated fats (see opposite), although your intake of some fish should be limited as they contain mercury, which could be harmful to your baby (see p.96).

Fats

Fats contain vitamins and contribute to the healthy development of cells. However, although fats make a useful contribution to overall nutrition, their intake needs to be limited. Choose healthier unsaturated fats, found in foods such as fish and some types of oil, over unhealthy saturated fats found in full-fat dairy products and meat, or trans fats found in processed foods.

Omega 3 fatty acids Studies suggest that the development of the baby's nervous system may be boosted by omega 3 fatty acids, the richest source of which is found in fatty fish. Avoid fish high in mercury (see p.96); opt instead for fish such as salmon and sardines, which are good, safe sources of omega 3 fatty acids. Wild salmon is very rich in omega 3, but farm-raised salmon is also a good source. Other sources include omega 3-enriched eggs, flaxseed, flaxseed oil, walnuts, rapeseed (canola) oil, and omega 3 supplements and antenatal vitamins containing omega 3 fatty acids.

Dairy products

These are an important component of the diet as they provide a good supply of proteins and fats, as well as calcium and some vitamins. Calcium is essential for the healthy development of bones and teeth. Opt for low-fat dairy products and semi-skimmed milk. Aim for 2–3 servings each day, a typical serving being 30g (1oz) of hard cheese, or 200ml (⅓ pint) milk.

Vitamins and minerals

In pregnancy, you need to ensure a rich supply of vitamins and minerals, as these are important for your own health and for your developing baby. They support the healthy functioning of body systems and contain antioxidants, which protect the body against the effects of harmful chemicals called free radicals.

Eating a healthy, balanced diet is of paramount importance in pregnancy to help you cope with the extra demands on your body and to provide your developing baby with essential nutrients. By eating a wide variety of healthy foods, you will ensure that you and your baby receive the correct balance of nutrients. Include a range of foods each day from each of the major food groups (see opposite), eat lots of fresh fruit and vegetables, and drink plenty of water to avoid constipation.

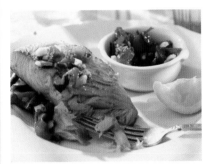

Include 2–3 portions each day of protein-rich foods, such as fish, lean meat, chicken, pulses, cheese, and nuts, to ensure the healthy growth of body structures.

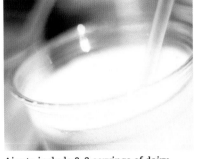

Aim to include 2–3 servings of dairy products each day. Ideally, these should be low-fat products, such as semi-skimmed milk and low-fat cheese and yogurts.

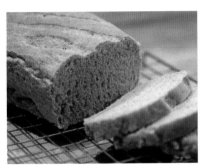

Have 4–6 servings daily of unrefined carbohydrates, such as brown rice and wholewheat breads and pasta, to keep up energy levels and ensure a supply of fibre.

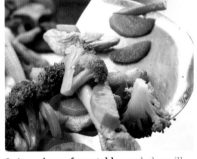

3–4 servings of vegetables each day will ensure a good supply of essential vitamins and minerals. Try to eat different coloured produce and don't overcook vegetables.

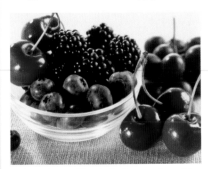

4–5 portions of fresh fruit every day will provide a wide range of vitamins and minerals, many of which contain important protective antioxidants.

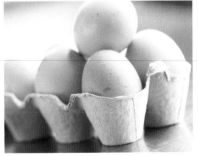

1–2 servings daily of iron-rich foods, such as eggs or dark green leafy vegetables, will help to maintain healthy iron levels during pregnancy when demands are increased.

Your pregnancy diet

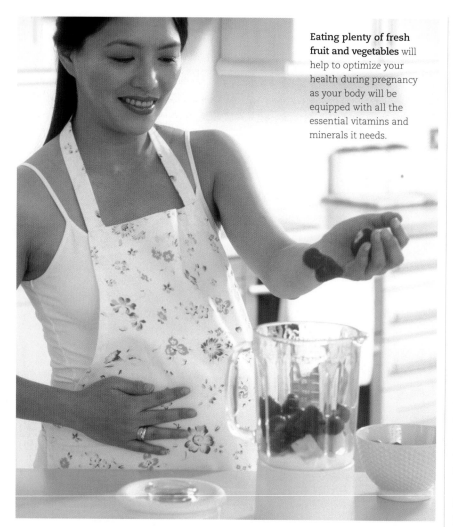

Eating plenty of fresh fruit and vegetables will help to optimize your health during pregnancy as your body will be equipped with all the essential vitamins and minerals it needs.

Good sources of the most important vitamins and minerals are given below. As long as you eat a varied diet that includes plenty of fruits and vegetables, you should be getting all you need, with a couple of exceptions. It can be hard to obtain enough iron through your diet to meet the demands of pregnancy. Your iron levels will be checked during pregnancy and supplements may be recommended. You'll also need a folic acid supplement before conceiving and in early pregnancy (see right).

Vitamin A This is important for healthy eyes, skin, and hair. It's found in orange fruit and vegetables, such as apricots, peppers, carrots, and tomatoes.

Vitamin B This contributes to the healthy functioning of body systems, and helps the body to fight infection. Good sources include bananas, milk, wholegrains, cheese, and cabbage.

Vitamin C This aids the absorption of iron and helps to fight infection. Rich sources include citrus fruits, kiwis, peppers, broccoli, and spinach.

Vitamin D This helps the absorption of calcium. Food sources include eggs and dark green leafy vegetables, and it is also obtained from sunlight. Women with limited exposure to sunlight, who are housebound, predominantly covered when outdoors, or from Africa, South Asia, the Middle East, or the Caribbean should take a 10 microgram vitamin D supplement daily.

Vitamin E This vitamin contains antioxidants and keeps skin, hair, and muscles healthy. Good sources of vitamin E include nuts and seeds.

Folate and folic acid Studies have shown that sufficient amounts of the B vitamin folic acid, or its natural form folate, can help to reduce the risk of neural tube defects, such as spina bifida, by up to 50 per cent. In these defects, the embryonic neural tube fails to close properly during the first four weeks of pregnancy, leading to incomplete development of the brain and spinal cord. Folate helps the neural tube to close and pregnant women are advised to eat a folate-rich diet. Foods high in folate include dark green leafy vegetables, pulses, and fortified cereals. It may not be possible to get sufficient folate through diet alone, so women are also advised to take a folic acid supplement of 400 micrograms daily before conception and during the first trimester.

Iron This is needed for haemoglobin production in red blood cells. Sources include meat, fish, chicken, eggs, dried apricots, spinach, and broccoli.

Calcium This is essential for healthy bones and teeth. Sources include dairy products, eggs, fortified cereals, and leafy green vegetables.

Zinc This helps maintain a healthy immune system. Sources include bananas, seafood, and nuts.

A vegetarian diet
A vegetarian diet, and vegan diets where dairy products are excluded, can be safe and healthy during pregnancy as long as you ensure a good balance of nutrients and sufficient protein (see p.126). Babies born to vegetarian women

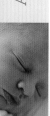

generally have a healthy birth weight, although vegans do need to be vigilant about obtaining adequate protein, as well as reliable sources of vitamin B12 and zinc. Vegans can meet their vitamin B12 needs by including foods such as yeast extracts, vegetable stock, veggie burgers, textured vegetable protein, soymilk, vegetable and sunflower margarines, and breakfast cereals (see p.121).

A low GI diet

Glucose, the product of carbohydrates, serves as the primary fuel for your growing baby. A new concept in nutrition is the glycaemic index (GI), which looks at how much a food will raise the level of glucose in the bloodstream. Foods that release glucose gradually, such as unrefined carbohydrates (see p.14), and thus have a low GI, appear to be healthier.

Benefits of a low GI diet Evidence suggests that a low GI diet has health benefits for both the mother and baby. Maternal carbohydrate intake can affect glucose levels in the bloodstream, which in turn can affect the baby's growth. Higher glucose levels, even those in the normal range, can make for a bigger baby – above the 90th percentile (the top end of a baby's growth chart, see p.284). There are health risks later in life linked to a high birth weight, such as obesity, diabetes, and heart disease. One study found that women who consumed a low GI diet had infants that were a normal size, but had less body fat than those from women who consumed a high GI diet.

A low GI diet can also help to control glucose levels in mothers with gestational diabetes (see p.473), in turn reducing complications of labour and birth associated with this condition.

Your calorie intake

You should aim to eat around 2,100–2,500 calories a day, increasing this by around 200 calories in the last trimester, which is equivalent to a banana and a glass of milk. Your energy needs may vary depending on your pre-pregnancy weight and your activity levels.

Gaining the correct amount of weight in pregnancy has benefits for mother and baby. You're more likely to return to your pre-pregnancy weight if you gain weight within the recommended guidelines (see p.99). Gaining too much weight is linked with bigger babies, which carries future risks to the baby's health (see above). Conversely, gaining too little weight is also not ideal for a baby's future health.

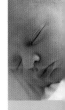

Exercising safely

Staying fit in pregnancy has many benefits for you and your baby and increases your stamina for labour and birth.

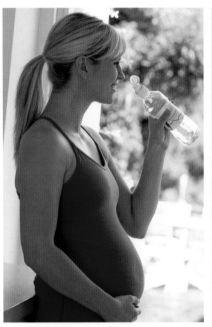

Stay well hydrated by drinking plenty of water before, during, and after your workout.

If you had an exercise programme before you became pregnant, you can continue with this in the first trimester as long as you have the all clear from your doctor or midwife. You may need to adapt your programme later in pregnancy.

If you didn't have a regular exercise programme before, now is the ideal time to adopt a new, healthier way of life from which you will reap the rewards for years to come. If you do start exercising now, build up gently; listen to your body and do only what feels comfortable.

Regular gentle exercise is much better than intense irregular bouts of exercise (which aren't advisable in pregnancy), as your body responds more positively to consistent, moderate exercise.

How exercise helps

As well as increasing your energy levels, exercise helps you to maintain a positive outlook and feel confident about your changing body image. Exercise can also ease common pregnancy discomforts such as nausea, leg cramps, swollen feet, varicose veins, constipation, insomnia, and back pain. By keeping muscles strong and toned, exercise makes it easier for your body to cope with changes in posture during pregnancy. There is also evidence that increased fitness helps to shorten your labour and your postnatal recovery time, and to lessen your overall anxiety about the birth.

Food for fuel

A nutritious, balanced diet is vital in pregnancy. If you're exercising too, eating well to keep energy levels balanced is doubly important. Eat regular, nutritious meals, ensuring that your calories come from wholesome, fresh foods, and avoid high-calorie sugary snacks.

DOS AND DON'TS

Exercise is safe in pregnancy as long as you follow the simple guidelines listed below. As your pregnancy progresses, you will probably need to adapt and moderate your exercise programme.

Do:
- Warm up and cool down properly.
- Drink enough water before, during, and after exercising.
- Wear comfortable clothes that don't restrict your rib cage.
- Exercise regularly and consistently.
- Adjust your expectations; pregnancy is not a time to go for personal bests.

- Build your strength, but do this gradually. Focus on your back, shoulders, chest, and lower body.
- Practise pelvic floor exercises (see p.69) daily to maintain pelvic floor tone.
- Breathe properly while exercising, especially when lifting weights.
- Protect your back when getting up from a lying position: roll onto your left side and sit up using your legs.
- Avoid exercises that feel awkward or uncomfortable.
- Focus on posture and alignment.
- Stop at once and seek advice if you experience severe localized pain, vaginal bleeding, or general unwellness.
- Eat frequent small meals and snacks to maintain energy and avoid your blood sugar levels falling.

Don't:
- Exercise in a hot or humid environment.
- Do jerky or bouncy moves or twist or rotate your abdomen.
- Lift weights that are too heavy.
- Do sports where you risk falling, such as skiing or horseriding.
- Overstretch: the pregnancy hormone relaxin can make you feel more supple than you are.
- Exercise to exhaustion. If you're tired, decrease the intensity or duration. Have an hour's rest to each hour of exercise.

Sex and relationships

You may find that you and your partner need to adapt to the emotional and physical changes that accompany pregnancy.

In a low-risk pregnancy, sex is perfectly safe, although your levels of desire may fluctuate throughout pregnancy. Most women report that their interest in sex is the same or slightly reduced in the first trimester. In the second trimester, it varies from woman to woman, and in the third trimester libido often falls.

Sex during pregnancy

During the first trimester, the hormonal changes that cause nausea, vomiting, and tiredness can naturally result in a reduced interest in sex. However, other pregnancy changes may increase your desire, such as an increased blood flow, which produces swelling in the clitoris and labia and extra vaginal secretions. In the second trimester especially, vaginal lubrication and intensity of orgasm can increase, which may be accompanied by gentle contractions that harden the abdomen; these are normal and nothing to worry about. Many women find that their libido falls towards the end of pregnancy as a bigger bump makes sex more awkward and uncomfortable, and they may also feel increasingly anxious about the birth.

How your partner feels Men have a range of feelings towards sex in pregnancy. While some find their partner's new, fuller shape particularly sensuous, others feel apprehensive about sex, fearing that they may harm the baby. Some feel a combination of these emotions. Unless there are concerns about the pregnancy (see right), it's generally thought that sex won't cause harm, as your baby is well protected by the amniotic fluid and your uterus, and the mucus plug sealing the cervix protects against infection.

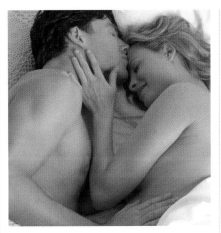

Embracing the changes that accompany pregnancy can enhance your relationship during pregnancy and after the birth.

When to seek advice

Some women experience vaginal bleeding after sex in pregnancy. This is most likely to be harmless and is often caused by the increased blood flow to the cervix in pregnancy, which can cause it to bleed on contact with your partner's penis. If this is the cause, the bleeding should settle after the birth. However, as there are other possible causes, report any bleeding to your midwife or doctor.

Apart from the size of your bump causing discomfort during sex, some women experience pain during sex towards the end of pregnancy as the baby moves further into the pelvis; or they may find that the contractions that can accompany orgasm become increasingly uncomfortable. These symptoms are unlikely to be a cause for concern, but it's worth mentioning them to your midwife for reassurance.

There are some circumstances in late pregnancy when intercourse may not be safe. This can be the case if you've had a

WHAT TO DO

An intimate pregnancy

During pregnancy, tiredness, feelings of insecurity about your new shape, and concerns about the safety of sex can all take their toll on your relationship. Allowing yourself time to adjust and keeping the channels of communication open will help you and your partner to enjoy this new stage in your relationship.

Talk to each other about your feelings and be aware that, for both of you, levels of interest may fluctuate.

If your bump makes some positions uncomfortable, experiment with alternative ones that accommodate your size, such as side-by-side, rear entry, or woman-on-top positions.

Enjoy other ways to maintain intimacy apart from intercourse, such as touching and massage.

previous premature labour or risk factors for premature labour, such as a weak cervix, or if you have placenta praevia (see p.212), or leakage of amniotic fluid, which can mean your waters have broken.

If you have any concerns, don't be afraid to ask your midwife for advice. Being able to enjoy sex in pregnancy will help you and your partner to feel close during this time of transition. Indeed, psychologists have found that couples who enjoy sex in pregnancy are more tender towards each other and communicate better after the birth.

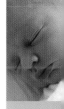

Illnesses and medications

Knowing how to manage illness and what medications are safe to take is important to protect your own and your baby's health.

Whether you have a pre-existing medical condition, or acquire an illness or infection during pregnancy, always consult your doctor before taking medication or before stopping any prescribed medication.

Pre-existing conditions

If you have a condition such as high blood pressure or diabetes prior to pregnancy, your pregnancy will be classified as high risk and you'll need to be monitored carefully. If you become pregnant while taking medication for a condition, don't stop taking it, but consult your doctor as soon as possible. You may find that your existing medication is safe, or you may need to change to another type of medication. The most important thing is to control your condition during pregnancy to minimize the risks to you and your baby, which will usually mean continuing with your medication.

Diabetes If you have diabetes and are planning to conceive, you need to get advice on how to manage your condition. Many hospitals have diabetic "preconception" clinics, where you can discuss the best way to control your blood-sugar levels and talk about how diabetes will be managed in pregnancy. Women with diabetes are advised to take a 5mg supplement of folic acid daily for three months before trying to conceive and for the first three months of pregnancy. This is a larger dose than the 400 micrograms of folic acid daily recommended for non-diabetic women (see p.16), the reason being that diabetes increases the risk of a baby having problems such as

spina bifida, which folic acid protects against. Babies born to diabetic women also have a greater risk of other problems, such as having a large birth weight, respiratory problems at birth, jaundice, and low blood sugar at birth.

As soon as you're pregnant, you should be referred to a specialist obstetric/diabetic antenatal clinic, where you'll receive extra care. You will have more frequent antenatal visits, additional scans, and extra blood tests to monitor your blood sugars. You will probably need around four insulin injections each day; the dose usually increases steadily through pregnancy until just before the delivery. The better your blood-sugar control, the less likely you or your baby are to experience problems during pregnancy.

As diabetic women have an increased risk of late-pregnancy problems such as pre-eclampsia (see p.474) and stillbirth, you may be advised to have an induction of labour a week or so before your due date (see p.432).

Once in labour, your blood-sugar levels will be closely monitored, and you will probably be given an insulin and sugar drip. Your baby's blood-sugar levels will be closely monitored, too, for 24 hours after the birth. After the delivery, your insulin dose will be reduced to pre-pregnancy levels; if you're breastfeeding, the dose may be reduced even further.

Epilepsy If you have epilepsy, it's very important to discuss pregnancy with your doctor before you become pregnant, as certain drugs carry a small risk of causing harm to the developing baby. Nonetheless, it's also important that your epilepsy is controlled, so your doctor will aim to ensure that you're on

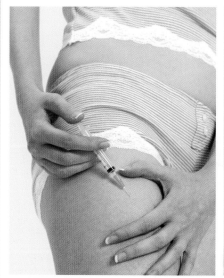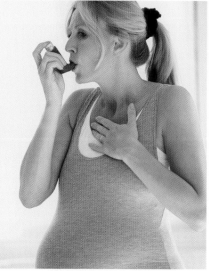

Diabetes is controlled with daily insulin injections in pregnancy. As the skin on your abdomen becomes taut, you may find it easier to inject into the fatty tissue of the thigh (left). **Continuing with asthma medication** is important to keep symptoms under control in pregnancy (right).

the lowest possible dose of medication before you get pregnant. When you are pregnant, the anomaly scan (often referred to as an anatomy scan) at around 20 weeks (see p.214) will check for problems such as cleft palate, which are slightly more common with certain medications. If your condition worsens in pregnancy, contact your doctor.

Systemic lupus erythematosus

This is an autoimmune disorder that can affect many parts of the body, including the kidneys, joints, skin, nervous system, heart, and lungs. The condition is more common in women, and particularly in those of childbearing age. Some women find that the symptoms for this condition ease during pregnancy, however for some they can worsen. It's important to control the condition during pregnancy as it can affect the developing baby, with an increased risk of miscarriage, poor growth, premature labour, and stillbirth. Most medications for lupus are safe to use during pregnancy, but some aren't, so you need to check with your doctor whether you need to change your current medication. From around 32 weeks, your baby will be closely monitored and his growth and wellbeing will be checked. If there are concerns about you or your baby, labour may be induced early, or you may have a planned Caesarean section.

High blood pressure If you have high blood pressure that requires medication, check with your doctor that the medication you are on is safe to use during pregnancy. It's important to continue taking your medication so that your blood pressure is controlled during pregnancy, because high blood pressure can be dangerous both for you and your baby. Your doctor or midwife will check your blood pressure frequently, and will test your urine for the presence of protein, because high blood pressure and protein in the

COMMON WORRIES

I'm asthmatic. Can I use my inhalers during pregnancy?
It's essential that you keep asthma under control in pregnancy, which means continuing to use your inhalers, as the risks from uncontrolled asthma are greater than any risk from taking asthma medication. If asthma is uncontrolled, it can mean that not enough oxygen gets to the baby, leading to a low birth weight and increasing your risk of premature labour (see p.431). One of the best ways to control asthma, in addition to taking medication, is to avoid triggers such as pet fur and dust mites. Use air filters, vacuum and damp dust, and use duvet and pillow protectors. Sometimes, pregnancy reduces the severity of asthma, but if you feel wheezier than usual talk to your doctor about reviewing your medication.

Homeopathy seems to be a popular therapy. How effective is it and is it safe?
Homeopathy works on the principle of treating like with like to stimulate the body's natural healing mechanisms. There has been debate about the efficacy of homeopathy and the scientific opinion is that there is insufficient evidence to show that homeopathy has any effect beyond that of a placebo. However, it is safe to use in pregnancy and remains a popular remedy for women during pregnancy and labour, with many reporting good results. It's used for common pregnancy problems such as nausea and heartburn and "kits" are available to use in labour (see p.401). If you wish to use homeopathy, consult a registered practitioner.

What's the verdict on taking herbal remedies and teas during pregnancy?
The general advice is to avoid herbal remedies as these are ingested, and although some are considered safe, others may cross the placenta and harm the baby. Many herbal teas, such as camomile or peppermint, are safe, but check the label before drinking a herbal tea. Other herbal remedies may be safe to take at a certain time; for example some recommend taking raspberry leaf tea in the last six to eight weeks of pregnancy as it's thought to make labour more efficient. If you wish to use a herbal remedy, talk to a registered practitioner first and consult your doctor.

urine are symptoms of the condition pre-eclampsia. Your doctor may also recommend additional scans to check that your baby is growing well.

Thyroid problems If you have an underactive thyroid gland for which you are taking thyroxine tablets, you'll need to have a blood test to ensure that your thyroid is functioning well and that you're taking the correct dose, as sometimes the thyroxine requirement increases in pregnancy. It's important that you are not lacking in thyroxine, as this may affect the baby. If you are being treated for an overactive thyroid gland, check with your doctor that you're taking an anti-thyroid drug that is safe in pregnancy. Your thyroid function will be monitored to check that your medication doesn't need to change.

Bowel disease Women with inflammatory bowel conditions, such as ulcerative colitis or Crohn's disease, usually find that their condition improves during pregnancy, although they may relapse after the baby is born. Although it's unusual for bowel conditions to cause major problems during pregnancy, it's important to check that you are not anaemic, which can be a side effect of some bowel conditions, and your doctor may recommend extra scans to check that the baby is growing well.

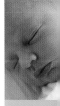

Exposure to chickenpox or rubella

Chickenpox in pregnancy can cause problems for the baby and can be severe in a pregnant woman, possibly leading to pneumonia. If you contract rubella for the first time in early pregnancy, this can cause miscarriage or severe problems in the fetus.

If you encounter chickenpox, contact your doctor or midwife who can check your immunity. If you aren't immune, your doctor may advise an injection to protect you from severe chickenpox.

Your rubella status is checked at the start of pregnancy. If you aren't immune, you can be vaccinated after the birth. Meanwhile you need to take extra care.

If you develop chickenpox or suspect rubella because of a rash, contact your doctor at once, but don't go to the antenatal clinic, where you may spread the infection to other pregnant women.

Infections during pregnancy

When you're pregnant, your immune system is slightly suppressed. This stops you rejecting the baby, who is genetically half the father's! This means that you may be slightly more susceptible to common problems such as colds, coughs, a sore throat, or food poisoning, and that the illness may last for longer.

Colds and coughs Most women get a cough or cold at some stage in pregnancy. However, ideally you should avoid cold medications as these can contain ingredients that aren't safe in pregnancy, especially in the first three months (see opposite). The exception is paracetamol, which you should take only if necessary. Steam inhalations ease congestion and hot honey drinks soothe a sore throat.

Flu If you catch flu during pregnancy, drink plenty of water and get lots of rest. Take paracetamol only if you feel it's necessary to ease discomfort. In the first trimester, it's important to bring down a high fever quickly as this can cause miscarriage: talk to your doctor about safe doses of paracetamol in pregnancy. Sponging with tepid water and sitting in front of a cooling fan can also help. Consult your doctor if your temperature continues after 24 hours. At present, flu jabs are recommended only for high-risk groups, including those with diabetes, chronic heart disease, or asthma.

Food poisoning and stomach upsets A severe episode of food poisoning can cause problems for you and your baby and could trigger an early miscarriage, so it's vital to practise good kitchen hygiene (see p.17). If you do develop food poisoning or a tummy upset, try to drink plenty of fluids, and if it continues for more than 24 hours, see your doctor (see also Gastroenteritis, p.468).

Thrush If you've an abnormal discharge, talk to your midwife or doctor as this may be thrush (candidiasis), which is common in pregnancy. If untreated, there's a chance it could be passed to the baby in a vaginal birth and the baby may need treatment. A swab may be taken to confirm the diagnosis, and a local antifungal remedy prescribed (see opposite). Eating natural yogurt may restore the bacterial balance in your vagina. Wearing cotton underwear and avoiding tight clothing is also advised.

Urine infections Many pregnant women get urine infections because the hormone progesterone relaxes all of the smooth muscle, allowing bacteria that normally live in your vagina to travel up the urethra (the tube that leads to the bladder) where they may cause an infection. The symptoms of a urine infection may be slightly different in pregnancy. You may have the classic symptoms of burning when urinating and frequent passing of urine, or you may have different symptoms such as back pain, lower abdominal pain, nausea, or vomiting. These are usually easily treated with antibiotics, most of which are safe in pregnancy.

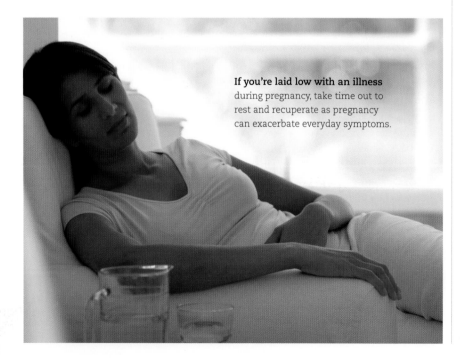

If you're laid low with an illness during pregnancy, take time out to rest and recuperate as pregnancy can exacerbate everyday symptoms.

Taking medications during pregnancy

During the first three months of pregnancy, the only safe over-the-counter medicine is paracetamol. Once you are past the first trimester, some other medications are considered safe, but always consult your doctor if you are in any doubt. The following provides guidance on medications used for treating common pregnancy complaints and minor illnesses.

Antacids Heartburn and indigestion are common problems in pregnancy, particularly during the third trimester when the increased size of the baby puts pressure on your stomach. The majority of antacids are safe to use during pregnancy, although you should avoid sodium bicarbonate as the sodium can be absorbed into the bloodstream. Consult your doctor or pharmacist about which ones are recommended.

Antibiotics Many antibiotics used to treat infection are safe for use during pregnancy. These include antibiotics containing penicillin, although there are safe alternatives if you're allergic to penicillin. The following antibiotics should be avoided during pregnancy:
■ Streptomycin. This can damage the ears of the fetus as it develops and may result in hearing loss in the baby.
■ Sulphonamides. These can cause jaundice in the newborn baby.
■ Tetracyclines. These drugs shouldn't be taken as they can affect the development of the baby's bones and teeth and can cause discoloration in the teeth.

Antiemetics If you have severe nausea and vomiting and natural remedies such as ginger or peppermint tea don't relieve the problem, your doctor may recommend an antiemetic medication that is safe to use during pregnancy.

Antifungal remedies You should avoid over-the-counter antifungal remedies, including oral remedies, for treating thrush. Consult your doctor, who can recommend a cream or pessary that is suitable for use in pregnancy.

Cold remedies Remedies for coughs and colds often contain a range of ingredients, such as caffeine, antihistamines, and other decongestants, many of which aren't safe in pregnancy. Read labels carefully before purchasing over-the-counter remedies and talk to your doctor or the pharmacist if you're in any doubt. Ideally, avoid all cold remedies and instead have steam inhalations and hot drinks. If necessary, take paracetamol for a brief period.

Diuretics It's normal to experience some swelling in the hands and feet during pregnancy, and you shouldn't attempt to deal with this by taking diuretics, including herbal diuretics. If you have sudden swelling in the face, hands, or feet, you should consult your midwife or doctor at once as this can be a sign of pre-eclampsia (see p.474)

Laxatives The first step in dealing with constipation is to take dietary measures by increasing your intake of fibre and drinking plenty of fluids. If this isn't enough, then over-the-counter laxatives are safe to take during pregnancy. Look for laxatives that contain bulking agents and avoid ones that contain senna, which is known to act as an irritant to the bowel.

Painkillers The general advice is to avoid all painkillers during pregnancy, especially during the first trimester. Before using a painkiller for a common problem, such as headache or backache, first try natural remedies: massage or a warm bath are often effective in relieving aches and pains. If these aren't sufficient, you can take paracetamol on a short-term basis. Aspirin and anti-inflammatories such as ibuprofen should be avoided throughout pregnancy. The painkiller codeine can sometimes be used for a short period to treat specific pain, but should only be taken on the advice of a doctor.

Rehydration solutions If you have a tummy upset resulting in a severe bout of diarrhoea that lasts for an extended period, your doctor may recommend a rehydration solution; these are safe to take in pregnancy.

Steroids If you have eczema, or find that this condition develops or worsens during pregnancy, your doctor may prescribe steroids such as hydrocortisone. While these are considered safe to use in pregnancy, avoid using them on a large surface area or for an extended period. Your doctor will provide advice and guidance on safe usage of steroid creams during pregnancy.

Steroid inhalers used to treat asthma are safe in pregnancy, and it's important to control your asthma while you're pregnant.

Oral steroids may also be prescribed for certain other conditions, and these may be safe to continue with under the guidance of your doctor. Anabolic steroids should not be taken during pregnancy.

Lifestyle hazards

Pregnancy can be beset with anxiety about potential hazards. Being aware of exactly what to avoid will help to allay fears.

Whether you're pregnant or are planning to conceive, now is the time to do a safety check on your social habits and home and work environment. Anything that could affect your wellbeing could affect your baby too, especially in the first trimester. However, don't become over-anxious. Instead, arm yourself with the facts so that you can avoid hazards, but also relax and enjoy your pregnancy.

Your social habits
The decision to have a baby may inspire you to review your social habits and, if necessary, make changes.

Alcohol consumption There is still no clear guidance on how much alcohol, if any, you can safely drink in pregnancy. It's unlikely that an occasional glass of wine is harmful, but the advice is that it's probably best to avoid alcohol when pregnant. What isn't in doubt is the damage caused to the fetus by excessive alcohol intake. Continuous heavy drinking in pregnancy can lead to a condition known as fetal alcohol syndrome. The effects of this on the baby include retarded growth, facial and joint abnormalities, and heart problems.

If there were a few occasions when you drank too much before you knew you were pregnant, try not to worry, but give up now. Many women also decide to give up alcohol while they're trying to conceive to optimize fertility.

Smoking Ideally, you should stop smoking before you get pregnant. If you're still smoking once you conceive, it's important to stop right away. If your partner or friends smoke, ask them not to smoke in your home or anywhere

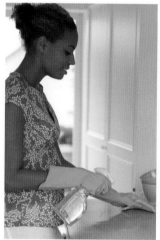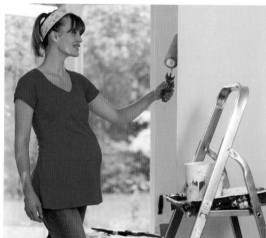

Wearing rubber gloves when using household cleaning products will reduce your exposure to chemicals (left). **Opt for "greener" paints** and keep rooms ventilated while decorating (right).

near you. Inhaled cigarette smoke interferes with the supply of oxygen to the baby, which can lead to a low birthweight and increases the risk of stillbirth or the death of a baby in the first month of life.

Recreational drug use As well as damaging your own health, recreational drugs can pose dangers for the fetus.

Heroin and cocaine are damaging both to a pregnant woman and her unborn baby. These drugs stunt fetal growth, affect the placenta, and can cause miscarriage or premature birth, as well as health problems in the newborn. Babies born to women who use heroin regularly will show drug withdrawal symptoms. A report on ecstasy linked the use of this in pregnancy to a rise in birth defects, such as limb abnormalities. The specific effects on the fetus of amphetamines and LSD are unclear, but it's safest to avoid them.

The direct effects on the fetus of the active chemicals in marijuana are not

clear, but smoking the drug involves the same risks as tobacco smoking.

Hazards at home
Many of us use chemicals daily in and around the home. As well as personal products, such as bath oils, deodorants, and hairsprays, we also keep dozens of other substances around the home, including cleaning fluids, detergents, bleach, and air fresheners.

When products are used in accordance with the manufacturers' instructions, there is little chance of them causing harm in pregnancy. However, minute traces of chemicals can enter the bloodstream, either through the skin or by inhalation, and cross the placenta. While there is no hard evidence to show that this has an ill effect, it makes sense to minimize the chances of chemicals reaching a developing baby.

When using products, wear rubber gloves to prevent skin contact and ventilate rooms. To avoid inhaling mists or vapours, choose non-aerosol products. Also, choose products recommended for their low environmental impact, as these contain fewer chemicals. Where possible, use natural alternatives to chemicals.

Painting and decorating It's important to stay safe while doing DIY. Don't climb up ladders or stand on tables to reach high places as your bump alters your centre of balance. Also, avoid skin contact or inhalation if you use oil-based paints, spray paints, paint strippers, floor varnishes, and sealant adhesives. Make sure rooms are well ventilated while decorating, and, ideally, get someone else to do the decorating.

Pets and infections Certain infections that could harm the fetus can be picked up from pets. The parasitic infection toxoplasmosis is spread through contact with cat faeces. It may produce flu-like symptoms, or no symptoms at all, and many unknowingly acquire immunity through previous exposure. However, although it rarely happens, acquiring toxoplasmosis for the first time in pregnancy can cause serious problems, such as miscarriage or birth defects. Other pets, such as dogs, cage birds, and turtles can carry salmonella bacteria. Salmonella infection doesn't directly harm the baby, but can make a pregnant woman ill.

Being scrupulous about hygiene helps you avoid such infections. Wear rubber gloves when handling a cat litter tray, cleaning cages where animals are kept, or disposing of dog faeces, then wash your hands (and the gloves) afterwards. Wear gloves also for digging or weeding in case animals have defecated in the garden. Or get someone else to do these tasks.

Toxoplasmosis and salmonella can also be contracted from eating undercooked or raw meat or eggs, so take care with kitchen hygiene and cooking (see p.17).

Workplace hazards
It's the legal responsibility of your employer to provide a safe environment.

In pregnancy, being aware of your rights can help protect you and your baby.

In recent years, women worried about whether working at a computer screen put their babies at risk. It's now clear that using a VDU (as well as photocopiers and printers) is safe. Some environments do pose possible dangers. If you work with hospital equipment, such as X-ray machines and scanners, inform your department that you're pregnant. Hospital regulations will ensure that, if necessary, you're given alternative duties.

Women employed in places such as hairdressers, manicure bars, laboratories, and craft workshops may be exposed to toxic chemicals. Also, inhalation of some dry cleaning solvents has been linked to miscarriage. It's up to employers to ensure ventilation and protection from hazards. If you're unhappy about conditions, talk to your boss or HR manager.

Standing on your feet all day and physical work that involves heavy lifting can be exhausting in pregnancy. If your work involves either of these, ask if it's possible to switch to less tiring tasks.

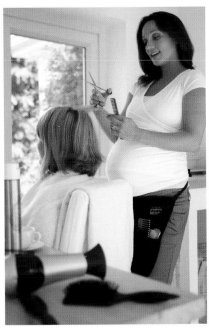

If your job involves handling chemicals, ensure that a risk assessment is done and that you are able to avoid harmful substances.

COMMON WORRIES

Is it safe to use a mobile phone during pregnancy? I've read that phones emit radiation.
The radiation emitted by mobile phones is "non-ionizing". This is not the same as the radiation received from X-rays, which can be harmful in large doses. There is no evidence to show that using a mobile phone is a health risk to either you or your baby.

I go swimming twice a week and love the feeling of having the weight taken off my bump! But is the chlorine in the pool bad for my baby?
In the past there has been some debate about whether it's safe to swim in chlorinated pools during pregnancy. However, most experts now believe that swimming in chlorinated water does not pose any health risks for pregnant women and their developing babies. You may find that the smell of chlorine adds to your nausea if you are suffering from morning sickness, although this is less of a problem in an outdoor pool. Try not to swallow the water, and shower when you come out of the pool. Swimming has great benefits during pregnancy. It has a low risk of injury while providing a good cardiovascular workout and improving muscle tone, so don't be put off by unnecessary worries.

Is it OK to use nicotine patches or gum while I'm pregnant?
Nicotine is known to decrease the blood supply to the fetus. This could affect the baby's growth, especially in early pregnancy. Although tobacco substitutes, such as patches, gum, and pastilles, deliver less nicotine to your body than smoking, you should never use them without seeking a doctor's advice. Ask at your local health centre for information on safer ways to beat cigarette cravings.

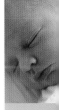

Skin, hair, and teeth

As well as affecting what happens to you internally, hormonal changes in pregnancy can also affect your external appearance.

Many women look and feel better than ever during pregnany, while others find that pregnancy has the opposite effect on their appearance. However pregnancy affects you, the changes will be temporary and you'll be back to your normal self soon after the birth.

Skin

You may find that your skin looks better in pregnancy due to hormonal changes, mild fluid retention, and increased blood flow. These can all result in smoother skin and are responsible for the famous "pregnancy glow". On the other hand, you may find that your skin gets drier and spottier and you may need to take extra care of it during pregnancy.

Skin also tends to darken during pregnancy, although the reason for this is unknown. One possible explanation is the increased levels of oestrogen and melanocyte-stimulating hormone, which stimulate skin pigmentation.

Stretch marks (striae gravidarum)

During pregnancy many women develop stretch marks, which can occur on tummies, breasts, hips, or legs. These initially appear as pink or purple lines and may be quite itchy. After pregnancy they fade into pale, silvery-white wrinkles. Nobody knows for sure why these occur, but they probably result from a combination of pregnancy hormones and your skin stretching. You're more likely to get stretch marks if you're very young, if you gain a lot of weight in pregnancy, or if you have a very big baby. There's less agreement about the role of other factors such as a family history, being very overweight before pregnancy or belonging to a particular ethnic group.

Many creams, lotions, and oils have been marketed for the prevention or treatment of stretch marks but none has been proven to work. Products containing vitamin E are often claimed to be effective, but studies carried out on such products are inconclusive. Commercially produced creams, lotions, and oils are safe to use and may help to minimize stretch marks by maintaining the elasticity of the skin; unfortunately, however, there is no guarantee that they will prevent them. The best advice is to avoid putting on excess weight and to drink plenty of water to keep the skin well hydrated.

Chloasma This describes the increased pigmentation of the cheeks, nose, and chin that affects around 50–70 per cent of pregnant women. You may reduce chloasma by using a protective high factor sunscreen cream and avoiding the use of photosensitizing skincare products. These are products that contain ingredients that increase your sensitivity to sunlight, such as quinoline or bergamot oil. Talk to your pharmacist about which products to avoid.

Hair and nails

Hair stays longer in the growth phase during pregnancy, meaning that your scalp hair is likely to grow and thicken. Not so welcome is the fact that facial and body hair may also increase. After the birth, many women find that they suddenly lose a lot of hair as the growth phase stops. You should find that your hair is back to normal within six months.

Fingernails may also change, often becoming stronger, although some

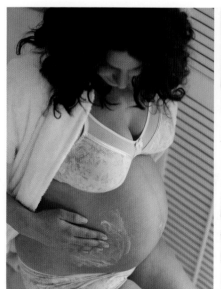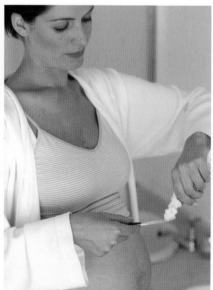

Applying moisturizing creams to relieve dry, itchy skin, or creams recommended to reduce stretch marks, is safe during pregnancy (left). **Taking good care of your teeth and gums** is important during pregnancy, when you're more susceptible to dental problems (right).

I am 18 weeks' pregnant and due to go on a beach holiday. My facial and body hair has grown and become very unsightly. How can I safely remove it?
You can safely tweeze, wax, and shave hair. Skin bleaching and hair removal creams are probably safe during pregnancy, but there has been insufficient research to be certain as they can be absorbed through the skin and their effects on the baby are unknown. Permanent hair-removal techniques, such as laser and electrolysis, are thought to be safe in pregnancy. Both techniques penetrate the skin no deeper than a few millimetres, so are unlikely to harm your baby.

I've been using topical cream to treat acne and I've just found out that I'm pregnant. Will it harm my baby?
Tretinoin belongs to a group of medications called retinoids that contain vitamin A, which has been linked to birth defects. Studies have looked at the effects of this cream in pregnancy and have found that babies whose mothers used it, even in the first trimester, had no increase in birth defects. However, doctors recommend avoiding tretinoin cream in pregnancy.

Another similar medication, isotretinoin, which is taken as a tablet, may increase the risk of birth defects and is therefore contraindicated in pregnancy.

I'm in the first trimester and due to attend my sister's wedding. Can I have highlights put in my hair?
Although the research into the safety of hair dyes if used in the first trimester may seem conflicting, the amount of chemicals used is small and it's unlikely that hair dyes cause harm. Also, if your hairdresser uses foil, the dye is kept off your skin.

I've heard that nail polish needs to be removed if you have a Caesarean section. Why is this?
Previously, women were encouraged to remove nail varnish before surgery. One of the reasons was that the "pulse oximeter", a device attached to your finger to measure the oxygen in your blood during surgery, may give lower readings if placed over nail varnish. However, the device works as intended with nail polish or long nails if it's mounted sideways on a finger. Therefore there's no need to remove your polish.

women find that they become softer and brittle. Nails may develop white spots or transverse grooves, but these are rarely anything to worry about and don't mean that you're lacking in vitamins.

Teeth
Pregnant women are more prone to tooth decay (dental caries), bleeding gums, and chronic gum infection (periodontal disease). Poor dental health not only affects you, but can also have an impact on your baby. Studies have linked infection of the gums in pregnant women to premature birth, and if a woman has ongoing tooth decay after the birth, her baby may acquire bacteria directly from her saliva, leading to tooth

decay in the child later on. It's therefore important that you take good care of your teeth during pregnancy and visit your dentist and dental hygienist regularly. Dental care during pregnancy and for a year after the birth is free.

Routine dental treatment and local anaesthetics are safe in pregnancy, but the Department of Health advises leaving the replacement of amalgam fillings until after the birth. Many worry about having their teeth X-rayed in pregnancy. The radiation exposure from dental X-rays is minimal and the risk to the baby probably negligible. However, dentists will only perform X-rays during pregnancy when it is unavoidable – if you need root canal treatment for example.

Beauty treatments and cosmetics

Hair and nail products Shampoos, conditioners, manicures, and pedicures are safe. Minute amounts of hair dye may be absorbed through the skin, but there's no evidence that this affects the baby. Chemical hair-straighteners and curlers are also thought to be safe.

Piercing Facial piercing or piercing the tummy button, nipples, or genitalia isn't advised as you're at a higher risk of infection. If you have a tummy piercing already, you can change a metallic ring for a flexible plastic retainer made from PTFE (polytetrafluoroethylene). Nipple rings can affect breastfeeding, so remove a ring before birth so the skin can heal. Vaginal or vulval piercings are best removed to avoid damage at birth.

Tanning Tanning beds aren't advised because of harmful UV rays. The beds can cause your body to overheat, which can harm your baby, and UV rays may break down folic acid. Tanning lotions are safe, but do a patch test first to check for allergic reactions.

Body wraps/hot tubs These raise body temperature, which is unsafe for you and your baby. Heat exposure from a hot tub in the first three months can increase the risk of spina bifida.

Facials The cosmetics used for facials are thought to be safe.

Botox The safety of this is debated as it contains a naturally occurring poison. As botox injections are localized it is probably safe, and women who've had injections before they knew they were pregnant have had no ill effects and neither have their babies. However, doctors advise against botox in pregnancy.

Skin, hair, and teeth

27

Travelling in pregnancy

Your growing bump need not put a stop to travel plans – just do a bit of extra planning to help your holiday run smoothly.

CHECKLIST

Trimester-by-trimester travel guide

Think about the implications of travelling at different times in your pregnancy when planning a trip.

1st trimester (weeks 1–12)
- Period of highest risk for miscarriage and development problems in the baby. Take extra care to avoid extremes of temperature and over-vigorous activities.
- Travel sickness could make morning sickness worse.
- Flying is safe, provided you have no pregnancy complications.
- Insurance is unlikely to be a problem.

2nd trimester (weeks 13–25)
- You are likely to be feeling at your best, and the chances of miscarriage or fetal development problems are greatly reduced.
- Flying is allowed, but check to see whether you need to carry a doctor's letter stating your due date.
- Check the dates for which you can be covered by travel insurance – they vary from company to company.

3rd trimester (weeks 26–40)
- Your bump is huge and travel may be very uncomfortable now.
- Most airlines will not allow you to fly after 36 weeks and some set an even earlier date.
- Insurers are unlikely to give you cover if you are within eight weeks of giving birth.

Provided your pregnancy is normal, going to faraway places is perfectly possible. However, discomforts such as extreme heat, high altitude, and makeshift accommodation may be less tolerable, and in some cases may compromise the safety of your baby.

The best time to travel

In the first trimester, you may find that morning sickness and tiredness lessen your enthusiasm for travel. Most women feel at their best in the second trimester and this is also seen as the safest time to travel as your risk of miscarriage is low, energy levels are increased, and your due date is still some way off. After 28 weeks, the size of your bump, fatigue, and the looming birth date are likely to make home seem the best place to be.

ADVANCE PLANNING

You've found your passport and put the tickets in your bag. However, when you're pregnant you may also need to take the following items:
- A note from your doctor or midwife stating your due date and giving you the all-clear to travel (this is essential if you're over 28 weeks' pregnant).
- Any special medical records regarding your pregnancy or general health.
- A list of numbers for healthcare facilities at your destination.
- Remedies for heartburn or other minor pregnancy problems, such as piles. You may not be able to buy your usual products abroad.

Making plans

A little extra planning is the key to successful travel in pregnancy. However tempting brochures look, think carefully before you book. How will you get there and how long will it take? Pregnancy adds to the stress of a long-haul journey. If you want to fly, check with the airline if you are actually allowed to get on the plane. Policies vary, but many airlines won't let you fly after 36 weeks. This is largely because of the possibility of a woman going into labour in mid-flight.

Taking precautions Avoid visiting countries where disease is a high risk factor. Protective drugs, such as vaccines and antimalarial tablets, aren't advisable in pregnancy or when trying to conceive. However, if you have to travel to an area

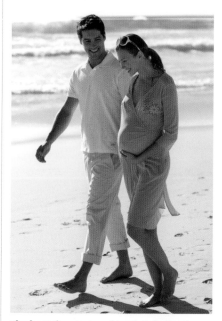

The best time to travel is often during the second trimester when nausea has abated and your bump is not yet uncomfortable.

where malaria is common, the advice is to take anti-malarial medication rather than risk infection. Look on the internet for information about an area's health hazards and local hospitals. If you have a condition such as diabetes that could cause complications, make sure you can get treatment while away.

Wherever you go, it is vital to take out travel insurance. Bear in mind that most companies do not provide cover if you're within eight weeks of giving birth.

Avoiding bugs

Pregnancy reduces the efficiency of your immune system, increasing your risk of an infection. When you're travelling, "tummy bugs" caused by contaminated food and water are more likely to strike.

If you're unsure about local tap water, buy bottled water (make sure the seal is unbroken) and use it when brushing teeth as well as for drinking. Avoid drinks with ice and don't eat salads or fruit you can't peel as they may have been washed in contaminated water. Fruit such as melon may have been injected with water to increase its weight and is best avoided.

Avoid outdoor stalls or cafés where food might have been prepared hours in advance. Try to find restaurants where food is freshly cooked and standards seem high. Be scrupulous about hygiene, and carry moist wipes in case handwashing facilities are inadequate.

On the journey

Sitting in a cramped seat for hours can cause your ankles and feet to swell. If you're travelling by car, stop every couple of hours to stretch your legs, have a snack, or find a toilet. On a train or aeroplane, keep your circulation moving with foot and ankle exercises, and every so often get up and walk down the aisle. Stay hydrated by drinking lots of water or juice, even if you do need to empty your bladder frequently. A few comforts, such as a cushion to tuck behind your back or a cooling water spritzer, can make a journey more bearable.

COMMON WORRIES

I am five months pregnant and about to go on a beach holiday. I know that too much sunbathing causes skin damage, but can hot sun also harm my baby? Experts are investigating a link between prolonged exposure to the sun and damage to the fetus. There is a possibility that ultraviolet rays could cause a deficiency of folic acid – a vitamin that helps to prevent defects in the baby's nervous system leading to spina bifida. Nothing is yet proven, but it's not worth taking the risk. Enjoy the sun in moderation but don't bake yourself or use sunbeds before you go on holiday.

I'm worried about flying because someone told me there is a high risk of DVT in pregnancy. Is this true? Deep vein thrombosis (DVT), the formation of a blood clot in a vein (often in a leg), is sometimes caused by long periods of immobility, such as sitting on a plane (see p.186). Although the risk factor is slightly increased in pregnant women, because their blood tends to clot more easily, the chance of you developing DVT is still very low. To minimize the risk even further, wear special support socks, which are designed to improve blood flow in the legs, and keep well hydrated.

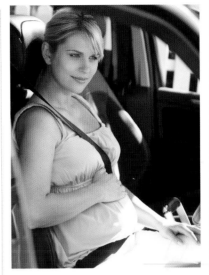

The position of your seatbelt may need adjusting to accommodate your bump.

Are car seatbelts and airbags safe to use in pregnancy? In the event of an accident, these appliances are far more likely to prevent injury than cause it – never travel without fastening your seatbelt. For comfort, position the straps above and below your bump rather than across it. Being hit by an inflated airbag will not hurt you or the baby, but to lessen the impact you should fix your seat as far back as possible.

Holiday activities

There are some activities to forego in pregnancy, such as water-skiing or horse-riding, where a fall could harm your baby. Scuba-diving is particularly dangerous because of the risk of air bubbles forming in the bloodstream. If you have children, ignore pleas to join them on white-knuckle park rides.

If you're used to exercising, there is no reason not to go swimming or walking, just don't overdo it – hiking up hills under a blazing sun could send your temperature soaring, which is a bad thing in pregnancy. In the first trimester especially, extreme heat can affect fetal development. You might also become dehydrated, which later on can increase the risk of premature labour.

Be cautious too about less energetic activities. Jacuzzis and saunas are best avoided as the heat could make you feel faint and may be harmful to your baby. An aromatherapy massage sounds like a treat, but some oils may be toxic to the baby, especially in the early months. If you want pampering, look for spas with treatments for pregnant mums.

In pregnancy, your skin becomes more sensitive to the sun, so whatever you're doing, be careful to protect against overexposure to the sun.

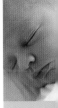

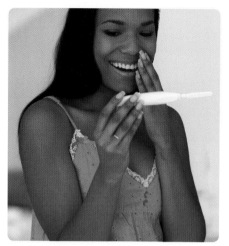 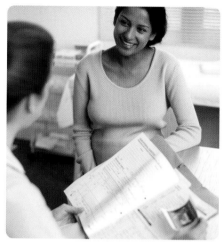 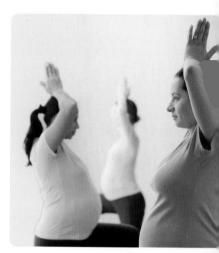

The 40 weeks, or 280 days, of pregnancy are a time of constant change as your body continually adapts to accommodate the new life growing inside you. This extensive chapter guides you through the physical and emotional changes you'll experience and offers reassurance, advice, and practical tips. Your baby's progress is charted in fascinating detail with scans and day-by-day insights into how your baby grows and develops within your uterus.

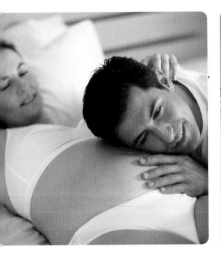
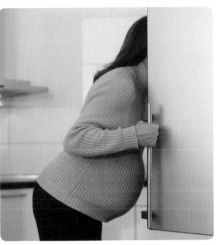
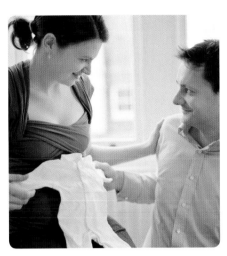

Pregnancy
day by day

Welcome to your first trimester

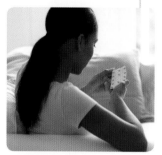

Preconceptual care A daily folic acid supplement before and during early pregnancy helps to protect your baby from spinal cord defects.

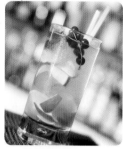

Avoid alcohol Drinking soft drinks rather than alcohol may help you to conceive; add fruit to drinks for extra benefit.

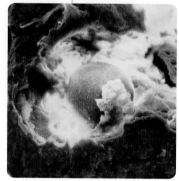

The release of an egg At ovulation, an enlarged follicle in the ovary ruptures to release the mature egg, ready to be fertilized in a Fallopian tube by your partner's sperm.

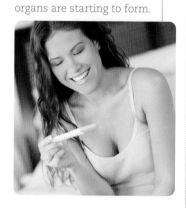

It's official! By the time you discover you're pregnant, your baby has reached the embryonic period and the brain, heart, and other organs are starting to form.

Early growth In the crucial first weeks, the baby's vital organs begin to develop and the neural tube, which becomes the brain and spinal cord, is forming.

At first, only you are aware of subtle body changes. By three months, changes may be visible.

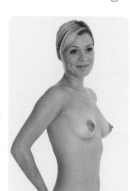
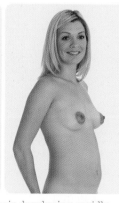

First trimester Your baby is developing rapidly and you may have a whole host of symptoms, but outwardly there's little sign that you're pregnant. **Starting to show** By the end of this trimester, your waistline may start to expand.

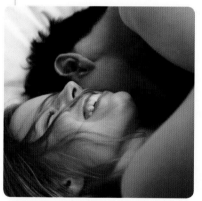

The path to conception Sexual intercourse timed to coincide with ovulation is most likely to lead to a successful pregnancy.

Facts and figures You have a 3.5 in 1,000 chance of having identical twins.

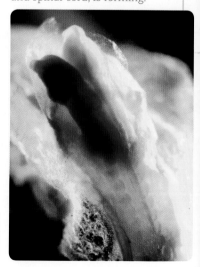

You're at the start of an incredible stage of life that will see your body undergo dramatic changes.

6	7	8	9	10	11	12

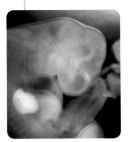

At 6 weeks bud-like structures can be seen on the embryo that will develop into your baby's limbs.

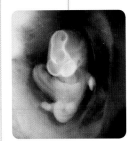

By 8 weeks the head has grown rapidly, giving an unbalanced appearance, and the limbs are lengthening.

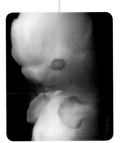

At 9 weeks the fetus is starting to have a recognizable form, with facial features beginning to develop.

Facts and figures At 7 weeks, your baby measures just 8mm from crown to rump.

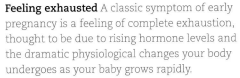
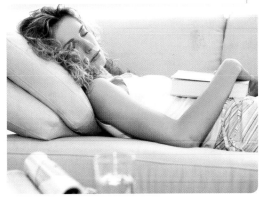

Feeling exhausted A classic symptom of early pregnancy is a feeling of complete exhaustion, thought to be due to rising hormone levels and the dramatic physiological changes your body undergoes as your baby grows rapidly.

Dating the pregnancy Between 10 and 14 weeks, a dating scan will confirm the gestational age of your baby. Your original due date may be revised as a result of this scan and the timing of future tests will be based on its findings.

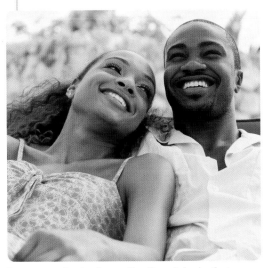

Parents-to-be As the realization sinks in that you're facing parenthood, you may discover a new dimension to your relationship and an enhanced sense of togetherness.

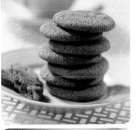
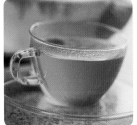

Soothing foods Early pregnancy can often be marred by nausea and vomiting, especially in the mornings; eating ginger biscuits or sipping a herbal tea can help to quell the symptoms.

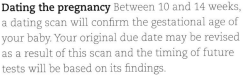
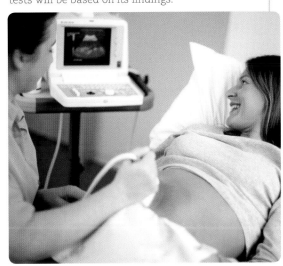

Your 1st week

THE 280-DAY COUNTDOWN BEGINS HERE – EVEN THOUGH YOU HAVEN'T YET CONCEIVED

It's business as usual for your body this week. You're having a period, so you know you're not pregnant. But if you conceive during this menstrual cycle, the first day of your period will count as the first day of pregnancy. It's a good idea to review your lifestyle and to make sure that you understand how everything works "inside". Knowing the facts may help to raise your chances of conceiving.

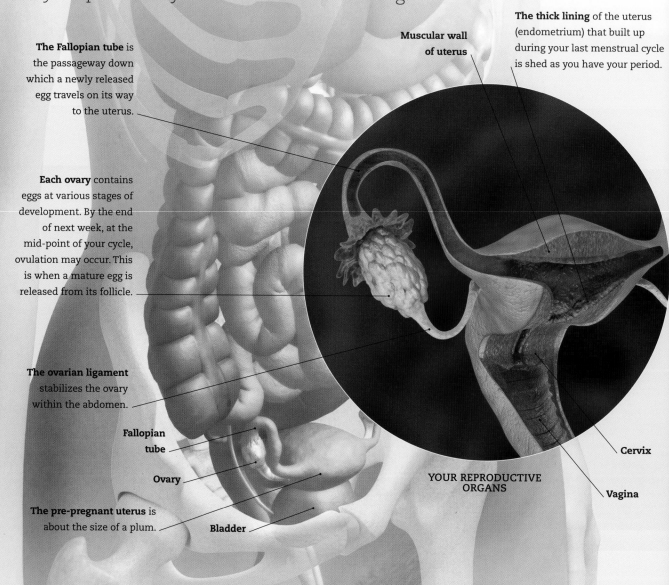

The Fallopian tube is the passageway down which a newly released egg travels on its way to the uterus.

Muscular wall of uterus

The thick lining of the uterus (endometrium) that built up during your last menstrual cycle is shed as you have your period.

Each ovary contains eggs at various stages of development. By the end of next week, at the mid-point of your cycle, ovulation may occur. This is when a mature egg is released from its follicle.

The ovarian ligament stabilizes the ovary within the abdomen.

Fallopian tube

Ovary

The pre-pregnant uterus is about the size of a plum.

Bladder

Cervix

YOUR REPRODUCTIVE ORGANS

Vagina

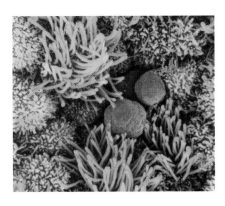

279 days to go...

WHAT'S HAPPENING INSIDE

The lining of the uterus builds up in the first two weeks of the menstrual cycle to prepare for pregnancy. The yellow and blue areas seen here are cells and the pink areas, secretions. If no pregnancy occurs, the lining breaks down and menstruation occurs.

This is day one of your period. If you are trying to conceive during this menstrual cycle, keep a note of this highly significant date.

Although this is officially the first day of your pregnancy, you won't conceive until around two weeks from now. This is classed as "day one" because once you conceive your pregnancy will be dated from the first day of your last menstrual period. It would be more logical to date pregnancy from the day of ovulation or conception, but, like most women, you're unlikely to know the day on which you ovulate, let alone conceive. You are, however, far more likely to remember when your last period started, especially if you're hoping to get pregnant and are keeping a record of your menstrual cycle.

While dating a pregnancy in this way can seem slightly baffling, it is a handy convention, and in fact your body is getting geared up for pregnancy from this date. In around 280 days, or nine months' time, you could be holding your newborn baby in your arms. Good luck and enjoy the journey!

FOCUS ON... NUTRITION

Take folic acid

Start taking this vital supplement now, from day one, if you haven't already. You should take folic acid as soon as you begin trying to conceive because it will be essential to your baby's development in the first few weeks of pregnancy (see p.16).

The amount of folic acid that has been shown to be effective is a daily supplement of 400mcg. A diet of foods rich in folate is also advisable so eat plenty of green vegetables, such as runner beans, spinach, and broccoli; pulses, such as peas, beans, and chickpeas; fortified cereals; and yeast extract, such as Marmite.

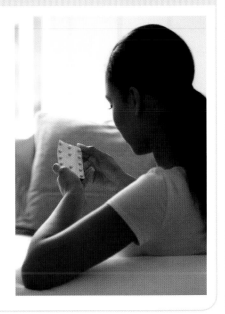

TIME TO THINK ABOUT

Having a baby

There's no perfect time to become parents, but you might want to bear in mind the following:

- While practical matters such as the state of your finances and the size of your house are considerations, remember that being parents is about much more than what you are able to offer your baby materially.
- This is a decision only you and your partner can make. Don't act on the advice of family members and friends.
- You might conceive immediately or it could take several months, so relax and don't have a set date in mind.

AS A MATTER OF FACT

Just 25 per cent of couples actively trying to conceive become pregnant in the first monthly cycle.

For 60 per cent of couples it takes nine months. So be patient and try not to get too stressed if you don't manage to conceive straightaway.

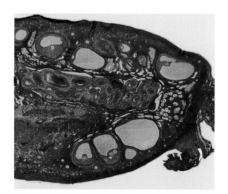

278 days to go...

WHAT'S HAPPENING INSIDE

Your eggs are already developing, as can be seen in this colour-enhanced cross-section of an ovary. The small white structures are immature follicles that contain eggs at different stages of development. Once a follicle matures, the egg will burst out.

By tracking your menstrual cycle and understanding how it works, you may increase your chances of conceiving.

This is day two of your period and day two of your complete menstrual cycle, which starts on the first day of your period and ends on the day before your next period. A full cycle is, on average, 28 days, but many women have a shorter or longer cycle.

Now may be the time when your period is at its heaviest, as the tissue and blood that make up the lining of the uterus (the endometrium) are shed. The average blood loss during menstruation is around 30ml (two tablespoons). While the lining is being sloughed off, the blood vessels in the uterus constrict, which can cause cramp-like period pains. As soon as your period has finished, an egg begins to mature within its follicle in one of your ovaries, ready to be released around mid-cycle. This is called ovulation (see p.49).

Meanwhile, the lining of the uterus starts to build up again under the influence of the hormones progesterone and oestrogen, ready to receive a fertilized egg. If the egg is not fertilized, hormone levels fall, the lining sheds, and the cycle begins again.

AS A MATTER OF FACT

Periods can synchronize in women who live or work together.

Scientists claim that pheromones (chemicals that trigger a biological response in someone) waft from one woman to another. Receptors in the nose detect these pheromones and a biological process takes place whereby one woman naturally adjusts her menstrual cycle.

CHANGES DURING THE MENSTRUAL CYCLE

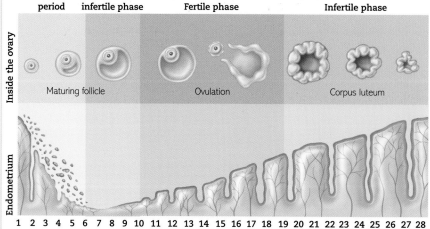

Menstrual period | Relatively infertile phase | Fertile phase | Infertile phase

Inside the ovary

Maturing follicle · Ovulation · Corpus luteum

Endometrium

1 2 3 4 5 6 7 8 9 10 11 12 13 14 15 16 17 18 19 20 21 22 23 24 25 26 27 28
Days of cycle

The monthly cycle of an egg as it grows to maturity inside an ovary is shown at the top of the chart. It is released from its follicle around day 14. The bottom of the chart shows the corresponding development of the lining of the uterus – shedding at the start of a period, then rebuilding in preparation for a fertilized egg.

The empty egg follicle (called the corpus luteum) secretes progesterone, which is a hormone that helps the endometrium to reach a thickness of about 6mm over the 28 days of the menstrual cycle, ready to receive a fertilized egg.

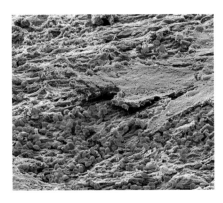

THIS IS DAY 3 OF YOUR MENSTRUAL CYCLE

277 days to go...

WHAT'S HAPPENING INSIDE

The lining of the uterus, known as the endometrium, can be seen here (pink structure) shedding during menstruation. This happens if a fertilized egg does not implant. The red dots are red blood cells, released when the blood vessels break down.

When you're trying to get pregnant, it helps to be aware of lifestyle and medical factors that can affect your menstrual cycle.

You may notice that the timing and volume of your periods differ. Your menstrual cycle can be affected by stress as well as by medical conditions, such as an overactive thyroid. In both these cases, periods can become lighter or irregular. If your periods are erratic, it can be difficult to predict when you might ovulate. Unpredictable or missed periods may mean that ovulation isn't occurring at all. If you know this to be the case because you're monitoring the signs of ovulation (see p.43), or using ovulation predictor tests (see p.43), do seek medical advice about your fertility.

You may be able to become pregnant naturally and easily despite problems related to your period, but some conditions that cause long, irregular, or heavy periods are linked to lower fertility. Heavy periods can be caused by conditions such as fibroids (see p.218), which can affect fertility. A higher than average level of blood loss can also make you anaemic, which is not the best start for pregnancy for you or your baby, so you may want to look at boosting your iron intake (see p.154).

Conditions causing painful periods can impact on fertility. Endometriosis is a common disorder that can make periods painful and cause discomfort during sex. If you have these symptoms, see your doctor who might arrange a scan or refer you to a specialist. In endometriosis, cells resembling those that line the uterus come to lie outside the uterus on structures such as the ovaries, the Fallopian tubes, and the walls of the pelvis. Endometriosis can be treated by laser surgery, which can boost a woman's chances of conceiving.

ASK A... DOCTOR

Should I monitor my menstrual cycle? Yes, monitoring your cycle is an important part of planning for pregnancy because it can help you to work out roughly on which day you're ovulating (see p.49) and thereby improve your chances of conceiving. It means you can ensure you have sexual intercourse at roughly the right time.

It's also helpful to note the length of your cycle, which may vary. The most important thing to note is that from ovulation to the start of your next period is always around 14 days, so when you get your next period you can work out roughly when you ovulated.

FOCUS ON... IVF

Stimulating egg follicles

IVF (in vitro fertilization) may be an option if you are having trouble conceiving. The first stage with this procedure is to stimulate the ovaries to produce many follicles, so that multiple eggs can be fertilized outside the body. Starting on around day three of your cycle, you will be given drugs to stimulate your ovaries. You will need to inject yourself (see right) or use a nasal spray to suppress the normal cycle, followed by injections of a follicle-stimulating hormone. Egg retrieval will then take place (see p.57).

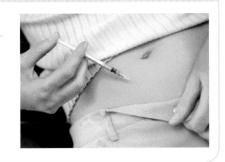

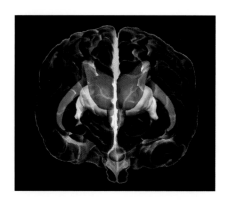

276 days to go...

WHAT'S HAPPENING INSIDE

In this coloured 3D scan of the human brain, the green central structure is the hypothalamus. In response to circulating oestrogen, this releases chemicals that prompt the pituitary gland (green area at bottom) to in turn release hormones that trigger ovulation.

Like many women, you may sometimes feel ruled by your hormones, and it helps to understand why they fluctuate.

The hormone build-up to ovulation starts right now in week one of your menstrual cycle. Your pituitary gland, which lies at the base of your brain, produces follicle-stimulating hormone (FSH). During your period, the level of FSH rises steadily, triggering the development of the follicles (around 15–20 each month) in each ovary. As well as containing each egg, the follicles produce oestrogen.

The hormone oestrogen circulates, affecting the pituitary gland and causing it to produce luteinizing hormone (LH) – this triggers ovulation (see p.49). This week your oestrogen levels are low and steady, but will rise dramatically later in your cycle.

Progesterone levels are low during your period, but start to rise several days afterwards and stay high for the second part of the cycle. Under the influence of progesterone, the muscles in the cervix relax, easing open the cervical canal. Changes also affect the mucus, which becomes more fluid, so sperm find it easier to swim through. It is progesterone that enables the lining of the uterus to thicken in preparation for implantation of the fertilized egg.

AS A MATTER OF FACT

Men get PMT too!

Scientists have confirmed there's a male version of PMT – Irritable Male Syndrome. Mood swings, temper tantrums, and loss of libido in men were found to be caused by falling levels of testosterone due to stress.

THE LOWDOWN

Fertility rites

Rooted in folklore, these fertility tips require a leap of faith and a good sense of humour!

■ **Use the moon.** Exponents of "lunaception" believe that women whose menstrual cycle aligns with the lunar cycle – so they menstruate during the new moon and ovulate when the moon is full – have more chance of conceiving. It's based on the theory that women's cycles are influenced by natural light.

■ **Dance around the Maypole.** Maypoles are thought to herald the arrival of spring and celebrate fertility.

CHANGES DURING THE MENSTRUAL CYCLE

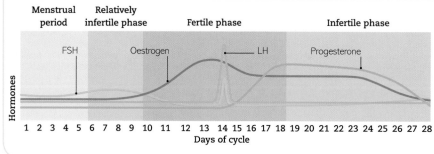

Menstrual period | Relatively infertile phase | Fertile phase | Infertile phase

FSH | Oestrogen | LH | Progesterone

Hormones

1 2 3 4 5 6 7 8 9 10 11 12 13 14 15 16 17 18 19 20 21 22 23 24 25 26 27 28
Days of cycle

There are four hormones at work during the menstrual cycle: FSH (follicle-stimulating hormone) causes the egg follicles to start developing in the ovary; oestrogen is produced by the developing egg and peaks just before ovulation; LH (luteinizing hormone) triggers ovulation; and progesterone thickens the lining of the uterus.

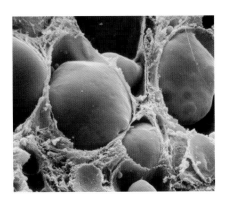

275 days to go...

WHAT'S HAPPENING INSIDE

This cross-section through the ovary shows several ovarian follicles. Between each follicle, the connective tissue can be seen. Each month about 15–20 follicles mature, but it is usually only one that will fully mature and release an egg.

Making some lifestyle changes is essential when you're trying for a baby, and cutting down on alcohol is a good start.

Even though it's still the week of your period, and some time before you ovulate, try to ensure you're in the best possible health to maximize fertility. One way to do this is to cut down your alcohol intake.

Heavy drinking can reduce the chances of conceiving and, if you do get pregnant, it can also affect your unborn baby's development. There is plenty of evidence that drinking beyond the recommended amounts is harmful. What's lacking, however, is evidence of the effects on conception and pregnancy of the occasional alcoholic drink, perhaps one or two glasses of wine once or twice a week. However, many women decide to err on the side of caution and stop drinking alcohol altogether while trying to conceive and in early pregnancy. Some find that morning sickness (see p.81) naturally puts them off alcohol.

Alcohol also affects male fertility, because it has adverse effects on the quantity and quality of sperm produced, and drinking large amounts can cause men to become impotent.

However, you may find an alcoholic drink helps you and your partner relax and puts you in the mood for sex, thereby increasing your chances of conception, so don't feel guilty about having the occasional glass of your favourite tipple.

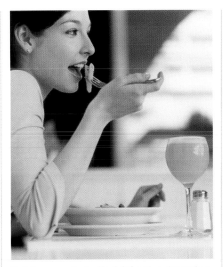

Opt for non-alcoholic drinks if you're trying to have a baby. A high intake of alcohol can adversely affect your chances of conceiving.

AS A MATTER OF FACT

Illicit or "street drugs" can harm your unborn baby.

You should try to stop using drugs before you conceive. However, if you regularly use drugs, or find it hard to manage without them, it is essential to get medical support. Ask your doctor for advice. He or she will be able to help and put you in touch with a support group.

TIME TO THINK ABOUT

Having medical checks

Before you try to conceive, speak to your doctor about the following tests:

■ **Rubella:** have a blood test to check you have antibodies against rubella (German measles). Being infected by the rubella virus for the first time in early pregnancy is associated with an increased risk of the baby developing an abnormality, as well as increasing the risk of miscarriage. If you were vaccinated against rubella as a child, your antibody level may be high enough to protect your baby. If it isn't high enough, you'll be offered an MMR (measles, mumps, rubella) jab and advised not to conceive for three months.

■ **Sexually transmitted infections:** go to a genito-urinary medicine (GUM) clinic for tests to rule out infections such as chlamydia, genital warts, and herpes. You may also want to consider having an HIV test. Women with HIV can still bear children, but may be prescribed a drug to reduce the chances of passing the infection to their child. A Caesarean may be recommended.

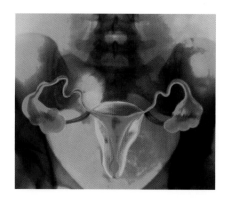

274 days to go...

WHAT'S HAPPENING INSIDE

In this artwork of the uterus, the green central structure is the pear-shaped uterus itself; the red part is the cavity of the uterus. The blue structures to either side are the Fallopian tubes, which each have an ovary, seen in pink here, at the end.

Eating well is an essential part of conception and pregnancy, so you and your partner should get into good habits now.

FOCUS ON... NUTRITION

Vital B vitamins

Your diet should include foods containing B vitamins (see p.16). Take a pregnancy multi-vitamin if needed.
- **B1** deficiency has been linked to failed ovulation and implantation.
- **B2** deficiency has been linked to infertility and miscarriage.
- **B5** is important for conception and fetal development.
- **B6** is essential for the formation and functioning of sex hormones.
- **B12,** with folate (see p.16), is essential to fetal development.

Take the time in this first two weeks of your cycle, before you ovulate, to look at what you eat on a daily basis – if you and your partner (see p.44) make some simple changes to your diet, it might just improve your chances of conception.

Use this opportunity to check your weight and your Body Mass Index (BMI) (see p.17), as a BMI of under 19 or over 24 could impact adversely on fertility.

If you're overweight, excess fat tissue may affect your metabolism and hormones and you may not ovulate as regularly, if at all. If you need fertility treatment, the chances of success are also lower if you're overweight, because you may respond less well to the drugs that stimulate ovulation. Once you're pregnant, being overweight can also cause an increased risk of complications, decreasing the chance of carrying the pregnancy to full term.

Weighing too little when you're trying to conceive isn't healthy either. Pregnancy takes its toll on a woman's reserves, so a little stored fat is a good thing for mother and baby. Being seriously underweight can affect ovulation and make periods irregular or absent, and conception unlikely.

Your BMI when you conceive is also a good indication of how much weight you should gain once you're pregnant (see p.99), so it's worth getting it checked at this point.

GET FIT AND FERTILE!

Regular exercise can increase your chances of conceiving by allowing your body to work at optimum levels. If you're fit and have a healthy lifestyle, you will reduce the level of toxins in your body and be less stressed, which makes it easier to conceive. Exercise will also regulate your energy and your blood-sugar levels, which assists the body in regulating the hormonal cycle – a key player in the reproductive process. Conversely, over-exercising can adversely affect the ovulation process and make conception more difficult.

The guidelines for exercising at this crucial time of conception are to continue weight-bearing exercise, such as walking, jogging, or aerobics, for 30 minutes five times a week at a moderate intensity. It is important to listen to your body – moderate means exercising within a comfortable range, where the exercise isn't too hard but is pushing your body enough to feel the benefits.

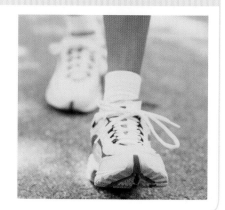

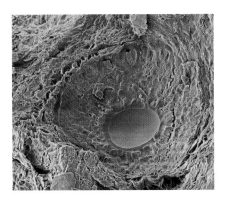

273 days to go...

WHAT'S HAPPENING INSIDE

Here an egg can be seen, in orange, developing in the ovary. The cells of the follicle, in which it is contained, can be seen surrounding the egg. At birth, baby girls have millions of follicles present in their ovaries.

When you're trying to have a baby, you need to take your age into account because your fertility will change as you get older.

In about a week's time you are likely to ovulate. At the start of puberty, you had about 400 immature eggs, or follicles, in your ovaries, and will have made no new eggs since then. In fact, your lifetime of eggs were there when you were born. It is possible to conceive from puberty until the menopause and doctors advise menopausal women to continue to use contraception for two years after their last period.

Women aged 20–24 are generally considered at their most fertile. For most women, periods continue until their early fifties, although the rate of fertility gradually lowers in the 30s, 40s, and 50s, and the rate of chromosomal abnormalities and miscarriage increases. Nonetheless, every year thousands of babies are born to women in their late 30s and 40s.

If you're hoping to start a family, it's safe to assume that fertility begins to fall off sharply after the age of 35. Your age also affects the quality of your eggs. In women in their early 20s, around 17 per cent of eggs have a chromosomal abnormality, but the figure rises to more than 75 per cent in women in their 40s. Chromosomal problems increase the chances of having a child with a disorder such as Down's syndrome (see p.476).

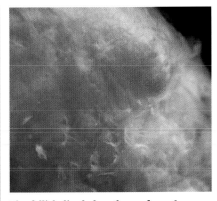

The follicle lies below the surface of the ovarian wall and protrudes just prior to ovulation. The follicle is most likely to rupture and release an egg mid-cycle, around days 13 and 14 of a 28-day cycle.

If you're concerned about your fertility, it is possible to have a blood test that can give an indication of your remaining ovary function so that you know how much reproductive time you have left. While some tests are based on levels of FSH (see p.38) and oestrogen, newer tests use other markers found in the blood, such as anti-Mullerian hormone (AMH) and inhibin B.

But conceiving depends on more than releasing an egg; it must travel down the Fallopian tube, be fertilized, implant, and the pregnancy be maintained. There's also the father's contribution to consider (see box, top right).

THE MALE BIOLOGICAL CLOCK?

A man can continue to make sperm more or less throughout his life, so you might not expect male fertility to fall significantly. There are plenty of older fathers around that seemingly prove this.

Recent research from France, however, found that men aged over 35 took a lot longer to get their partner pregnant. For those who conceived, there was a slightly higher risk of miscarrying. This is because sperm from older men is more likely to contain damaged DNA. So although older couples do conceive, it's a fact that men, like women, are past their peak fertility.

AS A MATTER OF FACT

Sperm have a long and perilous journey of 30–40cm (12–16in) to reach the egg.

This is why nature is bountiful when it comes to sperm, producing many millions with each ejaculation. On average each ejaculation produces 2–8ml of semen, with over 40 million sperm in each millilitre.

41

Your 2nd week

YOUR "FERTILE WINDOW" IS APPROACHING AND THIS COULD BE THE TIME YOU CONCEIVE

Towards the end of this week, one of the eggs in your ovaries is likely to have reached full maturity. Ovulation occurs as the egg, under the influence of hormones, bursts out of its follicle. If it meets a sperm, you may become pregnant. Now is the time to enjoy lots of sex with your partner, so go for it – as often as you like. If you have any anxieties about fertility, try to put them aside and relax.

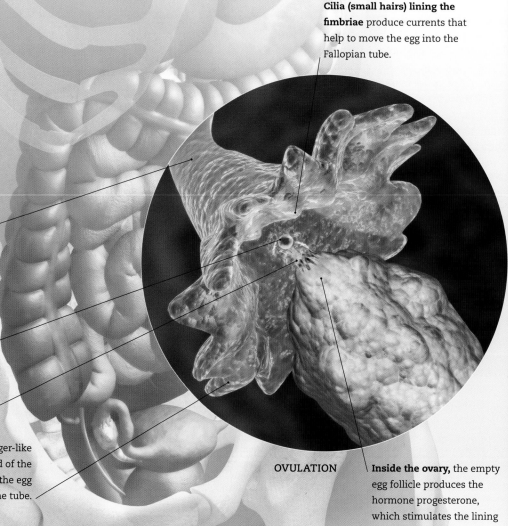

Cilia (small hairs) lining the fimbriae produce currents that help to move the egg into the Fallopian tube.

The wall of the Fallopian tube contracts and relaxes to draw the egg into the tube for its journey to the uterus.

The mature egg is released from its follicle and breaks through the surface of the ovary. To meet a sperm, and be fertilized, it must enter the Fallopian tube.

Fluid from the egg follicle is released with the mature egg.

Fimbriae, the finger-like projections at the end of the Fallopian tube, reach for the egg and sweep it gently into the tube.

OVULATION

Inside the ovary, the empty egg follicle produces the hormone progesterone, which stimulates the lining of the uterus to thicken.

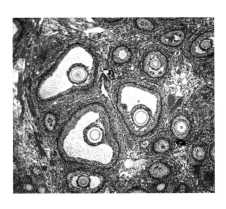

272 days to go...

WHAT'S HAPPENING INSIDE

Here, three developing ovarian follicles can be seen in white. The inner circle of each is the egg. Of the follicles shown, it is likely that only one will be fully mature at ovulation (see p.49) and release an egg.

By the end of this week you're likely to have ovulated. It's worth knowing the signs that indicate you're at your most fertile.

This is week two of your cycle.
You will probably ovulate by the end of this week, and will therefore be fertile. As sperm can survive for 5 days inside you and an egg lives for 12–24 hours after ovulation, the window for an egg to be fertilized is 6 days. However, as the day of ovulation varies from day 12 to day 16, the fertile phase is regarded as spanning 9 days. If you have regular periods, ovulation can be easier to track, but you may want to use other methods, such as looking out for natural signs (see box, right) or using an ovulation kit. Remember, however, the best way to conceive is to have sex regularly.

Although they are useful, testing kits are expensive and can be counter-productive because they make sex more clinical and less enjoyable. They work by testing the urine to detect a surge in LH, the hormone that triggers egg release.

Always follow the instructions given in the kit. After a positive test, you should ovulate 12–36 hours later. Results are about 99 per cent accurate but occasionally the result is falsely positive. Results can occasionally be falsely negative. If your test was negative, do another one the next day. Once you have a positive result, you can stop testing for that month.

ARE YOU OVULATING?

This week, look out for:
■ **Lower abdominal pain** at ovulation, called mittelschmerz (the German for "pain in the middle").
■ **Basal body temperature** (your temperature when you first wake in the morning) rising slightly.
■ **Cervical mucus** – the cervix produces secretions, which become wetter, clearer in colour, and stretchy, resembling raw egg white, just before ovulation. This indicates the start of your fertile phase.

CHANGES DURING THE MENSTRUAL CYCLE

Body temperature can be seen at the top of the chart, rising sharply straight after ovulation. The bottom section shows cervical secretions. These begin in the days leading up to ovulation, starting off moist and sticky, then becoming wetter and stretchy at your most fertile time.

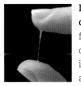

If you feel some of the cervical mucus with your fingers, you will find you can stretch it out. This is a sign that you are about to ovulate.

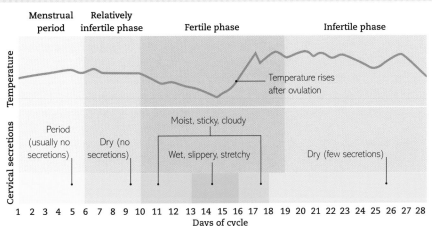

Menstrual period | Relatively infertile phase | Fertile phase | Infertile phase

Temperature

Temperature rises after ovulation

Cervical secretions

Period (usually no secretions) | Dry (no secretions) | Moist, sticky, cloudy / Wet, slippery, stretchy | Dry (few secretions)

1 2 3 4 5 6 7 8 9 10 11 12 13 14 15 16 17 18 19 20 21 22 23 24 25 26 27 28
Days of cycle

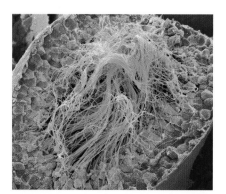

271 days to go...

WHAT'S HAPPENING INSIDE

In your partner's body, sperm are constantly being produced. Here the sperm cells can be seen: they consist of a head (green), which contains the genetic material, and fertilizes the egg, and a tail (blue), which propels the sperm along.

While you wait to ovulate, fascinating changes are occurring in your ovaries as your follicles mature to release an egg.

In the time leading up to ovulation, which will happen later this week, the most mature follicle moves to the surface of the ovary, ready to release its precious cargo. While you were having your period, around 15–20 follicles were developing in your ovaries.

Both of your ovaries contribute to follicle growth, but usually only one ovary brings a follicle to ovulation. Which ovary it is seems to depend on chance as ovaries do not operate a strict rota. As the follicles grow, they enlarge greatly, filling with fluid secreted inside the follicle. Some women release more than one egg some months (see p.49) and if both are fertilized, it will mean non-identical twins are conceived.

By the time of ovulation, the mature follicle will be about 2cm (1in) in diameter, while the egg is just about visible without a microscope.

To mature, follicles need FSH (follicle-stimulating hormone) produced by the brain's pituitary gland (see p.38), but their early growth doesn't appear to rely on it. It may, however, depend on other hormones and chemicals.

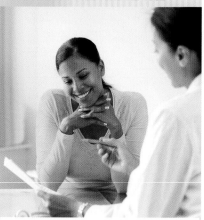

SPECIALIST MEDICAL ADVICE

If you have any ongoing medical problems, go to see your doctor before you start trying to conceive. Conditions such as diabetes, asthma, high blood pressure, heart trouble, a previous bout of deep vein thrombosis (DVT) (see p.186), thyroid conditions, sickle cell disease, and epilepsy can all impact on a pregnancy.

The effect will depend on the individual condition and specialist advice and care will be needed. If you're in any doubt about how your own medical history may affect a pregnancy, check with your doctor before you start trying to conceive.

FOCUS ON... DADS

Dads: your diet counts too

Since sperm take some weeks to mature, if you want to become a dad you should start eating a healthy diet at least three months before conception. There are dietary supplements, but most vitamins and minerals work better in the form of real food.

■ **Antioxidants** A diet rich in anti-oxidants, including vitamins A, C, and E, selenium, and zinc, helps prevent damage to sperm DNA.

■ **Selenium** may help sperm penetrate the outer layer of the egg.

Eat tuna, yeast, wheatgerm, wholegrains, and sesame seeds.

■ **Zinc** is present in large amounts in semen. Eat fish, lean meat, shellfish, turkey, chicken, eggs, wholegrains, rye, and oats.

■ **Manganese** is another element that could help male fertility. Eat leafy vegetables (including broccoli), carrots, eggs, wholegrains, and ginger.

■ **Essential fatty acids** may improve sperm motility. Eat oily fish, such as mackerel, salmon, and sardines, flaxseed and linseed, and kiwi fruit.

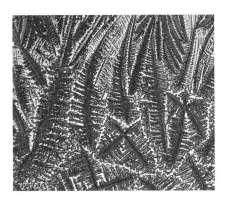

270 days to go...

WHAT'S HAPPENING INSIDE

As ovulation approaches, more cervical mucus is produced. Here it has crystallized to form a "fern leaf" pattern. Around the time of ovulation the mucus becomes clear, slippery, and stretchy, which makes it easier for sperm to swim through.

You may not mind whether you have a boy or a girl, but according to some theories you can influence gender.

Conceiving is all about having sex at the right time this week, but if you're hoping to have a child of a specific gender, the timing could be even more important. Some experts claim there is a link between when you have sex and the baby's gender (see below).

Recent research suggests that women who have a high calorie intake (especially if they eat that most phallic of fruit, the banana) are marginally more likely to bear a boy. Those who skip breakfast or have a low calorie intake are more likely to have a girl. One reason for this is thought to be that the extra calories consumed affect vaginal secretions and help to give the Y sperm, which makes baby boys, a vital boost.

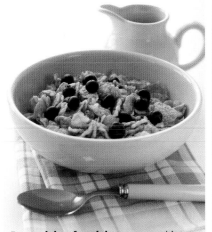

Research has found that women with high glucose levels, achieved by eating normally and not skipping breakfast, were more likely to conceive a boy.

AS A MATTER OF FACT

If you already have two same-sex children, you're 75 per cent more likely to conceive a child of that sex again.

Although the sex of the baby conceived is random, conceiving children of the same sex could be down to the fact that some men produce better quality X sperm, which makes baby girls, or Y sperm, which makes baby boys.

Statistically, couples who have two children of different sexes are less likely to try for a third child.

MAKING BABIES... BOYS AND GIRLS

The Shettles method, devised by Dr Landrum Shettles, is based on the fact that Y sperm (for boys) are smaller, faster, and less resilient than X sperm (for girls), and are less able to withstand an acidic environment in the vagina.

To conceive a boy, the Shettles method advises:
■ Timing sex as close to ovulation as possible and adopting positions such as rear-entry that promote deep penetration.
■ The woman should orgasm, ideally at the same time as the man, to make the vagina less acidic and favour Y sperm.
■ Drinking a cup or two of strong coffee just before sex to give Y-sperm an added kick.

The Whelan method, devised by Dr Elizabeth Whelan, suggests that having sex earlier in the cycle, some four to six days before ovulation, is more likely to result in a boy. Sex nearer the time of ovulation is more likely to result in a girl. Curiously, the Whelan way is more or less the opposite of the advice given by Shettles.

But what works? The mainstream medical view, supported by reports in journals such as the *New England Journal of Medicine*, is that the timing of sex has little or no bearing on gender. The possible exception is that having sex two days before ovulation may be slightly more likely to favour a girl.

Your 2nd week

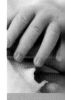

45

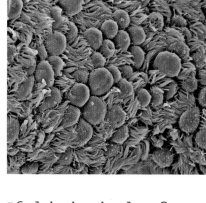

THIS IS DAY 11 OF YOUR MENSTRUAL CYCLE

269 days to go...

WHAT'S HAPPENING INSIDE

The lining of the Fallopian tube, seen here, has a moist mucous membrane. This contains cells (brown) that protect the tube's surface. The hair-like cilia (blue) move the eggs along the tubes following ovulation.

If this isn't the first month you've been trying to conceive, don't be too disappointed. It's normal for it to take some time.

Have you been trying for a baby for some time? It's hard to face the fact that we don't always conceive when we want to. This lack of success may be difficult to handle, especially if you're someone who has achieved in other areas of your life.

With reproduction, there's a large element of chance. Even for young women at their peak of fertility, the odds of conceiving in any one cycle are 50–50. It's not unusual to try for six months, or even 12 months, without success. Around 16 per cent of couples take over a year to achieve a pregnancy. So plan for conception over a longer time frame, say 12–18 months, unless you have any specific reasons to be concerned about your fertility or your health in general.

The main exception is if you are over 35. In this case, see your doctor after trying for about six months. The first step is likely to be a blood test for you, and a semen analysis for your partner. However, be reassured that if you are over 35, you may still get pregnant in the old-fashioned way. The average time taken for a 39-year-old woman to conceive is 15 months. But the snag is that if you do end up needing assisted fertility techniques, it all takes time.

STOPPING CONTRACEPTION

You can get pregnant as soon as you stop using some contraception.

■ **IUD (coil):** you can get pregnant if you have sex in the week before it's removed as sperm can live 3–5 days.

■ **Pill:** assume you're fertile immediately. Some women seem to be extra-fertile after stopping the Pill.

■ **Implants:** fertility can return immediately after removal of the implant, but some women find it takes longer. Occasionally periods can take three to nine months to become regular. This suggests that the effects of the hormone are still lingering, but you may still conceive.

■ **Injections:** irregular bleeding can continue for months, and you may not be able to conceive for several months either. However, as with implants, it's possible to get pregnant before your periods return properly.

■ **The intrauterine system (IUS):** you could get pregnant if you have sex in the week before removal of the IUS, but because the system contains progesterone, conception is less likely than with a regular coil (see left).

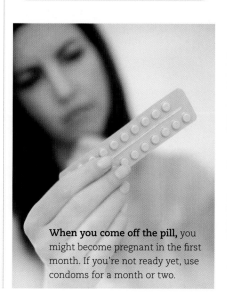

When you come off the pill, you might become pregnant in the first month. If you're not ready yet, use condoms for a month or two.

268 days to go...

WHAT'S HAPPENING INSIDE

This mature ovarian follicle contains a fluid-filled cavity (pale pink) known as the follicular antrum. At this stage, just prior to ovulation, one follicle has become much larger than the others, and it is this follicle that will rupture to release an egg.

As your hormone level rises around this stage of your cycle, so might your libido – it seems nature takes care of everything!

Oestrogen levels are rising and reach their peak today, based on a 28-day menstrual cycle. The rise in oestrogen from the follicles is what stimulates the release of the LH hormone (see p.38), which surges about 24 hours before ovulation. FSH (see p.38) from the pituitary gland starts rising later this week. Progesterone levels are low. There's no call for this hormone until the uterus lining needs to thicken. In fact, high levels would make the cervix hostile to sperm, so they would have trouble getting through to the uterus and the Fallopian tubes to fertilize the egg.

Women also produce the male hormone testosterone and this reaches a peak around ovulation. This hormone is responsible for libido in both sexes so, hopefully, you and your partner should find you're both in the mood for making babies at this time.

ASK A... DOCTOR

I had a miscarriage four weeks ago. Is it safe to try for another baby straightaway? There is no exact advice on when you should try again following a miscarriage. As a general guide, wait until you've had one menstrual period. This will help to date the pregnancy should you conceive quickly. However, your doctor may advise otherwise, especially if your miscarriage was linked with an infection. If you are waiting for tests because you miscarried, it makes sense to have these first.

You and your partner may need time to grieve for the lost pregnancy, so it is unwise to rush into trying to conceive again. Be reassured that the vast majority of women who had a single miscarriage go on to have a baby.

AS A MATTER OF FACT

Being stressed can affect your ability to conceive.

Perhaps it's no surprise that nature makes it more difficult to conceive in stressful circumstances. One reason might be that it reduces the ovary's response to the hormone surge at mid-cycle (see left). There is also a link between stress and the failure of fertility treatments, although the exact reason for this isn't known.

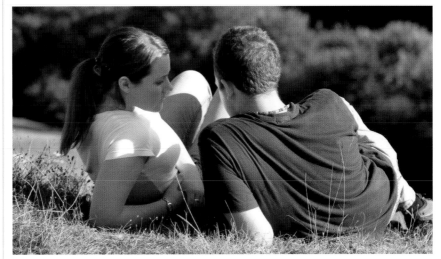

Miscarrying can be extremely tough and may put a strain on your relationship. It's worth talking about and working through your grief together before trying for another baby.

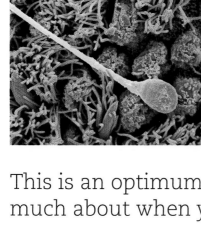

THIS IS DAY 13 OF YOUR MENSTRUAL CYCLE

267 days to go...

WHAT'S HAPPENING INSIDE

A sperm cell can be seen here inside the Fallopian tube. As sperm can stay active and alive inside you for up to three to five days, it's possible to get pregnant even if you don't ovulate until several days from now.

This is an optimum time to conceive, but try not to think too much about when you might be ovulating and just enjoy sex!

AS A MATTER OF FACT

Having an orgasm could boost your chances of conception.

One theory is that the female orgasm is an evolutionary device designed to waft semen into the cervix as the uterus contracts. If the woman climaxes up to a minute before her partner, or she doesn't orgasm, she will retain less semen than if she comes at the same time or after him.

Use the time around ovulation

to put some excitement and spontaneity back into your sex life. With all the recommendations and restrictions, not to mention old wives' tales, that supposedly maximize conception rates, it's easy to forget that sex is meant to be enjoyable. If you're hell bent on conceiving, then the fun can get forgotten. You might like to try different positions, times, or places for sex. If you and your partner aren't usually that adventurous, this is a good opportunity to try varying things a little.

Try to have sex every 24–48 hours. If your partner ejaculates regularly, it will encourage the production of quality sperm. The benefits of abstaining have been greatly overstated in the past. It is true that not having sex for up to seven days can boost the number of sperm, but research now shows that abstinence can impair their motility (swimming ability), especially if the sperm were already borderline. The longer the period of abstinence, the more marked the effect will be. So have fun and if you conceive that's a bonus!

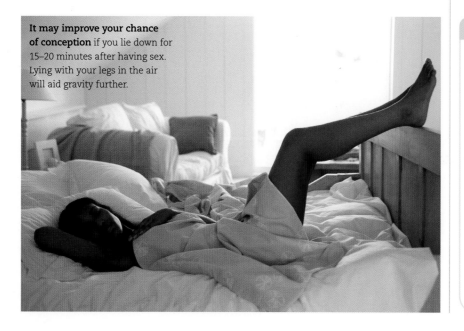

It may improve your chance of conception if you lie down for 15–20 minutes after having sex. Lying with your legs in the air will aid gravity further.

SEXUAL POSITIONS

It seems that how you have sex can affect the chance of conception. Positions that maximize penetration, such as rear entry, may work best as sperm is deposited as close to the cervix as possible – languishing too long in vaginal secretions can lead to a sperm's early death. If the man is on top, the woman could try placing a pillow under her buttocks to raise her pelvis and aid the movement of sperm towards the cervix. Woman-on-top positions may lead to leakage of sperm. Avoid using lubricants as they can adversely affect sperm.

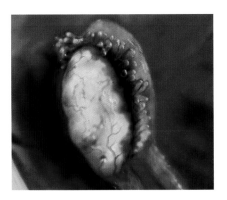

THIS IS DAY 14 OF YOUR MENSTRUAL CYCLE

266 days to go...

WHAT'S HAPPENING INSIDE

The ovary can be seen here at the end of the Fallopian tube. At around this time of the menstrual cycle, a follicle at the surface of the ovary releases an egg, which is swept into the tube by clearly visible finger-like projections called fimbriae.

You're highly likely to ovulate today, if you haven't already, and if egg meets sperm you may soon be pregnant.

Typically, ovulation occurs around day 14 but it can occur earlier or later. Ovulation is when an egg is released from your ovaries (sometimes two eggs are released – see box, below). LH rises thanks to oestrogen output from the growing follicles (see p.47), and it is this rise that triggers the events that now take place in the follicle. LH makes the egg inside the follicle become fully mature, ready for release and fertilization. This is the point at which the egg reduces its number of chromosomes (see p.54) from 46 to 23.

The follicle is rich with fluid by now. Just before ovulation, it is some 2cm (1in) or more in diameter and lies just below the surface of the ovary. If you could see the follicle, it would look like a blister about to burst. Next, the follicle produces enzymes that digest its outer layer, releasing the egg on to the surface of the ovary.

Once the egg is released from the follicle, it's soon swept into the nearest Fallopian tube by the finger-like projections that form the end of the tube, where it will hopefully be fertilized.

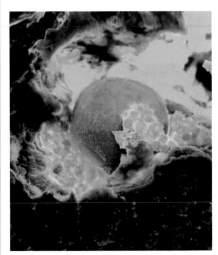

At ovulation, the follicle ruptures and the egg breaks through the surface of the ovary. Sometimes two follicles mature to this point, both releasing an egg.

FOCUS ON... RELATIONSHIPS

Pressure to conceive

If you're trying to conceive, you may have little else on your mind and this can put a strain on your relationship. With the goal of pregnancy in mind, it's easy to become clinical about sex. At this point, you and your partner may be regarding each other not so much as sex objects, but as components of a baby-making machine. Enjoyment can so easily get lost.

Understandably, you may find that your partner becomes aggrieved if he feels a pressure to provide sperm; the distress may have an adverse effect on a man's willingness and even ability to have sex. If this happens, it can lead to a downward spiral, which naturally makes conception less likely, and may cause discord.

Make an effort to be loving and work together rather than against each other. Consider taking a break; couples often conceive when they're away on holiday and more relaxed. Make sure you also enjoy some stress-free sex outside of your fertile window.

Conception

Pregnancy begins with conception, a complex process that involves the release of one or more eggs from the ovary, successful fertilization by a sperm in a Fallopian tube, and implantation in the lining of the uterus.

The release of an egg

Each woman is born with her full quota of follicles that contain immature eggs, some of which will mature and be released in her lifetime. Every month, follicle stimulating hormone (FSH), released from the pituitary gland, encourages a number of the follicles to ripen. These follicles in turn produce the hormone oestrogen, rising levels of which encourage the uterus to thicken and prepare for the implantation of a fertilized egg. As the eggs mature, the level of oestrogen rises and the pituitary gland receives a message to produce luteinizing hormone (LH). Every month, this surge in LH triggers one follicle (and sometimes more than one) to release a mature egg – the moment of ovulation.

Once the egg leaves the ovary, it enters the Fallopian tube, which lies close by, and starts to travel through the tube to the uterus. The Fallopian tube is just 10cm (4in) long and its lining has many tiny fronds that literally brush the egg in the direction of the uterus. Even so, the journey takes five days or more. In the course of this voyage, the fertilization of the egg takes place.

The journey of the sperm

During sex, the man releases an abundance of sperm – around 250 million at each ejaculation – into the vagina. Each sperm has a long tail to propel it, so it's well equipped to swim up to the Fallopian tube, where fertilization of the egg takes place. The whole distance, from the vagina through

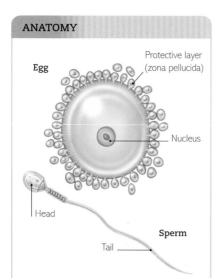

ANATOMY

Egg

Protective layer (zona pellucida)

Nucleus

Head

Sperm

Tail

The mature egg has a diameter of 0.1mm and is surrounded by a protective outer layer known as the *zona pellucida*. The far smaller sperm consists of a head, which contains the male genetic material and enzymes to help break down the egg's outer layer, and a tail that propels the sperm up the vagina and uterus to the Fallopian tube.

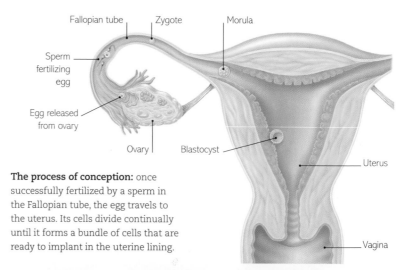

Fallopian tube | Zygote | Morula

Sperm fertilizing egg

Egg released from ovary

Ovary | Blastocyst

Uterus

Vagina

The process of conception: once successfully fertilized by a sperm in the Fallopian tube, the egg travels to the uterus. Its cells divide continually until it forms a bundle of cells that are ready to implant in the uterine lining.

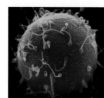

At fertilization, one sperm penetrates the egg. Once the egg and sperm have merged, they form a single cell called a zygote.

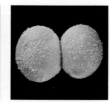

The zygote divides into two identical cells, and continues to divide as it travels down through the Fallopian tube.

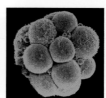

A morula – a bundle of around 16 cells – has formed by around three to four days after fertilization of the egg.

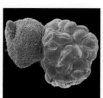

A blastocyst, a mass of up to 100 cells, hatches out of the egg's protective layer and prepares to implant in the uterus.

the uterus and up into the Fallopian tube, can be accomplished in hours. However, the sperm can survive in the vagina and uterus for 3–5 days, meaning there is a window of around 6 days in which fertilization can take place (an egg lives 12–24 hours after ovulation).

Not all of the millions of sperm make it as far as the Fallopian tube; in fact, most of them die, seep out of the vagina, or get lost along the way. Around just 300 sperm, only a tiny fraction of the number originally released, arrive at the site of the egg.

The moment of fertilization

Although many sperm cluster around the egg and try to penetrate its outer layer, only one of them will manage to burrow its way through the surface and fertilize the egg. Once this happens, the egg's outer layer thickens quickly to keep out other competing sperm, so that each egg can be fertilized by only one sperm.

Implantation in the uterus

By the time the fertilized egg reaches the uterus, it has grown from a single cell into a compact cluster of cells, called a blastocyst. This cluster attaches to the uterine lining very loosely at first, then more deeply and permanently. At this early stage, the blob of cells, which is more than just a fertilized egg, but not quite an embryo, is sometimes referred to as a "conceptus". Although its sex is already determined, it's not remotely baby-shaped yet. The cells produce enzymes that allow it to digest its way into the womb lining, and lie snugly below the surface.

Assisting conception

Some couples find that conception takes longer than anticipated. If you haven't become pregnant after two years of trying, your doctor may suggest fertility testing to identify if your fertility or that of your partner is suboptimal. If this is the case, you may want to embark on

How twins are conceived

At least one pregnancy in every 65 is a twin pregnancy. Twins are conceived in two ways, resulting in either identical or non-identical twins.

Identical twins occur when one fertilized egg splits into two separate cells. This type of twin is half as common as non-identical twins. Identical twins have the same genes and are the same sex, so they are very alike, although subtle differences in their environment can mean they're not always identical in every way. Identical twins are known as "monozygotic" twins, as they come from one "zygote", or fertilized egg. Triplets, quads, and higher multiples can be monozygotic too. However, triplets and more can arise from more complex combinations. For example, there may have been two fertilized eggs, one of which split into two.

Non-identical twins occur when two eggs are released at ovulation. Each twin's genes come from the parents, but the twins don't share the same mix of genes. Non-identical twins are also called "fraternal" twins, as they're no more alike than other siblings and can be of a different sex. They're also referred to as "dizygotic" twins, as they come from two separate "zygotes", or fertilized eggs. Non-identical triplets arise when three eggs are released instead of one. This is more likely to occur when ovulation is induced with drugs during fertility treatment (see below).

A fertilized egg divides into two

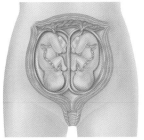

Identical twins that result from the division of one fertilized egg may share a placenta in the uterus. Occasionally, they also share an amniotic sac.

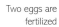

Two eggs are fertilized

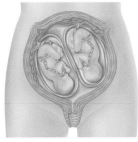

When two eggs are fertilized at the same time, non-identical twins are formed, each with its own placenta and amniotic sac.

fertility treatment to assist conception. The most popular treatment is in vitro fertilization, or IVF. This involves taking fertility drugs to help you produce more eggs. The eggs are harvested and fertilized with your partner's sperm in a laboratory (hence the term "test-tube baby"), and you're given hormone treatment to prepare the uterus to receive the fertilized eggs. If the quality of sperm is poor, a procedure called intra-cytoplasmic sperm injection, or ICSI, may be used, whereby a single sperm is injected directly into an egg and the fertilized egg is transferred to the uterus. Intra-uterine insemination, or IUI, involves putting sperm that have been sorted for viability directly into the uterus. This is used where sperm have poor motility, or there are problems with ovulation.

Your 3rd week

THIS IS THE WEEK A MIRACLE TAKES PLACE – YOUR BABY IS CONCEIVED

If you ovulated and the egg met a sperm, amazing things will happen fast. It takes just four days from fertilization for a single egg to divide into a ball of 58 cells. By the end of the week, this ball, called the blastocyst, will have reached the uterus, where it will start to implant in the lining. It will be a couple of weeks before you know whether you've conceived, but special hormones kick in now to help maintain the pregnancy.

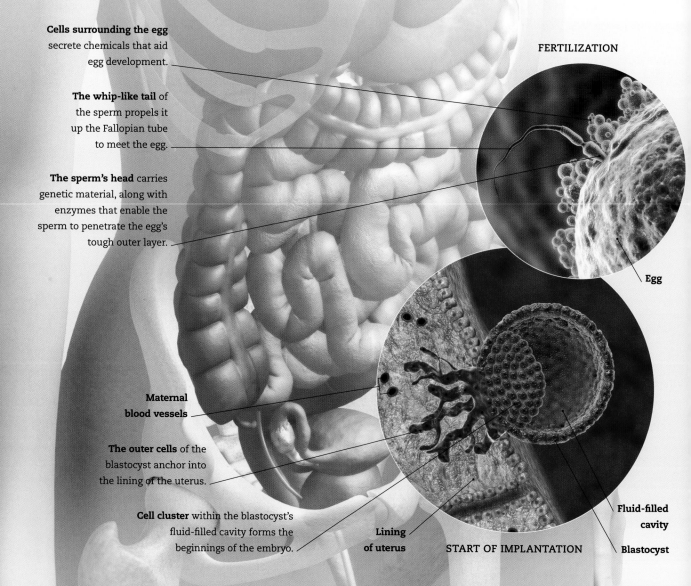

Cells surrounding the egg secrete chemicals that aid egg development.

The whip-like tail of the sperm propels it up the Fallopian tube to meet the egg.

The sperm's head carries genetic material, along with enzymes that enable the sperm to penetrate the egg's tough outer layer.

FERTILIZATION

Egg

Maternal blood vessels

The outer cells of the blastocyst anchor into the lining of the uterus.

Cell cluster within the blastocyst's fluid-filled cavity forms the beginnings of the embryo.

Lining of uterus

START OF IMPLANTATION

Fluid-filled cavity

Blastocyst

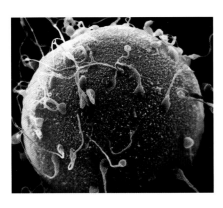

YOU ARE 2 WEEKS AND 1 DAY

265 days to go...

WHAT'S HAPPENING INSIDE

Here the egg is shown surrounded by sperm. Although only one sperm will fertilize the egg, several hundred are thought to be necessary to break down its defensive layers and enable fertilization to take place.

Your newly released egg will only survive 24 hours, but hopefully in that time it will meet sperm and be fertilized.

You are likely to have ovulated and your unfertilized egg now begins its journey. Once it has been released by the ovary, the egg is swept up by one of your Fallopian tubes and, moving in the direction of the uterus, comes to rest in the widest portion of the tube, awaiting fertilization.

It is no exaggeration to say that for each sperm released the chance of even reaching the site of fertilization is in the order of one in a million. Around 300 sperm reach the tube but only one will fertilize the egg. Once the sperm has penetrated, it triggers a reaction that

makes the surface impenetrable. Each sperm and egg contain 23 chromosomes, half of the total genetic material required. The egg will always contain an X chromosome but the sperm will carry either an X or Y chromosome and therefore determines the sex of the embryo. The sperm and egg chromosomes combine, forming the "zygote", and fertilization is complete.

A few hundred sperm survive the journey and encounter the egg in the Fallopian tube, but it is just one sperm that actually fertilizes the egg.

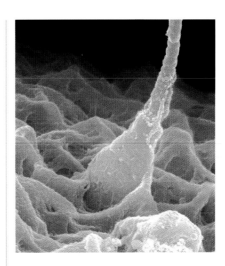

FOCUS ON... DADS

Fit but not fertile?

If you want to become a dad, there are many reasons why you should ensure you're in good shape, not least to support your partner as she prepares for pregnancy. However, while a couch potato lifestyle isn't desirable for men who want to conceive, it seems that pulling out all the stops at the gym might not be the best course of action either.

Researchers asked a group of fit young men to exercise intensively four times a week for two weeks.

Afterwards, their semen was tested and found to contain fewer sperm and lower levels of the hormones essential for conception. These hormonal changes were temporary and returned to near normal within a few days of the men resuming previous levels of activity.

The concern is that recovery might not be so fast among older men, or in those who have poor sperm counts and/or low hormone levels. So keep fit but don't overdo it.

AS A MATTER OF FACT

The hormones responsible for the production of sperm are released every 60 to 90 minutes. So a man is constantly producing sperm cells.

In theory, this means that a male is always fertile, but it takes sperm a 72-day period to fully develop. So, leading an unhealthy lifestyle during that time will impinge on the quality. For this reason, if you're trying to conceive, your partner should embark on a healthy lifestyle for three months to produce good sperm.

Genes and inheritance

The genes that parents pass on to their children at least partly determine their children's physical and mental characteristics. In some cases, an abnormal gene may be passed on, resulting in an inherited genetic disorder.

HOW GENES ARE PASSED ON

Through the generations

Through each generation, genes are shuffled and re-shuffled. Half of a baby's genes come from its father and half from its mother. The baby's parents in turn inherited half each of their genes from each of their

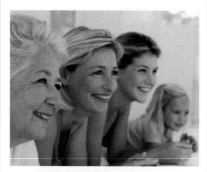

Genetic inheritance means that successive generations can share certain characteristics.

own parents. One quarter of each person's genes therefore come from the grandparents. So how does this happen? Instead of containing the full complement of 46 chromosomes, each egg and each sperm has just half, or 23, chromosomes each. When they meet at conception the chromosomes pair up to make up again the full complement that now forms the genetic blueprint for the new individual. One of the 23 pairs of chromosomes are sex chromosomes, so gender is also determined at conception. Each egg carries an X chromosome and each sperm either an X or Y. If two X chromosomes combine, the baby will be a girl; if an X and Y chromosome combine, the baby will be a boy (see right).

What are genes?

Genes are located on rod-like structures called chromosomes that are found in the nucleus of every cell in the body. Each gene occupies a specific position on a chromosome. Because genes provide instructions for making proteins, and proteins determine the structure and function of each cell in the body, it follows that genes are responsible for all the characteristics you inherit.

The full genetic instructions for each person, known as the human genome, is carried by 23 pairs of chromosomes, and consists of around 20,000–25,000 genes.

How inheritance works

At conception, the embryo receives 23 chromosomes from the mother's egg and 23 chromosomes from the father's sperm. These pair up to make a total of 46 chromosomes. Pairs 1 to 22 are identical or nearly identical; the 23rd pair consist of the sex chromosomes, which are either X or Y. Each egg and sperm contains a different combination of genes. This is because when egg and sperm cells form, chromosomes join together and randomly exchange genes between each other before the cell divides. This means that, with the exception of identical twins (see p.51), each person has unique characteristics.

How gender is determined Of the 23 pairs of chromosomes that are inherited, one pair determines gender. This pair is composed either of two X (female) chromosomes, in which case the baby will be a girl, or of one X and one Y (male) chromosome, in which case the baby will be a boy.

| Maternal grandmother | Maternal grandfather | Paternal grandmother | Paternal grandfather |

Mother

Father

Genes shared with maternal grandmother

Genes shared with paternal grandfather

Genes shared with maternal grandfather

Genes shared with paternal grandmother

Child

An egg always contains one X chromosome, while a sperm can carry an X or a Y chromosome. Whether your baby is a boy or a girl will therefore always be determined by the father. If a sperm carrying an X chromosome fertilizes the egg, the resulting embryo will be a girl. If a sperm with a Y chromosome fertilizes the egg, the resulting embryo will be a boy. In the male, both the X and Y chromosomes are active. In females, however, one of the two X chromosomes is deactivated early in development of the embryo to prevent duplicate instructions. This could be the X chromosome from either the mother or the father.

Gene variations Each gene within a cell exists in two versions, one inherited from each parent. Often these genes are identical. However, some paired genes occur in slightly different versions, called alleles. There may be two to several hundred alleles of a gene, although each person can have only two. This variation in alleles accounts for the differences between individuals, such as colour of eyes or shape of ears. One allele may be dominant and "overpower" the other recessive one (see box, right).

Why genetic disorders occur

Genes usually exist in a healthy form, but sometimes a gene is faulty. Genetic disorders arise either when an abnormal gene is inherited or when a gene changes, or mutates. Genetic disorders may follow a dominant or recessive pattern of inheritance (see right). They can also be passed on via the X chromosome. Such sex-linked disorders are usually recessive, which means that a woman can carry the faulty gene without being affected, because she has another healthy X chromosome to compensate. If a boy receives an affected X chromosome, he will be affected; a girl will be a healthy carrier like her mother. An affected male could pass on the affected gene only to his daughters.

Dominant and recessive genes

Genes come in pairs, and each gene in a pair may differ slightly. One gene may be dominant, and override the recessive gene. A recessive gene only has an effect if both genes are recessive. An example is eye colour, although there are more genes for eye colour than depicted here.

KEY

 Recessive gene for blue eyes

 Dominant gene for brown eyes

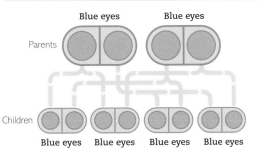

Two pairs of recessive genes
When both parents have blue eyes, as shown here, they will both have a pair of recessive genes for blue eye colour. All of the children will therefore have blue eyes as there is no dominant gene present to mask the recessive gene.

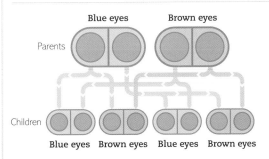

Recessive and mixed genes
In this example, each child will inherit at least one recessive blue eye gene from the parents. Depending on whether the other gene is dominant or recessive, the couple's offspring have a 1 in 2 chance of inheriting blue eyes, and a 1 in 2 chance of inheriting brown eyes.

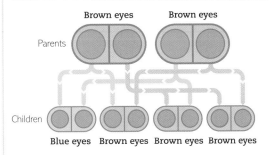

Two pairs of mixed genes
Here, each child has a 1 in 4 chance of inheriting two recessive genes and having blue eyes, and a 3 in 4 chance of inheriting a dominant gene for brown eyes. The brown-eyed offspring may have either a pair of dominant genes, or have mixed genes.

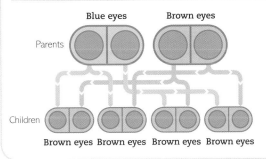

Recessive and dominant genes In this example, all of the children will have brown eyes. This is because each child receives a recessive gene from one parent and a dominant gene from the other parent. The dominant gene will override the recessive gene on each occasion.

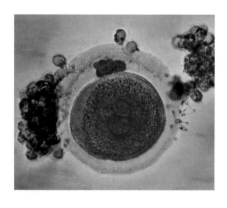

264 days to go...

WHAT'S HAPPENING INSIDE

Here a human egg cell 24 hours after fertilization is artificially coloured purple. Around the egg is a thick layer (yellow) that has now become impenetrable. The two red areas, or pro-nuclei, contain genetic material from the mother and father before it has fused.

When your egg has been fertilized, hormonal changes naturally occur to stop your normal menstrual cycle.

At this early stage following fertilization of your egg, the developing embryo will signal its existence to the pituitary gland in your brain and switch off your menstrual cycle. It does this by producing a new hormone, called human chorionic gonadotrophin (hCG). This hormone over-rides your usual monthly cycle and maintains the high progesterone levels that are essential for your pregnancy. The hormone progesterone (see p.38) is essential to an embryo's survival in the uterus, and therefore to your baby's wellbeing and development before birth.

Later, starting around weeks four to five, your embryo will make all the hormones needed to maintain its own life. Of course, its nourishment and shelter come from you, but even in the very early weeks of pregnancy the embryo behaves like an independent human, at least as far as its hormones and genes are concerned.

ASK A... DOCTOR

I've been doing ovulation tests, but they've all been negative. Does this mean I haven't ovulated this month? You may still have ovulated, even without a positive test. It's possible to miss the LH surge by chance. This is more likely if you don't test at the same time each day, or if you drink a lot of water.

Remember, too, that ovulation tests are imperfect, and it's possible to get a false negative. If you had other symptoms of ovulation, such as pain, or changes in your mucus (see p.43), it's likely that you ovulated anyway. However, if you have gone two or three months with consistently negative tests, then you might not be ovulating regularly. In that case, it's worth seeking medical advice.

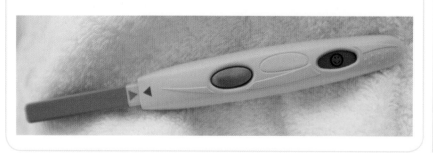

HEALTHY CONCEPTION

When you're trying to conceive, you'll find you are much more aware of your general health. As a rule, colds, flu, and other common infections are unlikely to affect your fertility or your unborn baby if you have conceived. Some infections and viruses, however, can have a more serious impact:
- **Shingles and chickenpox** (both caused by the same virus) are best avoided around the time of conception if you haven't had chickenpox before.
- **Food poisoning,** for example caused by listeria bacteria, can be harmful (see p.17).
- **Toxoplasmosis** can be contracted from handling cat faeces (see p.101).

AS A MATTER OF FACT

Too much testosterone can affect a woman's fertility.

Small quantities of testosterone are secreted from the adrenal gland and the ovaries. In low levels it may aid fertility, but too much can affect the menstrual cycle and lead to infertility.

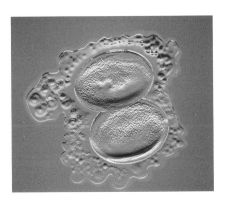

263 days to go...

WHAT'S HAPPENING INSIDE

When the two nuclei have pooled their genetic material to create a cell containing its full complement of 46 chromosomes – 23 each from the mother and father – the cell can start dividing. It is shown here at the first division, creating a two-celled body.

Vital cell divisions are now taking place as the fertilized egg begins its journey towards implantation.

The chromosomes from the sperm and egg joined over 24 hours ago. It takes around 30 hours for the resulting zygote to complete its first cell division. The zygote, at only 0.1mm in diameter, goes on to divide into 16 cells, forming a compact ball.

Cell division is such that the ball of cells is hardly any larger than the original zygote. The ball of 16 cells, now known as a "morula" (as it resembles a mulberry), travels towards the uterus, entering on day three to four after fertilization. Every cell within the morula is totipotent, meaning it is able to form any type of cell. From this point onwards the cells will lose this function as they start to specialize.

FOCUS ON... IVF

From eggs to embryos

Egg collection (see right) will be scheduled, following the first stage of IVF (see p.37). Not all follicles that were stimulated will contain eggs. Two days after egg retrieval, you will be given progesterone to thicken the uterus lining. Two to five days after fertilization, the most promising embryos are chosen to be transferred.

If you're under 40, you'll have one or two embryos transferred. If you're over 40, you may have up to three transferred. The aim is to achieve a pregnancy, yet limit the risks of a multiple pregnancy. Any leftover embryos can be frozen for future treatment cycles. Recent research suggests that frozen embryos are better than fresh ones – this may be because only the best embryos are selected for freezing and survive the freezing and thawing process.

The outcome of IVF depends to a great extent on the woman's age, but on average each cycle has a 20 per cent success rate.

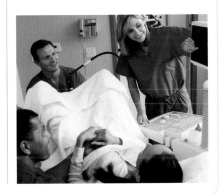

ASK A... DOCTOR

I've been doing ovulation tests. I've now ovulated, so do my partner and I need to keep having sex to make sure I conceive? You can't be sure that you've conceived already, so the usual advice would be to continue lovemaking. Even if you've been tracking your ovulation by monitoring your temperature or cervical mucus, or by using an ovulation kit (see p.43), you can't be sure exactly when it occurred. It won't be possible for you to pinpoint the exact time of ovulation.

Since the fertile window is several days, you may as well continue having sex for at least a couple of days after what you think is your most fertile time.

Furthermore, since sex says "I love you" more strongly than most other means of communication, it's good for both you and your partner to stay intimate at times you're not trying to conceive.

Remember also that abstention doesn't usually have the hoped-for effect of banking up and improving the quantity and quality of sperm. In fact, the opposite may happen (see p.48).

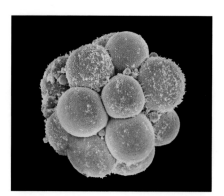

262 days to go...

WHAT'S HAPPENING INSIDE

This is an embryo at the 16-cell stage, when it has changed from a zygote into a morula. It is in the process of dividing into a hollow ball of cells – the blastocyst – which will eventually implant in the lining of the uterus.

Significant changes are taking place daily within your uterus and within just 72 hours from now, the fertilized egg will implant.

Around four days following fertilization fluid begins to collect within the morula (see p.57). This creates a separate outer cell layer, one cell thick, that encapsulates an inner mass of cells. The inner layer will become the embryo, and the outer layer the placenta (see p.76). The whole structure now consists of approximately 58 cells and is termed the "blastocyst".

The blastocyst spends several days within the cavity of the uterus before implanting. The morula had an impenetrable outer surface as it travelled, but this disappears as the blastocyst prepares for implantation.

ASK A... MUM

Why are people so interested in whether or not I've conceived? I certainly found that once I'd told people I was trying for a baby, they were inordinately interested in the process. It was difficult, especially in the week when I was waiting to find out if I'd conceived. The best way to deal with it is to respond by saying that you'll let people know if there's news. If you're struggling to conceive, telling people you're having difficulties should help to stop them from asking.

FOCUS ON... HEALTH

Fertility: the alternative approach

If you're having difficulty conceiving, or just want to improve your chances, consider using a complementary therapy. Always inform the practitioner that you might be pregnant.

■ **Reflexology** works by manipulating pressure points in the feet to improve energy flow to specific parts of the body. While there is plenty of anecdotal evidence that reflexology helps conception, this isn't currently backed up by scientific research. However, it may help to relieve stress, which can be a factor in couples who have problems conceiving.

■ **Acupuncture** (see right) works on the principle that problems such as infertility are caused by blockages in the body's energy flow or "chi". By inserting tiny needles into energy points that are linked to the reproductive organs, the flow is restored. In 2008, after reviewing seven studies of more than 1,300 women having fertility treatment, researchers concluded that acupuncture given around the time

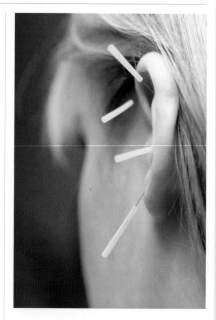

of embryo transfer increases the chances of pregnancy.

It's not as clear whether acupuncture can improve fertility in couples not undergoing treatment, but it is thought to boost male fertility by improving sperm health and reducing stress, a factor that can impede the chances of conception.

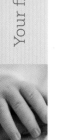

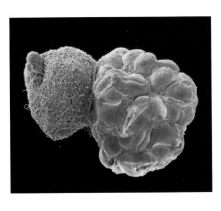

261 days to go...

WHAT'S HAPPENING INSIDE

This is an embryo at the blastocyst stage, five days after fertilization. It is seen hatching from the shell that originally surrounded the unfertilized egg. At this stage, the blastocyst has moved into the uterus and is preparing to implant.

While you're playing the waiting game, you may like to consider how you'd feel if there are two fertilized eggs waiting to implant!

Have you conceived, and might it be twins? Twins can be non-identical or identical and each type of twins is conceived differently (see p.51).

Non-identical (dizygotic) twins are the result of two separate eggs being fertilized by separate sperm. They may also occur as a result of IVF (see p.37) if two embryos are placed in the uterus.

Identical (monozygotic) twins occur when a single egg is fertilized by a single sperm and divides into two embryos. This split can occur at any stage up to nine days after fertilization and its timing is critical to the way the placenta(s) and amniotic sac(s) are formed. If the zygote (see p.57) splits within the first three days, two separate placentas and amniotic sacs develop. If the split occurs at blastocyst stage (see right), four to nine days after fertilization, the fetuses will share a placenta but have separate sacs; when the split occurs after day nine, the fetuses will share a placenta and a sac.

Having non-identical (fraternal) twins, which come from two separate fertilized eggs, depends a lot on family history. It's often said that twins skip a

The lining of the uterus, when fertilization occurs, becomes secretory to nourish an embryo. The lining prepares itself in the same way, no matter how many embryos implant.

generation, which isn't quite true. In fact, your chances of having twins are simply higher if you have a close relative with twins, but twins never become inevitable, however many members of your family have them.

Family history is most relevant with non-identical twins, and when the twins are on the mother's side. This makes sense because this kind of twin relies on a woman releasing two eggs in any one cycle (see p.49), which may be hereditary. However, for reasons that aren't clear, a family history of twins on the father's side can be important too. It may be that the male of the species can carry a gene that makes his daughter release more than one egg at a time when she ovulates.

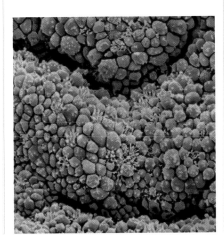

THE LOST TWIN

Twin conceptions may be more common than they appear.
Without knowing it, some women miscarry one twin in early pregnancy. It is sometimes possible to have symptoms of a miscarriage, yet, confusingly, the pregnancy then appears to continue until term, culminating in the birth of a completely normal singleton baby.

Nobody is quite sure how often this happens, or why. While around one birth in every 65–70 is a twin birth, research using scans in very early pregnancy suggests that at conception the figure is much higher. Some experts believe that 15 per cent of all births may start off as twins. Their loss could simply be nature's way of dealing with imperfections.

AS A MATTER OF FACT

The odds of having identical twins are about 3.5 in 1,000.

Some estimate that the chances of having twins after fertility-enhancing treatment is as high as 1 in 38.

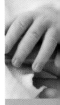

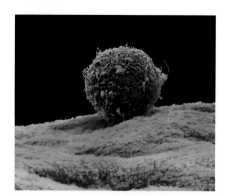

YOU ARE 2 WEEKS AND 6 DAYS

260 days to go...

WHAT'S HAPPENING INSIDE

The blastocyst prepares to imbed itself in the lining of the uterus – the endometrium. Once it is completely implanted – usually around seven days after fertilization – the pregnancy will become established.

Your reproductive organs undergo complex processes that will enable your body to maintain the pregnancy.

If you have conceived, the ball of cells known as the blastocyst that will eventually form the fetus will now be preparing to embed in the lining of your uterus, and the placenta will be starting to form.

Before this happens, however, there is another important change going on. After you ovulate, the empty ovarian follicle develops into a structure called the corpus luteum (which means, literally, "yellow body"). This small, fluid-filled sac becomes increasingly "vascular", developing blood vessels and beginning to produce the hormone progesterone. This is required to create mucus to allow your fertilized egg to survive, and build up the lining of your uterus, in which the blastocyst will soon imbed (see opposite).

The corpus luteum also produces a little oestrogen. By about 8–12 weeks of pregnancy, your placenta will take over the production of progesterone, but the corpus luteum continues to play a small role in hormone production until about six months, when it usually shrinks away.

ASK A... DOCTOR

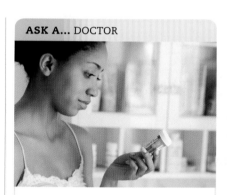

Should I stop taking medication in case I've conceived? Many medicines are safe to take, but some are not, or have not been fully evaluated. This last group includes many antihistamines for allergies, over-the-counter sleeping pills, and many painkillers (see p.23).

If you've accidentally taken an over-the-counter remedy that's not considered suitable for use in pregnancy, you're unlikely to have done any harm with just one dose. However, seek medical advice if you're concerned.

If you need to continue using a medicine in pregnancy, ask if it's safe to do so. While pharmacists are well-informed on all medicines, your doctor is the best person to consult on prescription-only drugs.

THE MIRACLE OF CONCEPTION

When you consider the multitude of events that have to fall neatly into place before a baby is conceived, it's hard to believe that anyone can become pregnant. No wonder they talk about the miracle of life!

To become pregnant the following have to happen:

■ **Your hormone balance** must be correct for the egg to develop.

■ **Ovulation must take place**: if you don't release an egg, there is no possibility of fertilization occurring.

■ **You need to have sex** at the right time in your menstrual cycle; sperm can last about three days in healthy cervical mucus, but if your timing is out, egg and sperm are unlikely to meet. In some cases there may be only two or three days each month when you can conceive.

■ **Your partner needs to produce** plenty of good, healthy sperm that can penetrate your cervical mucus to reach the egg.

■ **When the egg has been fertilized,** the blastocyst has to implant securely in the lining of the uterus.

■ **The right levels of the hormone** progesterone must be produced by the corpus luteum to maintain the pregnancy.

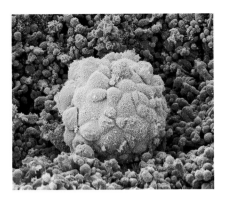

259 days to go...

WHAT'S HAPPENING INSIDE

The blastocyst is firmly embedded in the lining of the uterus. Once this has happened, the placenta (the temporary organ that supplies the growing embryo with oxygen and nutrients) will begin to develop.

It's a week since the egg was fertilized and it now implants in your uterus, where it will soon develop into an embryo.

Around seven days after fertilization, the blastocyst implants in the lining of the uterus. The outer cell layer, no longer protected, is able to attach to the lining of the uterus. The lining is now more receptive and has undergone changes that make it more "sticky" to aid attachment. The blastocyst erodes cells to sink beneath the surface of the uterine lining.

What was originally a single outer layer of cells now transforms into two layers. The outermost layer of cells creates space by eroding the lining, and it secretes hormones. These hormones inform your body that you're pregnant and stimulate the uterus to support the pregnancy rather than shed its lining in what would normally be your period.

The innermost cell layer will become the placenta and the amniotic sac that encloses the embryo. Within the blastocyst there is an inner mass of cells that will form the embryo.

STRETCH AND UNWIND

It can help to relax in this interim period, before you do a pregnancy test. Fill some time by getting in shape with these simple stretches. Getting into the habit of doing these exercises now will help your body cope with the increased demands once you know you're pregnant. Stretch before and after exercising to prevent muscle strain.

To do a back stretch, get on all fours and lower your bottom towards your feet while stretching your arms out on the floor in front of you. Lower your forehead as far as you can, keeping your neck and back aligned, and stretch your arms as much as you can. Inhale slowly and then relax your back and arms as you exhale. Inhale and exhale 10 times.

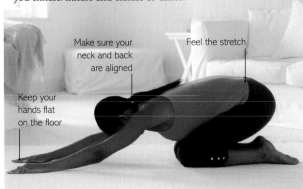

Make sure your neck and back are aligned

Feel the stretch

Keep your hands flat on the floor

To do a leg stretch, sit on the floor and stretch your left leg in front of you. Using your left hand take hold of your left foot for a few seconds. If you can't reach your toes, don't worry. Inhale to begin and exhale as you stretch. Repeat with your right leg.

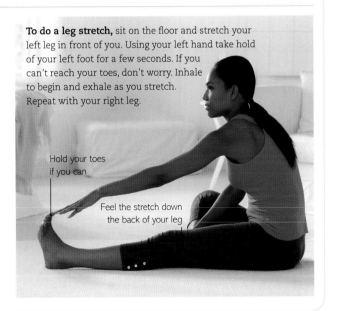

Hold your toes if you can

Feel the stretch down the back of your leg

Your 4th week

THIS WEEK, YOU'LL NEED A LITTLE PATIENCE AS YOU WAIT, WONDER, AND HOPE

The embryo-to-be, now securely implanted in the lining of your uterus, is starting to develop. Although you could do a home pregnancy test this week, you may end up disappointed or uncertain because at this stage a definite result is unlikely. It can be nerve-racking, wondering if an unwanted period is about to arrive and dash your hopes. Talk to your partner and share your feelings with him – he may be anxious, too.

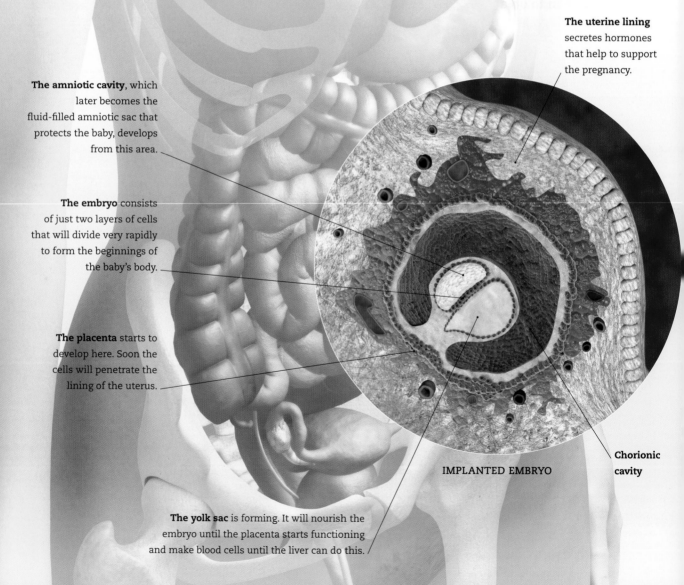

The uterine lining secretes hormones that help to support the pregnancy.

The amniotic cavity, which later becomes the fluid-filled amniotic sac that protects the baby, develops from this area.

The embryo consists of just two layers of cells that will divide very rapidly to form the beginnings of the baby's body.

The placenta starts to develop here. Soon the cells will penetrate the lining of the uterus.

IMPLANTED EMBRYO

Chorionic cavity

The yolk sac is forming. It will nourish the embryo until the placenta starts functioning and make blood cells until the liver can do this.

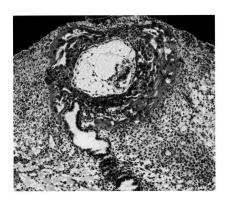

258 days to go...

YOUR BABY TODAY

This is a cross-section of the ball of cells embedded in the uterus at this early stage of pregnancy. It contains fluid in the centre and two areas of white cells with a darker streak of cells between them – these will form the embryo, now less than 0.5mm long.

Pregnancy hormones are being produced, but it may be difficult to detect them accurately, so it's best to wait before you do a test.

You might be keen to do a pregnancy test as you enter the fourth week of your cycle. Most women use over-the-counter home pregnancy tests (see p.71). These are simple to use and work by detecting the levels of hCG in your urine – this is the hormone that is produced as soon as the embryo implants in the lining of the uterus (see p.61).

There are home pregnancy tests that claim to detect a pregnancy six days before your period is due. But if you use one of these and test this early, your hCG levels (see above) may not be high enough to give a positive result, even though you might be pregnant.

ASK A... MIDWIFE

I'm worried about doing a pregnancy test as my partner is going to be disappointed if I'm not pregnant. Will this affect my chances of conceiving? Feeling under pressure to conceive is stressful, and this can affect the hypothalamus (see p.38) – the structure in your brain that governs your menstrual cycle. So your partner's avid interest may actually be counter-productive.

Be honest with your partner about how you feel. Explain to him that you share his enthusiasm for having a baby, but that you're feeling pressured, and that you're worried it will affect your ability to conceive. Conversely, if you aren't entirely sure that you are ready for a baby, now is the time to discuss this, too. Pregnancy is a life-changing event, and both you and your partner need to be fully committed, and also aware that it can, in itself, be stressful.

Have fun together and make sure the pressure to conceive doesn't take the fun and spontaneity out of your lovemaking (see p.49).

YOUR PREGNANCY DIARY

Trying for a baby is an exciting experience, so why not keep a written record – it's a good way to pass time in this interim period while you're waiting to take a pregnancy test. Rather than just noting down the dates of your period and signs of ovulation, use it to record the highs and lows so far.

Once you're pregnant, you can continue to use the diary to record your feelings: for example, your emotions when you saw the positive symbol on the pregnancy testing kit; how you broke the news to your partner and his response; what your baby's first kick felt like; the best and worst aspects of being pregnant. You may also find that letting off steam about your partner's foibles or your mother-in-law's idiosyncrasies is surprisingly therapeutic!

Besides providing a unique record of your pregnancy, keeping a diary can also help you in subsequent pregnancies: for example, you may find it reassuring to look back and find that nausea and vomiting was just a phase.

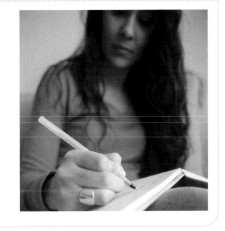

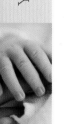

257 days to go...

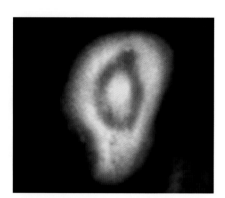

YOUR BABY TODAY

In this computer-generated image the entire blastocyst can be seen embedded in the lining of the uterus. The cells that will develop into the embryo are seen as the dark area in the 12 o'clock position.

Adopting a healthy lifestyle and improving your wellbeing are sensible measures now that you might be pregnant.

THE LOWDOWN

Cultural beliefs

Here's what some cultures believe:

■ **Hindu fathers** part the hair on their partner's head three times upwards from the front to the back to boost the development of the growing baby.

■ **In some countries,** there is great emphasis placed on protecting the unborn baby. In Thailand, the pregnant woman's abdomen may be painted to ward off evil spirits. It is also believed that giving gifts before the birth will attract evil spirits.

AS A MATTER OF FACT

There are at least 30 chemicals in cigarette smoke that can adversely affect fertility.

Because smoking reduces the rate at which cells replicate, it may cause most damage during the first days and weeks of pregnancy. As well as causing fertility problems in women, smoking can have negative effects on sperm and reduce testosterone in men.

Once your pregnancy is confirmed in the next week or so, you'll find you're bombarded with more health information than ever before. Is your diet well balanced? Could you cut back on the amount of salt, sugar, and fast food you eat? Are you eating plenty of fruit and vegetables, particularly green leafy vegetables, which are a good

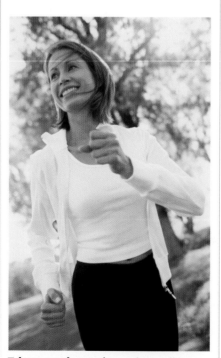

Take up gentle exercise, such as walking or swimming, as they are ideal before, during, and after pregnancy.

source of folic acid? Are you exercising enough and safely? Even though you don't know you're pregnant yet, it's worth being aware of the recommended advice and making some basic dietary and lifestyle changes. Turn to the section on pages 14–29 for some up-to-date information. It's also worth being aware of the early signs of pregnancy so you know what's normal.

If you have a pre-existing medical condition or are taking medication, seek medical advice.

FOCUS ON... YOUR HEALTH

Lifestyle changes

If you smoke, you should give up (so should your partner) for health reasons. Once you're pregnant, not smoking will reduce the risk of miscarriage, stillbirth, premature birth, low birth weight, and sudden infant death.

You should also cut down on or, better still, stop drinking alcohol altogether. The current advice from the Department of Health is to avoid drinking alcohol completely while trying to get pregnant and once you are pregnant, as safe levels are difficult to determine.

YOU ARE 3 WEEKS AND 3 DAYS

256 days to go...

YOUR BABY TODAY

The embryo has implanted into the uterus, and the entry point at which it buried into the lining of the uterus is now covered by a clot, shown here. The clot prevents blood loss and protects the embryo.

Try to stay busy to distract yourself from wondering constantly whether you're pregnant, and think positively.

ASK A... DOCTOR

I've done an early pregnancy test and have failed to conceive again, for the sixth month. Could it be because I have irregular periods?
Menstrual cycles that vary more than a few days in length from month to month are considered irregular. An irregular cycle can be troublesome when trying to conceive, but being aware of the signs of ovulation (see p.43) can help you to determine when you are approaching your short window of fertility.

Irregular ovulation and menstruation account for around 30–40 per cent of fertility problems. Many factors determine how fertile a woman is, such as her age, whether her cervical fluid is wet enough to sustain sperm, or whether her Fallopian tubes are open, but the most important factor is whether she ovulates regularly. Sometimes, a condition called anovulation occurs, in which there is irregular menstrual bleeding but no ovulation. If you don't release an egg each month, you won't have as many chances to conceive. You may be given drugs to stimulate egg production and boost ovulation.

Waiting for your period to start

– or better yet, not start – can be quite stressful when you're trying to conceive. If your menstrual cycle is irregular you may not know when your period is due and therefore may not know if you're late and potentially pregnant or not. The uncertainty is likely to make you anxious and every time you go to the toilet you will be dreading seeing that your period has started.

Whether or not you know you have fertility problems, the wait can be difficult. If you do get your period, the disappointment can be hard. The cycle of having your period, waiting for ovulation, hoping you're pregnant, and then finding out you're not can become very wearing month after month.

If you have been trying to conceive for a year with no luck then you should go to your doctor for tests. Or go at six months if you are over 35 or know that you may have fertility problems, such as blocked Fallopian tubes. Try confiding in a good friend about your problems so that you have someone to talk to, but try not to become obsessive and let it dominate all your relationships.

If you've only just started trying, remember there is only a one in four or five chance that you will conceive each month, so you're unlikely to get pregnant in the first month of trying!

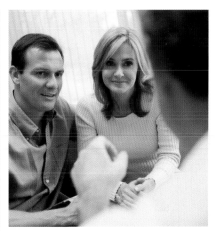

If you're aged over 35 and have been trying to conceive for six months, speak to your doctor about fertility tests. You should both go for checks because your partner's sperm will need to be tested, too. You will be given blood tests.

AS A MATTER OF FACT

Around a third of pregnancies in Britain could be accidental.

According to a paper published in the *British Medical Journal*, 31 per cent of women surveyed said their pregnancy was unplanned. This did not take into account women who conceived but decided not to go ahead with the pregnancy, which would make the figure even higher.

Your 4th week

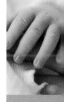

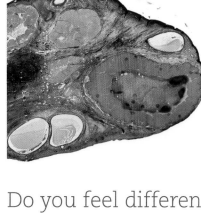

255 days to go...

YOUR BABY TODAY

To embed itself in the lining of the uterus, the embryo-to-be needs the help of progesterone, secreted after ovulation by the empty egg follicle, the corpus luteum (shown in pink in this cross-section of an ovary). Progesterone helps the lining thicken.

Do you feel different? You'll find yourself analyzing every twinge in your body as you look for signs that you're pregnant.

It's very early days and you're unlikely to have pregnancy symptoms yet – although you may have some light spotting (see opposite). Some women claim to "feel" pregnant, even before changes to their breasts are noticeable or before they start feeling sick. Some women say that they just "know". You may be very in tune with your body and may notice that it is changing even before you are able to take a test. Unfortunately, sometimes our minds can play tricks on us: you may want to be pregnant so much that you can sometimes convince yourself that you're feeling different. If you don't feel any different, don't worry, this is also completely normal.

Either way the only definitive way to know whether or not you are pregnant is to take a pregnancy test (see p.71). You don't need to go to your doctor to confirm your pregnancy as the tests that doctors use are the same as those bought over the counter. If the test is positive, you're pregnant!

FOCUS ON... NUTRITION

Diet ban

If you were dieting before you conceived, it can be tempting to carry on once you find out you're pregnant. Don't: if you're not overweight and you diet, your baby may become undernourished and is more likely to be premature and underweight at birth. Do, however, eat a healthy, balanced diet (see pp.14–17). Don't eat junk food when you're pregnant as this can increase the risk of your baby developing weight problems.

If you have a high BMI (see p.17), your doctor may give you the green light to lose some weight. Research indicates that obese women who lost weight, or whose weight stayed stable during pregnancy, were more likely to give birth to babies of a normal weight. In later life, their children were also less likely to suffer from diabetes and obesity.

In an ideal world, you should lose excess weight before conceiving, because obesity makes you more prone to diabetes and high blood pressure and means you're more likely to need a Caesarean section.

ASK A... NUTRITIONIST

Should I give up coffee in case I'm pregnant? The Food Standards Agency advises pregnant women to drink no more than 200mg of caffeine a day (that's two mugs of instant coffee, one mug of filter coffee, or two mugs of tea). Going without your caffeine fix is a good thing when you're pregnant, as research shows that, in high doses, it can increase the risk of miscarriage.

One study discovered that pregnant women who drank two or more cups of coffee (or its equivalent) were twice as likely to miscarry as those who gave up caffeine. Before you switch to decaff, note that decaffeinated drinks

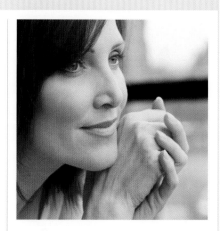

may raise cholesterol. The good news is that many women find they go off coffee in early pregnancy.

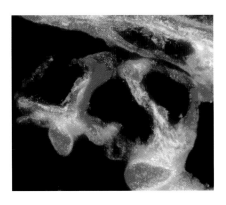

254 days to go...

YOUR BABY TODAY

The first stage of placental development – your baby's life support system – is shown here. The image shows nuclei (blue) within a continuous network of cells that will become the placental villi. At first the tiny villi are solid; later, they will contain blood vessels.

As the fertilized egg becomes completely embedded in your uterus, it may cause some light bleeding.

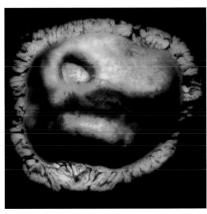

This computer-generated image shows the ball of cells – the blastocyst – as it appears situated within the uterus. The outer ring of interconnected cells that will eventually form the placenta is clearly seen.

AS A MATTER OF FACT

It is thought that around 50 per cent of pregnancies might miscarry before implantation.

Up to a third of pregnancies miscarry up to the fifth week and around a quarter will end in miscarriage between the fifth and seventh weeks (see p.94). Thankfully, the risk of miscarriage becomes much lower as the weeks go by, decreasing dramatically after the 12th week of pregnancy.

The ball of cells, known as the blastocyst, that will form the embryo has now completely embedded within the lining of the uterus and the lining has regenerated over it.

Unfortunately, in the complex process of conception, only about half of all fertilized eggs progress to become a blastocyst and only about half of these go on to become successfully implanted in the uterus.

When the blastocyst embeds, there may be some bleeding, known as "spotting". This often leads to confusion regarding the dating of the pregnancy, not least because it can occur around the time that you would normally start your period.

The colour of the blood can vary. In most cases it is pinkish, although bright red blood (fresh blood) can occur, as can brownish, old blood. As long as it is not profuse, the colour really doesn't matter. If the bleeding lasts for a short period, and you don't experience discomfort, it's likely that things are just fine, but do see your doctor for a checkup.

Around 25 per cent of women will experience some bleeding in early pregnancy, but most go on to full-term. However, in some cases, bleeding does mean a miscarriage is occurring so do always report the fact that you've bled to your doctor or midwife.

DOUBLING UP

In common with many parents, you probably thought long and hard about trying to conceive your second child. There's no ideal age gap between children, but consider:
The pros of a small age gap:
■ **You are in "baby mode"** and will be used to the routine and all aspects of babycare. You will have all the equipment you need from bottles through to a pram and cot.
■ **A two-year-old** might find it easier to accept his new sibling than a four-year-old who is much more conscious of having the sole attention of his parents.
■ **There will always be squabbles,** but children close in age tend to play better together.
The cons of a small age gap:
■ **It's tiring** looking after a one- or two-year-old while pregnant.
■ **It can put a strain on your body** to have pregnancies close together.
■ **If you have a second baby** before the first one can walk, you could be doing a lot of carrying, increasing the chance of backache.
■ **You won't have as much time** to get to know your first child before your second is on the scene.

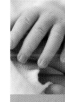

YOU ARE 3 WEEKS AND 6 DAYS

253 days to go...

YOUR BABY TODAY

This microscope view of an embedded blastocyst shows the amniotic cavity (semicircular white area at top), with the cells that will develop into the baby just below (dark oval at the 12 o'clock position). The yolk sac is the pink area below..

Complex changes are taking place inside your uterus to create a safe and nourishing environment for your unborn baby.

The ball of cells embedded in the uterus is already laying down the foundations for its future life as an embryo. At two layers thick, the germ cells form a flat disc that divides the fluid-filled inner part of the ball of cells into two chambers. The smaller of these fluid-filled chambers will become the amniotic sac. The larger chamber, lying closest to the future placenta, will become the yolk sac that supports the early embryo. The umbilical cord will eventually develop close to the smaller chamber. The inner germ cells have been developing at a slower rate than the rapidly expanding outer cell layers.

At first the umbilical cord is a simple stalk, containing no blood vessels but simply anchoring the embryo to the future placenta (see p.76), which will eventually become your unborn baby's lifeline.

AS A MATTER OF FACT

Newborns are getting heavier.

This is mostly due to improved diet and living standards. However, obesity in the mother is another factor – if the mother is overweight, there is an increased risk of diabetes (see p.473), which can increase the baby's weight.

ASK A... NUTRITIONIST

I'm hoping I'm pregnant, but I'm already worrying about the amount of weight I might put on, and am scared I'll never be slim again! These days, it is almost impossible to pass a newspaper stand without seeing the latest celebrity who has not only fitted straight back into her clothes after having her baby, but who actually weighs less than she did before pregnancy. However, this is concerning for health professionals, as a dramatic weight loss after the birth is not good for mother or baby.

The average weight gain during pregnancy is 11–14.5kg (25–32lb), if you have a Body Mass Index (BMI) (see p.17) within the normal range. Your baby and her support system will make up a good proportion of this, as will the increased pregnancy fluids, fats, and an enlarged uterus (see p.99). Much of this extra weight will be lost as soon as your baby is born. Also, after the birth, some of this extra weight provides nutrients for breastfeeding, which uses up to 500 calories a day.

The most sensible approach to controlling your weight during pregnancy is to eat a healthy diet and take gentle exercise to ensure that weight gain is not too dramatic. You should aim to eat around 2,100–2,500 calories a day, increasing this by 200 calories in the last trimester of pregnancy – the equivalent of a banana and a glass of milk.

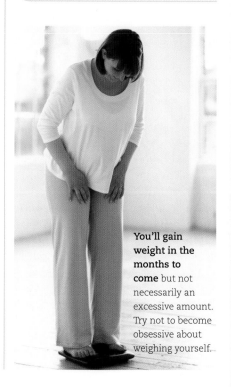

You'll gain weight in the months to come but not necessarily an excessive amount. Try not to become obsessive about weighing yourself.

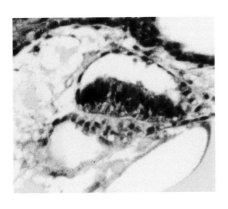

252 days to go...

YOUR BABY TODAY

This highly magnified image shows that the embryo consists of two layers of cells – those of the upper darker layer are more rectangular in shape and lie on the side of the amniotic cavity, and those on the lower layer lie on the side of the yolk sac.

Are you feeling irritable and tired, and are your breasts tender? Well, you might just be pregnant!

Nature has a strange way of working. You might feel low if you have your usual PMT symptoms and think it means that you haven't conceived, but in fact, there are many similarities between the symptoms of pre-menstrual syndrome or tension (PMS or PMT) and those of early pregnancy. This is because the hormones that cause PMT are raised in pregnancy and so can cause the same symptoms. In addition to this, you might be irritable and emotional even without having PMT, just due to the anxiety of wanting to be pregnant and waiting to see whether or not your period arrives.

While you are in the middle of this storm of hormones and raging emotions it can be difficult to remain calm. Talk to your partner about your emotions and anxieties – just expressing that you're finding things stressful can help you get through this tense time. Alternatively, confide in a female relative or friend, who might be able to relate to how you're feeling

Frustratingly, at this point it is still a waiting game; all you can do is try to be patient until you take your pregnancy test. If your period was due today – day 28 of your cycle – and hasn't made an appearance, you can do a test as early as today or tomorrow. Good luck!

FOCUS ON... YOUR BODY

Start squeezing!

It's never too early to start pelvic floor exercises and you'll be glad you did once you become pregnant. The pelvic floor is a broad sling of muscles that stretches between your legs and extends from the pubic bone in front to the spine at the rear. It holds and supports your bladder, uterus, and bowel in place and controls the muscles that hold closed the anus, urethra, and vagina.

Try these simple steps to tone your pelvic floor:

■ **First** try to locate your pelvic floor: sit on a chair and close your eyes – now visualize the sling of muscles stretching right across your body holding your uterus and bladder.

■ **Next** contract your pelvic floor muscles pulling inwards and upwards, hold for a count of five, then release. Repeat this exercise at least 10 times a day.

■ **Test:** if you're having trouble identifying the muscles, imagine that you are trying to stop the flow of urine; the muscles you feel contracting are those of the pelvic floor.

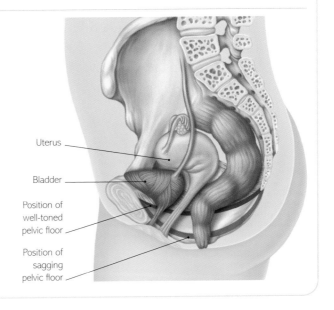

Uterus

Bladder

Position of well-toned pelvic floor

Position of sagging pelvic floor

Your 5th week

IF YOU HAVE NO PERIOD AND A POSITIVE TEST RESULT, YOU ARE PREGNANT!

When your pregnancy is confirmed, it's natural to experience a mixed bag of emotions – excitement, disbelief, joy, and anxiety. Everything is about to change forever for you and your partner. Give yourselves time to take in the big news. You may not feel pregnant yet, but momentous changes are taking place in the hidden world of your uterus. Step by step, the building blocks of life are being set in place.

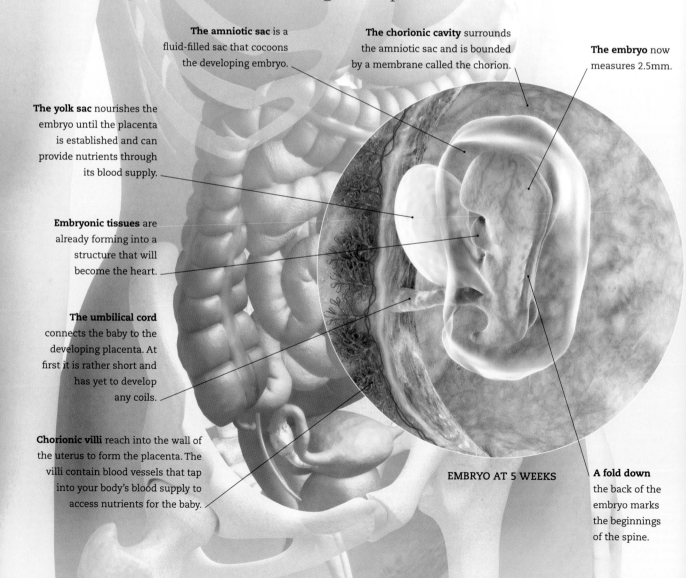

The amniotic sac is a fluid-filled sac that cocoons the developing embryo.

The chorionic cavity surrounds the amniotic sac and is bounded by a membrane called the chorion.

The embryo now measures 2.5mm.

The yolk sac nourishes the embryo until the placenta is established and can provide nutrients through its blood supply.

Embryonic tissues are already forming into a structure that will become the heart.

The umbilical cord connects the baby to the developing placenta. At first it is rather short and has yet to develop any coils.

Chorionic villi reach into the wall of the uterus to form the placenta. The villi contain blood vessels that tap into your body's blood supply to access nutrients for the baby.

EMBRYO AT 5 WEEKS

A fold down the back of the embryo marks the beginnings of the spine.

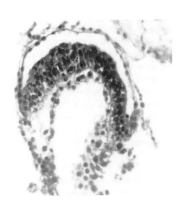

251 days to go...

YOUR BABY TODAY

This microscope view shows the cells that will become the baby in close up (darker curved area). These cells will repeatedly divide and multiply, becoming more and more specialized at each stage of their development.

The waiting is over. If your period hasn't started, take a home pregnancy test to find out whether or not you've conceived.

If you've missed your period
(assuming that your normal cycle is no more than 28 days and that your period is therefore late), you may want to do a home pregnancy test today.

A home pregnancy test, available at pharmacists and most supermarkets, contains a chemical that reacts if your urine contains the hormone hCG (human chorionic gonadotrophin). This is produced by an implanting embryo and will be found in your urine if you are pregnant. Levels of hCG are likely to be over 50mIU/ml on the day your period is due. With between 97 and 99 per cent accuracy, the majority of over-the-counter tests are sensitive enough to detect this amount, so they can be used on the first day of your missed period; some can be used earlier (see p.63).

The tests only turn positive once there is a certain level of the hCG hormone present in your urine: if you test too early, the result might be negative even though you are pregnant. Therefore, if you don't get your period but you had a negative result, test again after two to three days. If you are pregnant, the levels of hCG will have risen, giving a positive result.

If you get a positive result but your period starts anyway, it may be that you have suffered a very early miscarriage.

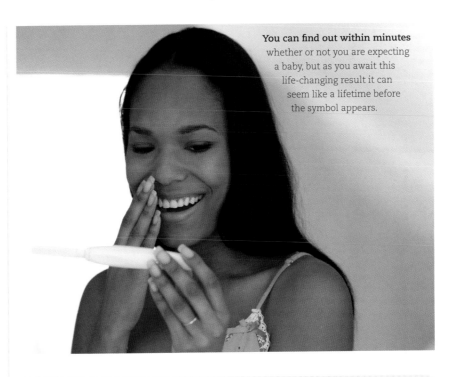

You can find out within minutes whether or not you are expecting a baby, but as you await this life-changing result it can seem like a lifetime before the symbol appears.

HOW TO USE A HOME PREGNANCY TEST

Always read the instructions, but most tests work as follows:
■ **You urinate on the stick** and leave it for a specified number of minutes.
■ **A symbol will appear** in the control window to indicate the test is working (if this does not appear, the test is faulty). If a symbol then appears in the results window, you are pregnant.

■ **It is advisable to do the test** first thing in the morning when your urine is most concentrated. By doing this, the hCG levels are likely to be detected more easily
■ **The results symbol** gradually fades, so read it after the specified time, not later. Do another test the next morning if you're unsure of the result.

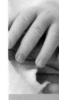

71

YOU ARE 4 WEEKS AND 2 DAYS

250 days to go...

YOUR BABY TODAY

The embryo until this stage of development has consisted of two layers of cells. Now, a third layer starts to become visible as a "bulge" between the two – this bulge can be seen in the centre of this image.

In this third week since conception, the forerunner of the brain and central nervous system is forming.

While you're busy coming to terms with being pregnant, there are incredible changes taking place inside you. The group of cells that will become your baby is currently shaped as a flat disc and undergoing significant development. A narrow groove begins to form down the middle of the cells. The leading edge of the groove is slightly wider, forming a circular "node". The outer edges of the node and groove are slightly raised.

The cells move from the rolled edges of these structures downwards into the groove to lie between the original two layers of cells. This creates three layers of cells, those on each outer disc surface and those sandwiched between them. The node and groove do not extend along the entire length of the disc.

At the head end, a separate groove forms. Called the neural groove, this ultimately forms the brain and spinal cord (the central nervous system). In four days' time, the disc will lengthen and widen at the end that will form your baby's head. In six days' time, the neural groove has folds on either side that will later meet to form the neural tube.

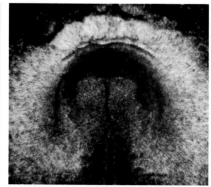

Shown here is the neural tube of an embryo in the early stages of pregnancy. The brain and spinal cord will develop from the neural tube. If the tube does not fully close, it can lead to birth defects, most commonly spina bifida.

ASK A... DOCTOR

I've been having difficulty getting pregnant and have now been diagnosed with polycystic ovary syndrome. What is this? This condition causes the ovaries to be bigger than normal and they produce a large number of small follicles that never grow to full maturity. As a result, no egg is released to be fertilized and periods are very irregular.

The condition is a common cause of fertility problems and treatments are aimed at stimulating ovulation and also reducing some of the symptoms, such as increased body hair. Polycystic ovary syndrome appears to run in families.

FOCUS ON... RELATIONSHIPS

"You're going to be a dad!"

It's the positive result you've been waiting for – hopefully! – but how do you share it with your partner? You could present him with an envelope containing your positive pregnancy test, or explain that you have a "special gift" for him but it won't be ready for about, oh, nine months. It shouldn't take him long to work it out! Ideally, choose a time when you are both alone and feeling relaxed so

that it can be a special moment. You may want to do another test with your partner just to make sure and also so that he feels involved.

Even if you're excited, and even if you can't get hold of your partner for a day, don't be tempted to tell your mum and close friends first. Your partner may be put out, understandably, if others know he's going to be a dad before he does.

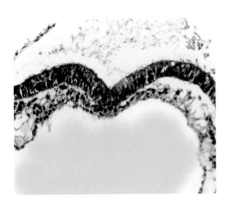

YOU ARE 4 WEEKS AND 3 DAYS

249 days to go...

YOUR BABY TODAY

As the embryo transforms from two cell layers into three, a groove develops along the back of the embryo. This groove (the dark area in the centre of this image) will develop into the embryo's neural tube – the forerunner of the brain and spinal cord.

Happy? Excited? But a little nervous? There is no greater life-changing event than finding out you're going to be parents.

SURPRISED TO BE PREGNANT?

If you're one of the few women who has become pregnant while using contraception, it is unlikely to have done your baby any harm, but depending on what you were using, here's what you should do:

- **Contraceptive pill:** stop taking it.
- **Contraceptive patch:** remove it.
- **Contraceptive implant:** see your doctor to have it removed.
- **Coil (intrauterine device or IUD) or intrauterine system (IUS):** visit your doctor without delay if you're using either as there's a small risk that the pregnancy could be ectopic (see p.93). Even if a scan shows that the pregnancy is not ectopic, the IUD or IUS should be removed: the risk of miscarriage is greater if it is left in place than if it is removed.
- **Contraceptive injection (Depo-Provera):** see your doctor if you conceive while using this. Research indicates that it won't affect the unborn baby, but you should not have any further injections.
- **Morning-after pill:** once an egg has implanted, the morning-after pill has no effect so it won't harm your baby. Do, however, see your doctor if you're concerned.

In the few days since you conceived, you may have experienced a whole host of different feelings. Even if you planned to get pregnant, it's perfectly normal for the initial elation to be replaced with some anxiety as the reality hits you that you are going to be a mum. You might also doubt the result of the test you've taken and not actually believe it until you begin to experience some of the early symptoms of pregnancy.

Your partner may react differently from you. If he doesn't appear as excited, don't interpret this as meaning that he is not happy about the news; not everyone deals with big events in the same way, and it might be some time before the reality of becoming a dad hits him. Withdrawing into himself may be his way of giving himself some time to process the information. Conversely, you may find he's actually more excited about the news than you!

Handling your feelings might be made more difficult by trying to keep the pregnancy a secret, for the time being. Most couples decide not to tell people until after the 12-week scan when the miscarriage risk is significantly decreased, but you may find that confiding in a few close relatives and friends will give you a much-needed outlet to talk about your feelings.

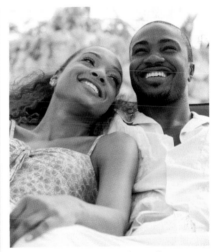

Discovering that you're going to be parents is a momentous occasion, and you and your partner are likely to experience a renewed closeness as a result.

AS A MATTER OF FACT

Pregnant women often try to connect with their baby through dreams.

You may find it difficult to bond fully with your baby and believe you're actually pregnant. A common dream in pregnancy is that you're swimming; it is thought to be a way of trying to "reach" the baby, who will soon be bathed in water (fluid) inside you.

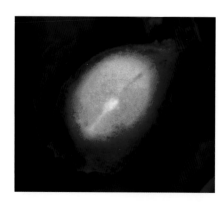

YOU ARE 4 WEEKS AND 4 DAYS

248 days to go...

YOUR BABY TODAY

The embryo, viewed from above here, has a subtle groove (the primitive groove) and a small central depression (the primitive node), both seen here in white. These changes start at what will become the base of the spine and progress towards the head.

You're probably eager to know when your baby will be born. The chart below will tell you the expected date of delivery.

Until you have a dating scan in a few weeks' time, your baby's due date will be calculated by counting 280 days from the first day of your last menstrual period – see chart, below. At the dating scan (see p.138), your baby will be measured and his age calculated. The scan date will then be used as it is considered to be accurate.

While you're bound to want to know the due date, try not to get too fixated on it. Most babies are born within about two weeks of their due dates but your baby will be considered to be born at term if you give birth between 37 and 42 weeks. So your estimated delivery date is just that, an estimate; your baby may be born earlier or later.

WHEN WILL YOUR BABY BE BORN?

To work out your expected date of delivery (EDD) – also known as the due date – you need to know when you started your last menstrual period (LMP) (see p.35).

Find your LMP date on the chart below to discover when your baby is expected. For example, if your last LMP was 13 January, then your baby will be due on 20 October.

January	1	2	3	4	5	6	7	8	9	10	11	12	13	14	15	16	17	18	19	20	21	22	23	24	25	26	27	28	29	30	31
Oct/Nov	8	9	10	11	12	13	14	15	16	17	18	19	20	21	22	23	24	25	26	27	28	29	30	31	1	2	3	4	5	6	7
February	1	2	3	4	5	6	7	8	9	10	11	12	13	14	15	16	17	18	19	20	21	22	23	24	25	26	27	28			
Nov/Dec	8	9	10	11	12	13	14	15	16	17	18	19	20	21	22	23	24	25	26	27	28	29	30	1	2	3	4	5			
March	1	2	3	4	5	6	7	8	9	10	11	12	13	14	15	16	17	18	19	20	21	22	23	24	25	26	27	28	29	30	31
Dec/Jan	6	7	8	9	10	11	12	13	14	15	16	17	18	19	20	21	22	23	24	25	26	27	28	29	30	31	1	2	3	4	5
April	1	2	3	4	5	6	7	8	9	10	11	12	13	14	15	16	17	18	19	20	21	22	23	24	25	26	27	28	29	30	
Jan/Feb	6	7	8	9	10	11	12	13	14	15	16	17	18	19	20	21	22	23	24	25	26	27	28	29	30	31	1	2	3	4	
May	1	2	3	4	5	6	7	8	9	10	11	12	13	14	15	16	17	18	19	20	21	22	23	24	25	26	27	28	29	30	31
Feb/Mar	5	6	7	8	9	10	11	12	13	14	15	16	17	18	19	20	21	22	23	24	25	26	27	28	1	2	3	4	5	6	7
June	1	2	3	4	5	6	7	8	9	10	11	12	13	14	15	16	17	18	19	20	21	22	23	24	25	26	27	28	29	30	
Mar/Apr	8	9	10	11	12	13	14	15	16	17	18	19	20	21	22	23	24	25	26	27	28	29	30	31	1	2	3	4	5	6	
July	1	2	3	4	5	6	7	8	9	10	11	12	13	14	15	16	17	18	19	20	21	22	23	24	25	26	27	28	29	30	31
Apr/May	7	8	9	10	11	12	13	14	15	16	17	18	19	20	21	22	23	24	25	26	27	28	29	30	1	2	3	4	5	6	7
August	1	2	3	4	5	6	7	8	9	10	11	12	13	14	15	16	17	18	19	20	21	22	23	24	25	26	27	28	29	30	31
May/June	8	9	10	11	12	13	14	15	16	17	18	19	20	21	22	23	24	25	26	27	28	29	30	31	1	2	3	4	5	6	7
September	1	2	3	4	5	6	7	8	9	10	11	12	13	14	15	16	17	18	19	20	21	22	23	24	25	26	27	28	29	30	
June/July	8	9	10	11	12	13	14	15	16	17	18	19	20	21	22	23	24	25	26	27	28	29	30	1	2	3	4	5	6	7	
October	1	2	3	4	5	6	7	8	9	10	11	12	13	14	15	16	17	18	19	20	21	22	23	24	25	26	27	28	29	30	31
July/Aug	8	9	10	11	12	13	14	15	16	17	18	19	20	21	22	23	24	25	26	27	28	29	30	31	1	2	3	4	5	6	7
November	1	2	3	4	5	6	7	8	9	10	11	12	13	14	15	16	17	18	19	20	21	22	23	24	25	26	27	28	29	30	
Aug/Sept	8	9	10	11	12	13	14	15	16	17	18	19	20	21	22	23	24	25	26	27	28	29	30	31	1	2	3	4	5	6	
December	1	2	3	4	5	6	7	8	9	10	11	12	13	14	15	16	17	18	19	20	21	22	23	24	25	26	27	28	29	30	31
Sept/Oct	7	8	9	10	11	12	13	14	15	16	17	18	19	20	21	22	23	24	25	26	27	28	29	30	1	2	3	4	5	6	7

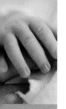

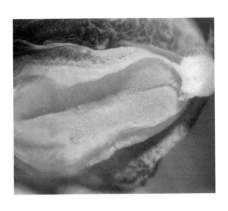

247 days to go...

YOUR BABY TODAY

The embryo, still less than 3mm long, now has a deep and narrow groove extending along its entire length. This groove will soon become so deep and its edges will curl over so much that it forms into a tube running along the length of the embryo.

Although there's lots of information to take on board, try to enjoy this time and remember pregnancy is a natural process.

ASK A... DOCTOR

I'm 40 and fighting fit. Will the doctors still see my pregnancy as potentially high-risk? Yes, any woman aged over 35 is categorized as high-risk, regardless of her health status. Although this can be frustrating, the reason for the close monitoring is that, statistically, women over 35 are more likely to suffer from complications during pregnancy, such as high blood pressure, miscarriage, and gestational diabetes; there is also an increased risk of having a baby with a genetic disorder, such as Down's syndrome.

Your doctor and midwife will simply want to keep an eye on you to be sure that your pregnancy progresses normally, and that both you and your baby remain healthy. By undergoing regular monitoring, any potential problems can be addressed and hopefully rectified early on.

Try not to see it as an intrusion. It's great that you're in good shape already, and if you continue to take care of your health and exercise regularly, you will reduce the risks of complications occurring.

No sooner than you found out you were pregnant, like most expectant women, you may have begun to worry about all aspects of your lifestyle and your unborn baby's health. To put things in perspective, remember that in generations gone by pregnancy was considered to be a natural event, and few women made lifestyle changes to accommodate the condition. So in the past, pregnant women were likely to carry on eating unhealthy foods, drinking alcohol, and smoking.

Furthermore, pregnancy tests tended to be much less accurate or sensitive, meaning that many pregnancies ended in early miscarriage without anyone being aware. For this reason, many of the problems now known to be risk factors for pregnancy complications or miscarriage were not analyzed or addressed, or fretted about.

Today, with the benefit of a great deal of research and precise monitoring of ovulation, conception, and pregnancy, women are very aware of what is happening inside their bodies, and are informed about the potential pitfalls. This is a mixed blessing: while it is important to avoid anything known to adversely affect your unborn baby, it is equally important to relax and enjoy the pregnancy, because stress is not good for you or your baby.

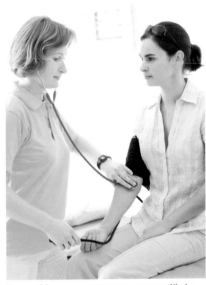

As an older expectant mum, you are likely to have more antenatal checks. High blood pressure can be a sign of pre-eclampsia (see p.474), which is a more significant risk for first-time pregnant women aged over 40.

AS A MATTER OF FACT

Pregnant women used to be advised to drink stout because it's a good source of iron.

Sadly, this is an old wives' tale as the iron content of stout is negligible. So, even though they're not as interesting, stick to your green leafy vegetables!

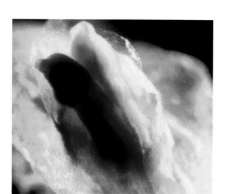

246 days to go...

YOUR BABY TODAY

The upper part of the embryo is shown here. There is still a wide opening along the back of the embryo that will gradually close over the next few days. The head and lower spine portions are the last to close.

The placenta – the structure that will become your unborn baby's lifeline – is forming.

Your pregnancy test result may be the only outward sign that you're pregnant, but there are many fascinating changes taking place inside you. The basic structures that will form the placenta (see p.127) are now in place. The outer layer of cells that originally entered the lining of the uterus is now coated with projections of placental tissue. It is the outer cells that are in direct contact with small lakes of your blood. The inner placental projections or fronds are termed "villi". Some villi anchor the pregnancy to your tissues and, from these, smaller free-floating villi arise. Later, further branches will appear and ultimately resemble the branching pattern of a fern leaf. The villi are still immature and have not established a blood supply of their own. It will be several weeks before the placenta is mature enough to supply all the oxygen and nutrients that your developing baby needs.

ASK A... MUM

I really wanted a baby, but now I have a positive pregnancy test result, I'm suddenly not so sure. Is this normal? I felt exactly the same at first and after chatting to friends discovered that lots of them had mixed feelings, especially at the beginning. I found a good way to overcome this was to focus on the reasons why I wanted the baby. I wrote these down. Then I tried to work out what I was really worrying about. Was it the thought of giving up some freedom? Financial worries? Concerns that I wouldn't be a good parent? This helped me to get things in perspective and realize I really did want the baby.

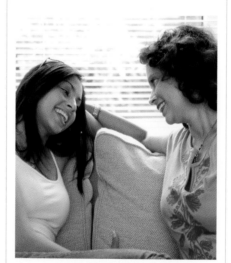

If you have any doubts while you're pregnant, try talking to a close female relative – perhaps your mum – or a friend. You're likely to find that they, at times, had similar doubts, but went on to enjoy pregnancy and being a mother.

TIME TO THINK ABOUT

As soon as you find out that you're pregnant see your doctor, who may carry out some routine tests and can explain your options for antenatal care (see below). The doctor will refer you for your first appointment with the midwife at about 8 to 10 weeks (see p. 122). Alternatively, you can refer yourself to a maternity unit.

■ **As home pregnancy tests** (see p.71) give such accurate and reliable results, most doctors rely on these for confirmation of the pregnancy and do not follow up with a blood test. You can, however, ask your doctor to diagnose your pregnancy if you haven't done your own test.
■ **Some doctors** take a urine sample to check for urinary tract infections, or anything that could affect the health of your pregnancy.
■ **A brief medical history** will be taken, noting down the number of pregnancies and births you have had previously and your family history.
■ **You may be weighed,** and have your blood pressure checked.
■ **Your doctor should explain** how antenatal care works and give you nutritional and lifestyle advice.

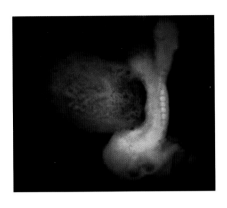

245 days to go...

YOUR BABY TODAY

The bulge at the lower part of this image will eventually become the baby's head. Segments called somites (seen as bright, round areas running down one side of the embryo), which will form the baby's spine, have started to develop.

At this important stage of development, the building blocks of your baby's spine are being laid down.

By the end of this 5th week individual elements that will form the embryo have begun to develop.

Starting at what will become the head end, individual segments, called "somites", form. Roughly three new pairs of somites appear every day and each forms part of your baby's spine as well as the muscles associated with each segment of the body. Eventually, there will be four somites at the head, eight in the region of the neck, 12 at chest level, five in the lumbar region, and five in the pelvic area.

Further somites develop in the baby below the pelvis but most disappear. In other mammals, these develop to form the tail.

FOCUS ON... YOUR BODY

Your metabolism

Regular exercise will increase your base metabolic rate, which is the rate at which your body burns calories. During pregnancy your metabolism will already be slightly elevated. When exercising your body will be encouraged to use up excess energy and fat stores, but will always keep enough reserve energy to facilitate the growth of your baby.

Exercise will also help your body to regulate blood-sugar (see p.92) and energy levels.

ASK A... NUTRITIONIST

I'm underweight. Could this affect my pregnancy? You may be more likely to suffer from nutritional deficiencies, which could affect the baby's health; you are also more likely to give birth prematurely, and have a smaller-than-usual baby, who is more vulnerable to health problems. You should discuss any eating issues with your midwife.

To gain weight, eat bigger portions and choose healthy foods that have plenty of protein, good-quality fats, and unrefined carbohydrates (see p.92). Opt for nutrient- and calorie-dense foods, such as avocados and full-fat dairy products; eat lots of leafy greens to ensure you are getting key vitamins and minerals (see pp.15–16). Eat healthy snacks, such as nuts, fruit, and seeds, and don't skip breakfast. Your doctor will refer you to a dietician, if necessary.

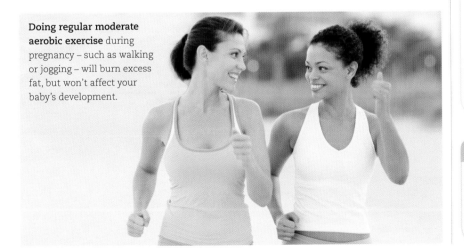

Doing regular moderate aerobic exercise during pregnancy – such as walking or jogging – will burn excess fat, but won't affect your baby's development.

ACTUAL SIZE OF YOUR BABY

At 5 weeks of pregnancy, the embryo is 2.5mm long.

5 weeks

Your 6th week

THIS WEEK YOU MAY NOTICE THE FIRST SYMPTOMS OF PREGNANCY – IF NOT, DON'T WORRY

Not all women start to feel pregnant this early on. Some experience a twinge of nausea or breast tenderness, while others notice no changes. Of course, it's natural to long for "proof" that your pregnancy is progressing, even if that happens to be morning sickness. But a lack of symptoms doesn't mean something is wrong; it's all really happening and your baby is going through some critical stages of development.

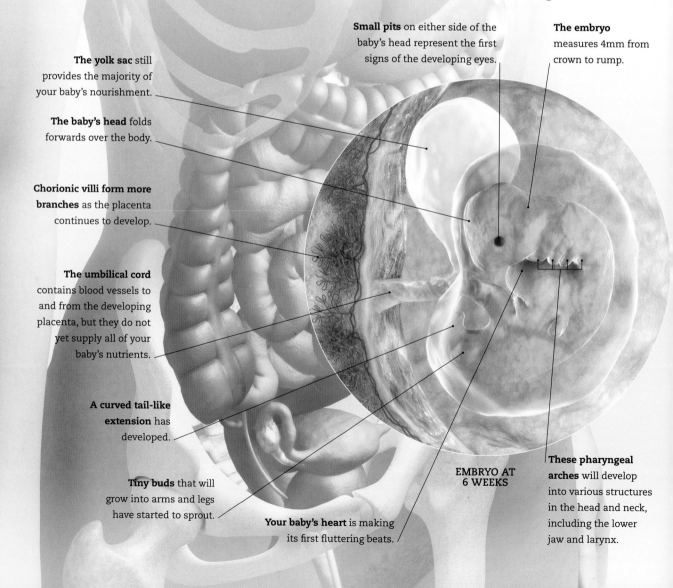

Small pits on either side of the baby's head represent the first signs of the developing eyes.

The embryo measures 4mm from crown to rump.

The yolk sac still provides the majority of your baby's nourishment.

The baby's head folds forwards over the body.

Chorionic villi form more branches as the placenta continues to develop.

The umbilical cord contains blood vessels to and from the developing placenta, but they do not yet supply all of your baby's nutrients.

A curved tail-like extension has developed.

Tiny buds that will grow into arms and legs have started to sprout.

Your baby's heart is making its first fluttering beats.

EMBRYO AT 6 WEEKS

These pharyngeal arches will develop into various structures in the head and neck, including the lower jaw and larynx.

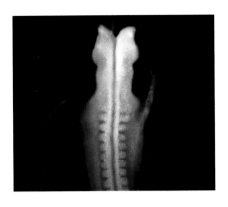

244 days to go...

YOUR BABY TODAY

The embryo now has 14 somites – the building blocks of your baby's musculoskeletal system. The first nine pairs are shown here. The upper part of the image shows the head end of the neural tube, which has now nearly closed.

If you've had no symptoms as you enter your 6th week, you may be on the lookout for signs that you are in fact pregnant.

You and your partner are probably the only people who know you're pregnant, and you may still be wondering if it's real. At this stage you may not have any symptoms at all, despite the rapidly changing and growing embryo inside you.

This absence of pregnancy signs is completely normal and is not a cause for concern. Try to remember that the majority of pregnancies are without any complications. It's normal for a healthy pregnant woman to have a wide range of side-effects or none at all. So don't worry if you're feeling great – in fact, count yourself lucky!

ASK A... NUTRITIONIST

Since being pregnant, I don't seem to have much of an appetite. Is this normal? It is common to go off food, especially if you have morning sickness (see p.81). You may no longer be able to stomach your favourite foods. If you're not eating much, it's important that what you do eat is nutritious. Choose nutrient-rich, dark green leafy vegetables and pulses, and fish (see p.96), which contains essential fatty acids.

AS A MATTER OF FACT

Up to 90 per cent of your supply of vitamin D depends on adequate exposure to sunlight.

Vitamin D helps your body absorb calcium, which is vital for the development of your unborn baby's skeleton. A daily 15-minute walk outside – with the sun on your skin – is sufficient; you can also boost your intake of vitamin D by eating oily fish, eggs, fortified cereals, and bread, and by taking supplements (see p.16).

EARLY ULTRASOUND SCANS

Some women will have an early ultrasound scan, but the majority of women will have one around the 12th week of pregnancy (see p.137). Early scans are usually undertaken vaginally, with a scanning probe inserted gently into the vagina. They are performed for the following reasons:

■ **If there is a history of multiple births** in your family (or you have used IVF or another form of assisted pregnancy), your doctor may wish to check the number of fetuses.

■ **If you've had a miscarriage in the past,** or show signs of cramping or spotting, or more profuse bleeding, a scan can be undertaken to check that there is still a heartbeat.

■ **To establish the cause of vaginal bleeding.** Your baby may be healthy, but fibroids or other conditions may be causing you to bleed. This will be addressed by your doctor.

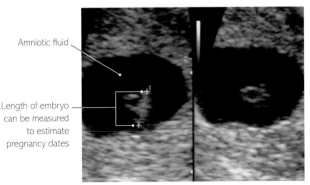

Amniotic fluid

Length of embryo can be measured to estimate pregnancy dates

Early vaginal scans do not show a great deal of detail. The sonographer waits until the embryo is in the correct position (left) to be measured.

Your 6th week

79

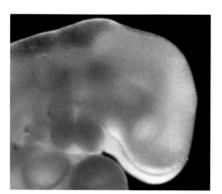

YOU ARE 5 WEEKS AND 2 DAYS

243 days to go...

YOUR BABY TODAY

The centre of this image shows the baby's developing heart (darker grey), a very primitive structure at this stage. The baby's head is to the right of the image. The embryo is almost completely transparent.

There won't be any visible signs of pregnancy on the outside for some time, but there are many changes taking place inside.

At this early stage, all your unborn baby's needs will be met by the yolk sac. Attached to the embryo by a connecting stalk, this essential balloon-like structure indicates the site of your pregnancy and can usually be seen through a microscope as early as this week as a sphere 3–4mm across. At first, the yolk sac is as large as the disc of embryonic cells that will eventually become your baby.

The yolk sac contains cells that perform a similar function to the liver. It releases several pregnancy hormones and produces the embryo's first red blood cells. After week 9 the liver will take over these functions as the yolk sac gradually disappears and the placenta takes over, by around the 10th week of pregnancy.

Over the next seven days, a primitive circulatory system develops, well before any blood circulates to the placenta in the 10th week. And, by the end of this week, using the highest quality ultrasound equipment, it is just possible to see the embryo's heartbeat. At this early stage, the heart is simply a tube.

AS A MATTER OF FACT

You should continue to take a 400mcg folic acid supplement daily until the 12th week of pregnancy.

This supplementation is in addition to a well-balanced diet that includes green vegetables and pulses. Many fortified cereals also contain folic acid, as do some fruits, such as oranges, papaya, and bananas.

If you can't stomach big plates of food, try eating a combination of small portions at mealtimes and as snacks.

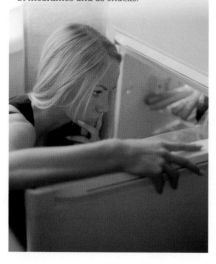

ASK A... NUTRITIONIST

Should I be eating for two?

Unfortunately, pregnancy is by no means a licence to eat anything and everything you'd like. "Eating for two" is a myth, and if you do so, you'll end up consuming too many calories and gaining too much weight. The best advice is to use your common sense. Studies show that pregnant women who eat according to their appetite naturally eat the proper amount and gain a healthy amount of weight.

Calorific needs in pregnancy vary greatly from woman to woman, depending on pre-pregnancy weight and physical activity. In general, energy needs increase by approximately 300–500 calories per day during pregnancy. In the first trimester, calorific needs are a bit less, more at the lower end of this range.

In the first trimester, when up to 80 per cent of women are nauseous or vomiting, getting enough calories can sometimes be a challenge. Like many pregnant women, you may feel most nauseous when your stomach is empty. One good trick is snacking. Eating five small meals rather than three large ones can be soothing to a nauseous stomach, while at the same time giving you the calories you need.

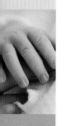

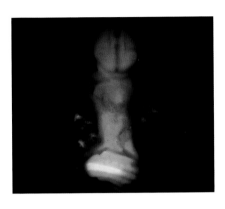

242 days to go...

YOUR BABY TODAY

A front view of the embryo: the head region is bent downwards so that the central nervous system can be seen. The tube-like structure in the head region is the developing spinal cord. The tail of the embryo is curving upwards.

Morning sickness is one of the most common and least welcome symptoms of pregnancy.

FOCUS ON... HEALTH

Ease the nausea

Unfortunately there is no definitive cure-all for morning sickness, though you could try the following natural remedies:

■ **Eat little and often** – having low blood-sugar levels may make the nausea worse so even if you feel sick, eating small snacks may help.

■ **Try eating a plain biscuit or cracker** first thing in the morning before you get out of bed.

■ **Stick to bland foods** such as cereal or toast and avoid eating fatty and oily foods.

■ **Try having foods and drinks that contain ginger** (see right) or peppermint.

■ **Drink plenty** if you are vomiting, to avoid becoming dehydrated. Put a bottle of water in the fridge and sip it gradually throughout the day. If you feel you are getting dehydrated, for example if your urine is getting very concentrated, you may need to see a doctor.

If the nausea or vomiting is too much to bear, then consult your doctor, who will be able to prescribe anti-sickness medications.

Feeling sick and vomiting are common symptoms of early pregnancy. There are various theories to explain why morning sickness occurs; one is that it's due to the rising levels of hCG (human chorionic gonadotrophin) hormone during the first trimester. Morning sickness, unfortunately, doesn't only happen before breakfast; in fact, it can happen at any time of day and more than once in 24 hours.

One of the greatest challenges of early pregnancy is keeping it a secret from colleagues. If you have to keep rushing to the loo to vomit, people are likely to become suspicious. They may

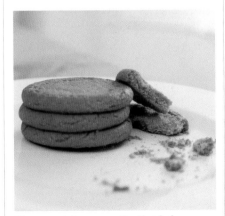

Ginger contains properties that help to ease nausea. Put a plate of biscuits on your bedside table, and nibble them before you get out of bed in the morning.

---

also notice that you look unwell or are more tired than usual. To help you handle this, you may want to tell one or two colleagues or your boss. You could ask them to keep it a secret for the time being. It's worthwhile keeping some face wipes, toothpaste, and a toothbrush in your drawer, together with any snacks that you have found help to ease your nausea.

If you're finding it difficult to handle your vomiting, or are worried you are vomiting too much, seek advice from your doctor. Rarely, the sickness can become more serious and require medical treatment (see p.111).

AS A MATTER OF FACT

Ginger has been shown in studies to help with pregnancy-induced nausea.

One study found that the decrease in nausea happened four days after including ginger in the diet daily; so don't give up if you don't get relief right away. Try crystallized ginger chews or tasty ginger biscuits; drink soothing ginger tea; and try cooking with fresh ginger. Be aware that most ginger ale does not contain real ginger, so is unlikely to ease nausea.

A changing world

The family is an ever-changing unit and has undergone some major shifts in the past two decades. Although times have changed, your role as a parent is the same as ever: to give your child consistent care, love, and loyalty.

THE STATISTICS

Changing family life

The statistics below give an insight into family life today.

■ **In the UK, 55 per cent of mothers of under fives work** (compared with around 25 per cent in 1975); in the US, 64 per cent of mums with children under the age of six work.

■ **About 25 per cent of children under five** with working mums are looked after full-time by dad and 30 per cent of working parents share childcare.

■ **Only 1 in 10 mums** stays at home full time with the children.

■ **Today, around 25 per cent of children live in** one-parent families, of which about 9 per cent have a single dad at the helm.

■ **In some parts of the UK about a third of all babies are** born to ethnic minority families – a figure that is similar in New Zealand and Australia. In the US, up to half of all children under five are from an ethnic minority.

■ **More than 41 per cent of babies in the UK are** born to unmarried women; in the US, 37 per cent of babies are born out of wedlock. This trend is echoed throughout the West, and the numbers are steadily rising.

■ **One in every 100 babies** grows up in a household with same-sex parents.

■ **About 100,000 under-13s** in the UK have a grandparent as sole carer.

The family today

Today, there are many varieties of family life. Although studies report on the problems of modern childhood, children are familiar with and tolerant of different cultures, and living and working practices.

Mature mums The number of new mums in the UK over 35 has doubled in the past decade, and the pregnancy rate in women over 40 has risen faster than in any other age group. The benefits are that older women are more likely to be settled, financially stable, and mature.

Single parenting Single mums in the UK have risen from 1 per cent in 1971, to 11 per cent in 2004. There's no doubt that children in single-parent families can be disadvantaged, but it's thought that much of this is due to financial constraints, and that those who have adequate socioeconomic resources do well.

Stepfamilies Stepfamilies are the fastest-growing family type. It's thought that at least 1 in 3 children will have a stepfamily situation within their lifetime. Siblings may be of wildly different ages, or of the same age.

Modern dads

Dads today are more involved in family life than those of previous generations. Some 96 per cent attend the birth (compared to 5 per cent in 1965), and over 70 per cent take time off after the birth. In the 1970s, dads of children under five devoted less than 15 minutes a day to child-related activities, compared to over two hours by the 1990s. Research shows that children whose dads spend

THE GENDER GAP

Boys versus girls

Historically, about 106 boys have been born for every 100 girls – a phenomenon believed to be nature's way of compensating for the fact that males are more likely to be killed through conflicts. But ratios are changing with girls outnumbering boys. One factor may be increased stress (women under stress produce more girls than boys). However, the most important contributor is now thought to be the number of gender-bending chemicals in our environment, such as synthetic oestrogens, PCBs (polychlorinated biphenyls), and pesticides.

considerable time with them achieve well educationally and at work.

Childcare

This is a necessity in most families. Studies show that good care outside the family has a positive impact on social skills, intellect, and language. UK grandparents provide 60 per cent of childcare. A good grandparent relationship provides stability, family values, and is thought to improve cognitive development.

Multiple cultures

Your baby will live in a multi-cultural society. This impacts on educational experience and friendships, and there's a strong chance a child will be looked after by someone from another culture at some point in her childhood.

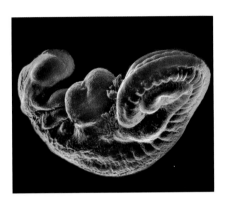

241 days to go...

YOUR BABY TODAY

This image shows just how curled up the embryo is at this stage. The head end of the embryo is on the left. The embryo now has 22 pairs of somites (building blocks of the musculoskeletal system) running along the back.

This is a crucial time for your developing baby as the neural tube, which will become the brain and spinal cord, is forming.

This week your baby begins to grow rapidly and will become much more recognizable as a baby over the next five weeks. There are three types of cell, each committed to a separate function. The first will form the skin and nervous system; the second forms blood vessels, muscles, and bones; the third forms the entire digestive system.

At this stage, it is the cells responsible for the spine and nervous system that are at work. Changing shape from a flat disc, the embryo starts to curl up. The edges of the groove that are already partially formed along the back gradually start to meet, closing and fusing to form a tube, which will become the brain and spinal cord. The last parts of the tube to close are at the very top of the head and finally at the base of the spine, two days later.

Taking care to get an adequate intake of folic acid (see p.35) in early pregnancy is essential to ensure that the neural tube closes completely, with no gaps.

TIME TO THINK ABOUT

Whether to tell

You're excited to be pregnant, but should you tell people yet?

■ **Most parents-to-be** wait to share their exciting news until after week 12 when the risk of miscarriage falls. You may, however, decide you want to confide in family and close friends. If they are people whom you would tell if you miscarried, then there is no harm in sharing your news.

■ **Legally, you don't have to tell** your employer yet. The latest date you should inform your employer is 15 weeks before the beginning of the week in which your baby is due (see p.255), but if you want time off for antenatal appointments before this, you'll need to explain why.

■ **Similarly, if your job** involves anything that could be a health and safety risk (for example, heavy lifting or working with chemicals), you must inform your employer early so your role can be adapted. It's also sensible to tell your boss the good news before office gossip about your expanding girth snowballs.

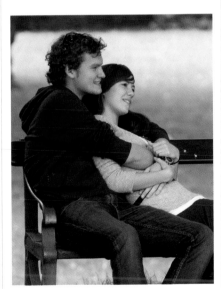

Not telling many people, if anyone, in the first few weeks will give both you and your partner time to come to terms with the news.

FOCUS ON... DADS

Keeping quiet

Your first reaction to finding out that your partner is pregnant might be to want to tell the world. After all, you may be excited or nervous and want to confide in people who you can trust. Think twice before telling lots of people (see box, left) and don't do so without talking to your partner. Of course, your partner may find it hard to hide some aspects of pregnancy, such as nausea and vomiting.

Most importantly, make sure that you are both in agreement that it is the right time to tell others.

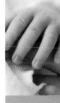

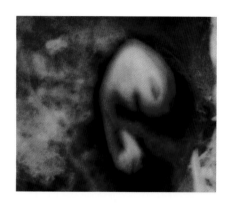

240 days to go...

YOUR BABY TODAY

This is a view of the right side of an embryo with the fronds of the chorionic villi in the background. The curled shape of the embryo is clearly demonstrated. The umbilical cord attachment to the early placenta can just be seen.

Are you feeling up one minute and down the next? Be reassured that this is a perfectly normal response to pregnancy hormones.

It may not happen quite yet, but be forewarned that you may become very emotional or irrational during pregnancy and suffer from mood swings. You may cry at things that had previously not affected you. This is due to a combination of your rapidly fluctuating hormones and the fact that pregnancy is a major life change.

Mood swings can be difficult for both you and your partner – try to keep communicating with each other and explain how you are feeling, no matter how irrational it may seem.

MORE VEG PLEASE!

Be creative to stimulate your appetite and get essential nutrients:

- **Try raw veggies** with a dip.
- **Throw in a few vegetables** when you make your morning smoothie (see p.135) – cucumber, celery, peppers, and carrots are mild in flavour, but deliciously nutritious.
- **Try grating** courgettes or carrots into soups, pasta sauces, and stews, or throwing a handful of squash, frozen peas, broccoli, asparagus, or green beans into a risotto.
- **Add vegetables** to a cheese sauce. If you cook them in the sauce, it will absorb all of the nutrients that would normally make their way into the cooking water.
- **Make your own pizza** topped with crunchy and colourful vegetables.
- **Choose vegetarian** dishes when you get a takeaway.

FOCUS ON... YOUR HEALTH

Tackling tiredness

Tiredness is a common pregnancy complaint and you might find you have a sudden loss of energy in the early stages as your body adapts to the changes caused by pregnancy. This often lasts throughout the first trimester, but after about week 13 you should start to feel more energized. When you're not resting, try to stay active.

Another cause of tiredness is anaemia. When you see your midwife you will be offered a blood test to check your iron levels, and if these are found to be low you will be offered supplements. To avoid anaemia, eat iron-rich foods, such as dark green, leafy vegetables, red meat, wholegrain cereals, and pulses, and drink prune juice. Vitamin C helps your body absorb iron, so try drinking fresh orange juice with meals. Limit caffeine intake (see p.66) as it inhibits iron absorption.

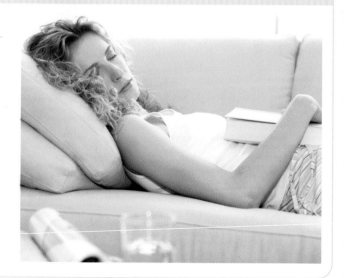

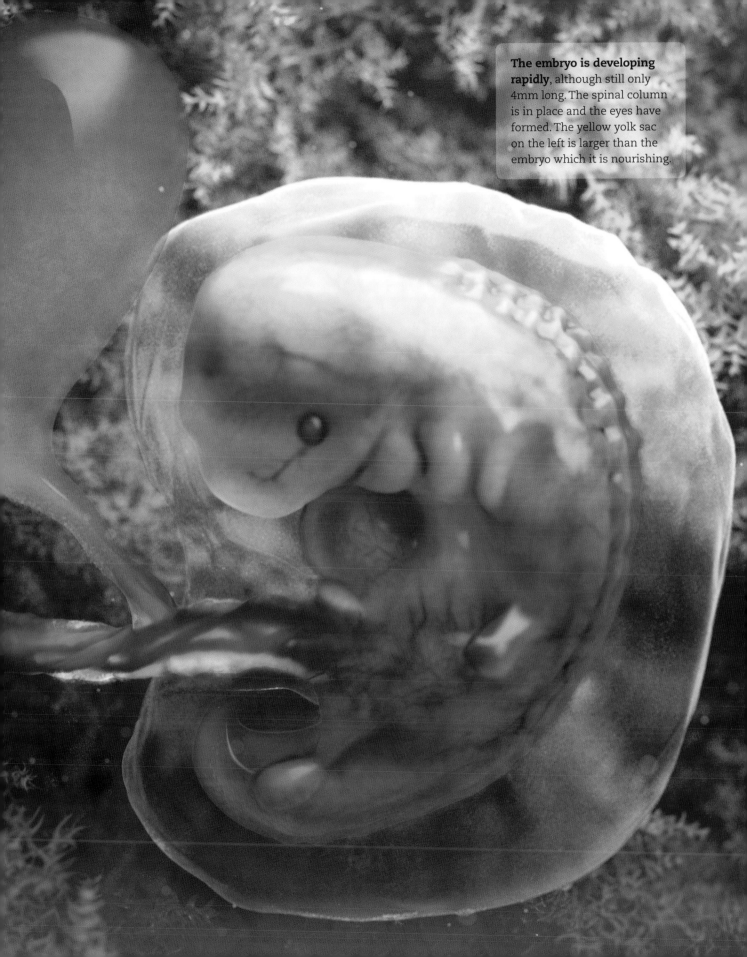

The embryo is developing rapidly, although still only 4mm long. The spinal column is in place and the eyes have formed. The yellow yolk sac on the left is larger than the embryo which it is nourishing.

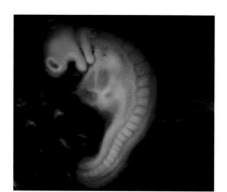

YOU ARE 5 WEEKS AND 6 DAYS

239 days to go...

YOUR BABY TODAY

Development in the upper body usually precedes that in the lower body – this image shows the bulge containing the heart and liver, and the very earliest sign of development of the upper limb buds, but as yet there is no sign of the lower limb buds.

The first change in body shape you may notice is a marked increase in your breast size, even at this early stage of pregnancy.

The first part of your body to change shape is likely to be your chest. Your breasts may increase in size quite rapidly, looking bigger and feeling heavier. They may also become quite tender to touch.

The nipples will change: the areola (the darker skin around the nipple) may become darker in colour and your nipples may tingle. As your breasts get bigger, you might notice blue veins appearing. All these breast changes are due to the hormone oestrogen.

AS A MATTER OF FACT

Each breast will increase, on average, by 5cm (2in) and 1.4kg (3lb) during pregnancy.

That is why it is important to wear the right bra, even in the early stages of pregnancy.

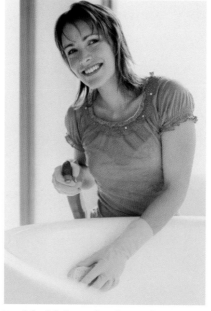

Read the labels on cleaning products carefully to make sure they are not toxic, and always wear rubber gloves. Pregnancy can be a good time to ask your partner to clean the bathroom!

ASK A... MIDWIFE

How can I ease the soreness in my breasts? Wearing a supportive bra can help with both the feelings of heaviness and the soreness in your breasts, which are common in pregnancy. If your breasts are very tender at night, try wearing your bra during the night while you sleep as this may help. Try to avoid sleeping on your front if this causes discomfort. You may find that rubbing in a cream containing aloe vera or camomile is soothing.

FOCUS ON... SAFETY

Detox yourself

Once you know you're pregnant, it's only natural to want to keep your baby safe, so...

Take care when you're cleaning. Studies suggest there may be a link between pregnant women using bleach and spray air fresheners, and babies developing asthma. Plus, commercial oven cleaners contain toxic chemicals that experts believe could damage unborn babies.
- Don't use "toxic" products.
- Keep rooms well ventilated.
- Steer clear of fumes.
- Wear gloves.
- Make your home sparkle with a solution made of bicarbonate of soda, distilled white vinegar, lemon juice, and essential oils.

Get someone else to clean your cat's litter tray (or if that's not possible, wear rubber gloves and wash your hands afterwards). Cat faeces may contain parasites that can cause toxoplasmosis (see pp.17 and 101), an infection that could harm your unborn baby.

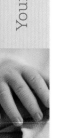

Your first trimester

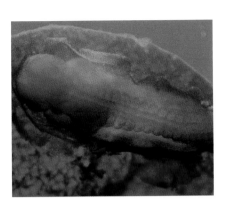

238 days to go...

YOUR BABY TODAY

Here the back of the embryo can be seen lying over the yolk sac. The opening overlying the developing brain has now closed (left side of image) and this will be followed two days later by closure of the opening at the base of the spine (out of view).

By the end of this sixth week, one of your baby's major organs – the heart – is rapidly developing and circulating blood.

Your developing embryo may still be tiny, but is undergoing rapid and complex development.

The heartbeat is now more easily recognized on an ultrasound scan. The heart continues to form from a simple smooth tube which, as it becomes more muscular, loops, folds, and divides to form four chambers. On the left side the upper chamber (left atrium) takes in blood from the lungs. From here blood passes through a one-way valve (the mitral valve) into the main left pumping chamber (the left ventricle). This then pumps blood out of the heart to the body along the main artery (the aorta). On the right-hand side of the heart, the upper chamber (right atrium) collects blood returning from the body and passes it through a one-way valve (tricuspid valve) into the right main pumping chamber (right ventricle). This pumps blood to the lungs and the cycle continues.

At this stage of development, the circulation is very basic with the heart tube simply sending blood around the length of your baby. No blood travels from your baby's circulation to the placenta (see p.127).

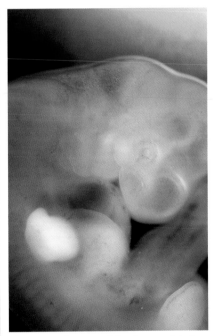

It's at an early stage of development, but the developing heart can be seen here as the dark red area. It lies just above the larger, slightly paler red area, which is the liver. Below the liver is the umbilical cord.

ACTUAL SIZE OF YOUR BABY

At 6 weeks, your baby's crown to rump length is 4mm.

5 weeks   6 weeks

HAVING A MISCARRIAGE

Whenever it happens, a miscarriage can be devastating. It is normal to experience grief, shock, and even a sense of failure, and you may also feel anger or a sense of injustice, especially if friends and family all seem to sail through pregnancy without any problems. Well-wishers may suggest that the miscarriage was "for the best" or "nature's way" but this can be cold comfort when you feel raw.

The most important thing you can do is take time to grieve. Get some support from friends or family, even if you don't feel like talking; exploring your emotions is an important part of the healing process. Your partner may be equally distressed, but is likely to show his grief differently, and while he may seem unscathed by the experience, he will also need support. Try not to feel disillusioned. Many, many women experience one or more miscarriages, and go on to have healthy pregnancies – and babies. Remember, too, that miscarriage is not your fault, no matter what you did before your pregnancy was confirmed. Give yourself time to heal and reflect and come to terms with this loss.

Your 7th week

SET YOURSELF SOME FITNESS STANDARDS TO SEE YOU THROUGH YOUR PREGNANCY

Getting in shape now will stand you in good stead as your pregnancy continues. Keeping active is important, so work up a daily exercise routine to strengthen your muscles and reduce fatigue – but listen to your body and don't exhaust yourself. This week your baby's vital organs, including the lungs and gut, start to develop. Your baby's head already looks too big for his body as the brain rapidly enlarges.

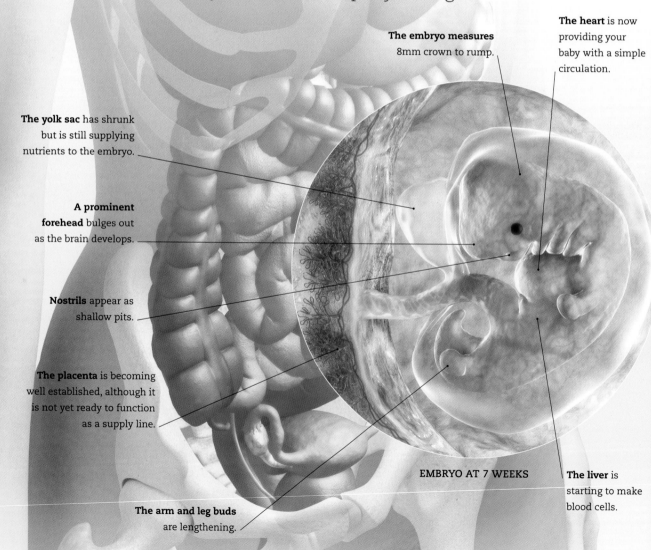

The embryo measures 8mm crown to rump.

The heart is now providing your baby with a simple circulation.

The yolk sac has shrunk but is still supplying nutrients to the embryo.

A prominent forehead bulges out as the brain develops.

Nostrils appear as shallow pits.

The placenta is becoming well established, although it is not yet ready to function as a supply line.

The arm and leg buds are lengthening.

EMBRYO AT 7 WEEKS

The liver is starting to make blood cells.

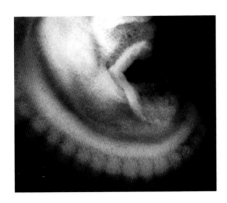

237 days to go...

YOUR BABY TODAY

In this side view of the embryo the spinal cord is clearly curved as it begins to develop. The pale-yellow ridge-like structures along the back are somites – your baby's developing musculoskeletal system.

You may be spending a lot of time in front of the mirror trying to spot your bump, but it could be weeks yet before you show.

Like most newly pregnant women, you're probably on the lookout for a bump, but it's unlikely to make an appearance just yet. On average, the fourth month marks the greatest period of growth, with your pregnancy most definitely appearing as a rounded abdomen.

If it's not your first pregnancy, you might show earlier, possibly as early as eight to 10 weeks, as your abdominal muscles will be more relaxed. Conversely, women who have firm abdominal muscles may show later. If you are expecting twins or triplets, you can expect to show even earlier.

ASK A... DOCTOR

Can having sex in pregnancy harm the baby? Unless you have been told by your doctor to avoid sex because of specific problems, such as a history of miscarriage or unexplained bleeding, then sex is safe at any stage. Enjoying intimacy with your partner is beneficial to your relationship.

Your baby is cushioned in fluid in the amniotic sac inside your uterus and protected by a plug of mucus at the cervix. Even deep penetration isn't harmful.

STRENGTHEN YOUR ABDOMINALS

It's safe to do abdominal exercises lying on your back during your first trimester. Towards the end of the first trimester, or when you start "showing" (see left), you should stop doing abdominal exercises on your back (see p.250 for other exercises you can do at this point).

When you are doing abdominal exercises, it's important to breathe correctly: remember to inhale to start and exhale on each effort.

The purpose of abdominal exercises is to strengthen core muscles. The deep transverse abdominis muscle that runs horizontally across your body is vital for core stability and strength as your baby develops. The rectus abdominis muscle that runs vertically down your body is the muscle that will stretch during pregnancy and weaken, so it's vital to keep the transverse muscle strong to help your posture and support your spine.

The sooner you begin to strengthen the transverse abdominis, the better. In the first trimester, one of the exercises you can do to strengthen this muscle is shown below.

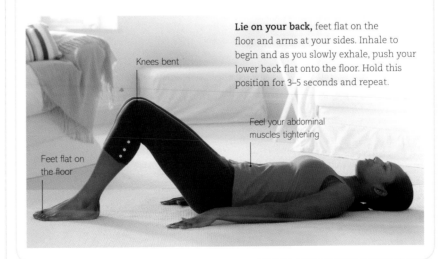

Knees bent

Feet flat on the floor

Feel your abdominal muscles tightening

Lie on your back, feet flat on the floor and arms at your sides. Inhale to begin and as you slowly exhale, push your lower back flat onto the floor. Hold this position for 3–5 seconds and repeat.

Strengthening and toning exercises

Exercises that strengthen your muscles will help you to deal with the additional demands of pregnancy and to cope better during labour and birth.

The exercises shown are sometimes called "functional movement enhancers" because they increase the strength of the muscles that you use for everyday functions such as walking, carrying, lifting, sitting, and standing. The workout can be used alongside walking, swimming, or other cardiovascular exercises and can be done three to four times a week.

Warm up March on the spot, swinging your arms back and forth. Continue for 3–5 minutes until your muscles are warm.

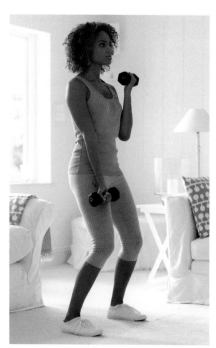

Biceps curl The biceps is an important muscle for carrying and lifting. You can use 1–2kg (3–5lb) weights for this sequence if you're a regular exerciser. Stand with feet hip-width apart, knees slightly bent, back straight, and arms at your sides. Breathe in, then exhale as you bend one elbow, raising your hand to shoulder level. Alternate arms until you've done 20 curls each side (40 in total). If you find this easy, try doing a total of 60 curls.

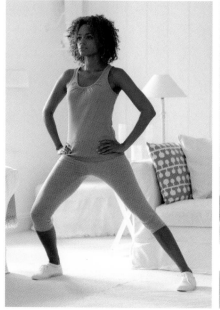
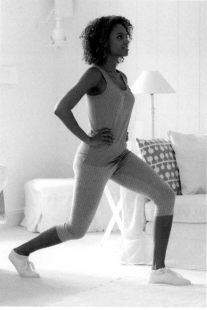

Side lunges (left) These (and the foward lunges, right) strengthen the abdominal and thigh muscles. Start with hands on hips, legs hip-width apart. Step one leg out to the side, bending the knee. Keep the other leg straight. Step back to the starting position, keeping the tummy pulled in and torso straight. Do 10 lunges on each leg. **Forward lunges** (right) Start with hands on hips, feet hip-width apart. Step one leg forwards; bend the opposite knee towards the floor, allowing the heel to lift off the floor. Return to the starting position. Do 10 lunges on each leg.

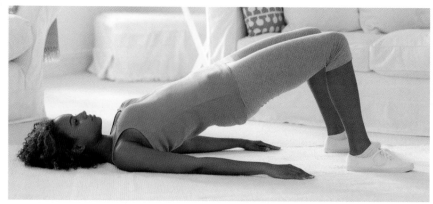

The bridge This exercise works your bottom, hamstrings, and inner thighs, and builds strength in your lower body to support your growing belly. Lie on your back with your legs bent and your feet flat on the floor, knees slightly apart. Raise your hips (this relieves pressure on your back and is safe to do in the first trimester). Keep your hands on the floor next to you, arms straight. Slowly bring your knees together while clenching your bottom; open and close your knees 10 times. Slowly lower your hips and roll onto your side to end.

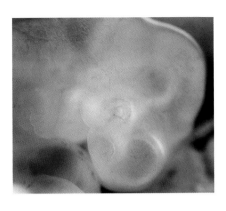

YOU ARE 6 WEEKS AND 2 DAYS

236 days to go...

YOUR BABY TODAY

The first recognizable facial feature to be formed is the eye, visible as a small circle within a larger one in the centre of this image. The larger grey areas are the fluid-filled chambers of the underlying brain.

Try not to dwell on your lifestyle before you realized you were pregnant, but do start making changes now.

Have you only just discovered you're pregnant? Not all women realize they are pregnant straightaway, especially if it wasn't planned. If you've only just found out, it's natural to be concerned about things that you did before you knew, such as drinking alcohol or taking drugs. You may be worried that you've harmed your unborn baby. Use your pregnancy as an opportunity to assess your lifestyle and improve your health.

Because of how pregnancy is dated (see p.35), your baby is still only a little over four weeks old. If you have not been taking folic acid (see p.35), start taking supplements from today.

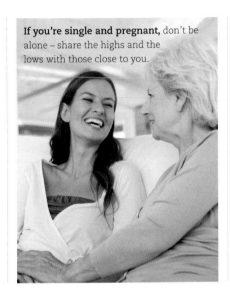

If you're single and pregnant, don't be alone – share the highs and the lows with those close to you.

TIME TO THINK ABOUT

Antenatal care

The options for antenatal care in the UK are outlined on p.102, but they do vary from area to area. Whatever your type of care, any ultrasound scans, investigations, and tests are likely to take place at a hospital. Your other options are likely to be:

- Shared care
- Midwifery care
- Consultant-led care
- Independent midwives

GOING SOLO

The prospect of being pregnant and single, especially if it wasn't your choice, can be tough. Make sure you:
- **Look after yourself:** plan a healthy diet, and an exercise routine. Get as much rest and restful sleep as you can. Ask a friend to spur you on or get online and seek support from other single pregnant women in your area – you will have a ready-made support network after the birth.
- **Ask for help** from family and friends. You will probably find they

are delighted to be involved in your pregnancy and are willing to come to antenatal appointments and classes with you: you may want to consider asking one of these people to be your birth partner.
- **Discuss support and access** with your baby's father (if appropriate), and if you can't agree, seek legal advice. You and your baby will benefit if an amicable arrangement is reached, and the sooner you start talking, the easier it will be after the birth.

- **Organize support** for after the birth. A survey found that grandparents who are actively involved in their grandchildren's lives contribute positively to their wellbeing. If you don't have family close by, try to build a network of other support that will see you through the early weeks.
- **Start thinking early** about your career options for after the birth. You don't have to make any decisions, but it helps to know some of the choices you may have to make later.

Your 7th week

91

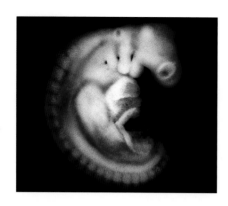

235 days to go...

YOUR BABY TODAY

The eyes begin life as shallow depressions, one on each side of the developing face. This image shows an early eye (circular area with darker centre), together with the curve of the pale yellow somites of the developing musculoskeletal system.

Needing to urinate frequently is, unfortunately, one of the unwanted side-effects of pregnancy.

ASK A... DOCTOR

Why do I have so much saliva in my mouth now I'm pregnant?
Called pytalism, excess saliva is caused by increased hormone levels. Don't try to keep the saliva in your mouth; if you find yourself drooling, spit into a tissue or small cup. Place a towel on your pillow. Sucking lemon wedges or ice cubes may help. Pytalism usually subsides in later pregnancy.

Are you spending a lot of time in the bathroom? As well as having to deal with symptoms such as nausea and vomiting (see p.81), if you're like the majority of pregnant women, you'll also need to pass urine more frequently. It means you're unlikely to want to be too far away from the nearest toilet.

It can feel as though your bladder cannot hold much urine so you may feel the need to go to the loo not long after you've just been, during the day and at night. This is because there is more blood being pumped through the kidneys so you produce more urine. As your uterus grows, it puts pressure on your bladder so it cannot expand as much as normal and will feel uncomfortably full earlier than usual. This can last throughout pregnancy, though you're most likely to experience it in the first and third trimesters.

If, however, you're concerned about the amount of urine you're passing, and/or you develop pain or stinging while passing urine, you may have developed a urinary tract infection and should see your doctor straightaway.

FOCUS ON... NUTRITION

Get carb loading

Make carbohydrates part of your balanced diet, but make sure you choose the right ones. Refined carbohydrates, such as white bread and white rice, are very quickly broken down, releasing a large amount of glucose into the bloodstream. This is quickly used up and then glucose levels fall rapidly. This fluctuation in glucose levels has been associated with diabetes, obesity, and heart disease, and recent data suggests it is not the optimal environment for adult or fetal health.

Unrefined carbohydrates, such as wholewheat bread and brown rice, break down more slowly, releasing glucose steadily and leaving you fuller. This can prevent the hunger signals that follow a rapidly digested meal and help with weight control. Your baby is constantly drawing glucose from your bloodstream, so a steady release of glucose leaves you both with plenty of fuel on an on-going basis. New research has found that babies exposed to a diet based on unrefined carbs may have more lean body mass and less body fat, though still a healthy birthweight. This will make them less likely to be overweight later in life.

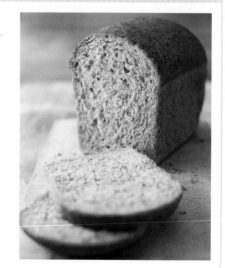

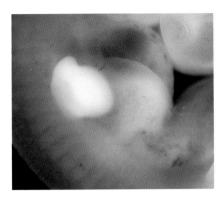

234 days to go...

YOUR BABY TODAY

The early limb bud that will form your baby's right arm can be seen here (white area). The upper limb buds appear before the lower limb buds. At this early stage, the hands and fingers are not yet developed.

Your baby's lungs won't be fully developed until late in pregnancy, but the foundations are being laid down right now.

ECTOPIC PREGNANCY

Pregnancy sac with embryo   Fallopian tube

In an ectopic pregnancy, the embryo develops outside the uterus, usually in a Fallopian tube.

An ectopic pregnancy can cause abdominal pain on one side and irregular vaginal bleeding. Some women get shoulder-tip pain, thought to be caused by internal bleeding. An ectopic pregnancy can rupture the Fallopian tube causing severe pain. Emergency medical attention is essential.

If an ectopic pregnancy is suspected, you will be given a scan. Sometimes the pregnancy will naturally regress; if not, medication or surgery will be necessary.

In this 7th week of pregnancy, your baby's lungs are starting to develop. This begins with a small lung bud branching out from the upper part of the tube (oesophagus) between your baby's mouth and stomach. This lung bud forms the main windpipe or "trachea", which then divides into two main branches (bronchi) that will eventually form your baby's right and left lungs. These bronchi continue to branch into smaller tubes, a process that will be repeated many times.

Your baby's gut is also starting to develop, from the mouth downwards. At the beginning of this week, his future digestive system consisted of a simple tube, closed at each end, that lay along his entire length. The tube remains closed but the oesophagus has now started to separate from the trachea and connect to the stomach. The swelling that will become your baby's stomach forms around the centre of his body, but undergoes a 90-degree rotation to lie more on the left-hand side.

Buds arise from the duodenum (the first part of the bowel that leaves the stomach) that will form the pancreas and bile duct to the gall bladder.

In just a couple of weeks, your baby will have all its major organs and body systems.

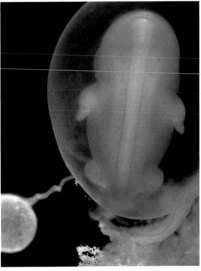

The embryo is safely cocooned in the fluid-filled amniotic sac. The yolk sac can be seen in the bottom left-hand corner, attached by what is now a very fine thread; its function is gradually replaced by the placenta.

AS A MATTER OF FACT

Music therapy is a highly effective way to reduce stress.

A study found that pregnant women who listened to music that mimicked the human heartbeat had reduced stress levels compared to those who did not receive the treatment.

Miscarriage

Miscarriage is the spontaneous loss of a pregnancy before the fetus is mature enough to survive outside the womb. Miscarriage is common, affecting 15–20 per cent of pregnancies, with the majority occurring in the first 12 weeks. Late miscarriage, after the first trimester, occurs in about 1 per cent of pregnancies.

DIAGNOSIS

Types of miscarriage

Different terms are used to describe miscarriage, depending on what is found during an ultrasound scan or an internal examination.

■ **Threatened miscarriage** is the term given to bleeding early in pregnancy when the cervix remains closed. In this case, the bleeding stops after a few days, and the pregnancy is likely to continue.

■ **Inevitable miscarriage** occurs when there is bleeding and the cervix is open, meaning that the fetus will be lost. If the pregnancy is less than eight weeks, the bleeding may be like a heavy, painful period. After eight weeks, the bleeding may be considerably heavier.

■ **Incomplete miscarriage** occurs when there is bleeding and the cervix opens, but the uterus doesn't expel its entire contents and some pregnancy tissue is left behind.

■ **Complete miscarriage** is when there is bleeding, the cervix opens, and the uterus expels all the pregnancy tissues.

■ **Missed miscarriage** is less usual. There may be no miscarriage symptoms, but the fetus stops developing and dies and the miscarriage isn't diagnosed until the routine scan at around 12 weeks.

Why miscarriage happens

An early miscarriage is usually due to a problem such as a chromosomal or structural abnormality in the fetus. It may also be caused by a fibroid (a non-cancerous growth in the uterus), an infection, or an immune system disorder. Miscarriage occurs more commonly in older women, in smokers, and in multiple pregnancies.

If you miscarry, it's important to know that it wasn't linked to anything you did, such as exercise, sex, or travel. Also, there is no evidence that rest reduces the risk of a threatened miscarriage going on to become inevitable (see box, left).

What will be done

If you bleed in early pregnancy, contact your doctor or midwife who will arrange for you to have a viability scan. Most hospitals have early pregnancy units where you can be seen promptly. If a scan shows a healthy fetal heart, the chance of miscarriage is reduced. If there is no heartbeat, or no developing baby, the doctor will assess if you've had a complete or incomplete miscarriage (see box, left). A complete miscarriage doesn't require treatment. If the miscarriage is incomplete, you'll be offered medication to hasten the miscarriage, or a procedure to scrape the uterus. Medication means that you avoid a general anaesthetic and risks such as infection or, rarely, damage to the uterus. Its disadvantage is that you may bleed more heavily and for longer. Discuss the options with your doctor.

If you have three or more miscarriages in a row, known as "recurrent miscarriage", your doctor may organize tests to see if there is a cause. It's unusual to discover a cause, but some rare abnormalities of the blood clotting system are associated with miscarriage.

After a miscarriage

Your period may be delayed by 6–12 weeks. Once the bleeding stops, there is no medical reason not to try to get pregnant again. However, the usual advice is to wait for at least three months before trying to conceive again so that you feel both emotionally and physically prepared for another pregnancy. Your partner also needs to feel that the time is right. Talking to a close friend, a family member, or a counsellor can help you come to terms with your loss.

LATE MISCARRIAGE

Pregnancy loss after the first trimester

Losing a pregnancy after the first trimester is much more unusual than an early miscarriage. After 24 weeks, a pregnancy loss is referred to as a stillbirth. There are several reasons why late pregnancy loss may occur, including infection; uterine abnormalities or abnormalities in the baby; and a weak cervix. If you have a late miscarriage, your doctor will discuss the possible causes with you and, if a cause is identified, whether anything needs to be done in a future pregnancy.

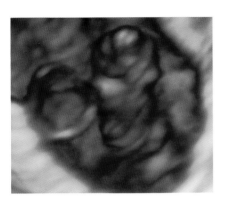

233 days to go...

YOUR BABY TODAY

This 3D ultrasound scan shows the embryo and its yolk sac, attached to the wall of the uterus. The yolk sac provides nourishment for the embryo until the placenta is fully functional, and produces blood cells until the liver can take over this role.

By this stage, you may have experienced bouts of dizziness – it's all part of your body and brain adjusting to the pregnancy.

THE LOWDOWN

Being a teetotaller

Your baby's health is the most important consideration, so before you've announced your pregnancy, you may need to take discreet steps to avoid drinking alcohol.

■ **Buy the first round** and get yourself a fizzy mixer and ice and a slice without the spirit. Once everyone else has had one drink, they're less likely to notice that you're on the wagon. For the next round, say you're pacing yourself and ask for a mixer.
■ **Claim you're detoxing** or hungover and order a juice or a Virgin Mary.
■ **Discreetly swap your full glass** with your partner's empty one.

AS A MATTER OF FACT

Exercising regularly can help you to sleep more deeply.

Insomnia is common in pregnancy, due to anxiety or difficulty in getting comfortable. Exercise is a destresser and will tire you out, increasing your chance of a good night's sleep.

If you feel lightheaded, especially when you get up from lying down, take extra care. Dizzy spells are common, especially as your pregnancy progresses and you get bigger, since your heart has to work harder against the forces of gravity to get blood to the brain.

Try to stand up very gradually, in stages, from lying to sitting to standing. Dizziness can also occur if you have been standing for a long period of time, as blood may collect in your legs. Keep moving to encourage the blood to be pumped back to your heart.

Alternatively, you may feel dizzy due to low blood-sugar levels. Other symptoms of low blood sugar include feeling sweaty, shaky, and hungry. Even if you're feeling or being sick, try to eat little and often to ensure that your blood-sugar levels remain stable.

If you regularly feel dizzy, speak to your doctor, who will carry out some basic health checks.

KEEP ON MOVING

The last thing you may feel like doing is exercising, but it can play a significant role in alleviating and preventing pregnancy symptoms. Although a jog through the park or a walk to the shops may not sound as inviting as a cozy nap on the sofa, exercise is invigorating and the effects will last. Try to think of it as being active, rather than "exercising".

If after completing a physical activity you feel even more fatigued, decrease how hard and long you exercise. Always listen to your body. As you become fitter and your pregnancy progresses, these feelings of fatigue should diminish, usually by weeks 12–14.

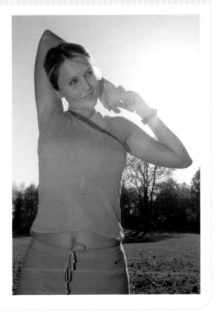

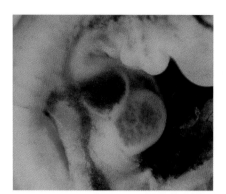

232 days to go...

YOUR BABY TODAY

At this stage of your baby's development, the heart is a tubular structure, visible in the centre of this image. It is, however, already providing your baby with a very simple circulation.

What will become your baby's tiny arms and legs are beginning to develop during this seventh week of pregnancy.

It will be some weeks before your baby – still an embryo – becomes recognizable as a human fetus. At the end of this seventh week, however, there are four simple limb buds, each slightly flattened at the end where, over the next two weeks, a hand or foot will form.

With the exception of muscle tone, which comes much later on in the pregnancy, all stages of your baby's upper limb development precede any developments in his lower limbs.

The eyes are the first recognizable landmarks to form on the face. At this stage, the eyes consist of two simple surface indentations, which then develop a second indentation within the first; the inner one will become the lens and the outer the eyeball. Your baby's eyes are wide apart and his ears and nose have yet to form.

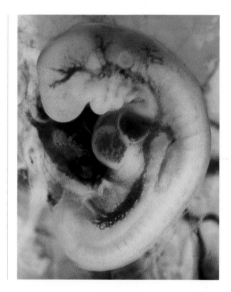

At this stage of an unborn baby's development, the circulatory system is at a very primitive stage. The upper dark bulge shown here is the heart, and beneath it lies the liver, where blood cells are starting to be made.

ASK A... DOCTOR

Can exercising increase the risk of miscarriage? There is no evidence to suggest that, as long as you're healthy and have been given the all-clear from your doctor, exercise will put you at a greater risk of having a miscarriage. In fact, the benefits of doing regular moderate exercise while you're pregnant far outweigh the risks to you and your baby.

The most important factors at this stage of your pregnancy are to exercise at the same level you did prior to being pregnant. Do not attempt any new high-impact and strenuous activity or take up a new sport. Follow the guidelines that are set out on page 18.

FOCUS ON... NUTRITION

Know your fish

Fish is packed with essential nutrients that are good for your baby's development (see p.169), so aim to eat at least two portions a week, including a portion of oily fish.

You do, however, need to be careful of consuming high levels of mercury, present in some fish, as it can harm an unborn baby's nervous system.

■ **Don't eat fish** that are at the top of the food chain as these are highest in mercury. These include shark, marlin, and swordfish. Eat no more than two fresh tuna steaks a week (weighing about 140g/5oz cooked or 170g/6oz raw) or four medium-size cans of tuna a week (140g/5oz when drained).

■ **Limit oily fish** to no more than two portions a week. Oily fish includes fresh tuna (canned tuna does not count as an oily fish), mackerel, salmon, sardines, and trout.

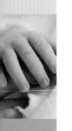

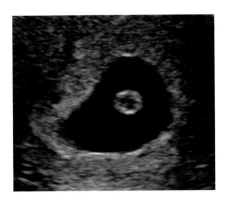

231 days to go...

YOUR BABY TODAY

This early vaginal ultrasound scan shows the first signs of pregnancy: the black central area is the fluid-filled cavity in which the baby (not visible) is developing. Within this is a small circular area, which is the yolk sac.

As your baby's body continues to develop, it won't be long before some very tiny movements will be visible on a scan.

While you're coping with early pregnancy symptoms, your tiny embryo is tightly curled in your uterus. There is a short portion at the lower end of the spine that in other species goes on to develop into a tail. This portion will soon start to disappear as more recognizably human features appear.

The ends of your baby's limb buds have flattened, like paddles, and next week will begin to form short digits that will become your baby's tiny fingers and toes. At first these are fused together – then, like the rest of the skeleton, the digits grow around a soft framework of cartilage that will gradually harden into bone. As the upper limb buds lengthen, your baby's elbows will begin to form.

Your baby's eyes continue to develop but won't be fully formed until around week 20; his nostrils now appear as two shallow nasal pits.

ASK A... MIDWIFE

Help! I'm pregnant again and my little boy is only 12 months old. How will I cope? Pregnancy can be exhausting, particularly in the first trimester, when your body is adjusting to the new demands placed upon it. Having a toddler to contend with at this time makes it all the harder.

Find quiet activities to enjoy with your toddler and leave the rough and tumble to someone else. Take time to nurture yourself, sleeping when your toddler naps, or just settling down on the sofa while he watches a DVD. Don't feel guilty about putting your feet up: it's important to take a step back at this stage and remember that your most important job right now is "growing" your baby.

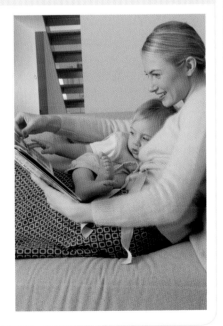

THE LOWDOWN

Good friends

Keeping your pregnancy quiet in these early weeks is difficult. Whether you want to tell people you're expecting is a matter of personal choice, but there's a good reason to keep it quiet for the time being (see p.83).

You may, however, need to talk to someone (other than your partner), so confide in a friend. Choose someone who will indulge your need to discuss everything – from pregnancy symptoms to birth fears and baby names. The ideal candidate will find your food cravings and 4am trips to the loo riveting... and provide bowls of ice cream and gherkins, as well as advice around the clock.

ACTUAL SIZE OF YOUR BABY

At 7 weeks, your baby's crown to rump length is 8mm.

5 weeks   6 weeks   7 weeks

Your 8th week

YOUR MOOD MAY SWING FROM HIGH TO LOW AS HORMONES AND EMOTIONS TAKE HOLD

You're probably beginning to feel different, even though you don't look pregnant. You may feel a bit low and irritable at times; this is largely due to the changing levels of hormones in your body. You may sometimes have mixed feelings about being pregnant, however much you long for a baby. If the idea of going on holiday appeals, opt for short journeys and a safe climate, and take extra care of yourself.

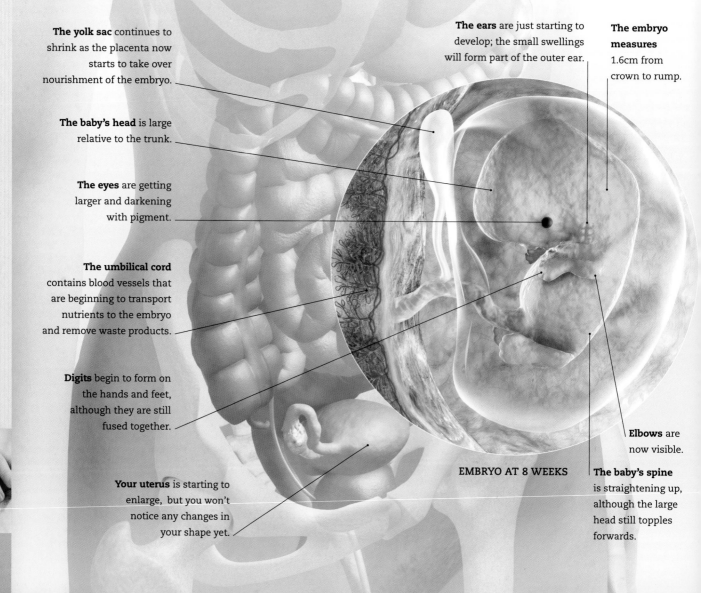

The yolk sac continues to shrink as the placenta now starts to take over nourishment of the embryo.

The baby's head is large relative to the trunk.

The eyes are getting larger and darkening with pigment.

The umbilical cord contains blood vessels that are beginning to transport nutrients to the embryo and remove waste products.

Digits begin to form on the hands and feet, although they are still fused together.

Your uterus is starting to enlarge, but you won't notice any changes in your shape yet.

The ears are just starting to develop; the small swellings will form part of the outer ear.

The embryo measures 1.6cm from crown to rump.

Elbows are now visible.

EMBRYO AT 8 WEEKS

The baby's spine is straightening up, although the large head still topples forwards.

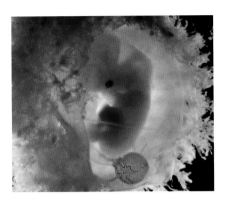

230 days to go...

YOUR BABY TODAY

The fronds that will form the early placenta can be clearly seen on the right here. At the bottom and separate from the embryo is the yolk sac, which is becoming ever smaller as its role is taken over by the placenta.

As your body begins to change shape, you may start to worry about gaining too much weight.

You're supposed to put on weight during pregnancy and while this is not a time to overeat, neither is it a time for faddy or restrictive diets. By eating sensibly and exercising moderately, you should gain a healthy amount of weight during pregnancy.

How much weight you should gain depends on your starting weight. If you are underweight when you become pregnant, you should put on more weight than someone who's overweight.

This starting weight is calculated by working out your BMI (see p.17), which is a measure of weight in relation to height. It's a useful tool to work out approximately how much weight you should gain during your pregnancy.

If your BMI falls within the normal range, then your recommended pregnancy weight gain is 11–14.5kg (25–32lb). If your BMI is in the underweight category, you should gain 12.5–18kg (27.5–40lb). If you're overweight, your

pregnancy weight gain should be 7–11kg (15–25lb). Women in the obese category should gain approximately 7kg (15lb). Women carrying twins should plan to gain about 16–20kg (35–44lb).

As a rough guide, an ideal weight gain is no more than 2.2kg (5lb) in the first trimester; no more than 5.5–9kg (12–20lb) in the second trimester; and no more than 3.5–5kg (8–11lb) in the third trimester. Remember not all of this weight gain is fat (see box, below).

HOW MUCH WEIGHT WILL YOU GAIN?

Over the 40 weeks of pregnancy, you are likely to gain very little weight in the first trimester and then experience a steady weight gain of around 750g–1kg (1.5–2lb) a week.

In the final few weeks of pregnancy, it's normal to gain a few more pounds. Remember that all figures given are averages and the amount you gain will depend on many individual factors;

where weight is gained can also differ from woman to woman. Always consult your midwife or doctor if you're concerned about any aspect of your weight gain or diet.

Weight gain chart

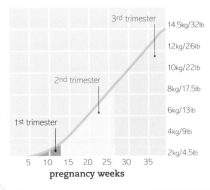

Components of weight gain

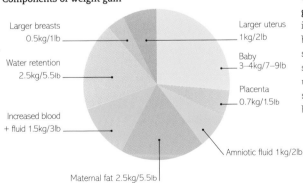

Larger breasts 0.5kg/1lb
Water retention 2.5kg/5.5lb
Increased blood + fluid 1.5kg/3lb
Maternal fat 2.5kg/5.5lb
Larger uterus 1kg/2lb
Baby 3–4kg/7–9lb
Placenta 0.7kg/1.5lb
Amniotic fluid 1kg/2lb

The weight you'll gain during pregnancy is a combination of your baby and her support system, the increased size of your breasts and uterus, essential fat stores, and additional bodily fluids and blood.

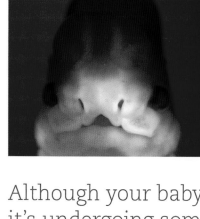

229 days to go...

YOUR BABY TODAY

Your baby won't look recognizably human yet but, as this image shows, the lower lip and jaw are formed; the upper lip is not yet complete, and the mouth appears very wide. The external ears are developing low down at the jawline and the eyes are wide apart.

Although your baby's brain is still very simply formed, it's undergoing some remarkable changes.

This is a really important stage of development for your baby.
At this time, her brain is a hollow structure, which is joined to the spinal cord, but it's now starting to fold and form five distinct areas.

The lowest part, or hindbrain, is the first part to grow rapidly and will become structures known as the pons, medulla, and cerebellum. These structures are the most primitive areas of the brain and determine many basic actions that we do without conscious effort, such as breathing and keeping our balance.

Above this is the midbrain that conveys signals from the hindbrain, peripheral nerves, and spinal cord to the forebrain. This part of the brain consists of the thalamus – involved with emotions and sensory perception – and the two cerebral hemispheres, both

quite smooth at present. Each hemisphere contains a fluid-filled chamber and within that the cerebrospinal fluid is produced.

At the 11–14 week scan (see p.139), brain development checks will be carried out to confirm that the baby has normal early cerebral development.

AS A MATTER OF FACT

Fish really is brain food!

Research found that six-month-olds whose mothers had consumed high amounts of fish during pregnancy scored better in mental development tests. However, only varieties low in mercury should be eaten (see p.96).

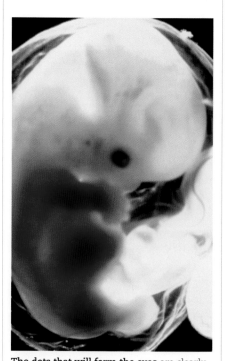

The dots that will form the eyes are clearly visible now. At the side of the head, a deep cleft can be seen between the front and back of the brain; this is normal at this stage.

ASK A... DOCTOR

I'm eight weeks' pregnant and have had some bleeding. Should I be concerned? Bleeding in early pregnancy is common. If the bleeding is light, and not accompanied by abdominal cramping or pain, then it's unlikely that there is anything wrong. However, always consult your doctor or midwife if you have bleeding at any stage of pregnancy to rule out any complications.

Bleeding in early pregnancy can sometimes be due to a cervical ectropian, which is when the surface of the cervix becomes "raw". This results from hormonal changes and is not harmful to the baby. Sexual intercourse can aggravate a cervical ectropian, causing bleeding.

Bleeding in late pregnancy may be more serious as it can be due to the placenta partially, or totally, detaching from the wall of the uterus, known as placental abruption, or to a low-lying placenta (see p.212). If you have a mucus discharge tinged with blood in late pregnancy, this may be a "show" (see pp.391 and 411).

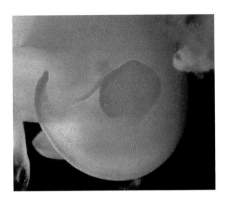

228 days to go...

YOUR BABY TODAY

At this stage, the embryo's "tail", shown curving up on the left, is starting to disappear. The somites of this area of the musculoskeletal system will eventually form the four fused bones of your baby's coccyx – the lowest part of the spine.

You may be thrilled and excited about having a baby, but it's natural to have mixed emotions at times.

Your emotions may fluctuate – one minute you're laughing and the next you're irritable and shouting, or crying. You might be confused that at a time when you should be happy, you often feel tense and tearful. Be reassured that this is a normal and temporary part of pregnancy.

Don't be too hard on yourself as these changing moods are caused mainly by pregnancy hormones, which is something out of your control. They are the same hormones that cause the symptoms of PMT – rapid mood swings, crying, and irritability – that you might have experienced before.

Be kind to yourself during these down times and do what works best for you, whether it's taking time out to be alone or sharing your feelings with others.

AS A MATTER OF FACT

Up to 70 per cent of pregnant women sometimes have symptoms of depression.

While one woman hardly has any mood swings, another could suffer for weeks, especially in the first trimester.

FOCUS ON... SAFETY

Protect yourself

Toxoplasmosis is a disorder caused by a parasite that can harm a developing fetus. Symptoms may resemble those of glandular fever, with a raised temperature and/or swollen glands in the neck.

It can be spread through cat faeces. However, it can also be spread from under-cooked meat. Thus, in addition to avoiding changing cat litter, use some caution in the kitchen. Beef, pork, and lamb need to be cooked well. Avoid cross-contamination in the kitchen when preparing foods. Be certain to clean chopping boards and utensils well with hot, soapy water after preparing meat.

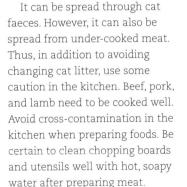

When you're having a down day, remember that these negative feelings will pass; mood swings are a normal part of pregnancy.

ASK A... MIDWIFE

I'm struggling to cope with my wife's mood swings. Are these normal? Yes, your partner will be emotional and all you can do is be as supportive, patient, and understanding as you can.

At this early stage of pregnancy, her changing hormone levels may cause mood swings and unexpected emotional responses. Sometimes things that have never been a problem, such as hearing a particular piece of music, might make her cry, or she may snap at you over something trivial. With her emotions out of kilter, she's likely to be as frustrated and confused by this behaviour as you are. Until it passes, just bide your time, bite your tongue, and give her a hug.

Antenatal care options

Throughout your pregnancy, you will be looked after by a midwife, doctor, or obstetrician, or a combination of these. The aim of your antenatal care is to monitor you and your baby so that problems can be identified and managed.

Your care during pregnancy

Early in pregnancy, you will need to think about who you would like to look after you during pregnancy, labour, and the postnatal period. You will also need to consider where you want to give birth as this will influence your choice of care provider. The main options are set out below, although these may vary depending on where you live. When you attend your booking-in appointment (also sometimes called the "first-contact" appointment) at about 8–10 weeks (see p.122–3), you'll be given information about the antenatal services you can access in your area. The antenatal checks carried out at your booking-in appointment will also form a risk assessment and help to establish the best choice for your antenatal care.

Types of antenatal care

The majority of your care will usually be provided by a midwife. At your booking-in appointment, she will tell you about the antenatal services in your area.

Traditional midwifery care With this type of care, the midwife you meet at the booking-in appointment provides most antenatal and postnatal care, but may not be involved with your labour, unless you book a home birth.

Shared care Your care is shared between your general practitioner (GP) and the midwife, or team of midwives, so that antenatal appointments alternate between the two. Some women may also have some of their care with a hospital-based obstetrician.

Team midwifery care You can expect one to two midwives, or a small team of midwives, to see you through your pregnancy, labour, and postnatal periods either at home, at your doctor's clinic, at a midwifery-led unit, or at hospital. You should meet all the midwives who form part of the team during your pregnancy.

Independent midwifery care Midwives who work independently of the NHS offer a package that includes antenatal, labour, and postnatal care that you pay for. The care is usually based in your home. If problems develop in pregnancy or labour, you may need to see an obstetrician, and your care may have to be transferred to hospital. An independent midwife can accompany you to hospital, but she may be unable to give you direct care once you've been transferred, and can only support you in an advocacy role. If you choose an independent midwife, you may want to know the level of experience she has in managing the complications that might occur during birth; what services are provided in the cost; if she works alone; what guarantees she offers for being at the birth; and who provides back-up in the event that problems develop.

Hospital-led care If your pregnancy is high-risk, for example you have a pre-existing medical condition, develop a condition in pregnancy, or are having twins or more, the majority of your appointments will be carried out in hospital under an obstetrician's care.

Where you give birth

This important decision doesn't have to be made at the booking-in appointment, but your midwife or doctor will discuss the options at this time. It's wise to be aware of the risks and benefits of your choice. If you have a pre-existing problem, or one develops in pregnancy, this must be factored into the decision.

At home This is the preferred choice for women who want to give birth in familiar surroundings. If you choose a home birth, you'll be more likely to know the midwife who will be with you in labour from your antenatal appointments. Evidence suggests that women who have a home birth are less likely to have intervention in labour.

YOUR OPTIONS

Informed choice

Being able to choose the type of care you receive is one of the most important aspects of pregnancy and childbirth. Make sure that you have the most up-to-date, evidence-based information available so that you can make informed decisions. The care you receive should take account of any special needs you have, such as a disability, or cultural or religious beliefs. You should be able to discuss the options with your midwife or doctor and feel free to ask them whatever you wish, to change your mind, and know that your preferences, regardless of the recommendations made by the midwife or doctor, will be taken into account.

You can choose to have a home birth at any stage in pregnancy. However, it's only advised for women who are low risk, with no pre-existing problems. You should consider the length of time it will take to transfer to hospital if problems develop in labour.

In a midwifery-led unit These units provide a home-like setting. They are led by midwives with no obstetric input and have facilities such as birthing pools. The aim is to have less stringent time frames on labour. As with home births, women are likely to have less intervention. Some units are next to or part of an obstetric unit so that if necessary you can be transferred to hospital quickly. This option is only recommended for low-risk pregnancies.

In hospital Some women prefer to give birth in hospital with doctors and medical equipment close by. Also, some women need specialist care and input from obstetricians because of existing conditions or problems that develop in labour. In this case, the obstetrician and the midwife will work closely together. Other specialists may need to be involved, for example if a woman has diabetes or a heart condition.

Your care providers

During pregnancy, labour, and the postnatal period you will be looked after by a range of professionals.

Midwives provide the vast majority of care for women in pregnancy, labour, and the postnatal period. They are specially educated and trained in the care of mothers and babies in low-risk pregnancies. They are also trained to recognize when problems may be developing and then work within obstetric teams where an obstetrician is the lead professional. Some midwives undertake extra training so that they can offer services such as ultrasound scanning, reflexology, and aromatherapy. Midwives often have support from healthcare assistants or maternity support workers who take blood, do routine observations, assist with breastfeeding, and undertake administrative tasks.

General practitioners (GPs) may alternate antenatal appointments with midwives.

Obstetricians provide a highly skilled service for high-risk women who had pre-existing medical problems or for women who develop problems in pregnancy. An obstetric team consists of consultants, who are the lead clinicians, followed by other doctors with a range of different clinical experiences.

Paediatricians are doctors with special training in the health of babies and children. All babies born in hospital have a newborn check by a paediatrician or specialist midwife before being discharged.

Neonatologists specialize in the care of newborns with problems.

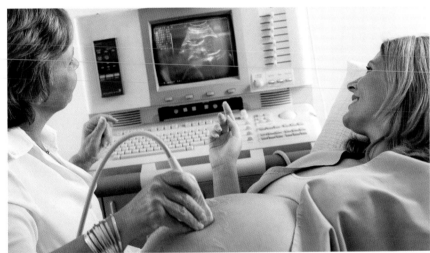
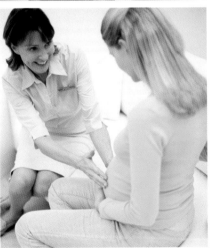
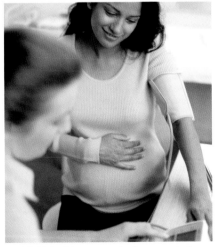
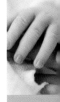

Routine scans are carried out at hospitals; women with high-risk pregnancies have most of their care here (top). **Midwives provide care** both at home and at doctors' clinics (bottom left). **GPs hold antenatal clinics** and may share care with midwives (bottom right).

Antenatal care options

103

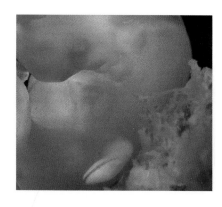

227 days to go...

YOUR BABY TODAY

The upper and lower limb buds that will form the legs and arms are clearly visible by now. The baby's head is still curled over the chest, but the beginnings of ears can just be detected as raised areas at the base of the head.

Your baby's facial features are beginning to develop and over the next few weeks will become much more defined.

AS A MATTER OF FACT

According to one study, eating apples during pregnancy could reduce the risk of your child developing asthma.

Following a Mediterranean diet may have the same effect. Researchers found that the babies of mothers who ate plenty of fish, olive oil, fruit, and vegetables were up to 30 per cent less likely to wheeze as well as 50 per cent less likely to develop skin allergies.

Your baby has ears! Low down, near the jaw line, the ears form, each arising from six small mounds, fusing together to give your baby her unique and individual ear shape. As the face and jaw forms and your baby's neck extends, moving away from the chest wall, the ears will migrate upwards; they will come to lie at the same level as her eyes by about 12–13 weeks.

The lips and nose are now beginning to take shape. To form the upper lip, two separate ridges of tissue grow from each side of your baby's face to fuse with the small piece of tissue in the midline extending downwards beneath the nose (the grooved part of the upper lip).

At around this stage, your baby's small and large bowel lengthen. Because they have insufficient room to expand inside the still very curled-up embryo, the intestines appear as a bulge on the surface of the abdominal wall. This bulge is covered by a membrane, into which the umbilical cord becomes attached. The bowel will continue to grow in this embryonic sac until 11–12 weeks when it will be reabsorbed into the abdominal cavity, leaving just the surface attachment of the cord.

FOCUS ON... SAFETY

Cooking with care

Scrupulous food hygiene is important in pregnancy for a number of reasons. First, your immune system is under extra pressure during pregnancy, making you more susceptible to food poisoning. Second, there's a risk that food-borne illnesses can affect the health of your baby, so it pays to be cautious. Do the following:
■ **Wash your hands carefully** and regularly, with hot water and soap. Make sure they are completely dry before preparing food, as bacteria spread more easily on damp skin.
■ **Keep food in your fridge** until you plan to prepare it, and cook it thoroughly before serving.
■ **Serve food piping hot,** as germs can multiply in lukewarm conditions.
■ **Refrigerate leftovers** straightaway, and reheat them well, only once.
■ **Thoroughly clean your hands,** implements, and work surfaces.
■ **Set the correct temperature** on your fridge and freezer.

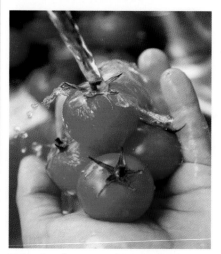

Make time for preparation and take the precaution of washing all fruit and vegetables. Keep raw foods away from cooked foods.

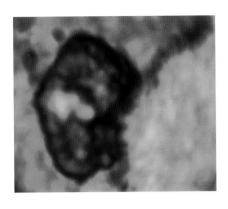

226 days to go...

YOUR BABY TODAY

This ultrasound scan of the baby in side view shows that the head (at top) is relatively large compared to the rest of the body. The lighter, elongated area at the centre of the baby's darker body is an upper arm bud.

Life goes on even though you're pregnant, but make sure you seek the right help if you're becoming overtired.

ASK A... DOCTOR

I'm going on a pre-booked holiday to a tropical climate. Can I have vaccinations now that I'm pregnant? In principle, it's a good idea to avoid travelling to parts of the world where there is a high risk of disease unless you really need to. Local healthcare might not be adequate and food and water may be contaminated, which pose dangerous risks.

If it isn't possible to change your destination or postpone your holiday, be aware of the following:
■ **Oral vaccines** to protect against yellow fever, typhoid, polio, and anthrax, for example, are contraindicated during pregnancy, although your doctor may decide that if you need to travel, the risk of having the vaccine is lower than the risks associated with contracting the disease.
■ **Some vaccines** (polio and typhoid) are safe when given by injection. Mefloquine tablets, taken to prevent malaria, are considered safe after week 16.
■ **It's safe to have a tetanus** vaccination if you're pregnant; check whether yours is up to date.

You may find work a strain at times. If you have symptoms, such as fatigue, and still haven't told colleagues you're pregnant, it can make for a stressful and difficult day. If you've told some colleagues, or your boss, you're expecting it may be easier but you might feel you have to prove you can still do your job as efficiently as before.

Travelling can be tiring so explore the possibility of doing more flexible hours, so that you can commute when it's less busy. Be reassured that even though you aren't feeling your best, your unborn baby is unlikely to be affected. Do, however, take care of yourself.

If you find that you're struggling to cope with your workload, consider speaking to your boss (you can ask him or her to keep your pregnancy a secret until you are ready to tell), or someone in the human resources department, to give yourself a little breathing space. If you have colleagues who are close friends, lean on them for support in these early weeks.

ARE YOU NESTING ALREADY?

There's nothing like a new arrival to inspire you to get all those DIY jobs done around the home. For most women, the nesting bug occurs in the later weeks of pregnancy, but if you're itching to get your house in order before then, do make sure you exercise a little caution.

First of all, avoid putting yourself and your baby at risk: don't stand on tall ladders, and don't bend and crouch for long periods as this may affect your circulation. Avoid contact with oil-based paints, polyurethane (used for flooring), spray paints, white spirit, and other paint removers, and avoid inhaling plaster dust.

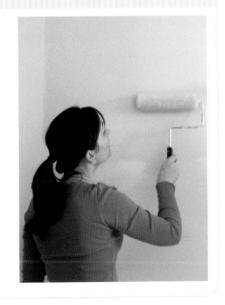

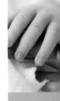

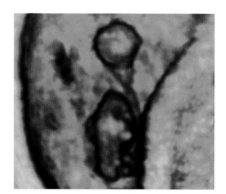

225 days to go...

YOUR BABY TODAY

The yolk sac can be seen floating like a balloon in the amniotic cavity on its fine stalk. As the embryo has drawn nutrition from the yolk sac it has gradually reduced in both size and importance. Meanwhile the placenta (on the right) is becoming established.

If you're booking a holiday, take into account that you may not feel up to travelling on a long journey.

BREATHE EASY

Exercise can help to keep breathlessness at bay, and increase the efficiency of your heart and lungs (cardiovascular system), helping you to cope with the physical demands of pregnancy now and in later months.

A cardiovascular workout involves increasing your heart rate for at least 20–30 minutes. However, pregnancy is not a time to start training for a marathon; stick to moderate-intensity workouts. A way to test if you are exercising at the right level is to talk while you are working out (see p.161) – if you can't, lower the intensity.

Try doing interval training, which involves alternating five minutes of cardiovascular workouts with five minutes of toning for the upper body (see p.196). Breathe out as you lift the weights, and in as you relax.

Breathing deeply allows oxygen to travel to your vital organs and helps the cardiovascular system to function effectively. During pregnancy, it's important to avoid taking short, shallow breaths and to focus on expanding your rib cage and filling your lungs with air.

You may have booked a holiday before you found out you were pregnant, or you might just feel like getting away. If you're feeling tired and have nausea and vomiting, however, you may not feel up to travelling too far.

One advantage of going away is being able to spend quality time with your partner and fully embrace the fact that you're going to be parents.

Wherever you're going on holiday, make sure your travel insurance company is aware you're pregnant and check the medical facilities at your destination. If you have any antenatal notes at this stage, take them with you. Airlines tend not to accept pregnant women on to flights once they are past 34 weeks, though different airlines have different guidelines (see p.28).

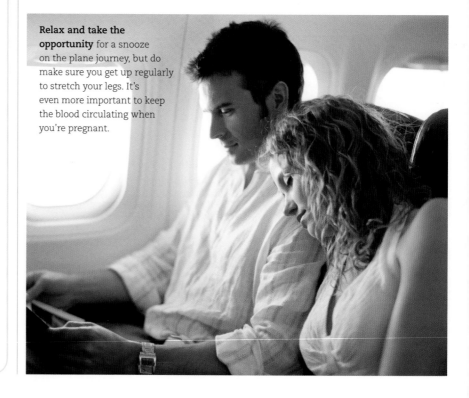

Relax and take the opportunity for a snooze on the plane journey, but do make sure you get up regularly to stretch your legs. It's even more important to keep the blood circulating when you're pregnant.

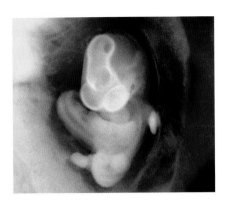

224 days to go...

YOUR BABY TODAY

The head is disproportionately large at this stage. In the centre of this image, the underlying structures of the brain can be seen: the forebrain has divided into two and these two halves will become the two cerebral hemispheres of your baby's brain.

You're no doubt already wondering if you're carrying a boy or a girl, but the physical signs of gender aren't apparent yet.

Although the sex of your baby was determined at the moment of fertilization, it will not yet be apparent whether the embryo is male or female.

At this stage of development, the external genitalia have exactly the same appearance on an ultrasound (almost non-existent). In a girl, no uterus or tubes have formed internally. The ovary in a female embryo and testes in a male embryo are currently just ridges of tissue, without any of the characteristics of either reproductive organ.

Incredibly, your baby's heart has already developed, with four chambers beating at about 160 beats per minute. The common tube leaving the heart has divided into the two main blood vessels: the aorta takes your baby's oxygen-carrying blood to her body and the pulmonary trunk takes her blood to the lungs. Valves within the heart ensure that the blood only travels one way and all of the major blood vessels are now established.

Your baby's eyes appear open because the eyelids have just started to appear and have yet to fuse. In reality, they won't properly open until week 26. Pigment is just starting to accumulate within the retina of the eye. The developing lens is supplied by a single blood vessel in the optic nerve, which will later disappear.

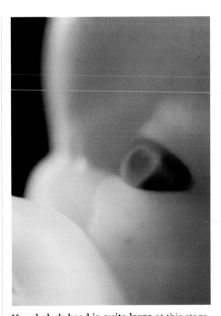

Your baby's head is quite large at this stage of development, due to rapid underlying brain expansion, giving the impression of an overhanging forehead. Her head is curled over her body with her chin on her chest.

ASK A... DOCTOR

I'm eight weeks' pregnant and have an ear and throat infection. Will I be allowed to take antibiotics? You may be prescribed antibiotics by your doctor as there are some that can be taken during pregnancy. Penicillin-based antibiotics are usually prescribed, or if you are allergic to these your doctor will be able to offer safe alternatives.

Never take antibiotics that have not been prescribed specifically for you. The following antibiotics should not be taken during pregnancy:

■ **Tetraclines** taken during pregnancy can adversely affect the development of an unborn baby's bones, and may cause some discoloration of the enamel on the baby's teeth.

■ **Streptomycin** can cause damage to the ears of the developing baby and result in hearing loss.

■ **Sulphonamides** can cause jaundice in the baby.

ACTUAL SIZE OF YOUR BABY

At 8 weeks, your baby's crown to rump length is 1.6cm.

6 weeks

7 weeks

8 weeks

Your 9th week

YOUR BABY HAS HANDS AND FEET, AND HIS BONES ARE GROWING

During this week, your baby starts to make tiny movements. You won't be aware of this, but it's exciting to think about. On the downside, you could be in the throes of nausea and sickness. However, many women find that the nausea starts to lessen from now on. There are various self-help measures you can take to relieve the sickness, but if it's making life miserable, talk to your doctor or midwife.

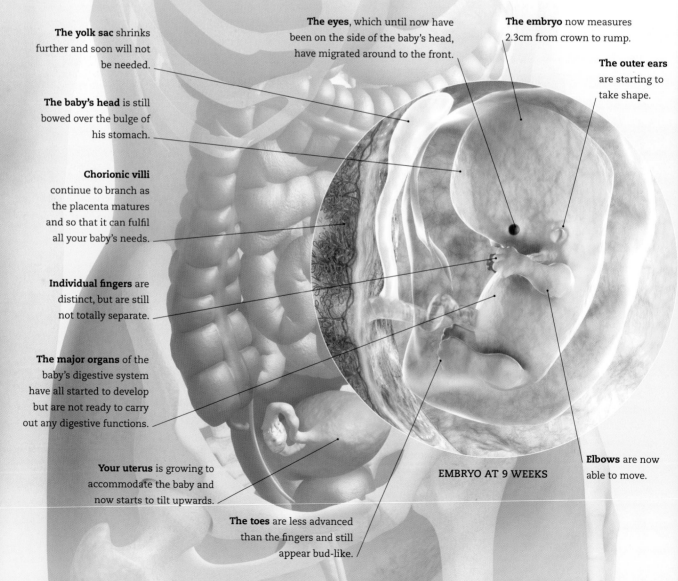

The yolk sac shrinks further and soon will not be needed.

The baby's head is still bowed over the bulge of his stomach.

Chorionic villi continue to branch as the placenta matures and so that it can fulfil all your baby's needs.

Individual fingers are distinct, but are still not totally separate.

The major organs of the baby's digestive system have all started to develop but are not ready to carry out any digestive functions.

Your uterus is growing to accommodate the baby and now starts to tilt upwards.

The toes are less advanced than the fingers and still appear bud-like.

The eyes, which until now have been on the side of the baby's head, have migrated around to the front.

The embryo now measures 2.3cm from crown to rump.

The outer ears are starting to take shape.

EMBRYO AT 9 WEEKS

Elbows are now able to move.

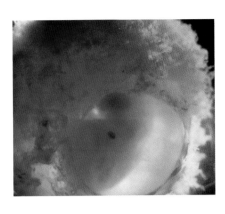

223 days to go...

YOUR BABY TODAY

The fetus can just be seen within the amniotic sac. The fronds (white area) on the surface of the sac make up the placenta and at this stage surround nearly all of the amniotic sac. At this point in the pregnancy the placenta is much larger than the fetus.

Not all pregnant women have cravings, but many women do experience a change in their food preferences.

When it comes to being pregnant, it seems your body instinctively knows what you like to eat. Experts are not sure how this can happen but it seems your body has natural protective mechanisms; certain foods are not good for the developing baby so your body turns you away from them; or your body is deficient in certain nutrients, so craves foods that will provide them.

Suddenly you can't stand the thought of food and drinks that you have always loved and find yourself craving things you never previously liked, or you long for bizarre combinations of foods. Aversions and cravings are often associated with nausea. It's common to go off fatty foods as the smell alone can make you feel sick. You may start to dislike the taste or the smell of coffee or tea, cigarettes, and alcohol.

It is common to crave strong-tasting foods such as pickles, which may be due to the fact that your taste buds change during pregnancy. What's termed "pica" is an unhealthy craving for bizzare items (see p.121).

You should try to eat healthily, but there are a few foods that should be avoided (see p.17). Otherwise eat whatever combinations you desire – and don't worry about the strange looks you might get in the sandwich shop!

ASK A... NUTRITIONIST

Should I stop adding salt to my food? There is no need to limit salt intake but don't have in excess of the recommended 6g (0.2oz) a day.

During pregnancy, your blood and other bodily fluids expand almost 50 per cent, an expansion that requires extra water and salt. The majority of salt in the diet comes from processed foods, not from the salt pot or the salt you add in cooking. To manage your intake, eat whole foods you cook yourself and add your own salt to taste.

FOCUS ON... DADS

Satisfy her cravings

If it's a mum-to-be's responsibility to play host to baby for nine months, it most definitely falls within your dad-to-be's job description to see that your partner gets everything she needs. A word of warning: cravings usually occur the minute the local shop has closed, or in the evening when you're relaxing. Forget the dill pickles and tubs of ice cream you've been told to expect. Instead, be prepared for a last-minute dash to the chippy for a pickled egg, a trek to a 24-hour supermarket that carries organic beef-flavoured crisps, beetroot, or a chocolate doughnut.

You can help by preparing meals and snacks some of the time: if your partner is presented with healthy food lovingly prepared by you, she may be less likely to reach for any unhealthy food she craves.

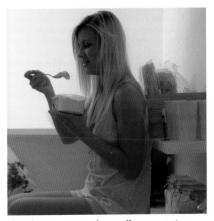

If an ice cream craving strikes, try to have one spoonful, not the whole tub. Team it with fresh fruit for a healthy combination.

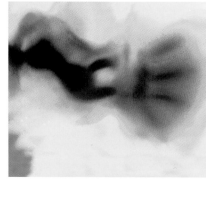

222 days to go...

YOUR BABY TODAY

The baby's hands (one of which is seen here) and feet are gradually developing and they are formed of cartilage, not bone, at this early stage. At right, the fused rays of the hand plate that will become the fingers can be seen.

Who will your baby look like? His unique facial features are beginning to take shape this week.

If you were to have an ultrasound scan this week, it would be possible to recognize several of your baby's facial features.

His eyelids fuse and will remain closed until around the 26th week. The lips have already formed and with the surrounding skin will have the greatest concentration of nerves. The muscular tongue arises from the base of your baby's mouth, but it will be two weeks before the first taste buds appear. The hard palate that forms the roof of the mouth arises from two "shelves" that start to grow, one each side, beneath the tongue; these shelves will lift upwards to join horizontally, allowing the tongue to drop down into the mouth. Once they have joined together, the septum of the nose grows downwards to meet them.

Your baby's tiny tooth buds are in place and this is critical to adequate jaw development. One branch of tooth buds will form the first milk teeth and a separate branch will eventually form the permanent teeth. The milk teeth develop slowly and it will not be until the sixth month of pregnancy that they acquire their hard enamel coating.

The embryo is still very curled up, with the head resting on the chest. Over the next two weeks, as the jaw and neck grow, the head will gradually lift.

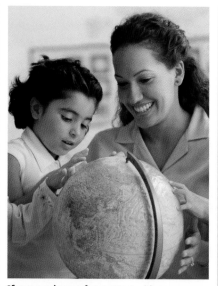

If you are in regular contact with young children while you're pregnant, it's even more important that you check your immunity to childhood illnesses.

CHILDHOOD ILLNESSES

Having immunity against common infectious illnesses will protect your unborn baby. You may have natural immunity from having conditions such as chickenpox and slapped cheek syndrome as a child. You will almost certainly have been vaccinated against mumps and measles, so your unborn baby will be protected from these.

If you are unsure about your immunity or medical history, or think you may have been in contact with any of these infections, contact your doctor or midwife immediately for further advice (see p.22). He or she will be able to do a checkup and provide reassurance.

ASK A... DOCTOR

I work for a dry cleaner. Could the chemicals harm my unborn baby?
Concerns about dry-cleaning chemicals stem from research showing that women who operated dry-cleaning machines had a higher risk of miscarriage. If touched or inhaled, some organic (carbon-containing) solvents used in dry-cleaning machines can pass through the placenta and some are thought to increase the risk of miscarriage or birth defects.

Talk to your employer to find out how your duties can be changed for the duration of your pregnancy to limit your contact with organic solvents and industrial chemicals.

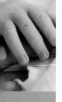

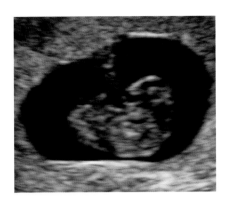

221 days to go...

YOUR BABY TODAY

In a matter of days, your baby's eyes have developed from slight ridges to clear depressions, on each side of the face. The face is developing rapidly at this stage, and your baby's heartbeat would be seen on an ultrasound scan.

It's a few weeks before the hormone responsible for nausea and vomiting subsides, but these will pass soon.

You may be wondering when you'll wake up and no longer feel sick. HCG (human chorionic gonadotrophin) levels, which may be responsible for feelings of nausea, will begin to fall in about three weeks' time and most women begin to feel better then. For some women the sickness may continue beyond this time.

You may have just started to feel nauseous or your sickness may have begun weeks ago and now be worse, but by around week 12 you should be over the worst. Nausea that happens daily, especially if it is associated with tiredness, can be very wearing so try to remember that it's temporary.

It's normal to have some morning sickness and you should be able to keep some foods and fluids down. However, for a small minority of pregnant women – about 1 per cent – the vomiting is severe, occurring regularly and lasting over a period of weeks. This more serious form of morning sickness is called hyperemesis gravidarum and can lead to dehydration. Hospital treatment with intravenous fluids and anti-sickness drugs may be required to rehydrate you.

Seek advice from your doctor if you're concerned about the amount of times you're vomiting or if you're struggling to keep fluids and food down.

FOCUS ON... HEALTH

Fit – not sick

If you're feeling particularly nauseous, try going for a brisk walk in the fresh air while concentrating on your breathing and posture. Sometimes taking frequent sips of water helps these feelings, and will allow you to exercise for longer. Regular exercisers may find that nausea is absent during exercise, although it may resume after the session.

Extreme nausea and vomiting can be a sign of over-exercising. Always drink water before, during, and after any physical activity.

ACUPRESSURE WRISTBANDS

A simple solution to help relieve feelings of nausea is to wear acupressure wristbands. Available from pharmacists, these bands have been clinically tested in the treatment of pregnancy-induced nausea. Unlike anti-nausea drugs, they don't give any side-effects and are easy to use.

The elasticated bands, one worn on each arm, work by applying pressure on the Nei Guan acupressure point (known as P6). They can be washed and reused as necessary.

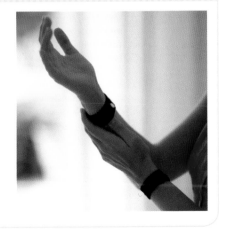

AS A MATTER OF FACT

About 70–80 per cent of pregnant women suffer from nausea and vomiting.

If you are one of the 20–30 per cent who don't, be thankful. You may get anxious if you're not feeling sick because it is such a common symptom, but don't worry and just count yourself lucky.

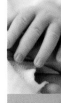

Your baby's life support system

The placenta links your baby's blood supply to your own and carries out all the functions that your baby can't perform for himself. The placenta is rooted to the lining of your uterus and linked to the baby by the umbilical cord.

HOW SUBSTANCES ARE EXCHANGED IN THE PLACENTA

Inside the placenta

The placenta contains a huge network of tiny projections called chorionic villi that branch out from a thin membrane, the chorion, and contain fetal blood vessels. The chorionic villi are bathed in maternal blood within the intervillous space. Each villus is only one or two cells thick, which allows the transfer of gases and nutrients between the mother and the baby, while ensuring that the two circulations never come into direct contact. Through the process of diffusion, oxygen and nutrients such as glucose, your baby's primary source of energy, pass from the mother into the fetal circulation, and waste products from the baby are picked up and carried away in the mother's bloodstream. The chorionic membrane also acts as a protective barrier, preventing many harmful substances and infections from reaching the baby.

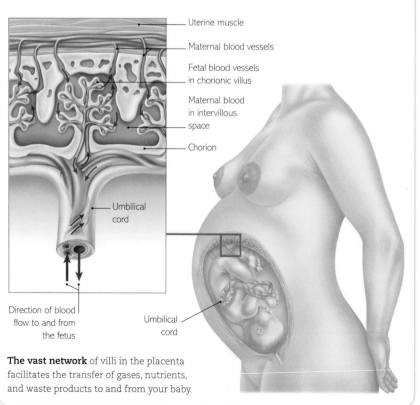

Uterine muscle

Maternal blood vessels

Fetal blood vessels in chorionic villus

Maternal blood in intervillous space

Chorion

Umbilical cord

Direction of blood flow to and from the fetus

Umbilical cord

The vast network of villi in the placenta facilitates the transfer of gases, nutrients, and waste products to and from your baby.

How the placenta develops

The placenta forms from cells in the embryo shortly after the egg implants in the lining of the uterus. Early placental growth is rapid, and at the beginning of the first trimester, the placenta is larger than the baby. However, the baby's growth catches up by 16 weeks, and by the end of pregnancy the baby is almost six times heavier. The final weight of the placenta is between 350g (12oz) and 700g (1.5lb). Once its structure is complete at the end of the first trimester, it takes on many important functions for the rest of the pregnancy (see opposite).

Growth after the first trimester The placenta grows throughout the second trimester. By the third trimester, growth slows, but placental efficiency continually improves as extra villi (through which substances are exchanged, see left) grow and increase the available surface area of the placenta by nearly fourfold. Cell layers also become thinner so that substances can be exchanged efficiently.

Placental blood flow is massive and many of the changes in your circulation are designed to meet its needs. By term, a 10-fold increase in placental blood supply results in a fifth of your circulation supplying the placenta with up to half a litre of blood (almost a pint) each minute.

The ageing placenta The placenta ages towards the end of pregnancy, especially after 40 weeks. However, at least 60–80 per cent of its function would need to be lost before there were any signs of problems with blood flow in the umbilical cord.

The role of the placenta

The placenta fulfils many essential roles that help sustain your pregnancy and enable your baby to grow and develop.

The exchange of substances The placenta transports substances to and from your baby, acting as your baby's lungs, kidneys, and digestive system.

To obtain oxygen, the baby's blood cells grab oxygen molecules from your own haemoglobin (the oxygen-carrying subtance in blood). Fetal haemoglobin has a modified structure that makes it bind readily to oxygen. Your baby requires twice as much oxygen, weight for weight, as you need, so the transfer of oxygen needs to be efficient. The placenta's enhanced blood supply, large surface area, and the characteristics of fetal haemoglobin all ensure the efficient transfer of oxygen from mother to baby.

As your haemoglobin gives up oxygen, it accepts carbon dioxide molecules. Your lungs breathe out air rich with the baby's carbon dioxide as well as your own and the cycle begins again.

To grow and develop your baby also needs amino acids, the building blocks for proteins, and minerals such as calcium and iron, and these all pass from your circulation via the placenta to the baby.

Protecting your baby The placenta protects your baby from infections and harmful substances. As your baby hasn't encountered any external threats he doesn't yet make protective antibodies, known as immunoglobulins, that can identify threats, such as viruses or bacteria. Instead, he is reliant on the transfer of immunoglobulins from your circulation via the placenta and into his circulation. This means that you are able to protect your baby in the uterus from illnesses such as chickenpox. After your baby is born, the immunglobulins he acquired from you will eventually be lost, which means that later as a child he becomes susceptible to chickenpox.

The umbilical cord

The umbilical cord, which connects your baby to the placenta, contains three vessels: two arteries, which carry blood from the baby to the placenta, and one vein, which carries blood to the baby. The blood in the arteries contains waste products, such as carbon dioxide, from the baby's metabolism. Carbon dioxide is transferred across the placenta to your bloodstream and then to your lungs, where it's breathed out. Oxygen is transported from red bloods cells in your circulation, across the placenta to the baby in the umbilical vein. As well as oxygen, the umbilical vein transports nutrients from the placenta to your baby.

The vessels in the umbilical cord have a protective coating called Wharton's jelly, and the cord is coiled like a spring so that the baby is free to move around. The coiling pattern of the cord has usually established itself by week nine and is usually in a counterclockwise direction. However, the cord can coil later, and sometimes isn't established until 20 weeks. The baby's movements seem to encourage the cord to coil.

The cord is usually attached to the centre of the placenta, although sometimes it's attached near the edge. Very occasionally, it divides into its separate vessels before finally entering the placenta. The cord is usually 1–2cm (less than 1in) in diameter and 60cm (23in) long, which is twice the length needed to ensure that there are no problems at delivery.

After delivery, the cord vessels close by themselves. The arteries close first, helped by their thicker muscular walls. This prevents blood loss from your baby to the placenta. The umbilical vein closes slightly later (starting at 15 seconds, but only completed by 3 or 4 minutes). This allows blood to continue to return to your baby during the first few minutes of life. As a result, many feel that a slight delay before clamping the cord can be beneficial to the baby. There are no nerves within the cord, so cutting the cord after delivery is a painless procedure for your baby.

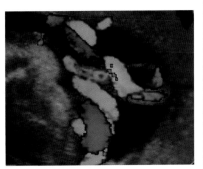

This Doppler scan shows the blood vessels in the umbilical cord. Blood flows through a single vein (blue) and two arteries (red).

Hormone production The placenta produces hormones, such as oestrogen and progesterone, that are vital to your baby's wellbeing and lead to many of the changes in your body during pregnancy.

Heat transfer A baby's high metabolic rate generates heat. The placenta's big surface area and high blood flow disperses heat, controlling the baby's temperature.

AS A MATTER OF FACT

Some harmful substances can cross the placenta.

For this reason, it's important that you protect your baby by taking medical advice before you use any type of medication during pregnancy.

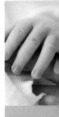

Your baby's life support system

113

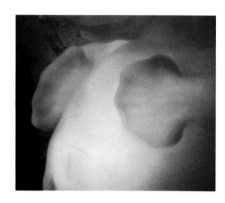

220 days to go...

YOUR BABY TODAY

In the upper limb buds, the flat expansion that will form the hand can be identified. The fingers are becoming more distinct and there will now be the first signs of movement at the elbows.

Your baby's bones are beginning to develop – and they will continue to lengthen from now until his teenage years.

FOCUS ON... NUTRITION

Good mood foods

If being pregnant gets you down at times, try a dietary boost. Happy, relaxed people tend to have high levels of serotonin, a brain chemical that is produced when you are consuming protein-rich foods. So eat meat (especially turkey), fish (see p.96), pulses, and well-cooked eggs (see p.17).

Eating foods that are rich in vitamin B, such as bananas and avocados, can also help to increase your serotonin levels.

You won't be aware of your developing baby's activities inside the uterus for some months yet, but the fact that his elbows are forming allows him to make some small movements; the wrists do not yet move.

Your baby is looking more human by the day. His vertebrae and ribs are now in place, and his fingers are gradually lengthening. His body is less curled up than it was a few weeks ago.

The skeleton will gradually calcify and harden. With the exception of the cranial skull bones, all your baby's bones have a soft cartilage core that will later be reabsorbed as it is converted into hard bone. This process of hardening, known as ossification, starts in so-called primary ossification centres during the next five weeks of your pregnancy. Within these primary centres, specialized cells form spongy then hard bone as calcium salts are laid down. Within the hard bone is red bone marrow, which in later weeks will become the main producer of the baby's red blood cells.

Secondary ossification centres develop in the second trimester at the ends of each of your baby's bones.

The portion of bone between the hardening primary and secondary centres is known as the growth plate. This plate is responsible for the continued lengthening of your unborn baby's bones.

MORE CHEESE PLEASE

Tired of being told what you can't eat? It is a common myth that eating cheese harms the unborn baby. Only blue cheeses and those with a mould-ripened crust, such as brie, chèvre, and camembert, are potentially dangerous because they increase the risk of listeria (a rare bacterium that can attack the baby, see p.17).

All other types of cheese pose no danger and are regarded as a good source of calcium.

So, while there are some cheeses you should avoid eating, you can enjoy all of the following:
- Hard cheese, such as Cheddar and parmesan
- Feta
- Ricotta
- Mascarpone
- Cream cheese
- Mozzarella
- Cottage cheese
- Processed cheese, such as spreads.

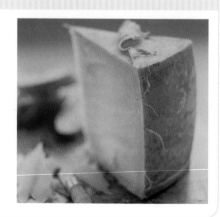

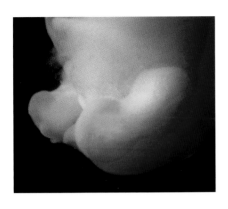

219 days to go...

YOUR BABY TODAY

The development of the baby's lower limbs always lags slightly behind that of the upper limbs. At this stage, the toes are not distinct and the legs are not yet bending at the knee.

It's understandable that your pregnancy will be on your mind. Try to find ways to communicate this to your partner.

At a time when you want to feel close to your partner, you may find that your relationship is changing, and it may be quite fraught with issues. Often men say that their pregnant partners are more sensitive or now react to things differently and that this can be difficult for them to handle.

Your relationship will inevitably change – going through pregnancy together is momentous – but so long as you keep communicating, you will be able to support each other. Being united now will stand you in good stead for the first year of parenting.

During the early stages of pregnancy, your partner may find it hard to relate to the fact that you're expecting a baby; the physical changes to your body won't be that visible at this stage and he is yet to see his baby on a scan. Conversely, you will be very aware of the pregnancy as you'll be undergoing many physical and emotional changes.

Your partner may need more time than you to adjust to the idea of becoming a parent. He may be concerned about practical issues, such as the changes to your lifestyle and the financial implications of having a baby. Talking openly to each other can help to ease anxieties for you both. Remember, that although many changes are happening to your body, your partner does have feelings and this is a big life change for him, too. If you've told your family and close friends about the pregnancy, all the attention may be on you. Your partner may be feeling left out and this is something that often gets worse as the pregnancy progresses and after the baby arrives.

Take time to find out your partner's concerns and look for ways to involve him more in the pregnancy, if that's what he wants. If you have a good support network of friends, encourage him to spend time with male friends who have been through the expectant dad experience.

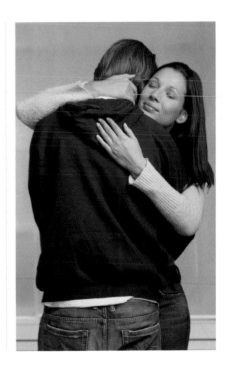

Support each other as you both go through the different emotions attached to becoming parents. Don't lose sight of your relationship and be understanding of each other's needs.

ASK A... MUM

I'm worried we won't have space in our small flat, but is a house move advisable while I'm pregnant? It's not advisable to deal with those sorts of pressures while you're pregnant. We started the process but thankfully it fell through, as it was proving quite stressful. We stayed in our flat until our baby was one and it was fine.

Remember that small babies have very few needs, other than being fed, loved, changed, and stimulated, and much of the paraphernalia that you think you need is unnecessary. If you have room for a cot, a buggy, a drawer for your baby's clothes, and a corner for toys, you'll be fine in a small space for the time being.

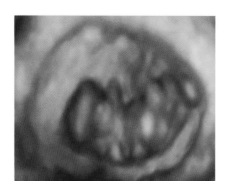

218 days to go...

YOUR BABY TODAY

This 3D ultrasound scan shows a baby lying on its back, in exactly the same orientation as the image opposite. It is just possible to pick up the limb buds on an ultrasound scan taken at this stage.

You don't have long to go until you have your booking-in antenatal appointment and will meet one of your midwives.

In a couple of weeks' time, you will have your booking-in appointment (see p.122–3) with the midwife. If you haven't been given a date for this yet, contact your doctor now to arrange it. You will be given a choice of hospitals. Before making a decision, chat to women you know locally who have had their babies at those hospitals to find out about their experiences. For example, some hospitals may have a birth centre attached, and have a less medically managed approach to childbirth.

Start thinking now about the kind of questions you want to ask your midwife. It's worth writing these down. Also make a note, in advance, of the key details of your medical history and any pregnancy symptoms.

TACKLING COLDS

Cold remedies contain a variety of ingredients, including antihistamines, that are best avoided in pregnancy. Check the label and talk to your doctor or pharmacist before taking any.

Try natural remedies, such as steam inhalations, before resorting to medicines, or take paracetamol at the lowest effective dose for the shortest possible time.

ASK A... PANEL ABOUT HOME BIRTH

It's my first pregnancy. Can I have a home birth?

Midwife: if you're in good health with no complications, giving birth at home is an option. Many women enjoy the experience of giving birth at home, and there is less likely to be unnecessary medical intervention, which can sometimes result in complications. Labour also appears to progress more rapidly and steadily, without the interruption of being transported to hospital.

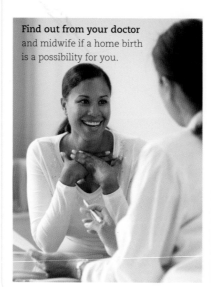

Find out from your doctor and midwife if a home birth is a possibility for you.

Obstetrician: there is no problem with this in general, but take advice from your doctor and midwife. You should avoid taking risks. If there is a history of long or complicated labours in your family, your baby is breech or very small, there are issues about the location of the cord or the placenta, you are very overweight or unfit, or you suffer from conditions such as diabetes, it might be worth erring on the side of caution. If you have your baby in a hospital, quick and early intervention can take place if needed. You do have a right to have a home birth; however, it is sensible to listen to the experts. Delivery of a healthy baby is the most important thing.

Mum: I had my first baby at home, and it was wonderful. I was nervous about what might go wrong, but my midwife reassured me that she would be monitoring me, and would get me to hospital if there was a problem. She also explained I could change my mind if I didn't think things were going well, and go into hospital for the birth (and an epidural!).

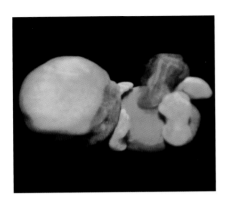

217 days to go...

YOUR BABY TODAY

The baby's hands can be clearly seen here but the fingers are still fused at this stage. The fingers will be completely separate in just one week's time and wrist movement is just about to begin.

By the end of this ninth week, your baby's digestive system is rapidly developing but won't function properly for some time.

Your baby is developing apace inside the uterus. The simple tube forming his gut has undergone most changes at the upper end. Now the lower part dilates as the single tube then divides into what will become the rectum at the back and then the bladder and urethra at the front.

Although the mouth is open to the amniotic fluid, there is still a membrane in place, which will disappear in one to two weeks' time. The lower bowel is not yet mature and does not move material along its length.

The remainder of the large bowel and small bowel is still lengthening. The duodenum is the first part of the small bowel and it is still a solid tube. The pancreas, gall bladder, and liver have formed as buds leading off from the upper small bowel, but none are yet contributing any digestive function.

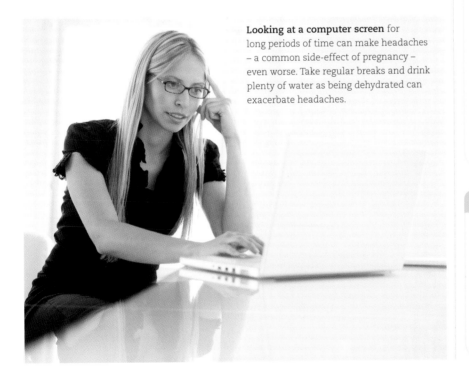

Looking at a computer screen for long periods of time can make headaches – a common side-effect of pregnancy – even worse. Take regular breaks and drink plenty of water as being dehydrated can exacerbate headaches.

ASK A... DOCTOR

Since I've been pregnant, I've had terrible headaches. Could computer work be the cause?
Tension headaches and migraines are common in pregnancy, probably due to fluctuating hormones, and it is not uncommon to have severe headaches with prolonged computer use. This could be due to eye strain and the fact that you are immobile, which can cause tension.

Take even more breaks from your computer screen now that you're pregnant. You'll probably find you need more toilet breaks anyway. If this doesn't help, ask if you can do tasks that don't require computer use for a short time. Headaches are often worse in the first trimester.

ACTUAL SIZE OF YOUR BABY

At 9 weeks your baby's crown to rump length is 2.3cm.

7 weeks

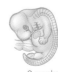

8 weeks

9 weeks

Your 9th week

117

Your 10th week

YOUR BABY'S MAJOR ORGANS ARE IN PLACE, BUT NOT WORKING YET

This is your baby's last week as an embryo; next week she'll be known as a fetus. Her major organs are in place, although by no means in full working order. There's a long way to go yet and her body systems will continue to mature for the rest of pregnancy, and beyond. The most noticeable difference to your body will be in your breasts. You may well have gone up a cup size – or more.

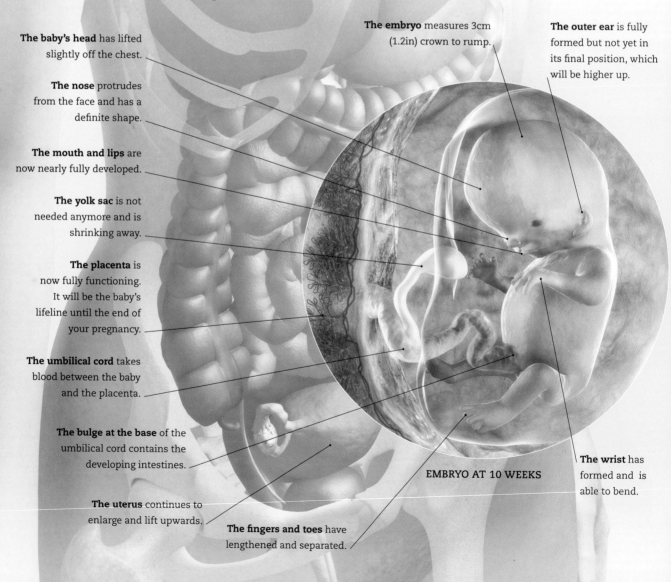

The baby's head has lifted slightly off the chest.

The nose protrudes from the face and has a definite shape.

The mouth and lips are now nearly fully developed.

The yolk sac is not needed anymore and is shrinking away.

The placenta is now fully functioning. It will be the baby's lifeline until the end of your pregnancy.

The umbilical cord takes blood between the baby and the placenta.

The bulge at the base of the umbilical cord contains the developing intestines.

The uterus continues to enlarge and lift upwards.

The embryo measures 3cm (1.2in) crown to rump.

The outer ear is fully formed but not yet in its final position, which will be higher up.

The wrist has formed and is able to bend.

EMBRYO AT 10 WEEKS

The fingers and toes have lengthened and separated.

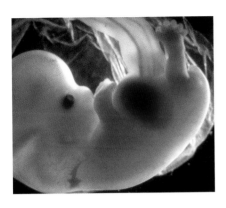

216 days to go...

YOUR BABY TODAY

Most of your baby's primitive organ systems are in place. The arms and legs have formed, complete with wrists and elbows, and have tiny fingers and toes; the retina of the eye, and the nose, can be seen. The large dark mass is the enlarged liver.

Your baby's welfare will be your main concern, but be reassured that, however you're feeling, she'll be getting sustenance.

You may be very conscious of your health and wellbeing at this time, but be reassured that even if you've felt unwell during this first trimester, your baby will have been taking what she needs from you: you have internal stores of various minerals and substances, such as iron, and will still be absorbing some nutrients from what you eat. However, if you're concerned about the amount of vitamins and minerals you're consuming through your diet, for the sake of your own health you could take an antenatal vitamin supplement. Remember, you should still be taking folic acid supplements and eating folate-rich foods (see p.35).

There is no cause for concern if you do not put on any weight in the first trimester, or even if you lose a bit of weight. The majority of weight gain takes place in the second and third trimesters (see p.99). However, if you're vomiting a lot and struggling to keep food down (see p.111), don't hesitate to see your doctor.

FOCUS ON... YOUR BODY

Your changing breasts

The changes you will be noticing to your breasts are caused by both an increased blood supply and a rise in pregnancy hormones, particularly in the first 12 weeks.

Before your pregnancy was confirmed you may have felt tingling sensations (especially in the nipple area) as the blood supply increased.

■ **As early as 6–8 weeks,** your breasts will have become larger and more tender and may have begun to look different on the surface, with threadlike veins starting to appear.

■ **At around 8–12 weeks,** the nipples darken and can become more erect.

■ **As early as the 16th week** of pregnancy, colostrum, the first milk, may leak from your breasts.

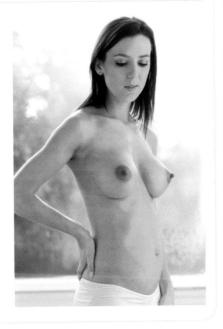

THE LOWDOWN

He's "pregnant" too

Can your partner ever really understand what you're going through? According to a recent UK study, some dads don't need a fake bump to empathize. Known as Couvade syndrome, symptoms experienced by expectant fathers ranged from morning sickness to backache, mood swings, and food cravings. Although, interestingly, often it was the woman claiming her partner had these symptoms.

Couvade is thought to happen because men are so deeply involved in the pregnancy, although some believe it could be jealousy (you're getting all the attention) or guilt that he's responsible for your condition and therefore your symptoms.

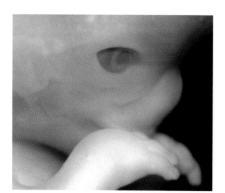

215 days to go...

YOUR BABY TODAY

The baby now begins to bend her wrists. The natural position is for the limbs to be slightly bent at all joints, especially in the early stages. There is a more distinct neck area as the baby's head is now slightly lifted off the chest.

The muscular diaphragm that will eventually enable your baby to breathe – and hiccup – is developing now.

As your baby's lungs develop in the chest, there is nothing to separate them from the stomach, liver, and bowel, in what will later become her abdominal cavity.

In adults, the chest is separated from the abdomen by the muscular diaphragm. The diaphragm moves downwards when we breathe, and the ribs expand outwards. This process allows air to enter the lungs.

Your baby's diaphragm forms from four in-folds of tissue. First seen at around this week of pregnancy, these folds gradually expand inwards, fusing together and closing the space by the end of this week.

In the centre of the diaphragm there are openings for the oesophagus to travel to the stomach, the aorta (the body's main artery), and the inferior vena cava (the body's main vein returning blood from the lower body). As pregnancy progresses, muscle fibres gradually strengthen your baby's diaphragm, which later allows her to make breathing movements.

The nuchal translucency scan is a screening test (see p.143). It measures the depth of fluid under the skin in the nuchal fold at the back of the baby's neck to assess how much fluid is present there. Excess fluid may indicate Down's syndrome. Nuchal translucency is the most accurate way to screen for Down's.

FOCUS ON... TWINS

Twin tests

If you're expecting twins or more, blood-based screening tests for Down's can mislead, as they rely on measuring the amounts of circulating AFP (alfa-fetoprotein) and other markers, which are present in much higher levels when there's more than one baby. That's why the most reliable screening test is the nuchal translucency scan at 11–14 weeks (see right and p.143).

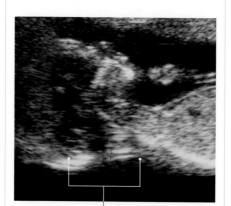

Red area shows the fluid under the skin at the back of the baby's neck

TIME TO THINK ABOUT

Screening and diagnostic tests

It's useful to be aware of the screening tests (see pp.142–3) and diagnostic tests (see pp.152–3) that will be on offer in the weeks to come. Your doctor or midwife will talk through the pros and cons of having each test. Some abnormalities may be detected at the 20-week scan.

■ **Screening tests:** these tests identify the "risk factor" for a particular condition, but do not confirm that your baby definitely has a condition. For example, a screening test for Down's syndrome may give your baby a risk factor of 1:200. This means that your baby has a 1 in 200 chance of being affected by Down's syndrome, but it does not mean that he actually has the condition.

■ **Diagnostic tests:** if screening tests reveal your baby has a high risk factor for a chromosomal abnormality, you will be offered a diagnostic test, such as amniocentesis or chorionic villus sampling, which gives a definite result as to whether or not a condition is present.

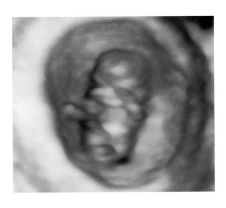

214 days to go...

YOUR BABY TODAY

The shoulders, elbows, and wrists are flexed leaving the hands in front of the face. It's far too early to be aware of them but several fetal movements will start to become apparent on an ultrasound scan at this stage.

You don't need to shop for a maternity wardrobe just yet, but it might be time to purchase some bigger bras.

If your normal bras are starting to feel a little uncomfortable, it's time to go for a fitting. If you have not done so already, get yourself measured professionally. Wearing a good and supportive bra during pregnancy is essential to prevent backache and sagging breasts.

Whenever you feel you need a new bra, get measured properly to ensure that you're wearing the right size. Although your breasts may be growing very quickly at this time, you should find that by the end of the first trimester the growth has stabilized. There is then unlikely to be much further breast growth until you're in your third trimester and after the baby is born.

Wearing underwired bras during pregnancy is not recommended as they can dig into the developing breast tissue and damage it, and may even cause problems with milk production; the wires digging into the skin can also be uncomfortable. Non-underwired bras with wide supportive straps, such as sports bras, are good in pregnancy.

Look for maternity bras that unhook at the front and double-up as nursing bras for after the birth. There are some very pretty and feminine styles available.

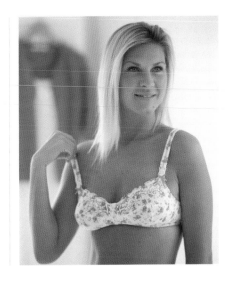

AS A MATTER OF FACT

Pica means craving inedible substances and comes from the Latin for magpie, a bird that scavenges indiscriminately.

If you like crunching coal or sniffing your hot-water bottle, you have pica. While licking the toothpaste is fairly harmless, you should resist eating toxic items such as chalk, glue, and soap. Pica could be a sign that your diet is deficient in some way, so seek advice. Taking an iron or vitamin supplement could help.

FOCUS ON... NUTRITION

Vegan needs

If you are a vegan and pregnant, you may have to work a little harder than most women to get the right nutrients. You need to make sure you obtain adequate vitamin B12 and as there are no natural sources of this, it needs to be obtained from fortified foods such as:
- Yeast extracts
- Vegetable stock
- Veggie burgers
- Textured vegetable protein.

You also need zinc. This is an important nutrient in pregnancy, necessary for growth, energy, and supporting the immune system. Zinc can be found in the following foods:
- Beans
- Pulses
- Nuts
- Seeds – pumpkin seeds are a particularly rich source.

Like most vegans, you probably already eat many of these foods.

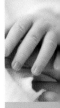

Your booking-in visit

Your antenatal "booking-in" appointment usually takes place between 8 and 10 weeks. At this visit, your antenatal notes will be compiled and you will have a chance to discuss any concerns or issues with your midwife.

At your booking-in visit, you will meet one of the midwives who will be handling your care. She will ask you questions about your past and present health, and about medical conditions in your family. You will also have blood and urine tests. Your due date will be estimated based on the date of your last menstrual period (see p.35).

Medical history

The midwife will take a full medical history to check if there are any health problems, which will help her to identify your pregnancy as high or low risk. If there is a problem, she will explain how this could affect your pregnancy.

If you have an existing condition, she'll discuss how your pregnancy may affect your health and whether or not your treatment needs to change. Inform the midwife of any medications you're taking; certain ones, such as some of those for high blood pressure, may need to be changed (see Illnesses and medications, pp.20–1).

You will also be asked possibly embarrassing, but important, questions about sexually transmitted diseases, past drug use, and terminations. It's important that you reveal your history so that your midwife can identify and prevent potential problems. If your partner is unaware of a past event and

you feel sensitive about this, arrange to tell the midwife when he isn't present and for the information not to be documented in your hand-held notes.

Family history

The midwife will ask about any health problems in your own and your partner's family. Some conditions can be passed on, and testing may be available to identify if your baby is affected.

Height and weight

A baseline height and weight measurement will be taken to calculate your body mass index (BMI) (see p.17). A low or high BMI increases the risk of complications and your midwife or doctor may monitor your weight gain.

Blood pressure

A baseline blood pressure measurement will be taken at your first visit. Blood pressure usually goes down at the start of pregnancy, rises around week 26, and by the 32nd week returns to its original pre-pregnancy value. So, if your initial blood pressure measurements are in the normal-to-high range, they are likely to rise to above normal during the third trimester and possibly need treatment.

Routine blood tests

You will be asked to provide a sample of your blood, which will be tested to screen for several conditions and to determine your blood group and immunity to certain infections.

Full blood count This is a screen for anaemia, which can be due to low levels of iron, folic acid, or vitamin B12. If

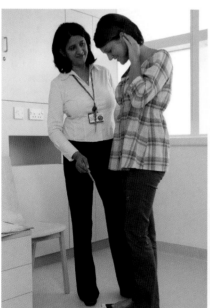
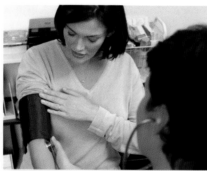
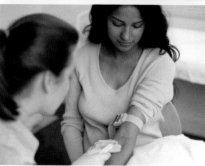

A baseline weight measurement is taken at your booking-in visit (left). **Your blood pressure** will be recorded at each of your appointments and any changes will be investigated (top right). **A blood sample** identifies your blood group and tests for a range of conditions (bottom right).

you're anaemic, you'll be advised to eat iron-rich foods (see p.18) and may need an iron supplement.

Blood group This determines your blood group (A, B, O, or AB) and whether you're rhesus positive (Rh+) or rhesus negative (Rh-) (see p.127). If you're Rh- and your baby is Rh+ you could develop antibodies against your baby's blood that cause anaemia in your baby. Your immune system is unlikely to come into contact with your baby's until labour so this isn't usually a problem with first pregnancies. To prevent problems in subsequent pregnancies, Rh- women are routinely given anti-D medication at 28 weeks and sometimes, too, at 34 weeks to stop antibodies forming. In addition, anti-D is given after any procedure such as amniocentesis (see p.153), or if you have vaginal bleeding.

Rubella This blood test checks your immunity to rubella. Rubella infection in pregnancy can cause serious problems for the baby. If you aren't immune, you can't be vaccinated in pregnancy, but will usually be vaccinated after delivery so you're protected in future pregnancies.

Hepatitis B This test identifies women who are actively infected with hepatitis B, a viral liver disease that can be passed to the baby during pregnancy and labour.

Syphilis The blood test checks if you have ever had syphilis. Active syphilis can cross the placenta and cause serious complications in your baby.

HIV You will be offered a test for human immunodeficiency virus (HIV). If you have HIV, you can reduce the chances of passing this on to your baby by taking anti-viral agents and not breastfeeding.

Sickle cell disease or thalassaemia You are tested to see if you are a carrier of sickle cell disease or thalassaemia, genetic disorders that affect the oxygen-carrying ability of red blood cells. These are most common in people of African, Hispanic, or Mediterranean origins. If you're found to be a carrier, your partner will need to be tested; if he, too, is a carrier there is a chance that your baby could develop the disease. In this situation, you will be offered counselling and the chance of an antenatal diagnosis.

Routine urine tests

Your urine is checked for protein, which may indicate infection or, less commonly, kidney disease. If protein is found, a urine sample is sent to the laboratory for culture to look for bacteria. Around 15 per cent of women have bacteria, but no signs of a urinary tract infection. If bacteria are found, you may need antibiotics to stop kidney infection, which is more common in pregnancy and can cause complications. If no infection is found, further tests will check your kidney function. Later in pregnancy, protein in the urine is a sign of pre-eclampsia (see p.474).

Getting your results

If all is well, you'll be given the blood test results at your next appointment. If there is any concern, the doctor or midwife will contact you earlier to discuss the results.

ADDITIONAL TESTS

Extra screening

Some additional tests may be offered depending on the clinic and your individual circumstances.

■ **Cervical cultures** As both chlamydia and gonorrhoea can be symptom-free, it's worth getting tested if you think you're at risk, as these can cause problems if passed on to your baby.

■ **Hepatitis C** You may be offered screening for this condition if your history puts you at a higher risk.

■ **Varicella** If you're unsure whether you've had chickenpox (varicella), a test can confirm whether you have immunity. If you're not immune and are exposed to the infection during pregnancy, treatment can prevent severe chickenpox in pregnancy.

■ **Toxoplasmosis** This identifies whether you've ever been infected with toxoplasmosis (see pp.17 and 101). Past infection protects you from infection in pregnancy, which could harm your baby.

FUTURE ANTENATAL CARE

What is coming up

If your pregnancy is low risk, you will have around 10 antenatal appointments for a first pregnancy and around seven for second and subsequent pregnancies. After the first contact visit and booking-in appointment, your next antenatal visit will be at around 16 weeks.

At each appointment, your midwife or doctor will carry out routine checks to assess your health and the wellbeing of your baby. These checks include taking your blood pressure and checking your urine for protein, the presence of which could indicate an infection that needs to be treated or, later in pregnancy, pre-eclampsia (see p.474). You won't be weighed regularly unless there are particular concerns that you're putting on too much or too little weight.

After around 16 weeks, the midwife will start to listen to your baby's heartbeat with an instrument known as a handheld sonic aid. From around 25 weeks, she will measure your abdomen to monitor the growth of your baby (see p.284).

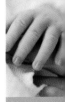

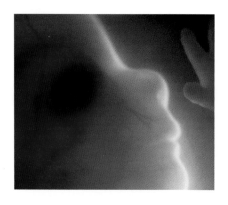

YOU ARE 9 WEEKS AND 4 DAYS

213 days to go...

YOUR BABY TODAY

The baby's facial features are becoming more distinctive by this stage. The very fine eyelids have now completely fused over the developing eye and will remain closed until approximately the 26th week of pregnancy.

Just as you get used to the idea that you're pregnant, you may discover that you're carrying more than one baby.

Do you have an instinct that you're having twins? Some women, even very early in pregnancy, suspect they're carrying more than one baby simply because they feel "more pregnant". Signs of a multiple pregnancy include highly sensitive breasts, and extreme nausea and vomiting and tiredness. In a multiple pregnancy, your uterus might also be larger than expected. Your doctor or midwife may be able to feel it rising into your lower belly from this week, instead of from 12 weeks as in a singleton pregnancy.

Whether or not you suspect anything, the first ultrasound scan (see p.138) will show definitely if you are carrying more than one baby.

(see p.138)

FOCUS ON... TWINS

The shocking news

The news that you're having two or more babies may not always be delivered with the greatest tact. For instance, the sonographer may look at the scan and say that "something needs checking". This sounds worrying, of course, but remember, he or she is only being cautious before giving you the life-changing news. The sonographer may also be checking your twins for size, to rule out any major problems. Once this is done, however, there are likely to be hearty congratulations.

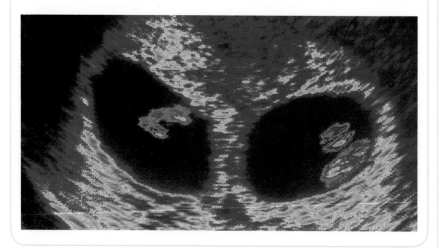

ASK A... MUM

I'm delighted we're having twins but how will I cope? I felt the same when I was expecting and had so many worries – "Will I be able to breastfeed two babies? How many nappies will I need?" At first, your head is likely to be spinning with these thoughts, as you get used to the idea of your twin pregnancy.

To give yourself time to come to terms with the news, you may prefer to keep it to yourselves for a few weeks. What you'll find is that family and friends react differently. Responses can range from pure joy (usually from thrilled grandparents) to envy or a bit of scaremongering (from friends and strangers).

We found it helpful to talk to others who were expecting twins or who were already parents to twins. Contact Tamba (see p.480) or your local twins support group, or look online for chatrooms.

(see p.480)

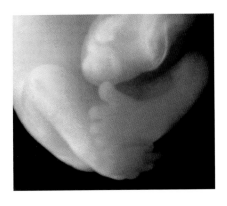

212 days to go...

YOUR BABY TODAY

The lower limbs are now held flexed at the hip and knee joints, and the legs may be crossed. The separate toes can be distinguished. Further growth of the thigh and shin bones will bring the foot length into proportion with the rest of the leg.

One of the downsides of pregnancy is being at greater risk of urinary infections, so you need to be aware of the signs.

It's important to be on the lookout for any signs of a urinary infection while you're pregnant. Although it's not very serious, and can be easily treated, it's a complication you can do without.

An infection may cause you to urinate more frequently, but this is also a symptom of early pregnancy so can be hard to spot. If, however, you also have stinging or discomfort when you actually pass urine, lower abdominal pain, or even blood in the urine, you may have developed a urinary infection. These infections are very common in women in general, because the urethra (tube that carries urine from the bladder to the outside) is very near the anus and so bacteria do not have far to travel to create an infection.

In pregnancy, there are high levels of the hormone progesterone; this relaxes the tubes of the urinary system making it even easier for bacteria to enter and infect the bladder or even the kidneys. It is very important if you have the symptoms of a urinary infection that your doctor tests your urine. In general, urinary tract infections are easily treatable in pregnancy. If there is an infection, you will be prescribed antibiotics that are safe to take (see p.23). The infection must be treated because, if left, it may cause damage to your kidneys.

FIGHTING FIT

If you were a regular exerciser before becoming pregnant, it is important to continue with some form of exercise. Stopping altogether, just because you're pregnant, would be a shock to your fit body.

There are some contraindications to exercising (see p.18), but if you have clearance from your doctor, take the following steps to ensure that you are continuing to exercise safely and effectively, and getting all the benefits from your programme without putting you or your baby at risk.

■ **Continue with activities,** such as running, cycling, and swimming, as long as you feel comfortable.

■ **Listen to your body** very carefully – look for signs that you should slow down or take a break.

■ **Take adequate rest** between workouts, and drink water before, during, and after all forms of exercise.

■ **Exercise at a moderate level** – you should be able to do the talk test (see p.161).

■ **Stick to low-impact** and low-risk activities (avoid sports that involve contact and the risk of falling).

■ **Wear the right clothing:** cotton will enable your body to dissipate heat, and a supportive sports bra is vital for your growing breasts, especially if you're running.

If you're used to cycling, continue to do so in early pregnancy. As you get bigger in later pregnancy, your changed centre of gravity might make it precarious.

Your 10th week

125

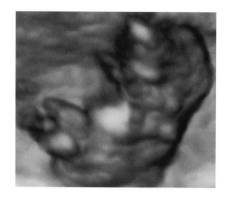

211 days to go...

YOUR BABY TODAY

The umbilical cord widens where it enters the baby's abdomen. This bulge is necessary to accommodate the bowel that is forming underneath at this stage of development. The bones of the head are not yet fully formed.

Your baby's organ systems are now present, in a basic form, marking the end of a major stage in development.

The embryonic period of development is complete tomorrow, and the fetal period will then begin. The development of the embryo has been characterized by three cell lines, each developing into its own types of tissues and organs, as it grew from a flat disc of cells into a human shape. Many of the changes have taken place concurrently, but it has been the heart, circulation, and nervous systems that developed initially with the development of the gut, limbs, and face following on.

During next week (your 11th week), your baby's kidneys and genital system will undergo their most rapid development. All your baby's organs need to mature fully, and many of them, such as the brain, lungs, and kidneys, will continue to mature throughout the pregnancy and after the birth.

Next week too, your baby's facial features will become more recognizable. The ears will take on their final shape, but they will not yet have moved to their final position.

The eyes, which began on the side of the face, start to move more centrally. The nose is visible, and the head achieves a more rounded contour.

FOCUS ON... NUTRITION

Veggie mum-to-be

A vegetarian diet can be safe and healthy in pregnancy. Lacto-ovo vegetarians, those who consume dairy products, usually have no trouble getting enough nutrients, though they should be careful to eat a varied diet rich in whole grains, beans, pulses, fruit, and vegetables, in order to obtain the proper mix of amino acids, vitamins, and minerals.

Vegetarians also need to obtain enough protein as vegetarian sources tend to be lower in protein than animal sources. An intake of 60g (2oz) of protein is needed daily in pregnancy, which means that vegetarians usually need to include a protein source in all three meals, and also eat a protein-containing snack.

In addition, vegetarians need to make sure that they obtain all 23 essential amino acids. Vegetarian proteins don't usually have all of these in any one source, but eating a variety of protein types at several meals will usually do the trick. It is not necessary for each meal to contain all 23, since the body can store them over several meals. If you're vegan, see p.121.

AS A MATTER OF FACT

A new non-invasive test to spot chromosomal disorders could soon be available.

This could simply require a sample of blood from the pregnant woman, unlike current tests that require a needle to be inserted into the uterus.

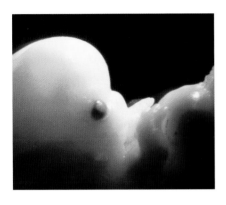

210 days to go...

YOUR BABY TODAY

The bones of the front of the skull are starting to grow over the baby's forehead and harden from cartilage to bone. The forehead is still very prominent and the top of the head still very flexible to accommodate the baby's rapidly developing brain.

The placenta is now fully formed and mature enough to start supplying all your baby's needs, although it will continue to grow.

FOCUS ON... NUTRITION

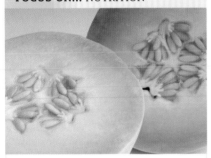

Refreshing melons

Staying hydrated is essential throughout pregnancy. A good tip is to eat fruit that is high in water. Water contained in fruit is easily absorbed into the body, because fruit contains natural sugars that draw water into the bloodstream. Melons – watermelon, cantaloupe, and honeydew – are naturally high in water. In addition, their mellow and less acidic nature makes them well tolerated in pregnancy.

In addition to helping you stay hydrated, melons supply you with extra folate, as well as other vitamins and nutrients. Try combining melons with cottage cheese or yogurt, sprinkled with granola, for a light meal, or blend them into a nutritious smoothie.

This is a milestone in your baby's development as the placenta takes over from the yolk sac to provide your baby with nutrients. Just like your baby, the placenta has needed to grow and develop a circulation to support the ever-increasing demands that are being placed on it.

One week after fertilization, the placenta formed a distinct inner and outer layer of cells that gradually

ASK A... DOCTOR

What is meant by rhesus negative? Red blood carries a positive or negative rhesus factor (Rh-factor). Problems arise if an Rh-negative woman carries an Rh-positive baby who has inherited the Rh-positive status from the father. If the mother's blood comes into contact with the baby's during delivery, she may produce antibodies against it.

This may cause problems in subsequent pregnancies when a mother's antibodies attack the cells of another Rh-positive baby, which can lead to severe anaemia and heart failure in the baby after the birth. You will be given injections to combat this.

penetrated the lining of the uterus, with finger-like fronds. You may have noticed a very slight bleed at this implantation stage (see p.67). More and more fronds spread out into the lining of the uterus, which itself undergoes a transformation process that enables each frond or villus to be bathed by small pools of maternal blood, enabling oxygen and nutrient transfer to take place.

Up until now, this blood flow has been limited by plugs of tissue, but at this stage of pregnancy these plugs begin to disappear. This means the placenta is sufficiently developed to withstand the pressure of maternal blood on each delicate villous. Villi will continue to branch out until around 30 weeks of pregnancy.

ACTUAL SIZE OF YOUR BABY

After 10 weeks your baby's crown to rump length is 3cm (1.2in).

9 weeks

10 weeks

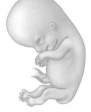

Your 11th week

YOU'LL NOW BE SETTING UP THE HEALTHCARE THAT WILL SUPPORT YOU OVER THE COMING MONTHS

Your baby is now unmistakeably human and is undergoing many sophisticated changes, such as development of the sense organs. To mark his new status, he's now called a fetus. If pregnancy hasn't seemed quite real to you so far, it soon will. It's time to get down to such practicalities as your first antenatal check. Procedures such as ultrasound scans and blood tests are about to become part of your normal pregnancy routine.

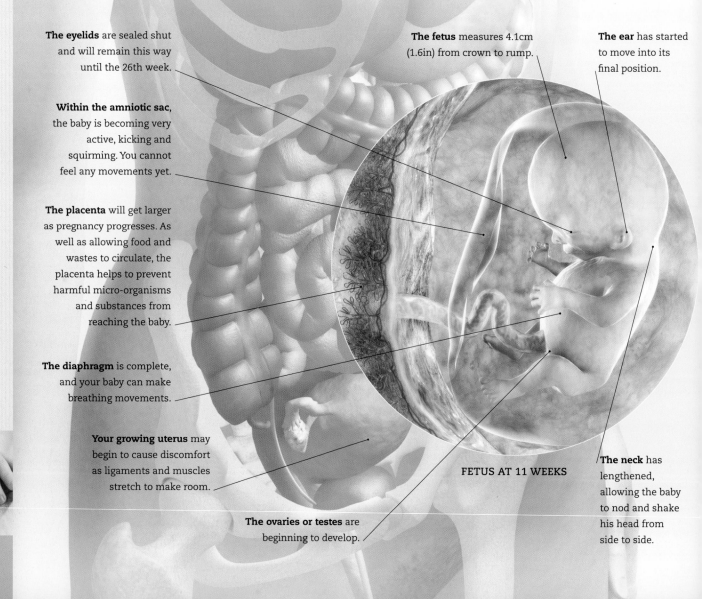

The eyelids are sealed shut and will remain this way until the 26th week.

Within the amniotic sac, the baby is becoming very active, kicking and squirming. You cannot feel any movements yet.

The placenta will get larger as pregnancy progresses. As well as allowing food and wastes to circulate, the placenta helps to prevent harmful micro-organisms and substances from reaching the baby.

The diaphragm is complete, and your baby can make breathing movements.

Your growing uterus may begin to cause discomfort as ligaments and muscles stretch to make room.

The fetus measures 4.1cm (1.6in) from crown to rump.

The ear has started to move into its final position.

FETUS AT 11 WEEKS

The neck has lengthened, allowing the baby to nod and shake his head from side to side.

The ovaries or testes are beginning to develop.

Your first trimester

128

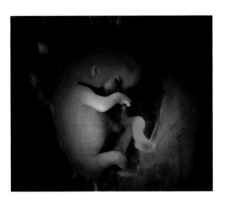

209 days to go...

YOUR BABY TODAY

In this side view of a fetus, the right ear and eye are just visible and the right hand and leg can be seen in characteristiclally bent positions. The reddish, tube-like structure, to the right of the image, is the umbilical cord.

A midwife starts to compile your pregnancy notes at your booking-in appointment, your most comprehensive visit with her.

You should have your booking-in appointment around now (see pp.122–3), and will meet one of the midwives who will be handling your care. The exact timing of this appointment will vary depending on where your antenatal care is taking place. Unless you have opted for an independent midwife (see pp.91 and 102), your antenatal team is likely to consist of several midwives and doctors who will look after you throughout pregnancy.

The purpose of this appointment is for a midwife to obtain your medical history, provide information, advise you on diet and exercise, and plan your care. It's also a chance for you to ask any questions you may have and discuss the schedule for appointments, blood tests, scans, and antenatal classes. You will be given booklets, information leaflets, and important contact telephone numbers.

The midwife will ask you about your medical history; your family's medical history; your partner and your partner's family's medical history; about any previous pregnancies you have had; and how this pregnancy has been so far.

Your answers will help the midwife identify factors that may affect your pregnancy – if there is a family history of pre-eclampsia (see p.474), for example. The midwife will also do some health checks, such as urine tests, at this and other antenatal appointments.

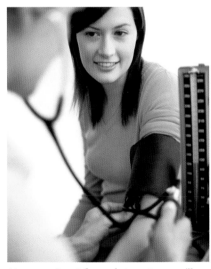

At your antenatal appointments you will undergo routine checks, including having your blood pressure taken. It's the midwife's job to look after your health throughout pregnancy.

ASK A... MIDWIFE

How should I decide which tests I want? Your midwife will give you lots of information regarding tests and it is up to you to decide whether you want them. There are two different types: screening tests (see pp.142–3) and diagnostic tests (see pp.152–3). The aim of screening tests is to work out the risk of there being a problem – based on the result, you may be advised to have a follow-up diagnostic test.

Most women opt to have the screening tests, but it's worth considering how far you would continue with the process. For example, if you had a high-risk result from the screening test, would you opt to have a diagnostic test? If you did, and the results of that were positive, would you want to continue with the pregnancy?

Such considerations are difficult but important. For example, if you know that, no matter what, you and your partner would want to continue with the pregnancy then you may decide not to have a test, or decide to have the test so that you can prepare yourself for a baby with potential problems.

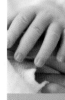

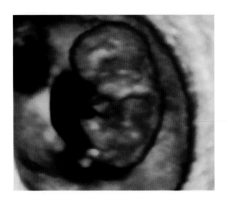

208 days to go…

YOUR BABY TODAY

The baby's head is just under half the length of his body. His limbs are still relatively short but the hands and feet can look quite big. Early basic trunk and limb movements are taking place but it's too early to feel them at this stage.

Will it be a boy or a girl? Significant changes are taking place that enable your baby's sexual organs to develop.

Hormones are influencing your unborn baby's development and the ovaries or testes now begin to form. The testes will gradually descend but their structural development won't be complete until your child hits puberty. The ovary will produce eggs (see p.226) but these will remain in the early stages of development.

A minute genital tube forms the external genitalia but each sex appears the same at this stage. This is not entirely surprising as the phallus is only 2.5mm long.

Your baby's bladder and rectum have now separated. The kidneys will take some time to develop fully: two buds grow up from the bladder to the tissue that will become the kidneys, one on each side. These so-called ureteric buds form the ureters – the tubes that transport urine from the kidney to the bladder. The ureteric bud must successfully fuse with the kidney tissue in the pelvis. As the ureteric buds expand upwards, the early kidneys developing in the pelvis will move upwards to lie in the abdomen.

ASK A… DOCTOR

I have hay fever. Can I take antihistamines? The potential effects of taking antihistamines in pregnancy aren't known, so it's best to err on the side of caution and not take them. However, if your symptoms are severe, see your doctor as there is one antihistamine available on prescription that can be taken during pregnancy.

FOCUS ON… TWINS

A shared support system

Non-identical twins are always in separate amniotic sacs with a placenta each. If your babies are identical (from one fertilized egg) they may share the same placenta and sometimes also the amniotic sac, with a single membrane called the chorion surrounding them. These are known as monochorionic twins and require greater monitoring. The arrangement of the placenta and amniotic sacs can be analyzed on an ultrasound scan.

When twins share a placenta, their circulatory systems may also be connected. This can cause one twin to receive too much blood, which can lead to heart problems; the other twin will get too little blood and will not grow at the correct rate. This is called twin-to-twin transfusion and happens in about 10–15 per cent of monochorionic pregnancies. The imbalance can sometimes be corrected by draining amniotic fluid from around the twin with the greater blood supply, or by using laser treatment to seal off some blood vessels in the placenta. An early delivery may be necessary.

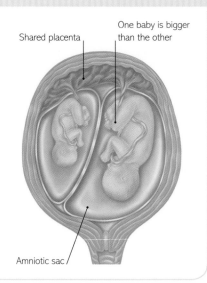

Shared placenta

One baby is bigger than the other

Amniotic sac

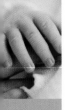

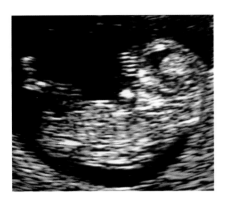

207 days to go...

YOUR BABY TODAY

This coloured 2D ultrasound scan shows a baby lying on his back with his head to the right. This is the ideal position when measuring the crown (head) to rump (bottom) length to accurately date the pregnancy: it simply measures in a straight line.

You may begin to get a few discomforts around your pelvis as your body begins to accommodate your growing uterus.

ASK A... NUTRITIONIST

I'm allergic to dairy products. What can I eat to make sure my baby gets the nutrients these provide? Dairy products are an excellent source of protein, calcium (which is required for the development of your baby's teeth and bones), some B vitamins, and a little iron. Full-fat milk contains vitamins A, D, and E. Eat foods that provide the same nutrients:
- **For calcium:** leafy green vegetables, particularly broccoli and kale; fish (see p.96) with soft, edible bones, such as salmon (tinned is fine), whitebait, and sardines; calcium-fortified soya milk.
- **For vitamin A:** brightly coloured vegetables, meats, eggs, and liver. Although most nutritionists do not recommend liver during pregnancy, if you aren't getting much vitamin A in your diet, a little will do no harm.
- **For vitamin D:** eggs. Vitamin D is also found in most fish (see p.96).
- **For vitamin E:** soya, vegetable oils, leafy green vegetables, and eggs. As long as you're getting plenty of these key nutrients from other sources, your baby's health will not be adversely affected.

Having a few niggly aches and pains during pregnancy is nothing to be concerned about. They occur because the ligaments and muscles of your pelvis are stretching to fit your ever-growing uterus. This can cause some discomfort but should be manageable.

If the pain you're experiencing does become crampy, like period pain, and there is any bleeding, or if the pain becomes very severe and constant, then you should go to the doctor or hospital to be checked over. You will be checked to rule out a miscarriage (see p.94) or an ectopic pregnancy (see p.93).

FOCUS ON... SAFETY

Bon voyage

Whether you're going on holiday or on a business trip, it's important to be prepared (see also pp.28–9):
- **Check you're fit to travel** – speak to your midwife or doctor.
- **Find out whether you need any vaccinations** and discuss these with your doctor (see p.105). It's advisable to avoid travelling to areas where there is a high risk of disease while you're pregnant if at all possible.
- **Get travel insurance** and make sure it covers you during pregnancy.
- **Carry your antenatal notes** with you at all times and stay within reach of medical help.
- **Don't stay seated** for long periods in transit and stay hydrated. Wear support socks to reduce the risk of DVT (see pp.29 and 186).
- **Wear adequate sun protection** if you're going to a hot climate.
- **Be careful** about what you eat, and drink bottled water.

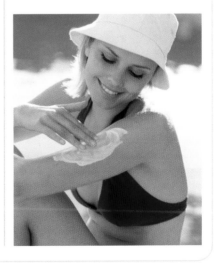

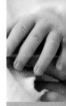

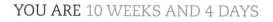

206 days to go...

YOUR BABY TODAY

The umbilical cord gradually becomes more coiled as the pregnancy progresses – as seen here on the left of the image. This coiling is thought to occur because of the many movements the baby makes.

Your baby's limbs are more developed now, enabling him to move, and his hands and fingers can be clearly seen on a scan.

Your baby takes on a more human form as his neck lengthens and his head is seen as separate from his body. The head is still about half the total length of your baby. The length of your baby can be measured on an ultrasound by measuring the distance between your baby's head (crown) and his bottom (rump). This is noted as the CRL (crown-rump length) measurement. The head is also measured: this is the biparietal diameter (BPD), which is the distance between the two parietal bones on each side of the baby's head.

Now that the neck is more developed and all the limb joints have formed, your baby can begin to make several movements. The completed diaphragm allows for breathing movements. In the gut, your baby's duodenum now opens up along its length, the small bowel starts to rotate and prepares to re-enter the abdominal cavity.

Within your baby's mouth, the hard palate has formed; the relatively large tongue means that it is easier for your baby to move amniotic fluid through the nostrils rather than through his mouth with each breath.

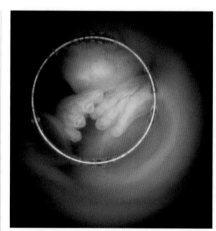

This endoscopic image, obtained by passing a fine light-emitting tube into the uterus, shows the hands obscuring the fetus's face.

TIME TO THINK ABOUT

Nuchal scan

At around 11–14 weeks of pregnancy, you may be offered a nuchal translucency scan (see p.143). This assesses the risk of Down's syndrome by measuring the depth of fluid in the skin behind your baby's neck.

■ **The nuchal translucency scan** is considered to be 80 per cent accurate. If your hospital offers you a blood test (PAPP-A – see p.142) with the scan, it becomes 85 per cent accurate. When the nasal bone is measured, the accuracy rises to 95 per cent; however, this test is not widely available.
■ **If the results** show a high risk, a further test (see pp.152–3) is offered.

FOCUS ON... TWINS

Double the trouble

As your body is growing two or more babies, there will be physical effects. But there is a positive side: if the symptoms are severe it is often a sign that the babies are doing well.
■ **During the first three months,** your heart has to work harder to pump additional fluid around your body, which can lead to a greater feeling of fatigue.
■ **Nausea and vomiting** can be more severe because you have higher amounts of pregnancy hormones.

Mention severe symptoms to your doctor if you're suffering, but remember these niggles aren't serious. You may be seen earlier if you suspect you're having twins, and will go on to have more antenatal appointments and ultrasound scans. You will be referred to an obstetrician, and may attend a multiple pregnancy clinic.

205 days to go...

YOUR BABY TODAY

The external ear is now more clearly seen as it makes its way to its final position. The eyes are also much closer to their final position and the neck continues to lengthen. The baby's hands often touch his mouth, providing important sensory feedback.

Healthy teeth and gums are essential in pregnancy, so brush thoroughly and go for regular dental appointments.

Make sure you're taking care of your teeth and gums. The hormone progesterone causes gum tissue to soften and it's therefore more likely to bleed when brushed and to become infected. Unfortunately, there is a link between gum disease and premature birth. The bacteria that cause periodontal disease release toxins into the mother's bloodstream, which reach the placenta and can affect the baby's growth. The infection can also lead to the production of inflammatory chemicals that can cause the cervix to dilate and trigger contractions.

You're entitled to free dental treatment on the National Health Service (NHS) throughout your pregnancy and until your baby's first birthday. It's safe to have a local anaesthetic injection while you are pregnant. If you need antibiotics to treat an infection, remind your dentist you are pregnant so that medications that are safe in pregnancy are prescribed.

If your dentist needs to take X-rays of your mouth, he or she will protect your baby by covering your tummy with a lead apron.

Make sure that you brush your teeth regularly, or even more often than usual, and ensure that you floss well. This will reduce the risk of your gums being infected.

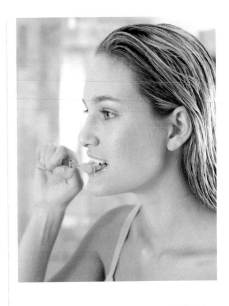

ASK A... DOCTOR

Why am I getting more vaginal discharge since being pregnant? In pregnancy, the layer of muscle in the vagina thickens, and cells lining the vagina multiply in response to an increase in the pregnancy hormone oestrogen. These changes prepare the vagina for childbirth. As a side effect, the extra cells mean that there is an increase in vaginal discharge, known as leucorrhoea.

If you feel sore or itchy in the vaginal area and the discharge is anything other than cream or white, or it smells, your doctor will need to take a swab to rule out infection.

Some infections, such as thrush, cause an abnormal discharge. They are common in pregnancy and are easily treated. Over-the-counter creams and pessaries, inserted into the vagina, are the most effective treatment for thrush. They are not harmful in pregnancy and one pessary often clears the problem. Don't take oral medication for thrush.

AS A MATTER OF FACT

A US study found that, on average, mothers with one child were missing two or three teeth, and those with four or more children were missing between four and eight teeth.

So the old wives' tale that "You will lose a tooth for every child" could have some basis in truth. There's no doubt that the hormonal changes occuring during pregnancy make gum disease more likely (see above).

Your 11th week

133

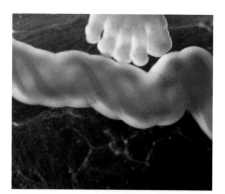

YOU ARE 10 WEEKS AND 6 DAYS

204 days to go...

YOUR BABY TODAY

This close-up of a fetus's umbilical cord shows the two spiralling arteries that carry deoxygenated blood from the baby to the placenta. The placenta also contains a vein that carries oxygenated blood from the placenta to the developing baby.

Has sex been the last thing on your mind, or have you noticed an increase in your libido? It seems all women are different.

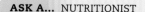

ASK A... NUTRITIONIST

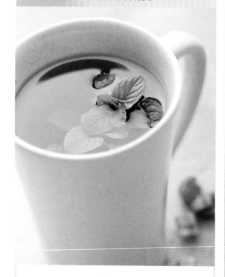

Is it safe to drink herbal teas?
Herbal teas do not contain caffeine, but limit choices to those that you know are safe, such as fruit, ginger, cinnamon, and camomile teas. Avoid raspberry leaf tea and esoteric herbs such as vervain which in high doses are uterine stimulants; they are best limited to the final weeks and during labour. Some teas may contain herbs not studied in pregnancy. Black and green teas contain caffeine, unless the packaging states otherwise.

Being expectant parents can bring you emotionally closer as a couple, but not necessarily physically. While some women find that their libido increases during pregnancy, often much to their partner's surprise, the majority find that their sex drive diminishes in the early weeks.

In the first trimester many women are affected by fatigue and nausea, and so the last thing they want to do is have sex. If this is the case then make sure you explain how you feel to your partner, so that he doesn't feel rejected.

Try to find other ways to stay physically connected with each other: perhaps you can still enjoy some aspects of foreplay, if not penetrative sex. If not, at least try to be affectionate to each other.

It may be your partner who's anxious about having sex. Many men worry about harming the baby through penetrative sex, although there is no chance of this happening.

Remember, if you do want to have sex, then unless a doctor tells you otherwise, it's safe to do so while you are pregnant.

FOCUS ON... YOUR BODY

Tackling spider veins

Spider veins (or spider naevi) are tiny red blood vessels that branch outwards, just under the skin. They are caused by an increase in the level of oestrogen during pregnancy. They usually appear on the face, upper chest, neck, arms, and legs. Often disappearing soon after birth, spider veins are not a cause for concern and can usually be covered with make-up. You can discourage spider veins by:
- **Upping your intake of vitamin C,** which helps to strengthen your veins and capillaries.

- **Avoiding crossing your legs,** which can exacerbate the problem.
- **Taking regular exercise** as it keeps your circulation moving.
- **Avoiding standing or sitting** for long periods, and elevating your feet when you do sit down.
- **Avoiding spicy food,** as some women have found that this helps to reduce spider veins.

If you suddenly notice the appearance of lots of broken veins on your skin, consider consulting your doctor or midwife.

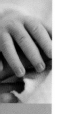

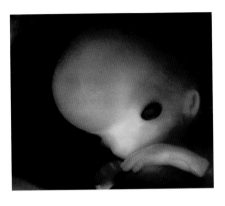

203 days to go...

YOUR BABY TODAY

The hands are often brought close to the face and the baby's neck has lengthened, which will enable him to flex it and make side-to-side movements. The baby's ear and eye are clearly visible on this scan.

The key organs that enable your baby to see, hear, and taste are rapidly developing now, and he's starting to move around.

SUPER-NUTRITIOUS SMOOTHIES

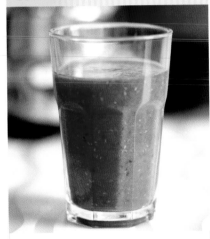

Smoothies are a simple way to stay hydrated and at the same time obtain some nutrients. The basic recipe for making smoothies includes fresh or frozen fruit, ice cream or yogurt, and juice to help blend it. Here are a few ideas:

■ **Strawberry/banana** – frozen strawberries, banana, non-fat vanilla yogurt, and orange juice.
■ **Raspberry/orange** – frozen raspberries, orange sorbet, non-fat vanilla yogurt, and orange juice.
■ **Blueberry/banana** – frozen blueberries, banana, non-fat vanilla yogurt, and orange juice.

Your baby will rely to a great extent on his senses inside the uterus (and once he's born), and key development is taking place now.

The ears continue to move up towards their final destination, but your baby can't hear at this stage. Hearing requires the middle and inner ear to structurally mature and the inner ear to complete nerve connections to the brain. Hearing will, however, be one of the first senses to develop and can be tested by seeing if the baby responds to the sound waves that reach him in the uterus. Judging when taste is established is harder, but taste buds have started to appear in the tongue.

Your baby's eyes have a lens and early retina but even if the eyelids were open the eyes would not yet be able to see light signals. The lens is solid and the optic nerve is not yet responding to signals from the retina.

More signs of bodily movement appear but although your baby is quite active he is too light for you to feel the kicks. However, you'll be fully aware of him in about two months (see p.213).

ASK A... DOCTOR

I had some bleeding after I exercised. Should I be worried?
If you experience vaginal bleeding during exercise with or without cramping, stop immediately and seek medical advice. It's unlikely that exercise is the cause, but you should be checked before doing any more exercise.

Bleeding in the first trimester may be due to a number of issues completely unrelated to exercise, but it's important to rule out any problems at the outset. Once you have the all-clear from your doctor, you can begin exercising again.

ACTUAL SIZE OF YOUR BABY

At 11 weeks your baby's crown to rump length is 4.1cm (1.6in).

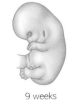

9 weeks

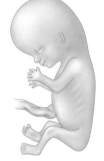
11 weeks

Your 12th week

AN IMPORTANT MILESTONE IS PASSED AS THE FIRST TRIMESTER ENDS

Yawning, arms and legs waving – your baby is on the go and you can actually see it happening. Most women have their first scan this week, and it's the big thrill of the first trimester. Up till now, you may have preferred to keep your pregnancy a precious secret. After the scan, you'll probably feel more confident about making an announcement, especially when you have the photos to prove there's really something happening!

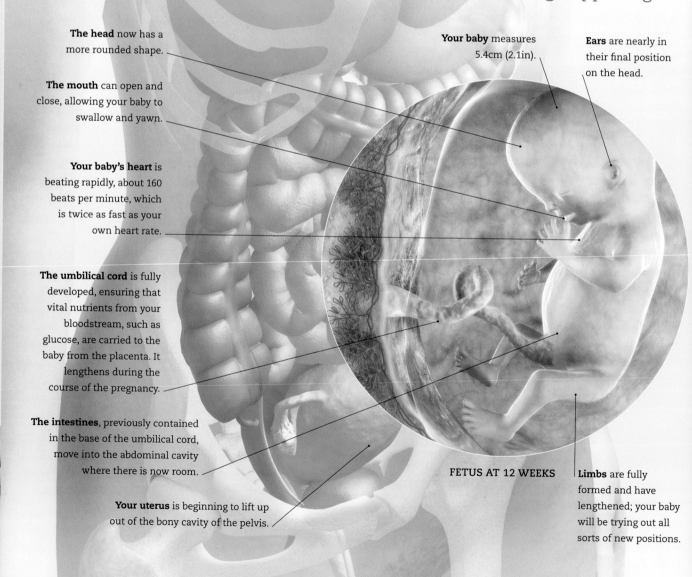

The head now has a more rounded shape.

The mouth can open and close, allowing your baby to swallow and yawn.

Your baby's heart is beating rapidly, about 160 beats per minute, which is twice as fast as your own heart rate.

The umbilical cord is fully developed, ensuring that vital nutrients from your bloodstream, such as glucose, are carried to the baby from the placenta. It lengthens during the course of the pregnancy.

The intestines, previously contained in the base of the umbilical cord, move into the abdominal cavity where there is now room.

Your uterus is beginning to lift up out of the bony cavity of the pelvis.

Your baby measures 5.4cm (2.1in).

Ears are nearly in their final position on the head.

FETUS AT 12 WEEKS

Limbs are fully formed and have lengthened; your baby will be trying out all sorts of new positions.

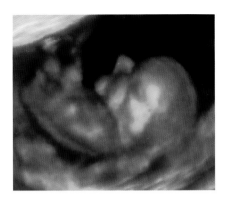

202 days to go...

YOUR BABY TODAY

Although on a scan it might look as though the baby is resting on her back, the fluid in the amniotic sac means that she is floating in a near weightless environment and can easily move into any position within the uterus.

In this final week of your first trimester, you'll probably have your first ultrasound scan and see your baby for the first time.

You and your partner have reached an exciting milestone.
You'll have a dating scan around now and see your baby; this may help you to feel closer to her. For many men, seeing the baby on the scan may be the first time the pregnancy becomes a reality.

At this scan, your baby's length will be measured (see p.139) and this will be used to work out her age. Up until about 14 weeks of pregnancy, all babies grow at around the same rate so irrespective of whether you and your partner are tall or short, until this time your baby will be the same size as others at this stage of development.

Working out your due date (see p.74) using the first day of your period isn't always accurate, especially if your menstrual cycle is long or irregular. The dating scan can give a more accurate expected date of delivery, but it by no means tells you for certain – very few babies arrive on their actual due date.

You may have the option of purchasing a scan picture of your baby. Don't be surprised to find yourself looking at it again, and again, and again! It's also a great way to share the news with others.

(see p.139) ... (see p.74)

FOCUS ON... DADS

It's really happening!

As a dad-to-be, going to your first scan will be a time of great excitement, but you may be anxious, too. It's normal for you and your partner to wonder if your baby is okay and to be desperate to hear that all is well.

The first scan may seem quite technical as it is used to detect your baby's heartbeat and take some measurements, but it's also very emotional. In reality, the first scan gives you the first look at this new life. It lets you see your baby moving around, with legs kicking and arms flailing, even though your partner can't feel these movements yet.

Perhaps, as a man, the biggest shock of the scan is the fact that it confronts you for the first time with the physical evidence that your baby really exists. Your partner is likely to be more used to the idea of pregnancy because she's carrying the baby, but the scan will make the pregnancy much more real to you, and you may be surprised at how emotional you feel.

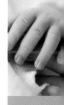

Your 12th week

137

Ultrasound dating scan

Your dating scan at 11–14 weeks can pinpoint the length of your pregnancy to within a five- to seven-day window. Such accurate dating helps to estimate your due date and determine the right time to perform tests later in pregnancy.

Your dating scan

The dating scan helps to establish accurately your baby's gestational age. This is particularly useful if you are not sure when your last menstrual period was, if you have irregular periods, or you became pregnant straight after you stopped using contraception such as the Pill. At this stage of pregnancy, your baby can be measured from crown to rump (from the top of the baby's head to its bottom). Accurate dating of your pregnancy is important not only for establishing your due date and the timing of screening and diagnostic tests, but also because it helps to avoid misdiagnosis of problems such as poor fetal growth (see p.284). Your due date may be revised at this scan if there is more than a five to seven day difference between your menstrual dates and the dates based on the crown–rump length.

A scan may be offered before 11 weeks if you have bleeding or pain to rule out the possibility of a miscarriage or ectopic pregnancy (see p.93).

How the scan is done During an ultrasound scan, high-frequency sound waves are emitted through the abdomen via a hand-held device called a transducer. As the sound waves hit solid tissue, they translate into an image that is viewed on a computer screen and interpreted by the sonographer.

You may be asked to drink plenty of water before this scan to raise the uterus and provide a clearer image. The sonographer will put some cold gel on your abdomen to maximize contact with the skin and will then move the transducer gently over the area.

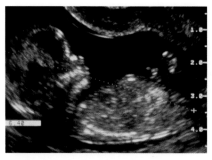

By 12 weeks the fetus has taken on a human appearance. The forehead, eye sockets, and small button nose are all visible in profile.

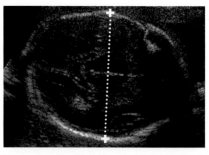

Measuring the diameter of your baby's head (the biparietal diameter) helps to assess your baby's growth and to date your pregnancy.

WHAT THE SCAN SHOWS

What can be seen on a dating scan?

As well as confirming your dates, your dating scan may reveal some other useful information.

■ **This scan will confirm whether** you have a single or multiple pregnancy (twins, triplets, or more).

■ **Uterine anomalies** can be seen, such as a double uterus although this is rare. Uterine fibroids (benign tumours) will also be identified.

■ **The scan may reveal an ovarian cyst** (corpus luteum) on the ovary that produced the egg. These are common and can persist in the first trimester.

■ **Fetal anomalies** may be seen, but most are diagnosed at the 20-week scan when organs are seen clearly (see p.214).

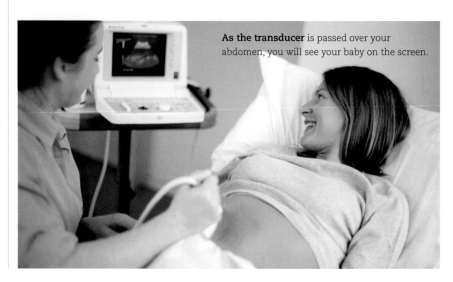

As the transducer is passed over your abdomen, you will see your baby on the screen.

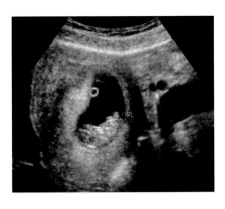

201 days to go...

YOUR BABY TODAY

This image shows the yolk sac at the 12 o'clock position with the placenta seen as a thickening to the lining of the uterus on the left. The baby is in the lower part of the uterus and is positioned lying on her back.

The dating scan is reassuring because it's an opportunity for your baby's progress and development to be thoroughly checked.

At your ultrasound scan, the pregnancy is dated according to your baby's length from crown (head) to rump (bottom) because she is – and will remain – quite curled up. This is known as the CRL (crown–rump length).

As your baby can flex her spine and stretch her neck, this measurement needs to be taken with your baby in a specific position so it can take some time to achieve. The measurement is used to estimate your baby's date of delivery and this may be different to the EDD you calculated (see p.74).

On this first ultrasound scan it should be possible to recognize all four limbs, the hands and feet, the spine, some aspects of brain development, the fluid-filled stomach, and the bladder. From now on your baby's kidneys will be producing small amounts of very dilute urine and the bladder will start to fill.

AS A MATTER OF FACT

Dating scans are only an estimate. The chance of delivering on your due date is only around 5 per cent.

So do keep the estimated due date in mind but don't expect your baby to abide by it!

ASK A... MIDWIFE

I've had quite a few pregnancy symptoms and don't feel as though my body is my own. How can I relax and enjoy being pregnant?
Not all women adapt well to pregnancy and for some dealing with the symptoms and worrying about issues such as weight gain makes them feel out of control. The best way to cope with these feelings is to embrace the changes and remain in touch with your body by exercising and taking time to focus on what is happening inside you. We spend most of our lives listening to all the things that happen on the outside, but very little time focusing on the inside.

Take a few minutes each day to practise deep breathing and relaxation and consider learning some pregnancy yoga and meditation techniques (see right).

The dramatic changes happening to your body may be mirrored in the wide swings of emotions and feelings you experience throughout your pregnancy. Some days you may feel excited and elated at the prospect of becoming a parent, and on others you may feel overwhelmed and anxious.

Perhaps the nine months' gestation period is nature's way of giving us time to get used to the idea of becoming a parent, and allowing us time to deal with our emotions and prepare for the birth. So try to relax, but if you're feeling really anxious speak to your doctor or midwife.

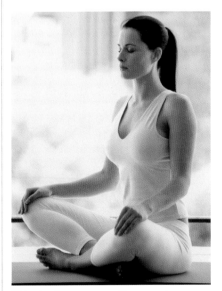

This simple yoga pose allows you to fully relax your body and mind. Consider joining a pregnancy yoga class as it's a great way to learn techniques and also an opportunity to meet other mums-to-be.

200 days to go...

YOUR BABY TODAY

As the baby floats in the amniotic fluid, her limbs are now more fully developed, allowing her to make many movements. The lips and fingers – which are now completely separated – stimulate sensory feelings.

Does your face resemble the pimply complexion of your teenage years? Don't worry, it's those hormones again, and it will pass.

Your skin is likely to change during pregnancy. Some women find that they develop spots or acne, due to the high levels of progesterone. Conversely, you may get dry skin, also due to pregnancy hormones. The dryness may become worse over your abdomen as your bump develops and the skin is stretched.

Freckles and moles may get darker. You may also notice tiny red lines on your chest or legs: these are called spider naevi (see p.134) and are due to the increased blood supply to the skin, which makes the vessels dilate and become more visible.

Other women find that the high levels of oestrogen mean that their skin is in a better condition than before they were pregnant. The "glow" of pregnancy is due to the increased blood supply that occurs in pregnancy, which gives you a rosy, healthy-looking complexion.

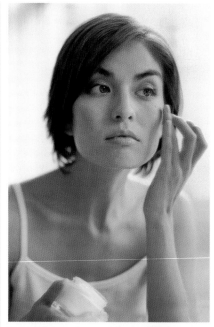

Your skin may become dry and flaky, on your face as well as elsewhere on your body. Using a good moisturizer should help.

TIME TO THINK ABOUT

Telling your employer

As soon as your employer knows you're pregnant, the employment laws that protect you will apply, so it's a good idea to tell him or her as soon as possible. Most parents-to-be wait until 12 weeks when the risk of miscarriage is lower.

■ **It's recommended** that you inform your employer in writing with details of your expected due date.

■ **Your employer** should conduct a risk assessment of your working environment. Any risks identified should be removed or, if this is not possible, alternative arrangements should be made for you.

■ **You can discuss** when your maternity leave will start, when you can take any outstanding holidays, and any other entitlements. If your baby is born early or your maternity leave starts earlier than planned due to illness, the arrangements can be altered at short notice.

■ **Your employer** should respect your right to confidentiality. If you wish the news to remain under wraps until a certain date, make this known.

ASK A... MIDWIFE

Since going to the scan my partner is very over-protective. Is this normal?
Your partner is now realizing his responsibilities and affection for the baby, and is showing these feelings by taking care of you. If you're finding that his cosseting of you is a little too much, you might want to discuss other ways he can feel involved in the pregnancy and prepare for the baby. Try to embrace his involvement and enthusiasm – it's a great way for you to strengthen your relationship and prepare for parenthood together.

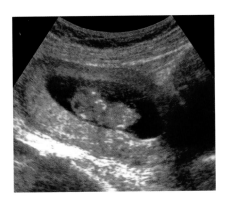

199 days to go...

YOUR BABY TODAY

The fetus can be seen inside the uterus on this coloured ultrasound scan. At this stage of development, the fetus measures approximately 5.4cm (2.1in) crown to rump and weighs around 14g (0.5oz).

By around this 12th week, the midwife might be able to hear your baby's heartbeat with a hand-held monitor.

At this stage your baby's heart beats at approximately 120–160 beats per minute, which is at least twice as fast as your own. The heart and its internal electrical conducting system are structurally complete but its external nerve supply is still quite immature. The nerves to the heart influence its rhythm, gradually slowing the rate as the pregnancy advances.

Your baby's heart is tiny and to maintain an adequate output it is unable to increase the amount of blood it pumps with each beat (as we can), but instead increases the number of times it beats each minute.

The abdominal cavity is large enough to hold the intestines. Whereas before they were bulging outside of your baby's body, they now fit into her abdominal cavity. Having started to rotate while outside the body, the bowel completes its final rotation in the abdominal cavity. Once inside, the bowel position remains fixed, and its diameter increases as the loops of bowel become hollow.

SMOKING: THE FACTS

If you've only cut down, rather than cutting it out, read on. Many smokers inhale more deeply when smoking less and their intake of damaging toxins increases. Here's how smoking affects your baby:

■ **The carbon monoxide,** nicotine, and other substances that you inhale pass from your lungs, into your blood-stream, and cross the placenta.
■ **Nicotine** makes your baby's heart beat faster as she struggles for oxygen, which can affect her growth rate.
■ **Smoking increases the risk** of miscarriage, premature birth, and low birthweight, and exposure to tobacco chemicals makes your baby more likely to suffer from conditions such as asthma and chest infections after the birth, which may be bad enough to warrant a hospital stay.
■ **There is also a higher risk** of cot death if you or your partner smokes. Your partner should stop too.
■ **If you live with a smoker,** you will be inhaling thousands of toxic carcinogenic chemicals that are released into the air around you from the burning end of the cigarette and the exhaled smoke.
■ **Several studies** have confirmed that passive smoking can damage the baby's health and increase the risk of miscarriage and premature birth.

FOCUS ON... TWINS

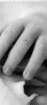

Feeding two?

If you're carrying twins, you're likely to have put on some weight by now, perhaps around 5kg (11lb). Early weight gain is usually a good thing, especially in your case, as this is a vital time for the formation and development of your baby's organs. As a rough guide, a good recommended weight gain is:

■ **For twins,** total weight gain of 16–20kg (35–44lb), preferably 11kg (24lb) by week 24, then a gradual increase until the birth.
■ **For triplets,** a total weight gain of 23–27kg (50–60lb), preferably 16kg (35lb) by week 24, then a gradual increase until the birth.
■ **For quads,** total weight gain of 31–36kg (68–79lb), ideally most of it by week 24.

Screening tests

Optional routine screening tests in the first trimester assess the risk of your baby having a chromosomal disorder such as Down's syndrome. If your risk is high, you will be offered a diagnostic test (see pp.152–3) for a definite result.

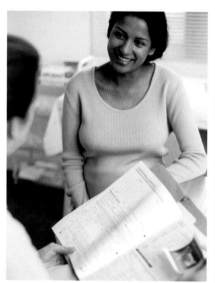

Your midwife will discuss in advance the available screening tests so you are fully informed before agreeing to any test.

What is screened for

Apart from Down's, screening tests also assess the risk of other chromosomal abnormalities, such as trisomy 13 and trisomy 18. Babies with these conditions have more severe mental and physical abnormalities than babies with Down's and seldom survive beyond a year. These conditions are rare, with each year around 1 in 10,000 babies born with trisomy 13 and 1 in 6,000 babies born with trisomy 18, compared to 1 in 800 babies born with Down's.

The "combined" test

The recommended screening test for Down's is the "combined test", which is performed between 11 and 14 weeks. The combined test is recommended because it has a high accuracy rate and the results are produced quickly.

The test uses a combination of a maternal blood test and an ultrasound of your baby. The ultrasound measures the thickness of the skin at the back of your baby's neck, called the nuchal fold (see box, opposite). The blood test looks at the levels of two chemicals: pregnancy associated plasma protein A (PAPP-A) and one of the pregnancy hormones, human chorionic gonadotrophin (hCG). The result of the blood test is combined with your age and the measurement of the nuchal fold. A mathematical formula is then used to calculate your baby's risk of Down's syndrome.

If you have your blood test before your ultrasound, you will usually receive your results immediately following your ultrasound. If you have your blood taken at the time of the ultrasound you will receive your results a few days later. Your baby's risk of Down's from the combined test may be higher, lower, or the same as her risk based on your age alone.

Cell-free DNA test

DNA is the genetic material we get from our parents that determines our characteristics such as eye colour as well as any genetic diseases. A blood test is increasingly becoming available that can detect DNA fragments, known as cell-free DNA, from your baby or the placenta floating in your blood.

Free fetal DNA can be found in maternal blood after 10 completed weeks of pregnancy. The test will detect 99 per cent of babies with Down's, 98 per cent of babies with trisomy 18, and 80 per cent of babies with trisomy 13, making it more accurate than the combined test.

UNDERSTANDING TESTS

Accuracy of screening tests

The detection rate for Down's, which used to be assessed on maternal age alone, has significantly increased as more screening tests have become available. The aim of screening tests is to provide a high detection rate for Down's and a low "false positive" rate. A false positive means the screening test indicated a high risk of Down's, but subsequent diagnostic tests gave the all clear, which means the mother will have been exposed to unnecessary testing.

Tests	Timing (weeks)	Detection rate	False positive rate
Combined test	11–14	85%	5%
Cell-free DNA test	After 10 weeks	99%	0.2%
Quadruple test	15–22	76%	5%
Triple test	16–18	69%	5%

Triple and quadruple tests

If your hospital doesn't offer a nuchal translucency scan, then a triple or quadruple test will be offered instead. These screening tests are carried out in the second trimester and assess your baby's risk of Down's syndrome from blood tests alone. The triple test, done at 13 to 22 weeks, measures levels of the hormones hCG, AFP, and oestriol. The quadruple test, carried out at 15 to 22 weeks, measures levels of inhibin A in addition to these three hormones.

A positive screen

It's important to remember that a positive result does not mean your baby has Down's syndrome. For example, if you have a 1 in 100 risk of Down's, your test will be "positive". However, the chance that your baby has Down's is low as your baby will be normal 99 times out of 100. Talking to your doctor, midwife, or a genetic counsellor can help you to understand your actual risk and decide if you want to have a diagnostic test such as amniocentesis (see pp.152–3) for a definite result. As diagnostic tests carry a risk of miscarriage, you need to weigh up the risks before deciding to go ahead.

Some research suggests that women are more likely to enjoy their pregnancy and birth and come to terms with the diagnosis if they know in advance that their baby has Down's. So don't assume that you should only have a diagnostic test to decide whether or not to continue your pregnancy.

If you have a positive screening test for another more severe chromosomal disorder, such as trisomy 13 or 18, your doctor will talk to you about the outlook for babies with these conditions – the majority of whom die early in life, sometimes within the first week – to help you decide what to do. In some cases these disorders are associated with abnormalities detected during the dating scan (see p.138), and the presence of these abnormalities

Nuchal translucency scan

An ultrasound scan, known as the nuchal translucency scan, is carried out between 11 and 14 weeks of pregnancy and is used to help assess your baby's risk of Down's syndrome. During this test, the sonographer measures the depth of fluid under the skin at the back of the baby's neck, known as the nuchal fold. If this measurement is high it indicates that excess fluid is present, which means that the baby has a higher risk of Down's syndrome. The measurement is then combined with the results of blood tests and the average risk based on your age, to give your baby's individual risk for Down's. If your risk is higher than 1 in 250, you will be counselled and offered a diagnostic test, such as amniocentesis or chorionic villus sampling, to give a definitive result (see p.152).

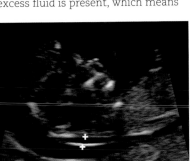

The small depth of fluid seen in the neck's nuchal fold in this scan means that the fetus has a low risk of being born with Down's syndrome.

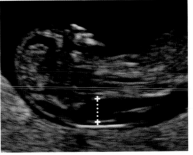

The thicker nuchal fold seen here indicates an increased risk of Down's syndrome in this fetus and a diagnostic test will be discussed.

combined with a positive test may confirm the diagnosis. Nevertheless, many women opt to have a diagnostic test before deciding whether or not to terminate their pregnancy.

Further screening Another option is to have a specialized ultrasound scan to look for Down's syndrome markers between 17 and 22 weeks. If the ultrasound doesn't show any signs of Down's, the risk of your baby being affected is reduced. However, a second trimester ultrasound is not such an accurate test for Down's as other screening tests and so you should only consider this path if you are strongly against having a diagnostic test such as amniocentesis, and feel that you don't need a definite diagnosis.

Should I have a diagnostic test?

Deciding on whether or not to go ahead with genetic, or diagnostic, testing (see pp.152–3) is a personal choice. Factors that may affect your decision-making process include:

■ **Your anxiety level** without knowing for sure, and how this will affect your enjoyment of pregnancy.

■ **Your fears about** pregnancy loss.

■ **What you would do if** you found out your baby had Down's syndrome or another condition such as trisomy 18.

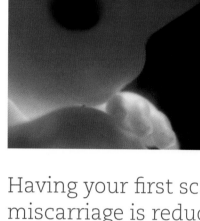

YOU ARE 11 WEEKS AND 5 DAYS

198 days to go...

YOUR BABY TODAY

At this stage the eye – not yet in its final position – still dominates the appearance of the face. The eye is not yet responsive to light and remains well protected behind the covering eyelid.

Having your first scan this week and knowing your risk of miscarriage is reduced now, should mean you can start to relax.

This can be a very positive time for you, especially if you've been anxious from day one of your pregnancy. The risk of miscarriage falls as your pregnancy progresses and by the end of this 12th week, it's no more than 1 per cent.

As you enter the second trimester, you should begin to feel better (see opposite), and this, combined with the knowledge that you have passed the most risky time, may help you relax. If you've been keeping your pregnancy a secret, you can also enjoy telling others.

FOCUS ON... SAFETY

Safe scans

Ultrasound has been used for years and is thought to be safe. Children who've been exposed to antenatal ultrasound do not have differences in speech, hearing, vision, or school performance, or an increased risk of cancer. However, ultrasound should only be carried out when necessary.

AS A MATTER OF FACT

Medical ultrasound has been used since the early 1960s.

However, the first discovery of high-frequency echo-sounding techniques, on which ultrasound is based, was as long ago as 1880 in Paris. In the early 20th century, ultrasound was used as a therapy tool and it was not until the 1940s that research began into its use as a diagnostic tool.

ASK A... NUTRITIONIST

I have a really sweet tooth. Is it okay to indulge this while I'm pregnant? While occasional treats of biscuits or chocolate are fine, processed foods usually contain hidden fats and sugars and provide few nutrients, so it's best to try to find healthier sweet alternatives to snack on, such as fresh fruit.

Always read food labels and look for alternative foods containing less fat and less added sugars. Just as you would consider carefully how you wean and feed your child, you should look after yourself in the same way while you're pregnant.

One of the best ways to curb your sweet tooth is to eat regular meals. This helps to steady your blood-sugar level and reduce sweet cravings. Try not to go longer than three hours without eating and, if you're hungry, have a healthy snack between meals, such as a chicken sandwich, a low-fat yogurt, malt loaf, or fruit, which can be fresh, tinned, or dried, such as raisins or apricots.

Try to drink about two litres of water a day, as perceived hunger is often really dehydration. Drinking a glass or two of water may stop you reaching for the biscuit tin.

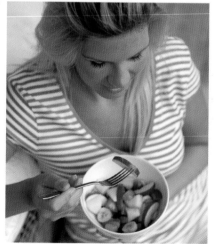

It's possible to satisfy sweet cravings with refreshing fruit. You may find that you feel better after eating a fruit salad than if you eat a bar of chocolate.

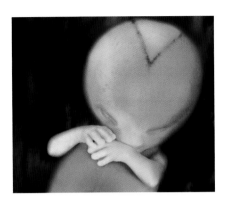

197 days to go...

YOUR BABY TODAY

The bones of the front of the skull have continued to expand and cover the head, protecting the delicate brain structures beneath. The soft spot in between the skull bones (centre) remains through pregnancy and into babyhood.

If you're finding you're out of breath when you get to the top of the stairs, accept this as a normal side-effect of pregnancy.

By the end of the first trimester it's normal to begin feeling a little breathless. This is because your heart and lungs are having to work much harder to supply your body with oxygen due to all the changes that are taking place to allow the baby to grow.

The amount of oxygen you need in pregnancy is about 20 per cent more than normal; some of this goes to the placenta (see p.127) and baby, and the rest to your other organs. To get this increased amount of oxygen you breathe faster and deeper, almost hyperventilating so you feel short of breath, especially when you exercise.

As your pregnancy continues, you may find that this shortness of breath, or feeling that you are not breathing very deeply, continues or worsens. As the baby grows, your uterus will expand upwards and your other abdominal organs will rearrange themselves to create more room. Your organs and uterus push up against your diaphragm so it becomes more difficult to take a deep breath; in order to get all the oxygen you need, you then have to breathe much faster. The hormone progesterone may also affect the rate at which you breathe.

If you have any concerns about breathlessness, don't hesitate to speak to your midwife or doctor.

FOCUS ON... HEALTH

Feeling better?

By the end of this trimester, many of the early pregnancy symptoms are likely to have passed.

■ **Nausea** may have begun to lessen and it can be a complete relief to wake up in the morning without feeling sick. Your appetite will return, and you can stop worrying about whether your baby is being properly nourished, which is often a common concern for women who suffer from nausea and vomiting. If your sickness hasn't passed yet, don't worry – for some women, it does last longer (see p.159).

■ **You won't need to pass urine** quite so often, which will be good news if you've spent an inordinate amount of time on the toilet. This is because your uterus is now moving up the abdominal cavity and therefore is placing less pressure on your bladder.

■ **The fatigue** that you may have felt in these early months is likely to have lifted, and you may be sleeping more deeply now that you're relaxing into your pregnancy.

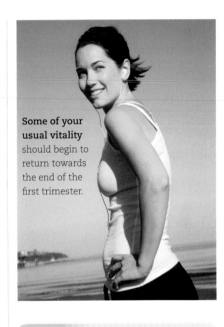

Some of your usual vitality should begin to return towards the end of the first trimester.

ASK A... MIDWIFE

I've gone from an A cup to D cup. Will this increase in size last forever? The majority of women who have had babies do report a permanent increase in breast size but it's unlikely to be to this extent! The effects of oestrogen cause fat to be deposited in the breasts and when your milk comes in after the birth your breasts will get bigger, but reduce again once you have stopped breastfeeding.

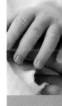

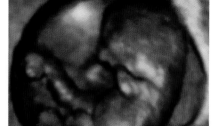

196 days to go...

YOUR BABY TODAY

Here the legs are crossed and the arms outstretched. The umbilical cord is short and thick at this stage, but will lengthen as the baby grows, and become much thinner with many coils.

You've reached the end of the first trimester and in this time your baby has developed from a ball of cells to an active fetus.

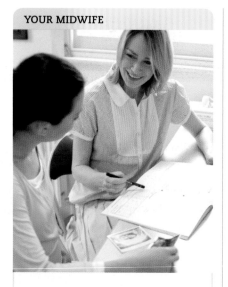

YOUR MIDWIFE

Most women develop a good relationship with their midwife, who can be a fountain of fantastic information, and a wonderful source of comfort and reassurance.

It's important that you are as honest as you can be with her. Like many women, you may be reluctant to reveal concerns, or to admit to unhealthy habits, for fear of being embarrassed or told off. It's very likely that your midwife will have heard it all before, and will be able to help and advise – and make a few tried-and-tested suggestions.

Your amazing baby can do so many things already, including being able to open her mouth and yawn, and swallow. Swallowing develops earlier than sucking. Your baby will be starting to swallow amniotic fluid but the more complex sucking movements cannot be identified until 18–20 weeks. Swallowing will encourage gut development. The amniotic fluid enters into the stomach not the lungs, which are protected now by the vocal cords and the higher pressure of the lung's own fluid. The amniotic fluid will later be excreted as urine when the fetal kidneys start to function.

After the stomach, the amniotic fluid will enter the small bowel. The intestinal walls are developing muscular layers but these do not yet contract in a co-ordinated way to move the fluid along the digestive tract. It will be 20 weeks before the structural organization of the gut is finally complete. Many digestive enzymes are starting to be released into the gut but these currently act as a stimulus to development rather than for the absorption of nutrients.

Your baby is reliant on a steady stream of glucose, which is stored as glycogen in the liver. This continues throughout pregnancy and at birth your baby will, for her size, have significantly larger glycogen stores than adults do.

The correct level of glucose in the mother is controlled by insulin secreted by the pancreas. The placenta, however, has little control over the amount it takes from your bloodstream and passes on. For this reason if your glucose level is very high, for example in poorly controlled diabetes, the baby will have high levels of glucose. To maintain a normal glucose level she will secrete insulin, but this will lead to increased fat deposition and weight gain.

ACTUAL SIZE OF YOUR BABY

At 12 weeks your baby's crown to rump length is 5.4cm (2.1in).

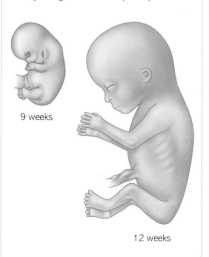

9 weeks

12 weeks

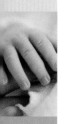

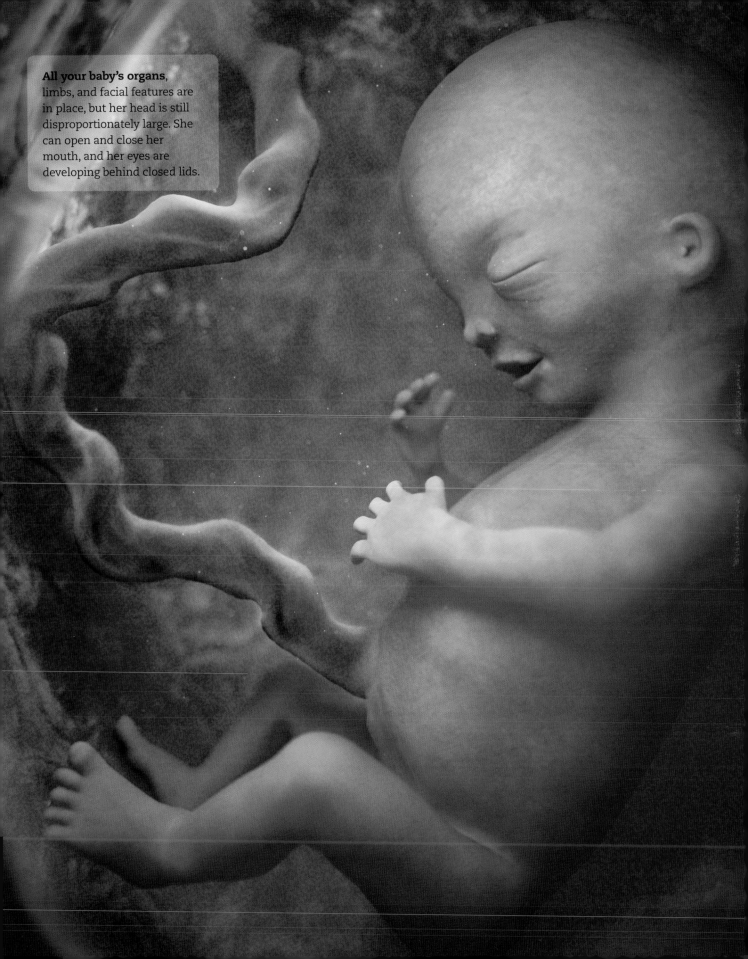

All your baby's organs, limbs, and facial features are in place, but her head is still disproportionately large. She can open and close her mouth, and her eyes are developing behind closed lids.

Welcome to your second trimester

| WEEK | 13 | 14 | 15 | 16 | 17 | 18 |

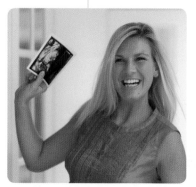

Spreading the word Safely past the first trimester, you will probably want to tell people your good news.

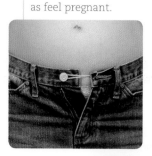

Visibly pregnant As your tummy expands and your waistline disappears, you'll start to look as well as feel pregnant.

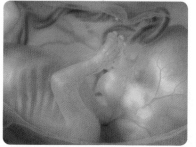

At 16 weeks your baby has taken on a definite human form. The body and limbs have grown substantially and a translucent layer of skin reveals underlying blood vessels.

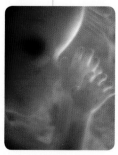

By 17 weeks the arms and hands are well developed; the fingers now move freely and start to grasp.

At three months your pregnancy becomes noticeable. By five months, there's no mistaking it.

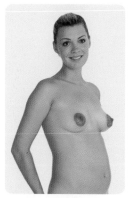
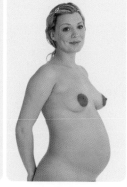

Second trimester As your pregnancy starts to show, you may feel renewed energy as the tiredness and nausea of early pregnancy fade.
Looking good By the end of this trimester, you'll look clearly pregnant as your baby steadily grows.

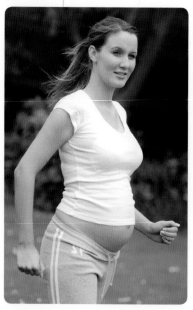

Feeling energized Regular exercise throughout pregnancy will positively benefit you and your baby in the months ahead and help prepare your body for labour.

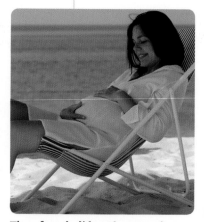

Time for a holiday The second trimester is the ideal time to get away from it all as your hormones settle down, energy levels lift, and labour is still a safe distance away.

Facts and figures Even in the womb, rhythmic movements such as walking send your baby to sleep.

Now your pregnancy starts to feel "real" as your body changes rapidly and you feel your baby move.

| 19 | 20 | 21 | 22 | 23 | 24 | 25 |

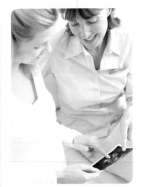

The 20-week scan Your baby's major organs are now clearly visible and will be studied in detail to ensure they're developing normally.

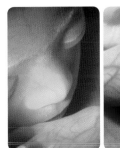

By 23 weeks your baby's facial features are distinct, with eyebrows and eyelashes visible. On the hands, fingernails start to grow.

Facts and figures At 21 weeks, your baby measures about 27cm (10.5in) from crown to heel.

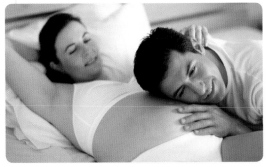

First flutters As your baby's movements increase and strengthen, your partner can begin to share in your pregnancy experience.

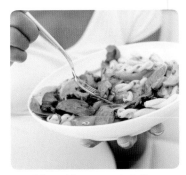

Nutritious bites A varied diet with plenty of vegetables benefits your own and your baby's health.

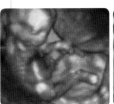 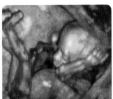 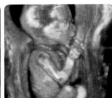

Your active baby Surrounded and cushioned by amniotic fluid, your baby is free to move around in the uterus without risk of being bumped or hurt.

Loud and clear By 24 weeks, your baby is able to hear sounds from the outside world and may react by moving around.

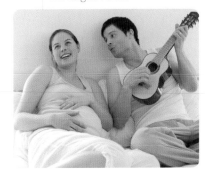

Exercise classes Antenatal exercise classes are tailored to meet your requirements in pregnancy and are also a great way to get acquainted with other mums-to-be.

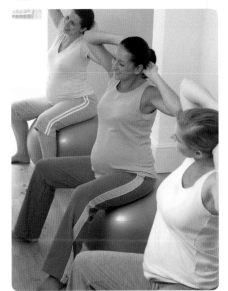

Your 13th week

AS YOU ENTER THIS SECOND TRIMESTER, YOUR BODY WILL SETTLE INTO PREGNANCY

For most women, any discomforts of early pregnancy start to disappear this trimester. The high levels of pregnancy hormones, which are thought to contribute to sickness, are subsiding, and fatigue should begin to diminish. Meanwhile, your baby floats peacefully in the amniotic sac. As he goes on growing, so the sac will expand to give him plenty of room to kick and stretch. His brain is developing at a rapid rate.

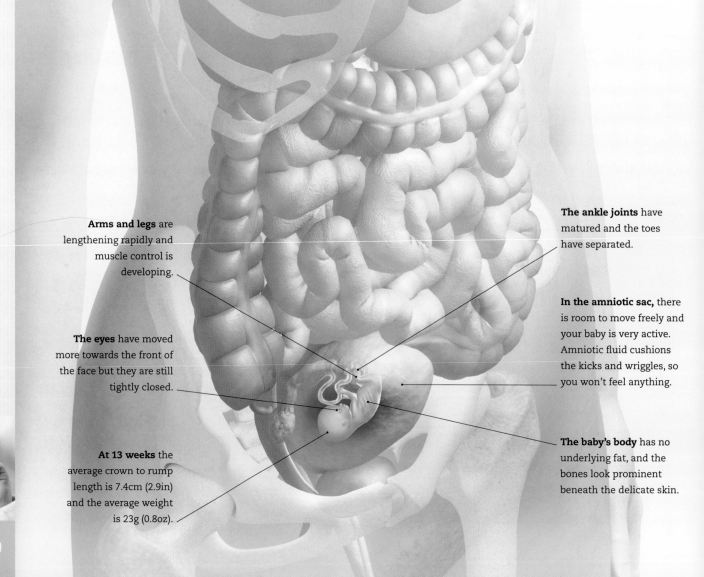

Arms and legs are lengthening rapidly and muscle control is developing.

The eyes have moved more towards the front of the face but they are still tightly closed.

At 13 weeks the average crown to rump length is 7.4cm (2.9in) and the average weight is 23g (0.8oz).

The ankle joints have matured and the toes have separated.

In the amniotic sac, there is room to move freely and your baby is very active. Amniotic fluid cushions the kicks and wriggles, so you won't feel anything.

The baby's body has no underlying fat, and the bones look prominent beneath the delicate skin.

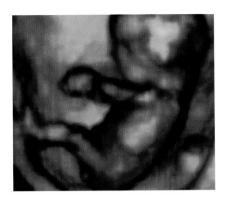

195 days to go...

YOUR BABY TODAY

This 3D ultrasound scan clearly demonstrates that the baby's arms and legs are now fully formed and much more in proportion with the trunk. All of the baby's joints are now formed, enabling a full range of movement.

This is a good time to start telling the important people in your life your exciting news – before they guess for themselves.

Now that you're in your second trimester and have had your dating scan (see p.138), you may want to start telling a wider circle of people that you're pregnant. You can feel confident doing this, knowing that the risk of miscarriage is reduced to no more than 1 per cent after the 12th week. Besides this, your bump will begin to show in a few weeks, if it hasn't already, so hiding the pregnancy will become difficult.

If you and your partner have been keeping the pregnancy a secret for the past three months, announcing it will be a huge release and it can be a positive experience to share the news with others. Do, however, be prepared for an onslaught of advice and people's tales of their pregnancy and birth experiences!

Sometimes letting others know that you're pregnant can be difficult. Be sensitive to other people's feelings: friends who also want to be parents, but are having difficulty conceiving, may find it difficult to share your happiness straightaway. It's preferable to tell these people face to face rather than them hearing it on the grapevine. Even if they don't react positively, and don't want to talk about your pregnancy all the time, give them time to come to terms with it at their own pace. Remember they can be sad for themselves while being happy for you.

TIME TO THINK ABOUT

Second trimester tests

If you haven't had a nuchal translucency scan (see p.143), blood tests will be offered this trimester to screen for Down's (see pp.142–3).

■ **The triple test** is carried out at 16–18 weeks. It measures levels of the hormones hCG, AFP, and oestriol.
■ **The quadruple test** is carried out at 15–22 weeks. It measures levels of inhibin A in addition to the hormones measured in the triple test.

FOCUS ON... YOUR BODY

Become a clothes cheat!

Although your clothes may be feeling a little tight by this stage, you probably aren't ready to wear voluminous maternity clothing just yet, so it's time to get creative! Simply bridge the gap between your button and button-hole with an elastic band (see right) or by sewing in an elasticated panel. Assuming he's bigger than you, try raiding your partner's wardrobe – his T-shirts, shirts, and jumpers can be ruched in with a low-slung belt.

Check what's in your wardrobe already: empire-cut dresses will see you through most of your pregnancy; looser smock tops can be layered over tight-fitting T-shirts; low-slung trousers can sit neatly under your bump, topped with an oversized shirt. The one item you might want to purchase is a pair of maternity trousers – something stretchy with an adjustable waist.

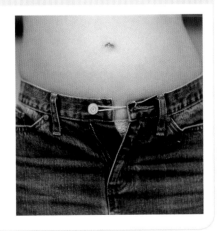

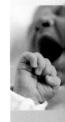

Diagnostic tests

If you've had a positive screening test for Down's syndrome or another genetic abnormality, you will be offered a diagnostic test, which gives a definitive answer as to whether or not your baby has an abnormality.

What are diagnostic tests?

Diagnostic tests involve taking a sample of either the placenta, the amniotic fluid, or fetal blood. The samples are then sent away and examined in a laboratory for chromosomal or genetic abnormalities. The two main diagnostic tests are amniocentesis and chorionic villus sampling, or CVS. As both of these tests carry a small risk of miscarriage (see opposite), you will need to consider carefully the advantages and disadvantages of the tests before going ahead with either of them.

Chorionic villus sampling (CVS)

Chorionic villi are fragments of placental tissue. As the placenta originates from the fertilized egg, the chromosomes in the cells that make up the placenta are representative of your baby's chromosomes. During CVS, a small amount of tissue from your placenta is removed and tested in a laboratory to reveal if your baby has a chromosomal disorder such as Down's syndrome or another trisomy disorder, such as trisomy 13 or trisomy 18. CVS is carried out between 10 and 12½ weeks' gestation and the results are usually available within 7 to 10 days. The procedure can also definitely identify your baby's sex, if you wish to know. If you don't want to have this information, make your wishes clear before the test. In 2–3 per cent of cases, the doctor will be unable to perform CVS due to the placenta's position. In this case, you may be asked to return for an amniocentesis at 16 weeks.

Amniocentesis This is the most common diagnostic test, carried out at around 15 to 20 weeks of pregnancy. The amniotic fluid around your baby mainly consists of your baby's urine and contains cells from your baby's skin and urinary tract. During amniocentesis, a number of cells are collected from the amniotic fluid. They are then sent to a laboratory and grown in a cell culture, until there is a sufficient number of cells to examine your baby's chromosomes and identify whether your baby has a chromosomal abnormality such as Down's syndrome. Amniotic fluid can also be tested for high levels of the substance alpha-fetoprotein (AFP), which could mean that your baby has a problem such as spina bifida. Sometimes, amniotic fluid is tested for signs of a bacterial or viral infection, which is thought to be a factor in premature births (see p.431).

HOW THE TEST IS DONE

Chorionic villus sampling

There are two ways of carrying out chorionic villus sampling. In the transabdominal method, a fine needle is placed through the abdomen to collect placental fragments. In the transcervical procedure, a thin tube (catheter) is inserted into the cervix. The method used depends on the position of the placenta and the doctor's training and expertise. During the procedure, ultrasound guidance is used so that the doctor can see the placenta's position.

CVS can also be carried out in a multiple pregnancy; in this case both the transabdominal and transcervical methods of collection may be used.

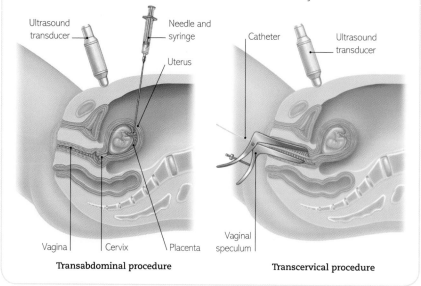

Transabdominal procedure — Ultrasound transducer, Needle and syringe, Uterus, Vagina, Cervix, Placenta

Transcervical procedure — Catheter, Ultrasound transducer, Vaginal speculum

Transabdominal procedure   **Transcervical procedure**

If, following the procedure, you experience severe abdominal pain, fever greater than 38°C (100.5°F), vaginal bleeding, or a large gush of clear fluid from your vagina you should call your midwife or doctor straightaway.

How you might feel

You may be concerned about the idea of a needle going through your abdomen, or a catheter into your cervix; however, the majority of women find that these procedures are not particularly painful. If you are having a transabdominal procedure, the needle usually doesn't hurt any more than it does when you are having a blood test. Some doctors use a small amount of local anaesthetic before the transabdominal procedure to numb the area, although the anaesthetic itself can occasionally sting. Although aferwards it's common to experience uterine cramps, similar to the cramps you feel during menstruation, rest assured that these cramps alone do not mean that you have an increased risk of miscarriage.

If your blood type is Rh negative (see p.127) you should receive an injection of anti-D after the procedure to prevent complications occurring during this and future pregnancies.

After the procedure

It's generally thought that being active after CVS or amniocentesis does not increase your risk of miscarriage. However, you may feel better if you don't exercise heavily right away; it's not necessary to remain in bed. In most cases, you should be physically able to return to work within a day or so after a diagnostic procedure, although some women may feel emotionally fragile and may not feel up to returning to work right away.

Getting the results

Usually, chromosomal results from diagnostic tests take around 1–2 weeks to return, and in some units may take as long as three weeks. If you have had your AFP level tested with amniocentesis (see opposite), the results for this are usually available fairly quickly, after around one to three days. If you've been tested for an infection, when you receive the results will largely depend on the type of infection. Bacterial cultures usually take around 24 to 48 hours to be returned, while viral cultures can take a little longer.

Comparison of CVS and amniocentesis

Before deciding on a diagnostic test, you may want to weigh up their pros and cons. Consider, too, that the risks may be reduced with a doctor who has expertise in a particular test.

CVS: the pros

- CVS can be done up to five weeks earlier than amniocentesis, so if an abnormality is found and you decide to terminate, this can be done in a safer, less traumatic way.
- As more genetic material is collected, the results may arrive sooner, decreasing the anxious wait.
- If you're nervous about a needle going into the abdomen, transcervical CVS means that you can avoid this but still have an antenatal diagnosis.

CVS: the cons

- The risk of miscarriage after CVS is higher than amniocentesis, at around 1 in 200 to 1 in 300. The miscarriage rate is the same whether it's done transabdominally or transvaginally.
- In the past, some women who had had CVS then had babies with limb abnormalities. It's now thought that most of these cases occurred when CVS was done before 10 weeks when the limbs were starting to form. The risk of limb defects without CVS is 1 in 1,700 and 1 in 1,000 with CVS.

Amniocentesis: the pros

- Amniocentesis is highly accurate and has the lowest risk of miscarriage at around 1 in 400.

Amniocentesis: the cons

- As this is done later than CVS and the results take longer, if you terminate you'll be induced and have a vaginal delivery.

Amniocentesis

During amniocentesis, the doctor uses ultrasound to locate an open pocket of amniotic fluid. Under continued ultrasound guidance, a thin needle is placed through the skin of the abdomen and then through the uterus and into the amniotic fluid. A small amount of the fluid is drawn up into the needle and an attached syringe. A local anaesthetic may be applied to your abdomen before the procedure to ease any discomfort.

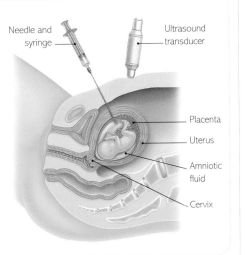

Needle and syringe

Ultrasound transducer

Placenta

Uterus

Amniotic fluid

Cervix

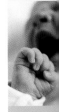

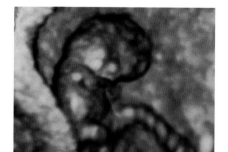

YOU ARE 12 WEEKS AND 2 DAYS

194 days to go...

YOUR BABY TODAY

In this ultrasound scan, the baby is seen floating in amniotic fluid, which provides plenty of space for him to move around in. Later in pregnancy, your baby will excrete waste products into the fluid, but his bladder is still tiny and kidney function not yet established.

The bag of amniotic fluid is your baby's home – it will keep him safe and free from infection until he is ready to be born.

Your baby is safely cushioned in the amniotic fluid. This surrounds him, gives him space to move and grow, and helps him to maintain a constant temperature.

The volume of fluid is only 1ml at seven weeks but is 25ml by this stage of your pregnancy. In about six weeks' time there will be around 60ml, with plenty of room for your baby to do lots of somersaults.

The amniotic fluid increases steadily until around 32 weeks of pregnancy, then stays constant until 37 weeks. It begins to reduce slightly thereafter by about 8 per cent per week.

Further on in the pregnancy, waste products excreted in your baby's urine will be absorbed from the fluid back into your bloodstream. At 37 weeks, your baby will urinate an astonishing one quarter to one third of his body weight every day. Compare this with your own production of 2–3 per cent body weight as urine.

Your temperature directly influences your baby's temperature. Temperature control is not an important requirement until later in pregnancy when your baby's high metabolic rate means that he needs to transfer heat to you in order to cool himself down.

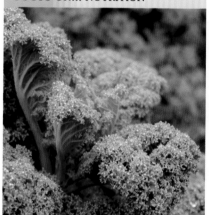

FOCUS ON... NUTRITION

Iron-rich foods

If you're suffering from pregnancy fatigue, try boosting your intake of foods that are rich in iron. Eat plenty of:
- Dark green leafy vegetables
- Red meat
- Wholegrain cereals
- Pulses
- Prune juice.

Vitamin C helps your body to absorb more iron from your diet, so try drinking fresh orange juice with meals, and limit your intake of coffee and other caffeinated drinks: caffeine inhibits your body's ability to absorb iron.

ASK A... NUTRITIONIST

My appetite has come back, but how many calories should I be eating at this stage of my pregnancy? Like many women, you're finding that the second trimester has brought relief from the discomforts of early pregnancy. As a result, you may have noticed you're less nauseous and have more of an appetite.

Calorific needs in the second trimester are approximately 2,100–2,500 calories per day, depending upon your level of physical activity. You shouldn't eat unlimited snacks, and when you do snack, opt for foods with nutritional value. For example, one banana has about 200 calories, and a handful (30g/1oz) of nuts about 180 calories. For a light 200-calorie snack, you can eat two pieces of wholemeal toast spread with a small amount of butter and jam; a small bowl of cereal with skimmed milk; or a small tin of soup with a slice of bread and butter.

If you're exercising regularly, you can of course increase your calorie intake without gaining excess weight.

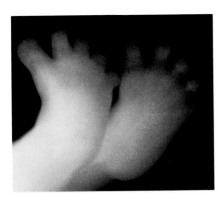

193 days to go...

YOUR BABY TODAY

The toes are now separate and are all the same length. The ankle joints are now mature enough to be working, although it will still be many weeks before you are likely to be conscious of any kicks.

As your uterus grows to accommodate your baby, you may begin to notice a few twinges around your pelvis.

There's a strong band of connective tissue in your pelvis, supporting your uterus. Known as the round ligament, this band has to stretch as your uterus expands, which can cause some discomfort. The pain is generally felt in the groin or lower abdomen and can be on either side. Although it starts in the pelvis, it may travel up to your hips. You may feel a short, sharp stabbing pain or a more prolonged, dull ache.

You will soon adapt and find sitting and lying positions that cause you the least discomfort. Paracetamol is safe to take during pregnancy, but you should take it at the lowest effective dose for the shortest possible time. Alternatively, try natural methods of pain relief, such as having a warm bath.

Round ligament pain is common in pregnancy and isn't a cause for concern. Do, however, see your doctor if sharp abdominal or pelvic pains don't resolve quickly or if your pain becomes crampy; if there is any bleeding; if there is a burning sensation when you urinate; or if you're feverish. If you're in any doubt, always seek medical advice.

The round ligaments, which help support the uterus, stretch as the uterus enlarges and pull on nearby nerve fibres and sensitive structures, causing discomfort.

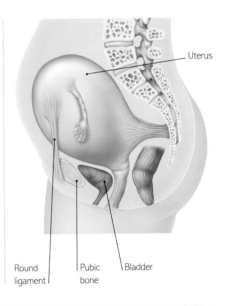

Uterus

Round ligament | Pubic bone | Bladder

FOCUS ON... TWINS

Carrying twins

If you're expecting twins, or more, it's good to know that most multiple pregnancies are straightforward and without complications. However, being pregnant with multiple babies is going to be more challenging for your body to handle than if you were carrying just one baby.

It's wise to know about the slightly higher risk of certain conditions that can occur. These include:

■ Placenta praevia (see p.212)
■ Polyhydramnios (see p.473)
■ Poor growth of one or more babies, which may be caused by twin-to-twin transfusion syndrome (see p.130)
■ Premature labour (see p.431).

The fact that any of these conditions can develop is the reason why you'll have more antenatal checks to pre-empt problems and minimize their effects.

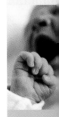

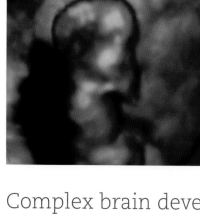

192 days to go...

YOUR BABY TODAY

By now the fetus's forehead is high and bulging, with visible joins in the plates of bone that comprise the skull. The eyes have migrated from the sides of the head at this stage of development.

Complex brain development is gradually enabling your unborn baby to become more responsive and mobile.

Your baby's brain is undergoing rapid development. The right and left cerebral hemispheres begin to connect. Each hemisphere controls the opposite side of the body, so the right side of the brain controls muscles on the left side of the body and the left side controls muscles on the right side of the body.

Motor fibres (those that control movement) mature first, so your baby can make increasingly complex limb movements. Sensory nerves (those that control feeling) mature later and are first present on your baby's hands and in his mouth. The brain matures quickly over the next three weeks and will be complete in around 10 weeks' time, as the rest of the upper and lower limbs and trunk achieve adult levels of sensitivity to stimuli. All your baby's nerves are very immature at this stage and he doesn't have any perception of position, pain, temperature, or touch.

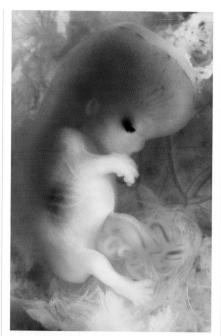

As your baby's brain develops, he is able to make larger movements with his arms and legs, but this activity won't be well co-ordinated at this stage.

FOCUS ON... NUTRITION

Yummy yogurt

For a calcium-packed snack, stock up on yogurt. Those with so-called "friendly" bacteria" are okay to eat during pregnancy and may help your digestion. Just make sure that the milk ingredients in your yogurts have been pasteurized to reduce the risk of infection with listeria (see p.17).

ASK A... MIDWIFE

I've been diagnosed with diabetes. How will this affect my pregnancy? Whether you develop diabetes in pregnancy (known as gestational diabetes), or have pre-existing diabetes, you will require special care from a diabetic healthcare team and a consultant obstetrician. This is because diabetes poses risks in pregnancy, particularly if there is poor control of blood-sugar levels.

All this can be managed with close antenatal care: your blood sugar needs to be well controlled as your insulin requirements will increase during pregnancy. You will also need to adapt your diet and may need insulin injections.

Pregnant women who are diabetic are at a greater risk of high blood pressure, blood clots, and pre-eclampsia (see p.474). If you have diabetic kidney disease, or diabetic retinopathy, a condition that affects the retina in the eye, there's a chance it will worsen during pregnancy. For your baby, there is an increased risk of congenital abnormalities and growth may be too fast or too slow.

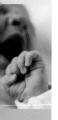

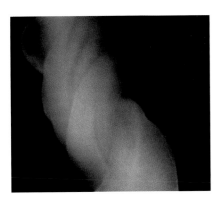

191 days to go...

YOUR BABY TODAY

This image is a close-up of your baby's umbilical cord. The umbilical arteries can be seen as they carry blood from the baby to the placenta. As there are no nerve fibres in the cord, your baby is unaware that this is happening – or even that the cord is there.

You and your partner will be developing your own special relationship with your baby.

At this point in your pregnancy, you won't be able to feel your baby move. It will also be a little while before your baby will be able to hear (see p.238) and recognize your voice and that of your partner, or hear other sounds, such as music. Nevertheless, some women still enjoy talking to their babies, feeling that it brings them closer to the baby, and it certainly does no harm! Do whatever feels natural for you, whether that is talking out loud or in your head.

You might want to think of an interim name for your baby. This might be "the bump" or "the bean" or an in-joke between you and your partner. It can be helpful to give your baby an identity because it's difficult to talk about him or her at this relatively early stage, and when you don't know the gender.

If you're still keeping the pregnancy a secret in some quarters, using a code phrase to refer to the pregnancy may be useful in some circumstances.

AS A MATTER OF FACT

Your baby's many different movements are vital for his development.

As your baby twists and stretches his body, flails his arms and legs, and moves his head, he is helping his skin to grow normally and his bones, muscles, and joints to mature.

ACTIVITIES TO AVOID IN THE SECOND TRIMESTER

The second trimester is generally when fatigue lifts, and you begin to feel more energetic. This is a great time to continue your exercise programme, making good use of your increased energy levels before you are too big and too uncomfortable to move and enjoy being fully active.

While you're encouraged to continue to exercise during the second trimester, there are some high-risk exercises that should be avoided. You should avoid any activity that potentially could cause you to fall, activities that involve a high degree of balance and agility, and specifically exercises that require lying on your back for extended

periods, or twisting of the upper body. Changes in your centre of gravity can increase the chances of stumbling and falling, risking injury to you and your baby.

The following activities are best avoided during your second (and third) trimesters:
- Vigorous exercise at a high altitude (unless you are used to it)
- Diving and scuba diving
- Road or mountain cycling
- Rock climbing
- Skiing, snow boarding, and waterskiing
- Ice skating/ice hockey
- Horseriding
- Bungee-jumping!

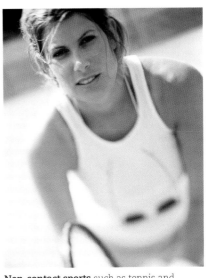

Non-contact sports such as tennis and badminton are ideal in the second trimester as there is a low risk of injury. Play opponents at a similar, not higher, standard to yourself so that you don't over-exert yourself.

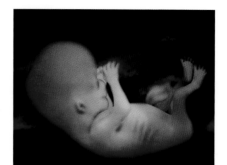

190 days to go...

YOUR BABY TODAY

The developing eyes are now facing forwards. The right eye, along with the baby's right ear, can be seen here. Your baby spends most of the time in a curled position, often with legs crossed, and hands close to the face.

It's never too early to start planning what you'll need to buy for your baby, even if you don't want to start shopping just yet.

Now that you're in your safer second trimester, you may be tempted to start buying a few baby items, unless you're superstitious and would prefer to wait. A good reason to start shopping in this trimester is that your energy levels should be at their pregnancy peak. In later months, you will find it too tiring to carry your bump, as well as your bags, around the shops and having a good browse may not be your favourite pastime.

Even if you're not shopping yet, start planning. Ask friends to recommend their favourite buggies, cots, slings, and car seats, then check prices so you can plan your budget. You might also find that family and friends offer second-hand goods you can buy or borrow.

If you purchase new baby clothes, leave the tags on and check the shop's return policy in case you have a baby who's too big for the newborn clothes or you decide against the items you've bought.

I've just told my parents I'm pregnant but they reacted very negatively because they don't approve of my partner. What can I do? First, give them time to come to terms with the news. Creating a baby with someone is the ultimate commitment, and marks an important life-changing event. For your parents, it is a signal that your partner isn't going anywhere, however much they might disapprove of him.

Once things have calmed down, suggest that your parents take the pregnancy as an opportunity to re-establish their relationship with your partner and wipe the slate clean. Reassure them that you and your partner very much want them to be a part of their grandchild's life, and that you'd rather clear the air now, so that there aren't any negative feelings and tension once your baby is born.

Remember that all is likely to be forgotten when your parents hold a much-loved grandchild in their arms, and as part of that baby will be your partner's that should help them to feel warmer towards him.

FOCUS ON... YOUR BODY

Managing hair growth

Changing hormones can play havoc with hair growth. To deal with any new unwanted hair:
- **Shave larger areas** and pluck out the odd stray hair.
- **Depilatory creams and hair-lightening bleaches** are probably safe to use but insufficient research has been carried out. They can be absorbed through the skin.
- **If you're waxing** or using a sugaring solution, be aware that your skin may be more sensitive.
- **Laser and electrolysis** treatments are safe as they don't penetrate the skin enough to be harmful.

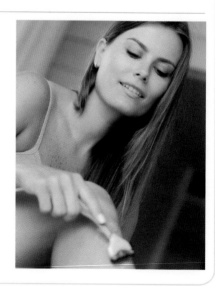

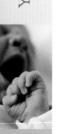

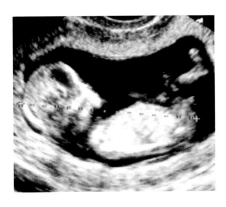

189 days to go...

YOUR BABY TODAY

This 2D black-and-white ultrasound scan is similar to the scan you may see and may be given. The baby is the central white area, and the amniotic fluid is black. This type of scan is the best way to measure your baby's length at this stage.

Your hormones have done all the hard work to establish your pregnancy and as they settle down, so should your nausea.

AS A MATTER OF FACT

Your immune system weakens during pregnancy to stop your body rejecting your developing baby.

This, unfortunately, makes you more prone to colds and bugs. As an added burden, pregnancy hormones can worsen a blocked nose and nausea.

Morning sickness usually subsides around the start of the second trimester. It's believed that the rapid hormonal changes required to establish and maintain the pregnancy in the early stages may cause the sickness. By this stage your pregnancy is well established and your baby's major internal organs and support system are fully formed, so these hormone levels start to stabilize. This may be why the nausea passes.

Furthermore, there is a theory that nausea is the body's way of protecting your baby from harmful substances in the early crucial stages of development, so you become naturally adverse to alcohol and junk food, for example.

If your nausea and sickness hasn't begun to subside by this stage don't worry as for some women it does continue into the second trimester. See your doctor or midwife if you are concerned about your level of sickness.

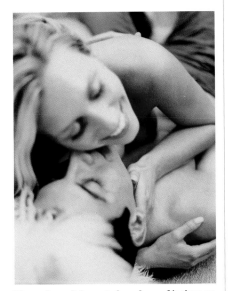

There doesn't have to be a loss of intimacy, even if you and your partner are having less sex. Take the time to be affectionate and show your partner you want to be physically close.

ASK A... MUM

My partner hasn't wanted sex at all since I've become pregnant. Will he ever fancy me again? Yes! Although it's difficult, try not to take his reluctance to have sex personally. When I was pregnant, my husband didn't want to have penetrative sex, and most of his fears centred around harming the baby or me. This was made worse by the fact that I'd taken a long time to get pregnant, and was also having a difficult pregnancy, with lots of nausea and sickness.

We spoke to our midwife and she was able to reassure my partner that he couldn't harm the baby in any way by having penetrative sex. She also told us that it wasn't uncommon

for either partner to experience a reduced sexual desire in pregnancy for a variety of reasons. Although many women experience an increased libido at this stage of pregnancy, the same may not be true for their partner.

It's important that you talk to your partner to find out his fears and explain your own thoughts and feelings. Don't let this issue cause an argument between you. Each couple is different and you will need to talk to each other to find your way through this problem.

You may also find it helpful to talk to someone who isn't so closely involved, such as your midwife, doctor, or a trusted friend.

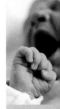

Your 14th week

THERE ARE SUBTLE CHANGES HAPPENING TO YOUR SHAPE THAT ONLY YOU WILL NOTICE

Your baby isn't big enough to give you an obvious pregnancy bump, but you'll definitely notice your waistline become thicker. At this stage of pregnancy, many women feel re-energized and have a strong sense of wellbeing. Healthy eating is very important, so be clued up about the best food choices. In particular, your body needs plenty of protein; and your baby needs it, too, to sustain her rapid growth.

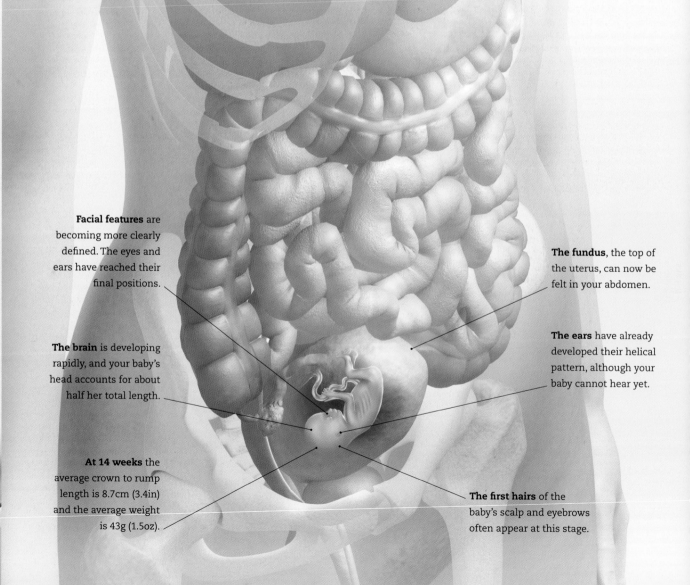

Facial features are becoming more clearly defined. The eyes and ears have reached their final positions.

The fundus, the top of the uterus, can now be felt in your abdomen.

The brain is developing rapidly, and your baby's head accounts for about half her total length.

The ears have already developed their helical pattern, although your baby cannot hear yet.

At 14 weeks the average crown to rump length is 8.7cm (3.4in) and the average weight is 43g (1.5oz).

The first hairs of the baby's scalp and eyebrows often appear at this stage.

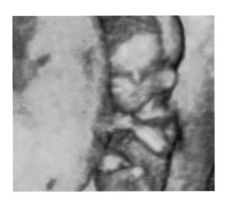

188 days to go...

YOUR BABY TODAY

It's easy to see where your baby's bones are on an ultrasound as they show up as brighter areas. Other features may be harder to see. If you have a scan and are unsure what you are looking at, ask your doctor or midwife to interpret it for you.

Relief, excitement, apprehension... it's normal to feel all this and more at this stage of your pregnancy.

While you're undoubtedly feeling better physically, and probably have lots more energy, you may still be up and down emotionally. This is completely normal.

This stage of pregnancy can be a very emotional time: reaching the second trimester is a pregnancy milestone and coincides with seeing your baby on the scan (see p.138). You know that, with the chances of miscarrying now being so minimal, you're really going to have a baby. However, like many pregnant women, you may find that the feeling of relief at reaching this stage is followed by occasional anxieties.

One good outlet for all this emotional energy is exercising, which you may find easier now you're over the first trimester fatigue. Exercise releases endorphins, the feel-good hormones, and so can improve your emotional as well as physical wellbeing, but always exercise safely (see box, below).

see p.138

AS A MATTER OF FACT

Exercising may reduce the time you are in labour.

Research has shown that women who exercise at a moderate to high intensity can cut their time in labour by up to three hours, and they tend to have less complicated deliveries than those who don't exercise.

LISTENING TO YOUR BODY

Check with your midwife or doctor whether there's any reason why you shouldn't be exercising; there are certain pregnancy conditions, such as placenta praevia (see p.212) and the risk of premature labour, that may preclude you from exercising.

When exercising during pregnancy, always use your common sense and look out for symptoms that may indicate you are exercising too hard. Aerobic exercise is often tracked by measuring the heart rate, but this is difficult during pregnancy as there is a natural increase in your heart rate, even at rest. So the most effective way to keep your exercise at a safe level is the talk test: you should be able to carry out a conversation while exercising. This will indicate that you are not exercising to exhaustion and potentially restricting the oxygen flow to your baby.

There are other symptoms that indicate you're exercising too hard or should not be exercising at all:
- Vaginal bleeding
- Dizziness and headaches
- Chest pain
- Extreme and sudden muscle weakness
- Calf pain and leg swelling
- Leakage of amniotic fluid.

If you suffer from any of the above symptoms, even momentarily, stop exercising and seek medical advice.

see p.212

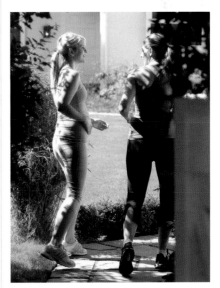

Rather than taking a gentle stroll, try walking at a brisk pace, but make sure you can still talk. This will ensure you're exercising at a moderate aerobic level.

Your 14th week

161

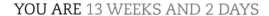

187 days to go...

YOUR BABY TODAY

This scan shows a cross-section of your baby's brain, with the two hemispheres clearly seen. From this point on, your baby's brain measurement from one side to the other, taken just above the ear, is used as a reliable indicator of her growth and development.

Even at this early stage of development, your baby has started to urinate, although in very small quantities.

Your baby's bladder now fills and empties every 30 minutes; she swallows the amniotic fluid, filters it through her kidneys, and then passes it as urine. The bladder volume is tiny at this stage, and even by 32 weeks it will only be 10ml, reaching 40ml by 40 weeks. Your baby produces very dilute urine, having only a limited capacity to reabsorb water in the kidney to concentrate the urine. However, the placenta performs most of the kidney functions until birth.

Your baby's blood system can now make and break down blood clots. The placenta has been able to form clots for some time, reducing the risk of bleeding.

A small number of white blood cells are now being produced by your baby but she is still relying on yours to fight infection. Her red blood cells contain haemoglobin that transfers oxygen to all the cells of the body. Before birth she has several forms of haemoglobin that differ from yours. These are more stable at a lower acidity and bind more easily to oxygen. This allows your baby's body to extract the oxygen in your haemoglobin for her own use.

The toes are now fully formed and separated, and their individual bones can be clearly discerned on an ultrasound.

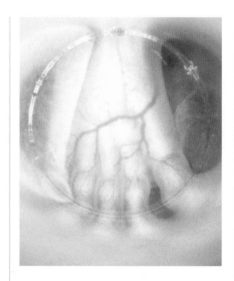

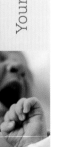

ASK A... DOCTOR

I'm expecting triplets. How will my antenatal care differ? All the usual risks of pregnancy are increased for women having more than one baby. This is partly because hormone levels are higher when there is more than one baby, and, in your case, it will be hard work for your body to carry and nourish three fetuses.

You can expect to be referred to an obstetrician, who will plan your antenatal care with you. You'll have more frequent checkups and scans to check the health and progress of your babies. Although many of the risks are outside your control, if you attend all your appointments and look after your health, it is likely that you will have three healthy babies.

With triplets, you will probably need to give birth by Caesarean section. The average pregnancy length for triplets is 34 weeks.

For more information about multiple pregnancy and details of local support groups, contact the Twins and Multiple Births Association (TAMBA) (see p.481).

TIME TO THINK ABOUT

Amniocentesis

This involves testing the amniotic fluid and is normally done at 15–20 weeks (see pp.152–3). It may be offered:

■ **Where there's** a family or pregnancy history of a genetic problem.
■ **To older women** who are more at risk of having a baby with a chromosomal abnormality.
■ **When a screening test** (see pp. 142–3) has shown there is a high risk of a chromosomal abnormality.

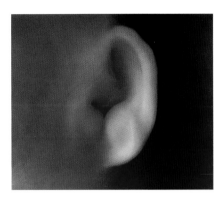

186 days to go...

YOUR BABY TODAY

It is surprising how much detail is already present in your baby's body. This close-up of an ear shows that its helical pattern of folds is nearly fully developed, although it is still too soon for your baby to hear anything.

Your waistline will be increasing and your body shape changing but your bump is unlikely to be very prominent for several weeks.

By week 14, if you stand in your underwear in front of the mirror, you will see a change in your body shape, but to the outside world you may not look very different. Women who have previously been pregnant tend to show earlier than those who are pregnant for the first time, as their stomach muscles have already been stretched once and so stretch much more quickly.

Women often say that this is the time when they look as though they have put on weight and feel fat, not pregnant! But it won't be long before your bump will be visible for the world to see.

If you're feeling uncomfortable and heavy, make sure you choose the right clothes. See page 151 for some tips on how to adapt your wardrobe without having to spend any money yet.

ASK A... MIDWIFE

Is it safe to use complementary therapies? Complementary therapies can help with some pregnancy discomforts. If you're seeing a practitioner, make sure that he or she is registered and experienced in treating pregnant women. "Natural" doesn't mean "safe"; only use therapies that are known to be safe in pregnancy.

USING ESSENTIAL OILS

Aromatherapy uses essential oils extracted from plant sources. These can be effective remedies for some complaints, but not all are safe in pregnancy (see below, right). Essential oils need to be diluted in carrier oil for massage, or alternatively can be added to a bath or diffused in a lamp or burner. Guidelines should always be printed on the label, so make sure you check these before use.

You can use:
- Lavender
- Roman camomile
- Rose
- Orange
- Bergamot
- Grapefruit
- Lemon
- Neroli
- Patchouli
- Sandalwood
- Spearmint
- Tea tree
- Vetiver.

Essential oils have not been tested on pregnant women for obvious reasons but, based on the properties they contain, the advice is to err on the side of caution and avoid those that are known to cause cramping or contractions, as well as those that thin the blood.

Don't use: basil; cedarwood; cinnamon; clary sage; cypress; clove; fennel; hyssop; jasmine; juniper; lemongrass; myrrh; parsley; pennyroyal; rosemary; sweet marjoram; thyme; peppermint.

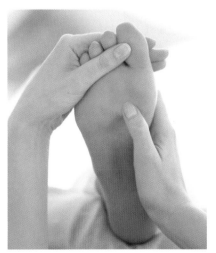

Reflexology is a complementary therapy that involves applying pressure to reflexes on the hands and feet. It's believed to help with morning sickness, backache, fluid retention, and swelling during pregnancy.

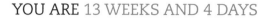

185 days to go...

YOUR BABY TODAY

Whether your baby's legs are crossed or uncrossed, it is very difficult to tell from an ultrasound at this stage whether your baby is a boy or girl: male and female look too similar to reliably tell them apart.

Your baby's central nervous system, consisting of the brain and spinal cord, now has all its basic components.

The core development of your baby's central nervous system has taken place, and it will now progress further using four overlapping processes. The number of nerve cells increases and their positions alter during migration – a process by which cells move to their final locations and develop specific functions. The connections between individual nerve cells become more organized, and the fibres become insulated.

The growth of the nervous system now enters its most active phase. Reflecting this, the head accounts for half of the entire length of the baby. Both the nerves and their supporting cells increase in number. Although most of the nerve cells are produced during pregnancy, the supporting cells continue to increase in number during your baby's first year. The supporting cells assist in the migration process, which is largely completed by 22 weeks.

ASK A... MIDWIFE

Can I carry on jogging? There's no reason why not if you were a regular runner before you became pregnant, but do take it easy – now is not the time to run a marathon!

You need to avoid becoming overheated so don't jog on hot days and drink plenty of water, regardless of the temperature. Wear a good sports bra to support your growing breasts. Whenever you can, run on soft surfaces, such as grass, to reduce the stress on your joints, especially your knees.

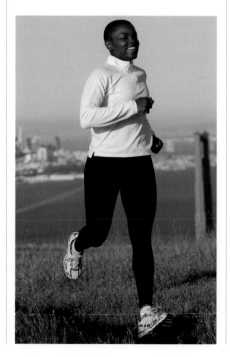

Jogging is a good aerobic activity during pregnancy in the early months, but is only advised if you're used to running. Don't take it up as a new activity in pregnancy.

Perfect pork

Pork is an excellent source of protein, vitamin B6, and zinc – which are all essential nutrients for pregnancy. Pork has a reputation as a fatty meat, but this is not deserved; it is probably due to the fact that some cuts can be fatty, such as spare ribs, bacon, and ham, but many cuts of pork have less saturated fat than beef.

The key to eating healthily is to look for the leanest cuts. These usually have the word "loin" in the name, such as tenderloin or top loin chop. Pork tenderloin is, in fact, lower in fat than skinless chicken breasts. A serving of pork should be approximately 85g (3oz).

Pork is healthy and delicious, and quick and easy to prepare. Sprinkle some salt on lean pork chops, grill, and serve with some apple sauce on the side; your craving for something both salty and sweet can be met in a healthy way. Always make sure that the pork is prepared on a separate chopping board from other foods and thoroughly cooked (see p.104).

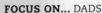

184 days to go...

YOUR BABY TODAY

At this stage the head, although still large, has a much more rounded shape than before and, as the jaw and neck lengthen, the chin moves away from the neck. An ultrasound now will show the thumb as distinct from the fingers.

It's only a minor pregnancy symptom, but nasal congestion can happen most days – and make you a snorer at night!

Is your partner nudging you in the night because you're keeping him awake? It's common for pregnant women to snore. This is largely due to increased swelling of the nasal passages, but it can also be caused by increased weight and the fact that you may roll over on to your back during the night.

Your stuffy nose is due to the increased volume of blood in your body while you're pregnant. This can cause congestion and make your ears feel blocked, too. Nosebleeds are also very common in pregnancy; some women find that every time they blow their nose they have a small amount of bleeding. This is because the blood vessels in the nose are very fragile, and with the increased volume of blood flowing through them, they tend to bleed more easily. However, the bleeding should be very light.

To treat a nosebleed, tip your head forward and pinch the middle of your nose (in the soft part) hard. It should stop quickly. If it doesn't, try an icepack on the nose to help the blood vessels constrict. In the rare situation of heavy bleeding, go to the hospital. Seek medical advice if you are getting heavy bleeding regularly.

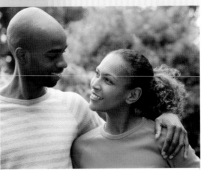

FOCUS ON... DADS

Looking forward

During the first trimester, you probably anxiously awaited developments in the pregnancy and supported your partner when the going got tough. Now that her early pregnancy symptoms, such as nausea and sickness and fatigue, are likely to have passed, and the risk of miscarriage is reduced, you may begin to feel differently about the pregnancy and your future.

As your partner starts to show increasing strength and vigour, and her body shape and small bump become noticeable, you may find that the reality of the pregnancy hits you. At this point your sense of trepidation will probably turn to optimism as you both look forward.

ASK A... NUTRITIONIST

Is it safe to eat peanuts or foods containing them during pregnancy? If you would like to eat peanuts or food containing peanuts (such as peanut butter) during pregnancy, you can choose to do so as part of a healthy balanced diet, unless you are allergic to them or a health professional advises you not to.

The UK government previously advised women to avoid eating peanuts in pregnancy or when breastfeeding if you, your partner, or your baby's siblings suffer from asthma, eczema, hay fever, or other allergies.

This advice has changed because recent studies have suggested that avoiding peanuts during pregnancy may be increasing the incidence of allergies, pinpointing countries where peanuts are a staple food and allergies relatively rare. The latest research also shows that there is no clear evidence to say if eating peanuts during pregnancy affects the chances of your baby developing a peanut allergy.

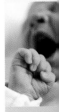

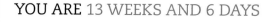

YOU ARE 13 WEEKS AND 6 DAYS

183 days to go...

YOUR BABY TODAY

In this coloured ultrasound image the baby is red and the placenta green. It is just possible to see the two crosses that measure the depth of fluid in the nuchal fold at the back of the neck (see p.143). Now is the last opportunity to measure this reliably.

Your baby is growing and getting stronger every day, and it's all thanks to her life support system – the placenta.

Your baby's rapid growth
continues and her weight will increase during the next three weeks from 43g (1.5oz) to 140g (4.9oz). Muscle and bone growth advances, but, although all joints are present, it will be three weeks before the skeleton begins to harden.

Your baby is now totally dependent on the placenta for her nourishment. Environmental factors have almost no influence on your baby's size at this stage; all babies up until around 20 weeks' gestation are the same size.

The placenta is larger than your baby and supplies all the nutrients she needs. To aid her growth, the placenta extracts amino acids from your circulation, giving her high levels. Amino acids are the building blocks of protein, from which muscles and organs develop.

FOCUS ON... NUTRITION

Protein plus

Protein is required for the development of the baby and placenta, as well as to fuel changes taking place in your body (see p.14). The protein requirement for pregnancy is 60g (2oz) daily, instead of the usual 50g (1.8oz). Include a source in all three meals daily. Protein sources include meat, poultry, fish, milk, cheese, beans, nuts, and seeds.

The best protein foods are those that are lower in saturated fat and cholesterol. Trim the fat off meat and eat one or two servings of fish (see p.96) or seafood. When choosing dairy products, pick skimmed milk and low-fat cheeses. These retain all the protein benefits of the full-fat versions. Nuts and seeds are rich in heart-healthy oils. Vegetarians need to eat a wide range of plant proteins to ensure they are getting adequate amino acids (see p.126).

The umbilical cord can be seen connecting this 13-week-old fetus with the placenta, which nourishes your baby. The incredible blood vessels of the placenta are clearly visible in the background.

Your second trimester

166

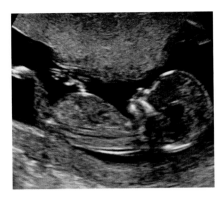

182 days to go...

YOUR BABY TODAY

This 2D ultrasound shows the profile of the baby particularly well. The nasal bone can just be seen at the bridge of the nose, as can bright echoes from the lower and upper jaws; the umbilical cord is rising from the centre of the abdomen.

It can be difficult to avoid information overload – everyone, it seems, will have advice to share with you.

ASK A... DOCTOR

Why are varicose veins common in pregnancy and what can I do to avoid getting them? Your blood volume increases up to 30 per cent during pregnancy, due to the added needs of your baby and your expanding body. In addition, the hormone relaxin (which is produced to soften ligaments and joints) also softens the walls of your blood vessels. The blood vessels relax and the increased blood and extra weight of the baby make you susceptible to varicose veins.

To reduce the likelihood of getting varicose veins:

■ **Avoid sitting or standing in one position** for prolonged periods: walk around regularly, moving your arms as you do so to increase the blood flow in your body.

■ **Exercise daily:** most forms of cardiovascular exercise will help to increase blood flow. Aquarobics is a good choice as the pressure of the water helps to increase blood circulation.

■ **Sleep with your legs slightly elevated** by placing a pillow under your bottom sheet at the end of your bed.

One side-effect of pregnancy all women have to deal with is conflicting information and advice. One article says to do something, while a friend says the exact opposite. It can be confusing and irritating. While you can choose to stop reading a newspaper or turn over to a different television channel, it's more difficult to avoid the unwanted advice of other women. Even more difficult is the advice from close relatives, such as your mother and mother-in-law. You'll need the support of your family and friends,

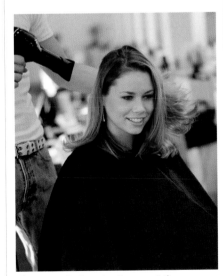

The second trimester is a great time to pamper yourself with a new haircut and colour. Your new hairstyle will complement your glowing skin.

so won't want to alienate them, but don't feel pressured to act in a certain way. Also don't reject everything straightaway – some of the advice may in fact be useful and accurate.

If someone is persistently advising you explain that you're overwhelmed by information and would rather not talk about the pregnancy at this time. Or listen to the person's advice, smile politely, and then do as you wish. You could subtly hint that you will ask for advice as and when you need it.

FOCUS ON... YOUR BODY

Style challenge

Give yourself a hair makeover.

■ **There is no evidence** that the chemicals in hair dyes are dangerous in pregnancy. Most permanent and non-permanent dyes contain chemicals that are unlikely to be toxic when used in the small amounts taken to dye hair, and only every few months.

■ **If you're worried** use natural dyes or stick to highlights, which don't expose the whole scalp to dye.

■ **When colouring your own hair,** do so in a well-ventilated space and always wear the gloves provided.

Your 15th week

START TALKING TO YOUR BABY – HE CAN HEAR YOUR VOICE

Like many pregnant women in the second trimester, you may now be reaping the benefits of the pregnancy "glow", as hormones improve the appearance of your skin and hair. Enjoy this time and the attention that often comes with it. Amazingly, your baby's ears have formed enough for him to hear you speaking. He'll recognize your voice – and your partner's – when he comes out into the world.

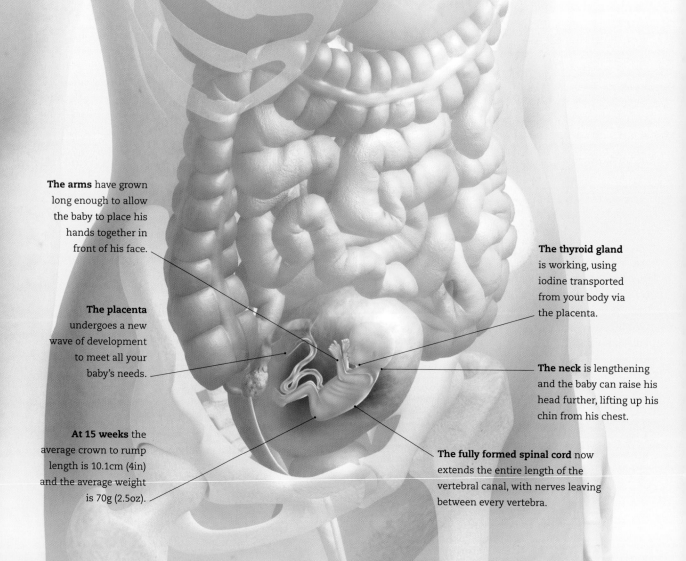

The arms have grown long enough to allow the baby to place his hands together in front of his face.

The placenta undergoes a new wave of development to meet all your baby's needs.

At 15 weeks the average crown to rump length is 10.1cm (4in) and the average weight is 70g (2.5oz).

The thyroid gland is working, using iodine transported from your body via the placenta.

The neck is lengthening and the baby can raise his head further, lifting up his chin from his chest.

The fully formed spinal cord now extends the entire length of the vertebral canal, with nerves leaving between every vertebra.

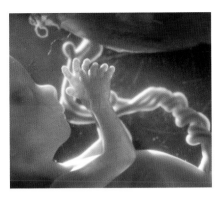

181 days to go...

YOUR BABY TODAY

At this stage, the fetus's forearms, wrists, hands, and fingers are all well differentiated. The eyes, which are visible as dark areas behind the sealed eyelids, have migrated inwards from the sides of the head.

Now that some pregnancy discomforts have passed and while you await your bump, you may feel strangely "normal".

You may not feel as though you are pregnant at the moment. The beginning of the second trimester is an interesting transition period: you know you're expecting a baby – you've seen the ultrasound scan – but you may not look or feel that pregnant, and you won't feel the baby move for several weeks yet (see p.213).

The physical reminders that were common in the first trimester – such as nausea and fatigue – may have greatly lessened or passed altogether.

Many women say they feel completely ordinary and find this strange because they think that they "should" be feeling something. Try to enjoy this time and keep looking at that scan picture if you need a reminder that your baby is there. You may long to feel normal once you hit the third trimester and some of that fatigue returns.

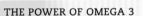

THE POWER OF OMEGA 3

It's a fact that what you eat could make your baby's brain and nervous system work better. Recent studies suggest that women who eat a diet rich in omega-3 fatty acids during pregnancy and breastfeeding may enhance their baby's language development, IQ, and cognitive development. These essential fatty acids may also decrease allergies in children of mothers who consume them during pregnancy and breastfeeding, and help to decrease postnatal depression.

Omega-3 fatty acids are found in oily fish. In fact, only seafood contains all three essential omega-3 fatty acids; essential because the body can't manufacture them.

Although fish is a main source of omega 3, you need to ensure you don't consume varieties that are high in mercury (see p.96). Salmon and sardines are two oily fish that are low in mercury yet rich in omega-3 fatty acids. Wild salmon is a particularly rich, and delicious, source of these healthy fatty acids.

Other non-seafood sources of omega-3 fatty acids are canola (rapeseed) oil, walnuts, flaxseed, and omega-3 enriched eggs. These sources contain only one essential omega-3 fatty acid, but it is still worth eating them. Note that flaxseed, which is also a great source of fibre, must be ground for the body to absorb it. Sprinkle it on cereal or yogurt.

FOCUS ON... DADS

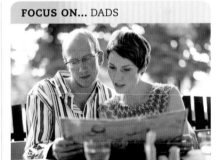

The two of you

Make the effort to set aside time for you and your partner to be alone together while she's pregnant. Whether it's an evening out once a week, or that weekend away you've been promising yourselves for an age, do it now! Remember, the second trimester is also a good time to go on holiday (see p.185).

It's common for there to be fundamental changes to a relationship when a baby arrives; some new fathers feel a bit pushed out, especially in the early weeks. By spending time together now, you will build a greater bond for when the baby is born and feel satisfied that you enjoyed lots of pleasurable time together during the pregnancy.

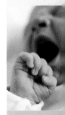

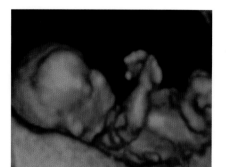

180 days to go...

YOUR BABY TODAY

In this 3D ultrasound scan, the baby is lying on his back. The arms and legs have lengthened and the baby is able to move them freely. His head is still relatively large compared to the trunk and the forehead bulges out.

He's well-developed on the outside, but complex changes are taking place as your baby's internal organs continue to mature.

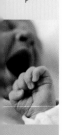

WORKING DURING PREGNANCY

The majority of employers are supportive when they find out an employee is pregnant, and hopefully this will be the case for you. However, should a problem arise, there is employment law in place to protect pregnant women:

■ **You can't be sacked** during pregnancy, unless you breach the terms of your agreement.

■ **You can't be made redundant** because you're pregnant or on maternity leave. However, if the reason for the redundancy is a legitimate one, unconnected with your pregnancy, it is allowed.

■ **Your employer** has extra responsibilities when you're pregnant, and these include ensuring that your workplace is safe. For example, you should be protected from handling or lifting heavy loads, standing or sitting for long periods of time, handling toxic substances, or working long hours.

■ **You're entitled** to a "reasonable" amount of paid time off for antenatal appointments.

■ **Symptoms of pregnancy** are considered an illness and can be a valid reason for sick leave.

Your baby's neck is growing, and he's now looking more and more like a human being. Internally, the thyroid gland first develops at the base of the tongue but gradually moves down to lie in the neck, overlying the trachea (windpipe). The thyroid gland is producing the hormone thyroxine, using iodine transported from your body across the placenta.

ASK A... DOCTOR

I've developed a dark vertical line down the middle of my tummy. What is this? This line is called the linea nigra, which occurs due to

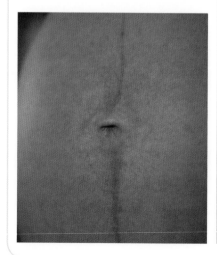

The baby's kidneys are starting to function. The nephrons in the kidneys are lengthening and maturing: these essential units enable the kidney to function by filtering the blood and eliminating waste from the body.

New nephrons will be produced up until the 37th week and the kidneys continue to lengthen by around 1mm a week during the entire pregnancy.

changes in skin pigmentation. It's extremely common, affecting 90 per cent of all pregnant women in some way or another, and is often more noticeable if you are darker skinned.

You may also notice a darkening of the skin around your nipples and a darkening of freckles, moles, or birthmarks. A few women may also experience brown patches on their face called chloasma or the "mask of pregnancy" (see pp.190 and 467). These changes are caused by the extra amounts of the hormone oestrogen during pregnancy, which affects the melanin-producing cells of the skin – these cells produce the pigment that darkens the skin. These colour changes are normal and will usually fade once the baby is born.

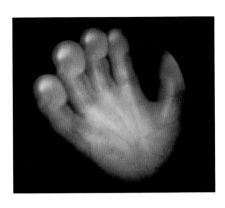

179 days to go...

YOUR BABY TODAY

The hands are well developed at this stage, but, as can be seen here, the skin is very thin and transparent, which means the developing bones of the fingers and the blood vessels can be seen.

Your baby's external sex organs are now visible and it may be possible to identify gender from an ultrasound scan.

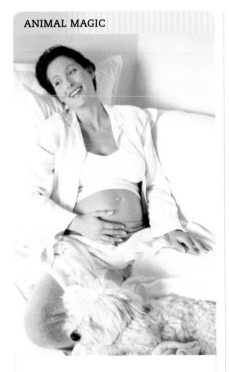

ANIMAL MAGIC

Do you share your home with a pet? Recent research shows that living with a cat or dog in early childhood may reduce the risk of your child developing asthmatic symptoms. The study found that children residing with cats were more likely to have allergy-related antibodies to felines. Never leave your baby alone with a dog or cat.

By around this point in the second trimester, the sex of the baby's external genitals has become apparent. When the genitals first began to form at around four weeks, they were the same in males and females. They consisted of a rounded bump called the genital tubercle and two ridges called labioscrotal swellings separated by a membrane. From around six weeks, differences started to occur, driven by the presence or absence of a male (Y) chromosome (see p.200). By the 14th week, in boys the genital tubercle has elongated to become the penis and the labioscrotal swellings have fused to form the scrotum. In girls the labioscrotal swellings remain separate, forming the labia (lips), while the genital tubercle forms the clitoris.

ASK A... MIDWIFE

How can I relieve my constipation?
Constipation is a common symptom of pregnancy, mainly because the hormone progesterone slows down your bowel function, making everything more sluggish. Many women exercise less than usual during pregnancy, which can also cause things to become blocked up. Finally, iron tablets, which may be prescribed for anaemia, are notorious for causing constipation.

There are, thankfully, many ways to relieve the problem:
■ **Eat more fibre:** ensure that you are getting plenty of fibre in your diet, in the form of fresh fruit and vegetables, and wholegrains, and drink plenty of water to aid the passing of your stools.
■ **Go natural:** studies have shown that psyllium husks, from the crushed seeds of the *Plantago ovata* plant, are an effective natural remedy.
■ **Try reflexology:** this has been shown to be an effective treatment: one study found that 85 per cent of women reported a positive result, and regular bowel movements. Visit a registered therapist, who is experienced in treating pregnant women, or do a little yourself at home. Try massaging the base of the heel of your foot, and the arch, pushing your thumb evenly and deeply into the tissue of your foot.
■ **Massage:** gently rub your abdomen with two drops of bergamot essential oil, blended in a tablespoon of light carrier oil, such as grapeseed.

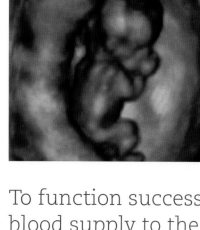

178 days to go...

YOUR BABY TODAY

In this image the placenta can be seen to the left of the baby. The placenta is still very much larger than your baby and is growing at a faster rate, preparing to meet the demands of your baby, who will later overtake it in size and weight.

To function successfully, the placenta needs a good maternal blood supply to the arteries in the wall of the uterus.

The placenta now starts a second wave of growth that will take almost six weeks. The outer layer of cells in the placenta move into the coiled, or spiral, arteries in the uterus, destroying their muscular wall. This causes the arteries to dilate, resulting in a low resistance to blood flow. Only those arteries beneath the placenta (80–100 vessels) are invaded by the placental cells in this way. If these cells move too deeply, they can fuse too tightly with the muscle of the uterus and have difficulty separating after delivery. If the wave of invading cells is inadequate, however, the low resistance to blood flow doesn't develop. This can increase the risk of the mother developing pre-eclampsia (see p.474), and cause the baby growth problems.

AS A MATTER OF FACT

It is a native Hawaiian belief that the placenta is part of the child.

It is a tradition to plant the placenta with a tree, which then grows alongside the child.

ASK A... MIDWIFE

I'm trying to stay out of the sun but is it okay to use fake tanning lotions? Fake tanning lotions are probably safe to use but they have not been tested on pregnant women so their effects aren't known. It may be better to err on the side of caution and go without a tan while you're pregnant. Bear in mind that fake tan does not protect your skin so, if you do wear it, you'll need to wear additional protection when you are out in the sunlight.

Do not, under any circumstances, take tanning pills. These are banned in the UK. They contain beta-carotene or canthaxanthin and can be toxic to your unborn baby, and also have been known to cause hepatitis and eye damage.

SLEEP REMEDIES

Even though you may not need to go to the toilet as much during the night as you did in the first trimester, and may not yet be suffering from too many aches and pains, sleep may still escape you in the second trimester.

You may find that during this life-changing time you may be having especially vivid dreams, which can disrupt your sleep. Even if you're feeling well, it's essential to get adequate sleep: after all, your body is working hard to create another life. To get more sleep:
■ **Eat a late-night snack** containing the amino acid tryptophan (see p.177), which is sleep-inducing.
■ **Place a few drops of lavender oil** on your pillow to aid sleep or use it in a bath (see right).

■ **Cut down on caffeine** (see p.66) and make camomile tea your bedtime drink instead.
■ **Have a bath before bedtime,** and add a few drops of relaxing lavender oil. Make sure the water isn't hot as this can stimulate rather than relax.

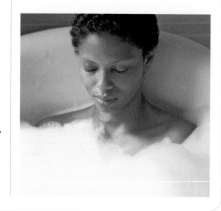

Your second trimester

177 days to go...

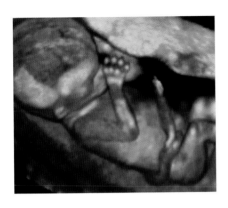

YOUR BABY TODAY

This 3D ultrasound shows the hands held up in front of the face. The knees seem "knobbly" with every bone clear to see on the scan. The soft spot on the baby's head can also be seen: this protects the brain while still allowing for its rapid growth.

You might receive some compliments, because at this stage of pregnancy you're likely to look glowing with good health.

The terms "blooming" or "glowing" are often used to describe pregnant women, especially during the second trimester. The ideal image is a woman with thick shiny hair and perfect skin that has a healthy blush.

The improved condition of your skin is thanks to the hormone oestrogen (pregnancy hormones can have positive effects, too!) and the increased blood supply to the skin; the many blood vessels just below the skin's surface give you a healthy glow, or at least stop you looking pale and tired. The glands also secrete more oil, giving your skin a healthy-looking sheen.

Again due to hormonal changes, your hair may look thicker. Less hair than normal falls out during pregnancy and hair grows more quickly. After the birth you may find that your hair appears to be falling out more than normal as you lose the hair that's built up during the nine months. Normal hair loss is about 100–125 hairs a day; after the birth you might lose 500 hairs a day.

If you don't feel you match this picture of good health, it may just be that you can't see it yourself, especially if you're still adapting to your pregnancy. If you're looking pale and feeling tired, speak to your doctor or midwife as you may be anaemic and need to boost your iron intake (see p.154).

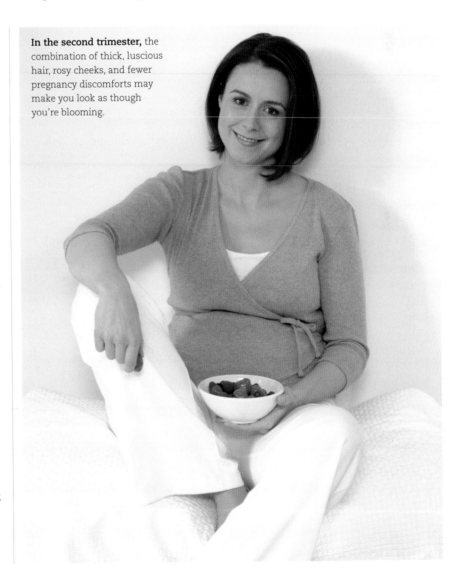

In the second trimester, the combination of thick, luscious hair, rosy cheeks, and fewer pregnancy discomforts may make you look as though you're blooming.

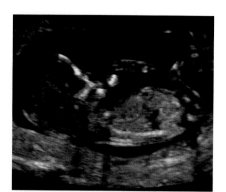

176 days to go...

YOUR BABY TODAY

Your baby is starting to swallow amniotic fluid more regularly: this enters the stomach (seen here as a dark circle in the centre of the abdomen). The tiny bladder is also visible as a black fluid-filled structure within the lower pelvis.

The neural tube, the basis of your baby's spinal cord, developed in the very early weeks; now the spinal cord is fully formed.

Nerves from your baby's spinal cord are linked to each set of vertebrae, but as your baby lengthens the spinal cord does not grow at the same rate, and the lower tip ends up lying at the mid-lumbar level, half way between the hips and lowest rib.

Below the mid-lumbar level, the nerves leaving the spinal cord have lengthened so that they still exit between the lowest vertebrae. In adult life, the cord will end slightly higher than in the newborn baby. Because the spinal cord does not extend the entire length of the vertebral canal, a fluid-filled space fills the lower portion.

By the end of this week, your baby is able to use fat as a source of energy. This isn't, however, an important source of energy because that need is met largely by glucose crossing the placenta from your bloodstream. Free fatty acids in your circulation easily cross the placenta to your baby and are used for organ growth, forming cell walls, making myelin

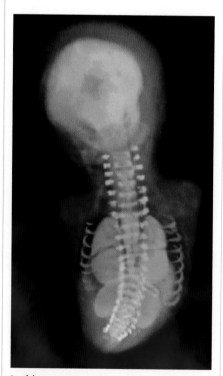

In this computer-generated image, the internal organs of the fetus can be seen. The skull, spine, and rib cage are also clearly visible. The lungs (pink) are protected by the rib cage; the kidneys (red) are below.

sheaths around nerves to insulate them, and for many other functions.

Cholesterol is not only supplied to your unborn baby via the placenta, but he is also forming it within his own body. For this reason, your cholesterol level bears little relation to your baby's, which needs to be high for your baby to produce fat, especially in the first few months of pregnancy.

AS A MATTER OF FACT

Your baby could be tuning in to your favourite TV show!

Research examined babies of mothers who watched *Neighbours* while pregnant alongside women who didn't. After the birth those babies who had been exposed to the music in the uterus became quiet and "paid attention" to the tune; the other group of babies ignored it.

ASK A... DOCTOR

When can my baby first suck his thumb? Ultrasound scans have shown unborn babies sucking their thumbs from as early as 12–14 weeks of pregnancy. However, this is likely to be a reflex at this stage as the brain does not have any conscious control over movement until the fetus is much more developed later on in pregnancy.

Some research has suggested that if an unborn baby shows a preference for sucking, for example, his right thumb, then he will prefer to lie with his head turned to the right after the birth. The same research suggested that this preference could be used to predict right- or left-handedness in the baby as he grows older.

175 days to go...

YOUR BABY TODAY

This profile view shows that the bridge of the nose is shallow and the eyes are still dominating the face. The jaw is lengthening and the chin held away from the chest. The hands (with outstretched fingers) are in a common position – close to the face.

It's worthwhile finding comfortable sleeping positions now; these will stand you in good stead throughout pregnancy.

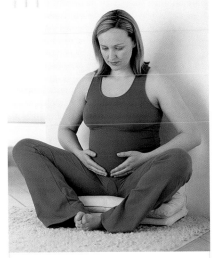

Quiet times

Times when you can focus quietly on your baby are precious bonding opportunities and a great way to relax. You may like to visualize your baby floating in the amniotic fluid.

Try this "butterfly" pose with the soles of your feet joined. Place your hands on your abdomen and massage your baby using different strokes. Think of your baby and shed your pre-occupations with each out-breath.

Your bump will be getting bigger by the day and, as a result, you may find it increasingly difficult to get comfortable when you're lying down, especially during the night.

You should avoid sleeping on your back in the second half of your pregnancy, so start practising some new positions now. This is because the weight of your uterus will press on the major veins that return blood to your heart, which may result in dizziness, low blood pressure, and possibly a reduction in blood flow to the uterus.

Ideally, lie on your left side (although it will do you or your baby no harm to lie on your right side) as this is actually good for you and the baby. It improves blood flow to the placenta and helps your kidneys eliminate fluids and waste products. Don't worry if you wake to find you're lying on your back: just roll onto your side and support yourself with pillows if necessary.

It's fine to lie on your front if you prefer (your baby is safely cushioned in the amniotic fluid), but the bigger you get, the more difficult this will become.

ASK A... MIDWIFE

My midwife is lovely but she's always in a hurry. How can I get her to answer my questions? This is a common problem. Antenatal clinics are often very busy, with lots of women for the midwife to see. As a result, most clinics allow only a 10-to-15-minute appointment for each woman – barely enough time to go through the basic physical checks. However, it is important that your questions are addressed and it may be helpful to write them down so that you remember what you want to ask. If your midwife doesn't have time to discuss the issues during your appointment, ask her to arrange to talk to you at a mutually convenient time. This could be in the form of a phone call, or another appointment at the clinic. Or she may be able to direct you to other sources of information such as books, leaflets, websites, or other healthcare professionals.

It's a crucial part of your antenatal care that you feel comfortable with your caregivers and are given the opportunity to discuss any questions you have or issues that arise, and this is recognized by the National Institute for Clinical Excellence (NICE) in their guidelines for antenatal care.

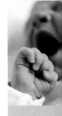

Your 16th week

THE BUMP STARTS HERE, ANNOUNCING YOUR PREGNANCY TO THE WORLD

Some days, you'll take huge pride in your emerging bump, on other days you may sigh for the loss of a trim figure. Enjoy your changing shape – you'll probably find that your partner loves it, too. For many couples, this can be a time of increased interest in sex. If you have any emotional or physical worries, there'll be an opportunity to discuss them with your midwife. Another antenatal check is likely to take place this week.

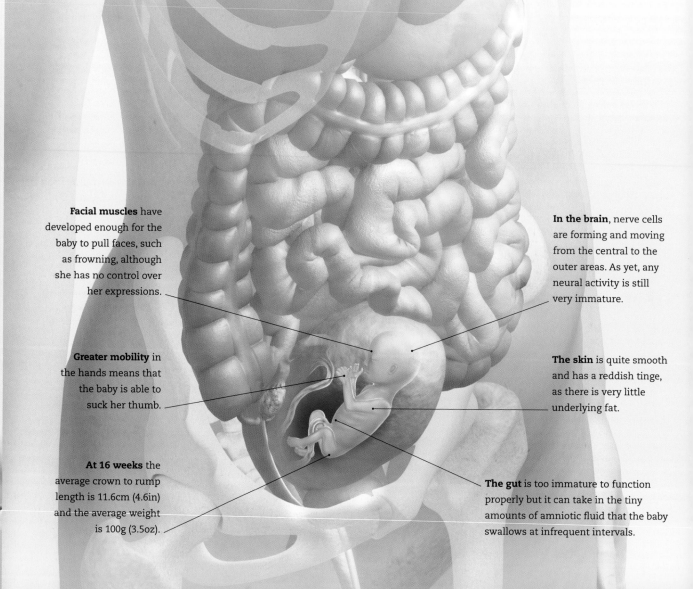

Facial muscles have developed enough for the baby to pull faces, such as frowning, although she has no control over her expressions.

In the brain, nerve cells are forming and moving from the central to the outer areas. As yet, any neural activity is still very immature.

Greater mobility in the hands means that the baby is able to suck her thumb.

The skin is quite smooth and has a reddish tinge, as there is very little underlying fat.

At 16 weeks the average crown to rump length is 11.6cm (4.6in) and the average weight is 100g (3.5oz).

The gut is too immature to function properly but it can take in the tiny amounts of amniotic fluid that the baby swallows at infrequent intervals.

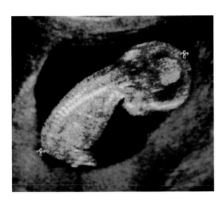

YOU ARE 15 WEEKS AND 1 DAY

174 days to go...

YOUR BABY TODAY

In this artificially coloured ultrasound scan of the baby within the uterus, the spine shows up especially clearly. The two blue crosses, at the top of the baby's head and at his bottom, indicate where the crown to rump measurement is taken.

Your bump may be clearly visible by this 16th week of pregnancy, and you'll be amazed at how quickly it grows.

At around this stage you may begin to "show", that is, instead of having a slightly bigger waist you develop a definite bump and start to look pregnant. You may begin to notice people's eyes are drawn towards your abdomen. If you'd rather keep the pregnancy quiet in some circles – for example, at work – wear baggy clothes.

While some women have neat little bumps positioned more to the front, others have bumps that are more spread out. The size and shape of yours will be individual to you, so try not to compare. There are old wives' tales that if you're carrying in front you're having a boy, and if you're carrying spread out over your hips you're carrying a girl, though this hasn't been proved.

If you haven't bought any maternity clothes, you may want to shop for some or adapt your clothes (see p.179).

AS A MATTER OF FACT

Twin bonding occurs well before the babies are born.

Advanced video technology has captured the special relationship between twins in the uterus. They have been seen to interact and even grasp each other's hands.

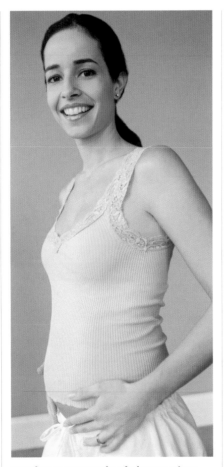

Your bump may not be obvious to others when you're wearing baggy clothes, but in tight-fitting ones it will be quite prominent. Although your shape changes gradually, some women find that their bump gets larger more quickly during some weeks than others.

ASK A... NUTRITIONIST

I keep waking up hungry in the night – what should I do? It is normal to get the night-time munchies during pregnancy, but annoying, especially if you're already having difficulties sleeping. Try to pre-empt night-time hunger by snacking on the right foods before you go to bed:

■ **Eggs, milk** (and therefore cheese, and yogurt, too), tuna, and turkey are good sources of the amino acid tryptophan, which encourages the body to produce the B vitamin niacin. This helps the production of serotonin, a brain chemical that has a calming effect and aids sleep.

■ **Eat slow-release carbohydrates,** such as wholemeal bread or pasta. So, for example, half a tuna, cheese, or turkey sandwich, a small amount of wholemeal pasta with some cheese, or a bowl of good-quality wholegrain breakfast cereal with some warm milk and honey will fill you up, while also helping you to sleep better.

■ **A handful of nuts and seeds,** or some plain yogurt with honey and fruit, are high in protein and will stop your stomach from rumbling.

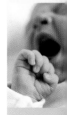

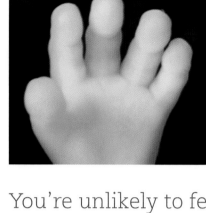

YOU ARE 15 WEEKS AND 2 DAYS

173 days to go...

YOUR BABY TODAY

The fingertips are prominent and the fingers still quite short. Each finger is separate and moves independently of the rest. This is the most comfortable position for the hand, with the thumb and fingers outstretched rather than curled into a fist.

You're unlikely to feel her move yet, but your baby is becoming increasingly active inside your uterus.

By now, your baby may be active for up to five minutes at a time. In the next few weeks, you may begin to feel some slight fluttering movements, particularly if this is not your first pregnancy (see p.193). You'll only be aware of those movements that cause your baby to make contact with the inner muscular wall of your uterus.

The placenta itself can act like a cushion absorbing the impact of all but the strongest of the baby's movements. For this reason, women with an anterior placenta (one lying on the front wall of the uterus – that closest to the skin) often feel the movements at a much later stage than those with a posteriorly sited placenta (one that lies closer to the back).

Your baby's brain is continuing to develop. The nerve cells that will form the outer grey matter start centrally within the brain, and need to move outwards to their final position. This process takes place in waves that occur from 8 to 16 weeks. The migration process is not complete until 25 weeks and electrical activity cannot be detected until 29 weeks. Even after this point, grey matter continues to mature and organize neural connections in the brain throughout the pregnancy. Your baby's body is now longer than her head for the first time.

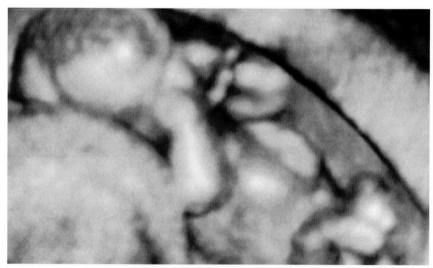

3D ultrasound scanning uses computer technology to produce more detailed images than conventional 2D scans. This scan shows a 15-week-old fetus in the uterus. At this stage all of the organs are formed, as are the vocal cords.

ASK A... DOCTOR

Can using sunbeds and jacuzzis harm my unborn baby? Although there's no evidence that sunbed or jacuzzi use harms the baby, it has been reported that a rise in the mother's temperature, which can happen while on a tanning bed, or in a hot tub or sauna, may increase the fetus's temperature. A temperature above 39°C (102°F) has been associated with spinal malformations in developing babies, and if a rise in temperature is maintained for long enough, it may cause brain damage. The temperature of the amniotic fluid can also increase and it is thought that an extreme rise in your temperature can cause problems with the flow of blood to the baby.

So limit sunbed and jacuzzi use, don't have hot baths, and be careful in hot climates (see p.185).

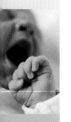

Your second trimester

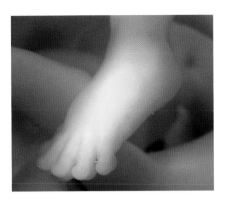

172 days to go...

YOUR BABY TODAY

Now the toes are lengthening and a gentle arch to the foot is beginning to take shape. Your baby can grasp her feet at will but has difficulty bringing them up to her mouth: this is not a problem a little later in pregnancy.

It's time for another routine antenatal appointment to ensure everything is progressing well with you and your baby.

You may be booked in for an antenatal appointment at around 16 weeks, and this is normally the first formal visit you'll have with the midwife following your booking-in appointment (see p.122).

Your urine will be tested, and your blood pressure measured. Furthermore, the midwife should be able to hear your baby's heartbeat (see p.188), which can be very reassuring.

Women who do not have the nuchal translucency scan (see p.143) at around 11–14 weeks, may be offered one of two blood tests, known as the triple test or quadruple test (see p.143), which are screening tests for Down's syndrome.

This appointment also offers you an opportunity to discuss any concerns you may have, and your midwife will report the results of the routine tests (see pp.122–3) you had at your booking-in appointment, or shortly thereafter.

If your blood test results show that your haemoglobin levels were low, you may be offered a prescription for iron.

(see p.122) (see p.188) (see p.143) (see p.143) (see pp.122–3)

AS A MATTER OF FACT

Maternity wear first appeared around the middle of the 19th century.

At this time a prudish society felt that pregnancy should be hidden. For this same reason, and for the wellbeing of mother and child, women were encouraged to stay in bed in the weeks leading up to the birth.

FOCUS ON... YOUR BODY

Does my bump look big in this?

You'll need to choose clothes that accommodate your growing bump, but that doesn't have to mean investing in a whole new maternity wardrobe just yet.

The following innovations will help to keep you comfortable and extend the life of your normal clothes for a few weeks at least:

■ **Pregnancy support pants:** these stretch with you and ease the strain on your lower back, while giving you a smoother outline.

■ **Trouser expander:** an elasticated belt that enables you to wear your jeans with a burgeoning bump. Alternatively, loop a hairband – or, for extra girth, a slice cut from a pair of tights – around the button, through the buttonhole and back.

■ **Belly band:** a wide band of stretchy fabric that you wear on your bump, to conceal the gap between your top and waistband.

■ **Bra extenders:** hook on to the fastening at the back of your bra to add up to 8cm (3in).

■ **Borrowing:** you can borrow clothes from your partner or friends who are slightly larger than you.

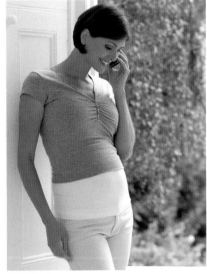

A belly band is a versatile item that covers your bump, enabling you to continue wearing some of your favourite tops.

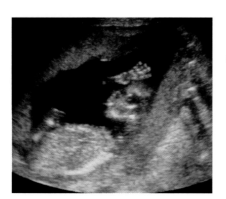

171 days to go...

YOUR BABY TODAY

In this 2D ultrasound, the top of the baby's head is in shadow, although the hand can be seen in front of the face. All the bones are growing and maturing at this stage of pregnancy.

Your baby's skin is still transparent and there is little fat lying beneath it at this stage of the pregnancy.

Your baby's skin is made from three layers. The outer layer is the epidermis, and beneath this lie the dermis layer, and the subcutaneous layer. The epidermis started as a single layer of cells but is now three or four cells thick. The most superficial layer of epidermal cells flatten but do not harden until much later.

The dermis is made from connective tissue comprising collagen (90 per cent) and elastin fibres that allow for stretch and resistance. Within the dermis are blood vessels and nerves that support the epidermis and provide sensory feedback. At first, the junction between the dermis and epidermis is smooth, but increasingly dermal ridges form and it becomes irregular.

At the same time your baby starts to develop hair follicles. There is no significant subcutaneous fat present at this stage and the skin is almost transparent. Fat plays a part in temperature control and acts as a barrier to the passage of water. These barriers are not yet in place so the skin is still very permeable.

AS A MATTER OF FACT

In the case of women who are at high risk of pre-eclampsia, low-dose aspirin throughout the pregnancy may be prescribed.

Pre-eclampsia (see p.474) causes excessive blood clotting and low-dose aspirin could help to counter this. Always seek medical advice before taking any type of medication during your pregnancy.

FOCUS ON... DADS

The "goddess" within

Your partner may have mixed feelings about her changing shape. She may at times appear to be a "pregnant goddess" who enjoys the fact that she's carrying a child. After all, there is nothing more female than being able to conceive and give birth. When she feels positive about this, she may seem strong and content.

However, at other times, rather than loving her bump she may feel down about gaining weight and losing her body shape. When some fashion magazines show extremely thin women as a symbol of "beauty", it is little wonder that the arrival of the bump can trigger a number of conflicting feelings in a pregnant woman, making her sometimes doubt her looks and knocking her self-esteem.

You can help your partner by steering her towards her more positive "goddess" side and reassuring her about her looks. It's worth reminding her that what she's doing is amazing and that you think she's absolutely gorgeous.

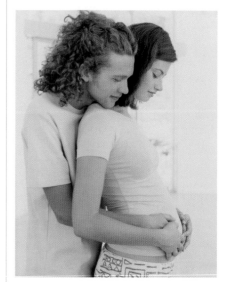

Boost her self-esteem: as her body changes shape, make her feel beautiful and wanted.

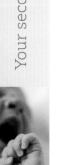

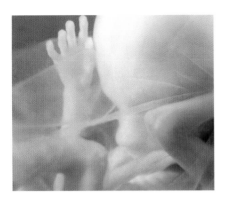

170 days to go...

YOUR BABY TODAY

Here the baby is seen within the amniotic sac. For the first time, her head is smaller than her body, marking another developmental milestone. Having a large, heavy head is not a problem in the near weightless environment of the uterus.

Your midwife may speak to you about writing a birth plan so she can get an idea of the type of labour and birth you want.

The purpose of a birth plan is to communicate your wishes for labour and birth to those who are caring for you. Writing a plan will help you to address different aspects of the labour, such as methods of pain relief and who you'd like to attend the birth. It also gives you a chance to ask questions about procedures such as induction and other types of medical intervention. Filling in a plan is also a useful way for your birth partner to be made aware of your wishes so that he or she can communicate these to the midwife or doctor while you're in labour.

Do bear in mind that circumstances may dictate that not all of your preferences are met, but there's more chance of you getting the labour and birth you want if you've thought it through and written down your views. Being as informed as possible about labour and your choices (see pp.302–3) will help you to prepare in advance.

ASK A... DOCTOR

I have dry eyes and am finding it hard to wear my contact lenses. What can I do? During pregnancy, hormonal changes may cause your eyes to feel dry, and you may experience burning, itching, and a feeling that there is a foreign object under your eyelid. This is common in pregnancy. Dry eyes can also occur after the menopause, when there are similar hormonal fluctuations.

The condition appears to be caused by a change in the composition and quantity of tears, leaving the eye dry and inadequately lubricated. The discomfort can be remedied with "artificial tears" (see right), available from an optician or pharmacist, and it usually disappears once the baby is born. In the meantime, limit the time you wear your lenses and wear your glasses more often, especially if you are looking at a computer screen for long periods of time.

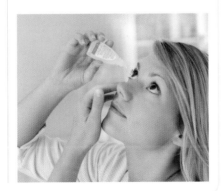

TIME TO THINK ABOUT

Your birth plan

Fragranced candles, womb music, and beanbags... or serious pain relief from the first contraction? Writing a birth plan is an opportunity for you to think about how you'd like your labour and delivery to go. Discuss your birth plan with your midwife and birth partner as early as this week, so you're all clear about your objectives (see pp.302–3).

■ **Write everything down:** your birth partner(s), pain-relief preferences, whether you'd like an active labour, and the environment you'd prefer to give birth in. You might know you want to give birth in hospital or at home, or in a birth centre, which offers a home-style setting with the back-up of medical technology.

■ **Be specific:** for example, you might like to use a birthing pool to labour in or want to give birth in an upright position. You might want minimal medical intervention.

■ **Be flexible:** labour doesn't always go according to plan and your baby's safe delivery is the most important thing.

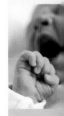

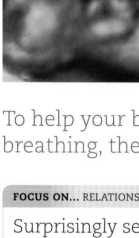

YOU ARE 15 WEEKS AND 6 DAYS

169 days to go...

YOUR BABY TODAY

The upper limbs are well differentiated into forearms, wrists, hands, and fingers; these develop at a faster rate than the lower limbs, a feature that continues even after the birth.

To help your baby's lungs expand and develop in preparation for breathing, the chest wall must be fully bathed in amniotic fluid.

Your second trimester

FOCUS ON... RELATIONSHIPS

Surprisingly sexy

You may be taken aback by a sudden increase in your libido. Often, in the second trimester, women find that they feel far more energetic and sexy. The increased blood flow to the pelvic area combined with an increased lubrication of the vagina means that, in theory, having sex can be better than ever.

High levels of progesterone and oestrogen make your breasts and vagina super-sensitive so expect to become more easily aroused during foreplay. You may also find that you orgasm more quickly than usual. The uterus tightens when you orgasm, so be prepared for this.

Your partner may be delighted by this up-turn in events, as well as approving of a beautiful rounded body to explore, but if he isn't responding positively, talk to him about how he's feeling.

In this close up the baby's left arm and chest wall can be seen. Because the skin is almost transparent the ribs are easy to see. They are very soft at this stage and still predominantly made of cartilage.

Your baby's lungs continue to branch and divide. The cells lining the airways constantly produce fluid that leaves the lungs when your baby makes breathing movements. The release of this fluid is regulated by the vocal cords within the larynx.

As well as fluid, the lungs have glands that produce mucus. Cells with tiny hair-like structures, known as cilia, have appeared that help to move the mucus. This production of mucus is important once the baby is born to prevent the constant flow of air from drying the lining of the lungs, to trap dust particles, and to act as a barrier to infection.

Because the gut is still very immature, the gradual increase in amniotic fluid is due to the relatively low frequency of fetal swallowing. By 37 weeks your baby will be swallowing almost a litre (1.75 pints), half of the total amniotic fluid volume, each day.

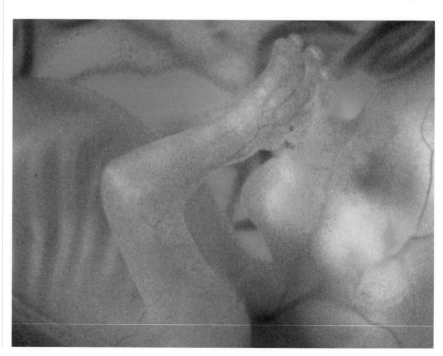

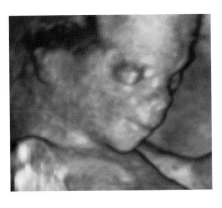

YOU ARE 16 WEEKS EXACTLY

168 days to go...

YOUR BABY TODAY

As your baby's skin starts to become more waterproof, the amniotic fluid is increasingly made from urine produced by your baby's kidneys and bladder. This urine does not contain waste products, as these are transported across the placenta.

It's natural that your partner will want to protect you and his baby, but you may need to help him get the balance right.

AS A MATTER OF FACT

Dads-to-be tend to have more vivid dreams than usual.

Pending fatherhood can make a man think about his own background and roots, and trigger dreams of parents and grandparents. As he becomes more protective and nurturing, he may even dream that he's pregnant.

Is your partner worried about you having a sip of wine or eating a tad too much chocolate, or is he constantly checking you're getting enough rest? You may find that your partner becomes very protective of you and his baby and while some women enjoy the attention, others find it irritating. If it bothers you, ask your partner why he feels the need to be so protective. If you can understand his feelings and concerns, it can help.

Take the time to explain to him how you feel, and if everything is going well and you're feeling great, let him know. Explain that pregnancy is not an illness and is a natural process, and reassure him that you're being well looked after by the midwife. For further reassurance, you could get him some reading material and involve him by inviting him along to an antenatal appointment. He may have particular questions he wants to ask the midwife.

STRENGTHENING YOUR LEGS

A strong and toned lower body can be achieved by doing the exercises shown below. Strengthening these muscles will make day-to-day tasks, such as walking and climbing the stairs, a lot easier as your baby grows. Strengthening your leg muscles can also help to prepare you for labour positions, such as squatting.

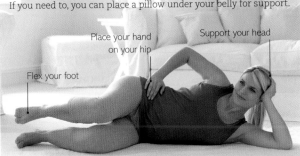

Lie on your side. Place both legs in front of your body, bent at the knee at a 90-degree angle. Slowly lift your top leg up and lower it to the starting position. Repeat 30 times, if comfortable. If you need to, you can place a pillow under your belly for support.

Place your hand on your hip
Support your head
Flex your foot

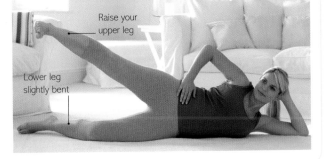

Lie on your side, with your lower leg slightly bent at the knee and top leg positioned at a 45-degree angle. Lift your leg slightly (about 10cm/4in), hold for 10 seconds, and then lower back to 45 degrees. Repeat 30 times, if comfortable.

Raise your upper leg
Lower leg slightly bent

Your 16th week

183

Your 17th week

YOUR BABY IS INCREASING HIS MOVEMENTS AND EVEN DOING SOMERSAULTS

Things are becoming lively in your uterus. Your baby has plenty of room to move around and he's making the most of it, stretching and turning. All the activity is good for his future physical and mental development. You might feel like some relaxation, so think about taking a break. The second trimester is usually regarded as the best time in pregnancy for travelling and getting out and about.

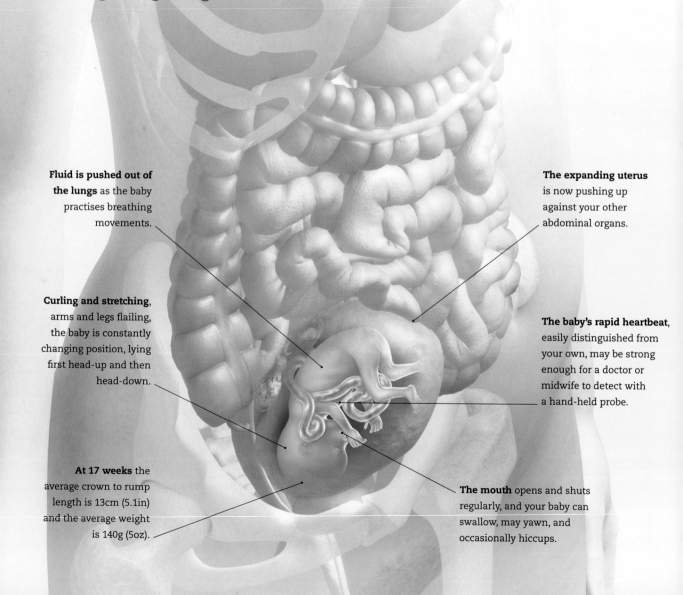

Fluid is pushed out of the lungs as the baby practises breathing movements.

The expanding uterus is now pushing up against your other abdominal organs.

Curling and stretching, arms and legs flailing, the baby is constantly changing position, lying first head-up and then head-down.

The baby's rapid heartbeat, easily distinguished from your own, may be strong enough for a doctor or midwife to detect with a hand-held probe.

At 17 weeks the average crown to rump length is 13cm (5.1in) and the average weight is 140g (5oz).

The mouth opens and shuts regularly, and your baby can swallow, may yawn, and occasionally hiccups.

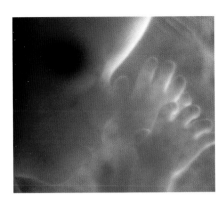

167 days to go...

YOUR BABY TODAY

At this stage of development, your baby's lips and mouth are well formed, and she can open and close her mouth and swallow. Inside her mouth, her taste buds are now mature, but she cannot taste anything yet because nerve connections are immature.

As this is considered a safe stage of pregnancy, with no, or few, symptoms to contend with, it's a great time to go on holiday.

At this time, you're likely to be over the sickness and fatigue of the first trimester and not over-burdened by, or uncomfortable from, a large bump yet. You can also rest easy knowing that your baby is developing well, with very little chance of a miscarriage occurring. Going on holiday is a great opportunity to spend quality time with your partner and pamper yourselves.

Do relax and enjoy yourself, but be aware of the extra health precautions you need to take during pregnancy (see below and pp.28–9). If you've had any complications, check with your midwife or doctor that it is safe to go on holiday.

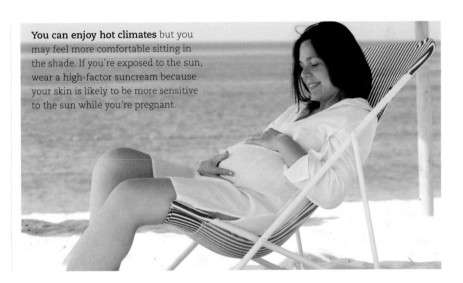

You can enjoy hot climates but you may feel more comfortable sitting in the shade. If you're exposed to the sun, wear a high-factor suncream because your skin is likely to be more sensitive to the sun while you're pregnant.

FOCUS ON... SAFETY

Enjoy a healthy holiday

If you go on holiday while you're pregnant, there are a few additional factors to consider, not least the fact that you might not have as much energy as you had before:

■ **Give yourself plenty of time** when you're trying to finish all those pre-holiday bits and pieces at home and at work; getting ready for a holiday can be stressful. Pack hand luggage for a flight sensibly so that you won't have to carry heavy bags with you.

■ **Plan a car journey carefully,** bearing in mind that you may need more toilet stops or snack breaks than usual.

■ **Be aware that sightseeing** will be more tiring than usual, so pace yourself and allow yourself to spend time in a cafe, just watching the world go by.

■ **If you're abroad,** drink bottled water – lots of it, especially if you're in a hot climate. Avoid having ice in your drinks as this tends to be made using tap water.

■ **Peel fruit** or wash fruit and vegetables with bottled water.

■ **If you get diarrhoea,** it's even more important than usual to drink plenty of water to replace the fluid you've lost. Don't take anti-diarrhoea medication but it is safe to take an oral rehydration solution, such as Dioralyte, which contains the correct balance of salts. If your urine is very concentrated and you can't keep fluid down, see a doctor.

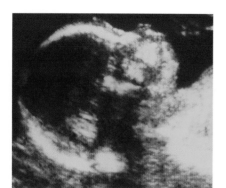

YOU ARE 16 WEEKS AND 2 DAYS

166 days to go...

YOUR BABY TODAY

In this coloured 2D ultrasound scan the baby is facing upwards. The skull bones reflect the ultrasound beam most effectively and show as bright areas. The curved frontal bone of the forehead is seen just above the short nasal bone forming the bridge of the nose.

Your baby is at his most mobile around about now, and he may even be doing somersaults in your uterus.

ASK A... DOCTOR

What is DVT and am I at increased risk of it when I fly?

DVT stands for deep vein thrombosis, a condition in which a blood clot forms in a deep leg vein. DVT partially or completely blocks the blood flow in the vein, causing pain and discomfort. The most serious form of DVT is a pulmonary embolism, when part of the clot breaks off and travels to the lungs, blocking a pulmonary artery. This can cause chest pain, shortness of breath, and blood-tinged phlegm to be coughed up. In severe cases, a pulmonary embolism can be fatal.

Pregnancy is considered to be a thrombotic condition, meaning it can lead to clots forming in blood vessels, so you are at increased risk of DVT even when you're not travelling by plane. Women who have previously had DVT or who are obese are more at risk of getting the condition.

Wearing support stockings (see p.225), drinking plenty of fluids, and moving around while flying can help to prevent DVT. If you've had blood-clotting issues in the past, avoid flying at all during pregnancy.

There are several ways in which your baby can now move: he can curl and stretch his trunk, move his head up and down and from side to side, and move his arms and legs independently. Regular chest wall breathing movements occur, along with occasional hiccups. The mouth can open and shut, and your baby can yawn and swallow amniotic fluid. He'll bring his hands up to the face and prefer lying on his side rather than back. He has plenty of space in which to move.

Your baby's taste buds first appeared at 10 weeks and by now have an appearance very close to that of a mature taste bud. They also have their own nerve supply, connected to a branch of the facial nerve. Because these neural connections have not yet matured, it is too early for your baby to be able to taste anything.

FOCUS ON... TWINS

How your babies interact

By now, you may be starting to feel your twin babies move. Contact between them probably began a few weeks ago, long before you knew

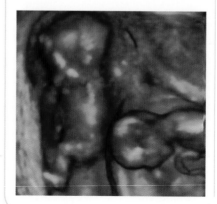

about it, and it becomes more complex as their brains develop. By this stage of pregnancy, a baby has the elementary brain circuits that help him feel the parts of his body and appreciate their position, so it's no wonder that your babies can now interact at a basic level.

Your babies will move around 50 times an hour and can touch each other, even though in all but a tiny percentage of cases they're in separate amniotic sacs so there's a membrane between them. Ultrasound studies show that twin babies make physical contact and sometimes react to each other's touch and pressure.

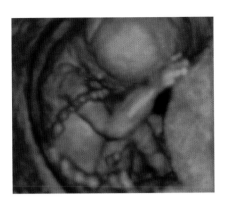

165 days to go...

YOUR BABY TODAY

This 3D scan is taken from a viewpoint above the baby's head and looking over the shoulder, but since the baby is curled up the face cannot be seen. The placenta is to the right of the image, with the umbilical cord over the baby's arm.

While you're pregnant, it's even more important to find ways to relieve stress and keep any worries in perspective.

RELIEVING STRESS

Learn to recognize the signs that you're stressed: you may feel your heart racing or a rise in your body temperature. When you know you're stressed, take action.

■ **Identify the cause** and try to keep it in perspective. Let go of the stress by breathing deeply and relaxing your muscles. Imagine blowing the stress away as you exhale.

■ **Stay busy –** sometimes having too much time to think can make you more stressed.

■ **Go swimming:** it's a great stress reliever and a fantastic way to stay in shape, too.

■ **Take time to relax,** especially if you have a lot on your mind or are juggling lots of things. Put your feet up, watch TV, read a novel, or think about your growing baby.

■ **Talk through your problems** with your partner or a close friend. If you're worrying about any aspect of your health or how your baby is developing, seek reassurance from your midwife or doctor.

■ **If work is an issue,** be honest with your boss or the human resources department and they may be able to help. Your most important job right now is to nurture your baby.

You may be pregnant and happy, but life goes on: you might still be working full-time, as well as running a home, and you're bound to have stressful days and times when you feel you can't cope. And, of course, you're still contending with those challenging pregnancy hormones that can cause some emotional ups and downs.

Like many women, you may become stressed about the big changes that are going to happen, and worry about factors such as finances, whether you'll be a good mother, and how your relationship will change. It's important to keep worries in perspective and maintain an emotional balance as being stressed isn't good for your health or that of your baby.

Find ways to destress (see left), including talking to others – your partner, friends, and midwife – about concerns.

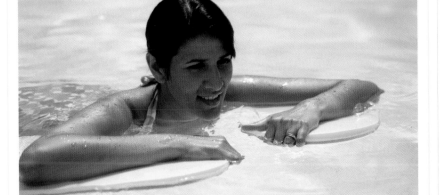

AS A MATTER OF FACT

A mother's stress can be transmitted to the fetus.

The level of the stress hormone cortisol in the amniotic fluid matches that in the mother's blood. Cortisol is thought to adversely affect fetal development.

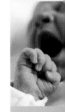

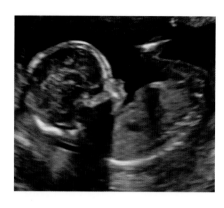

164 days to go...

YOUR BABY TODAY

In this 2D ultrasound, the baby's head is to the left, with the arms not visible, although the knee and lower leg can be seen. At this stage, details of the brain developing under the skull are becoming much more apparent.

Until you feel your baby move, hearing his heartbeat is the next best way for you to bond with him.

ASK A PANEL ABOUT... MONITORING YOUR BABY'S HEARTBEAT AT HOME

My partner is keen to hire a hand-held Doppler so we can listen to our baby's heartbeat. Do you think this is a good idea?

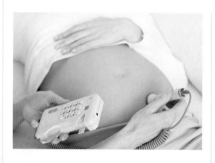

Doctor: Hand-held ultrasound Doppler devices, which allow parents-to-be to listen to the fetal heartbeat at home, are popular in the US and are now being offered to hire or buy in the UK. Parents are told they can listen to their baby "in complete safety as early as 10 weeks of pregnancy" and "any time they wish", implying there is no limit on frequency of exposure.

However, there has been no research into the effects of frequent scanning, which would be more than the baby receives during antenatal care. A Doppler is not a toy and using it in this way is an unnecessary risk.

Midwife: Using your own Doppler may help reassure you if you are very anxious about your baby's wellbeing, but it is just as likely to have the opposite effect if you can't pick up the heartbeat. Identifying different sounds takes practice and if you have difficulty finding the heartbeat (this happens to midwives, too!), it could be distressing. If you're worried about your baby for any reason, help and advice is only a phone call away.

Mum: I used a Doppler because I am a worrier and it really gave me peace of mind. I didn't use it very often and only when there was a good reason to. For example, at one stage of my pregnancy, I had an episode of bleeding and clots. After this, I was very worried about my baby's health and hearing his heartbeat really helped to calm me down, so it had benefits for the baby, too. I don't think a Doppler is a substitute for medical advice but it's a useful addition.

At this stage of pregnancy, your midwife may be able to hear your baby's heartbeat using a hand-held Doppler ultrasound machine. Because ultrasound waves do not travel well in air, gel is applied to the end of the probe or "transducer" as it is placed on your abdomen. This then detects the heartbeat and converts it into a sound that we can hear.

It's quite easy to distinguish your baby's heartbeat from your own as it beats almost twice as fast. However, your baby's heart rate peaked around five weeks ago and, since then, has slowed down as the nerves controlling the heart's rhythm have matured.

During the second half of pregnancy, the range of the heartbeat is between 120 and 160 beats per minute and will be responsive to many stimuli, as well as to your baby's activity.

AS A MATTER OF FACT

The baby's heart rate is not an indication of gender.

A study in the mid-1990s, using over 10,000 measurements, dispelled the theory that the speed of a baby's heartbeat predicted whether it would be a boy or a girl.

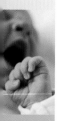

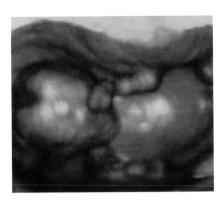

163 days to go...

YOUR BABY TODAY

The baby's face is partially obscured by the hand in this 3D image. Babies at this stage are small enough to fit onto the ultrasound screen, but beyond 20 weeks it is increasingly only possible to see a smaller part of the baby at any one time.

Ensuring you drink enough fluids is essential to good health in pregnancy, so carry your bottle of water everywhere.

Staying hydrated in pregnancy can be a challenge. Because of the hormonal changes taking place, some of the fluid you take in leaks into your body tissues, rather than staying within the bloodstream.

It's difficult to recommend an exact amount of fluid that should be drunk to keep you hydrated, since this depends on many factors, such as the foods you eat (some naturally contain water), your size, the amount you exercise, and the heat and humidity in the environment. Therefore, you need to listen to your own body to determine if you're adequately hydrated. One of the best ways to do this is to look at your urine. If it's clear to light yellow, you're adequately hydrated. If it's bright yellow or orange, you're likely to be dehydrated.

Drinking plenty of water is important. Sometimes, though, if you are nauseous, or just plain tired of drinking water, you may want to try other options for hydration, such as drinking juice or eating more fruit (see box, below). Remember that caffeinated beverages, such as coffee, are not hydrating; caffeine has a diuretic effect, which means that you will want to pass urine more often.

In the second and third trimester, dehydration in pregnancy can lead to premature contractions. This is because an anti-diuretic hormone is produced to help your body hold on to water. This hormone acts a lot like oxytocin, the hormone that triggers labour, causing contractions. Staying hydrated will prevent this from happening.

FOCUS ON... NUTRITION

Fabulous fruit

One great way to stay hydrated is to eat fruit. Many fruits are very high in water, especially melons, grapes, and strawberries. The water in fruit is very well absorbed in your body, because it comes partnered with sugar, which helps the water stay in your bloodstream.

In addition, fruit is highly nutritious and contains many of the vitamins and electrolytes that your body needs to stay in balance.

ASK A... MIDWIFE

Should I stop picking up my toddler while I'm pregnant? You may be experiencing some back pain and discomfort as your hormones begin to soften your ligaments. This means that your joints are less stable than usual, and injury is more likely.

Lifting your toddler will not harm your baby, but it may cause you discomfort, and you may be more likely to lose your balance. Ask your toddler to climb on to a chair so that you don't need to lift from a bending position. To lift from floor level, squat down and use your legs to bear the weight. Avoid bending, which strains your back. Encourage your toddler to get on to your lap for a cuddle.

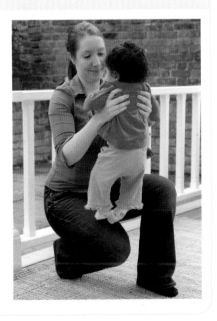

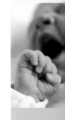

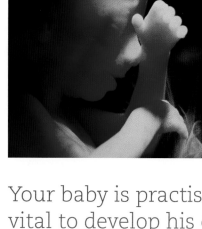

YOU ARE 16 WEEKS AND 6 DAYS

162 days to go...

YOUR BABY TODAY

Your baby often brings his hands to his face and sometimes sucks his thumb at this stage; however, the sucking action is not well co-ordinated and the thumb is likely to enter the mouth more by luck than design. The arms are now in proportion with the rest of the body.

Your baby is practising his breathing movements, which are vital to develop his chest muscles and enable his lungs to grow.

While he's in the uterus, your baby is practising his breathing movements and this also aids his lung development. When he breathes in, the diaphragm moves downwards and the chest wall moves inwards.

Each "breath" the baby takes lasts less than a second. Breathing might only happen occasionally at this stage and when it does it can be either regular or irregular.

Your baby might also open his jaw and swallow at the same time as making a breathing movement.

A single breathing movement with a large movement of the diaphragm may resemble a sigh.

For the chest wall movements to be effective, there must be adequate amniotic fluid (see p.182). This is especially true for the critical time of lung development, from 16 to 26 weeks.

By the 24th week of pregnancy, your baby will spend approximately three hours in a 24-hour period practising breathing movements, and around eight hours in a 24-hour period in the last eight weeks of pregnancy.

AS A MATTER OF FACT

When a pregnant woman smokes, it reduces the number of times her baby practises breathing movements.

In a *British Medical Journal* research study, the proportion of time that the baby practised breathing movements was found to fall within five minutes of the mother beginning to smoke her cigarette.

FOCUS ON... TWINS

Growth rate

While most unborn twins grow at much the same pace, from now on some don't.

Your babies are almost certainly developing all the right organs at the right time, even when there's a size discrepancy. If, however, a scan detects a growth difference between your twins, you'll have additional scans to monitor growth. Lesser degrees aren't usually a problem. Doctors aren't usually concerned unless there's a growth difference of more than 15 per cent.

ASK A... MIDWIFE

Why am I beginning to get brown patches on my face? As many as 70 per cent of pregnant women find the colour of their skin changes. You may notice brown patches appearing on your forehead, cheeks, and neck, known as chloasma or the "mask of pregnancy". Darker-skinned women may develop lighter-coloured patches.

Chloasma is caused by an increase in the production of melanin, the pigment that gives the skin and hair its natural colour. It will gradually fade after the birth. To minimize the patches, stay out of the sun as much as possible, use a high-factor

sunscreen, and wear a hat outdoors. Try covering larger patches with a tinted moisturizer or foundation and use a concealer on smaller patches.

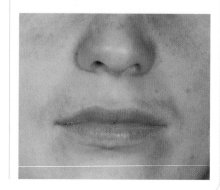

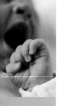

Your second trimester

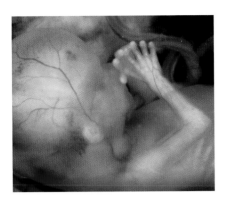

161 days to go...

YOUR BABY TODAY

Every part of your baby has an enhanced blood supply bringing nutrients for growth. Blood vessels are easy to see on scans as the skin is still quite transparent, with little fat yet deposited beneath the skin.

While your energy levels are at a peak, make the most of eating out but choose your meals wisely.

STRONGER NAILS

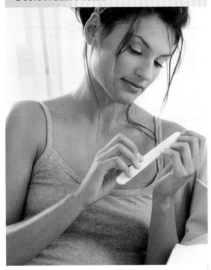

Your nails are likely to be stronger and healthier than ever, due to the hormonal changes that occur during pregnancy.

As your nails are in good condition, you can simply file them and they'll look nice even without nail polish. If you do decide to have a manicure, make sure it takes place in a well-ventilated room. Avoid using nail polishes that contain dibutyl phthalate (DBP), an ingredient that is linked to birth defects in animals.

Being pregnant doesn't have to cramp your lifestyle, and it's perfectly possible to eat out safely. You may, however, have to ask what's in particular dishes to avoid eating foods that aren't recommended during pregnancy, such as soft cheeses, shellfish, and raw eggs (see p.17).

Don't be afraid to ask questions about what exactly is in a dish and always request that your meat and fish are cooked to well done, to avoid any possible contamination. Check that all cheese and milk products, including yogurts, included in recipes, have been pasteurized.

You may find that fatty foods upset your tummy and cause heartburn (see p.194), and, if so, stick with foods that have been grilled or steamed, rather than fried. Beware of accompaniments such as pickles and chutneys that may not be entirely fresh. Pâtés and terrines should also be avoided.

ASK A... NUTRITIONIST

I'm a vegetarian but keep craving meat. Is this normal? When you're pregnant, it's common for your body to crave things that might be missing from your diet. You may be craving meat because you are low in iron or protein, for example, both of which are required in higher quantities during pregnancy.

When you're pregnant, it's particularly important to ensure that you're getting the nutrients you need. If you don't eat meat, you can get iron from wholegrain cereals and flours, leafy green vegetables, molasses, pulses, such as lentils and kidney beans, and dried fruit, such as sultanas, raisins, and apricots.

It helps to have a glass of orange juice, or another drink or food high in vitamin C, such as peppers and other citrus fruit, with your meals, as this encourages the absorption of iron.

Protein is also crucial to your baby's development. Pulses, wholegrains, nuts, seeds, eggs, and dairy produce all contain good quantities of protein. Try adding some quinoa – a protein-packed grain – to your diet. Quinoa is a great alternative to rice and is one of the few plant sources of protein that contains all the essential amino acids. It's also high in omega oils, which will encourage the development of your baby's nervous system and brain.

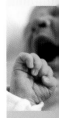

Your 18th week

YOU'LL FIND YOU'RE GAINING WEIGHT WEEK BY WEEK, WHICH IS PERFECTLY NORMAL

Not all the weight you're gaining is your baby. In fact, most of the increase is because parts of your body, such as your breasts, are getting bigger and your blood volume is increasing. You might want to think about booking antenatal classes now because they fill up quickly. They are a great source of information, as well as a good way to make friends and compare notes with other pregnant women.

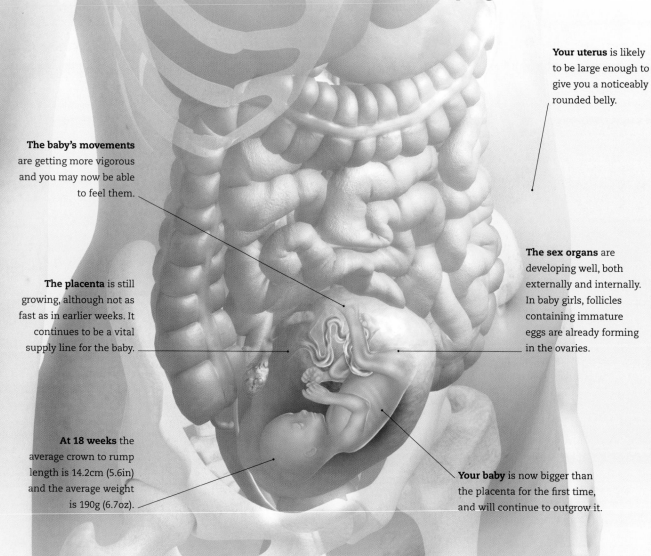

Your uterus is likely to be large enough to give you a noticeably rounded belly.

The baby's movements are getting more vigorous and you may now be able to feel them.

The placenta is still growing, although not as fast as in earlier weeks. It continues to be a vital supply line for the baby.

The sex organs are developing well, both externally and internally. In baby girls, follicles containing immature eggs are already forming in the ovaries.

At 18 weeks the average crown to rump length is 14.2cm (5.6in) and the average weight is 190g (6.7oz).

Your baby is now bigger than the placenta for the first time, and will continue to outgrow it.

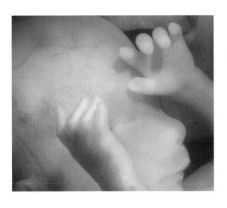

160 days to go...

YOUR BABY TODAY

Your baby's jaw continues to grow throughout the pregnancy, but at this time it can still appear to be quite short. The early tooth buds are hardening within both jaws and, just as with the other bones, calcium is being laid down to strengthen their structure.

Around this time, you may become aware of your baby moving, although for some women first movements are felt much later.

Although your baby is very active, she's not big enough for you to feel any but the strongest kicks on the walls of your uterus. "Quickening" is the term used to describe these first movements, which feel like tiny flutterings or bubbles in your lower abdomen. You may not notice them or not realize that they are the baby at first, as they feel similar to having wind.

If you've been pregnant before, you will be more familiar with the sensation and able to recognize it. First-time mums generally don't feel movements until a bit later, at about 18 to 20 weeks (see p.213), so don't worry if you haven't felt anything yet. The flutterings become more persistent and definite over time, and there will eventually be recognizable kicks and nudges.

Once you can feel the activity, you will become very conscious of them and may become aware of a pattern to them.

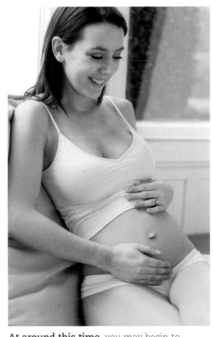

At around this time, you may begin to feel some slight sensations when your baby moves around.

That funny feeling

Was it wind, or did your baby move? The first time you notice your baby moving marks the start of a new chapter in the bonding process, and it seems it has always been the case, even in ancient times.

In many cultures, until the advent of pregnancy tests, "quickening" was the first conclusive evidence of pregnancy, and was viewed as the point at which human life began.

According to ancient Egyptian, Greek, American, and Indian beliefs, the first movement marked the moment when the soul entered the fetus. Aboriginals regard the location where the first quickening is felt as highly significant for the baby.

Being patient

It will be exciting when your partner tells you she can feel the baby move for the first time, and this is a great milestone of the pregnancy. However, when you touch your partner's bump, you may be disappointed to find that you can't feel anything at all. Just be a little patient as there will be plenty of opportunities later on in the pregnancy to feel the movements.

Babies move when they are asleep and awake.

The reason you are less likely to feel your baby move when you're active is that you are likely to be distracted yourself and miss some movement.

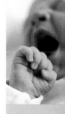

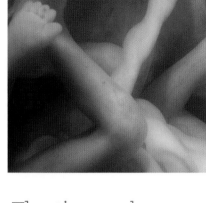

159 days to go...

YOUR BABY TODAY

Here, the baby's legs are in the typical crossed-legs position. The right arm is on the right side of the image. The limbs and umbilical cord appear to be in a tangle, but the umbilical cord is filled with a jelly-like fluid and does not become compressed.

The tiny embryo was once dwarfed by the placenta but now your baby has outgrown it and will continue to do so.

In the early stages of pregnancy, the placenta grew at a far greater rate than your baby. Your baby has now caught up and from now on will be larger than the placenta.

The structure of the placenta will change over the course of the next few weeks as the second wave of cells move into the spiral arteries in the uterus (see p.172). The placenta is currently at its thickest but as it continues to grow, albeit at a slower rate for a time, it thins out.

Your baby's more rapid growth means that at 140g (5oz) she is now heavier than the placenta and by the time she is full term she will be six or seven times its weight. Nutrients supplied across the placenta provide your baby with energy for growth, but growth is in part regulated by her own insulin production and insulin-like growth factors.

Although your baby has relatively high concentrations of growth hormone, which is responsible for growth after birth, this does not seem to play an important role in her growth during pregnancy.

FOCUS ON... HEALTH

Tackling heartburn

If you're battling with the burning sensation and sour taste of heartburn, try these solutions:
- Eat smaller meals, and ensure you chew your food well
- Avoid foods that aggravate your symptoms, such as spicy, rich, and fatty dishes
- Don't smoke or drink alcohol
- Drink milk
- Drink peppermint, ginger, and camomile tea
- Munch raw garlic
- Chew gum after eating
- Remain upright after meals; bending can increase discomfort
- Don't eat late at night
- Raise the head of your bed by 15cm (6in) and lie on your left side.

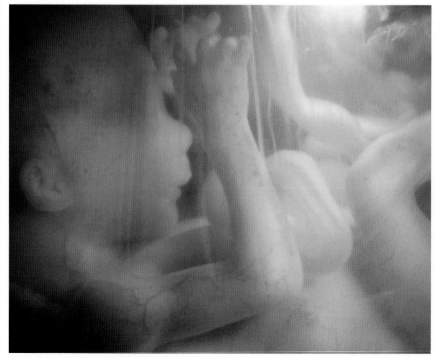

The baby is in a typical position, curled with knees and elbows bent. The blood vessels show up clearly as the skin is still quite transparent. The ear is well developed at this stage.

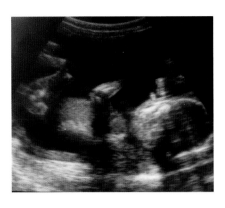

158 days to go...

YOUR BABY TODAY

Although the baby is lying on her side and the face cannot be seen, this image does show the leg and foot particularly well. Because 2D ultrasound only shows a "slice" of the baby, parts may appear to be missing, such as the arm here which stops midway.

It's normal and healthy for you to gain more weight in the second trimester than in the early months of pregnancy.

While you may have gained little weight in the first trimester, from the second trimester onwards you will gain weight each week. On average, women put on 1–2lb (approximately 0.5–1kg) per week from the second trimester to the end of pregnancy, though the weight gain tends to slow down in the last few weeks.

The amount of weight you should be gaining depends on many factors, not least your starting Body Mass Index (BMI) (see p.17). The target weight gains are detailed below.

Not all of the weight gained is the baby; in fact, the fetus makes up only a small part. The rest of the weight is accounted for by your growing uterus, amniotic fluid, breasts, and increased blood volume and fat (see p.99).

If you have any concerns about your weight, seek advice from your midwife. Your weight may not be checked routinely at your antenatal checkups, but your midwife will weigh you if she's concerned about the amount of weight you're gaining.

ASK A... DOCTOR

I keep having hot flushes. Is this normal? Many women experience hot flushes during pregnancy as a result of increased levels of the hormone progesterone. This encourages the blood vessels to dilate – suffusing them with blood, and heat. What's more, when you're pregnant, your metabolism increases, causing extra heat to be produced. That's not to mention the little heater that you have growing inside you.

Wear layers that can be speedily removed and avoid eating spicy foods, and drinking alcohol and caffeine, all of which can encourage hot flushes. Exercise can help by improving circulation, and yoga, and other relaxation exercises, can help you to keep cool and calm.

WEIGHT GAIN

Your target weight gain for the second trimester is no more than 5.5–9kg (12–19lb), which is about twice as much as the target for the first trimester. If, due to pregnancy discomforts, such as morning sickness, you had a difficult first trimester and did not gain much

Weight gain chart

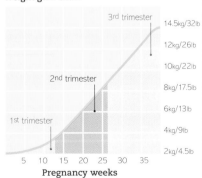

weight, this is a good time to increase your calories to try to make up some of the weight gain. If you gained too much weight in the first trimester, focus on staying active, and filling your plate with lower-calorie yet nutrient-rich fruits and vegetables.

Keep your target goal weight gain in mind. The recommended total pregnancy weight gain is 11–14.5kg (25–32lb) for women whose Body Mass Index (BMI) (see p.17) is in the normal range, between 20 and 25.

If at the start of your pregnancy you were overweight, your total weight gain should be 7–11kg (15–25lb). If you started underweight, you should gain a total of 12.5–18kg (27.5–40lb). If you're expecting twins, you should aim for a total gain of about 16–20kg (35–44lb).

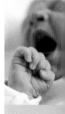

195

A safe workout

Alternating upper and lower body exercises keeps your heart rate up. Remember to get your doctor's approval before starting exercise programmes.

The following workout is effective and safe in the second trimester and can be done three to four times a week to maintain tone and fitness. For exercises with weights, use 2kg (5lb) weights.

Warm up Standing straight, step one leg to the side, then bring the other leg to meet it. Continue this step and touch movement for a minute. Then add an arm movement for one minute: with each step-touch, lift the arms to shoulder height then down. Next, with hands on hips, lift your left knee to your tummy. Alternate the legs for two minutes. Finally, stand straight and circle your left arm across the body and back to the side; repeat with the other arm. Continue for one minute.

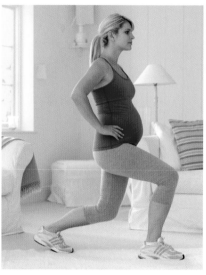

Forward lunge Stand with your hands on your hips. Step your right leg forwards, then with the left foot in place, bend your left knee towards the floor until the right knee is nearly at a right angle. Alternate each side until you've done around 30 repetitions in total. (After the second trimester, you might need to hold the back of a chair.) Keep your tummy pulled in, back straight, head up, and shoulders relaxed.

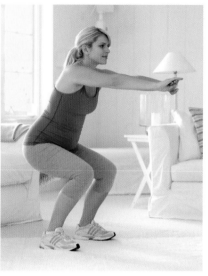

Squats Stand with your feet shoulder-width apart. With your arms stretched out in front of you to shoulder level, squat down, keeping your abdominal muscles pulled in and your feet firmly on the floor. Lower your bottom towards the floor then lift up to the starting point. Breathe out as you lower and in as you lift. Make sure your knees do not go over the end of your toes. Repeat 20 times.

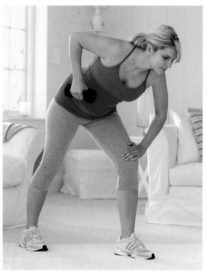

Forward pull-ups With a 2kg weight in your right hand, stand with your left leg in front of you and both knees slightly bent; slowly lower your upper body towards your left knee and rest your left hand on the knee for support. Start with your right arm straight down, then lift your arm up, keeping your elbow close to your body. Your elbow should end pointing to the ceiling. Repeat 20 times on each arm.

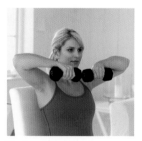

Upright row Sit on an upright chair or stand with legs slightly bent, feet hip-width apart. Hold the weights with your arms down in front of your body. Exhaling, slowly lift the weights to neck height, stopping under the chin. Then inhale and lower the weights to the starting point. Repeat 20 times.

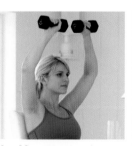

Shoulder press Stand or sit as in the previous exercise. Holding a weight in each hand, slightly bend your arms at the elbows and hold your hands above your shoulders. Then, while breathing out, slowly lift your arms towards the sky until they are straight. Repeat 20 times.

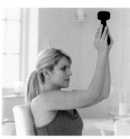

Pectoral lift Sit or stand as before. Hold your arms in front of you at shoulder height while holding a weight. Bend your elbows at a right angle, keeping the upper arms parallel to the floor. With the elbows together, gently lift your arms up and down. Repeat 20 times.

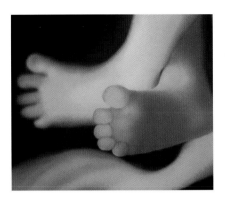

157 days to go...

YOUR BABY TODAY

The skin of your baby is extremely soft and smooth. The soles of the feet and toes are shown in this image and it is clear they are free from wrinkles. During the next week evidence of fingerprint and toeprint patterns will appear on the skin.

Although changes are taking place, your baby's lungs are still fairly immature and won't be fully developed until week 35.

Your baby's complex lung development is continuing.

To picture their growth and development, imagine the whole of the lungs as a tree: the trunk has developed (the trachea or windpipe), and this has branched into smaller and medium-sized branches (bronchi), but the twigs (bronchioles) holding the leaves (alveoli) have not yet formed. It is the alveoli that have walls so thin that they allow oxygen to be absorbed from the air in them and carbon dioxide to leave via the bloodstream.

From now until 28 weeks the "twigs" are forming that will hold the alveoli that will become filled with air after birth. These "twigs" will have a limited ability to transfer gases but the lungs will not be fully effective until the alveoli develop. The growth of the blood vessels that support the lungs closely matches the growth of the lungs themselves. These blood vessels will be essential for the transfer of oxygen after your baby is born.

After birth, all the blood that is leaving the right side of the heart will enter the lung circulation, but before birth, with the lungs filled with fluid and not used for breathing, only a small amount of blood (approximately 10–15 per cent) is directed to them.

STRETCHING SAFELY

Relaxin is one of the most important pregnancy-related hormones. As its name implies, relaxin relaxes the connective tissue, tendons, and ligaments in your body to allow the diaphragm to expand and create space for your baby to grow. It also loosens the ligaments and tendons enough to facilitate the opening of the birth canal for a vaginal delivery.

Relaxin affects most parts of your body and, as a result, your spine and pelvis will also feel less stable, so be aware of your posture and alignment when exercising.

■ **When standing,** always keep your hips in a neutral position. Don't move your hips to one side.

■ **Beware of hyper-extending** (arching) your lower back and rounding your shoulders.

■ **Keep all your movements slow** and controlled, and do not stretch beyond your comfort zone. The increased flexibility of your muscles and tendons could potentially result in over-stretching during activities such as yoga or Pilates.

Relaxin is also responsible for the relaxation of the circulatory system: the walls of the veins are relaxed, which sometimes results in varicose veins (see p.167). Doing cardiovascular exercise will help to increase blood flow and can reduce the occurrence of varicose veins.

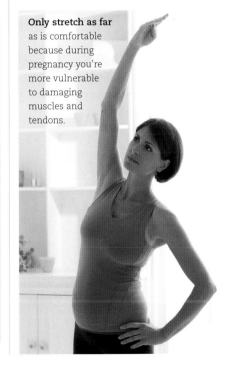

Only stretch as far as is comfortable because during pregnancy you're more vulnerable to damaging muscles and tendons.

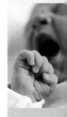

Your 18th week

197

156 days to go...

YOUR BABY TODAY

This image shows how much less obvious the soft spot on the top of the baby's head has become by now. The fingers show up well here, and as your baby increases in size, it becomes easier and easier for ultrasound to show this level of detail.

As your bump begins to grow and is more obvious, your pregnancy will become the main focus of people's attention.

Are you getting a little more attention than you would like?

Once your bump becomes very obvious, you may begin to feel that it and you are public property. Fascinated by your ever-increasing abdomen, some friends and family, or even strangers, may want to see your bump, touch it, or even kiss it. This can feel very strange because, as a rule, people tend not to go around touching each other's stomachs!

If you're uncomfortable about being touched, then you could politely ask people not to touch the bump, or simply move away. There are, however, some advantages to having people notice that you are pregnant: your bump acts as a warning for people not to jostle you in crowds and people tend to give you a seat on public transport.

Another unwanted intrusion might be that people feel entitled to ask you intimate questions regarding your medical history and about the baby. This may make you uncomfortable, especially if you tend to be a private person. People you have never met before might comment on your figure, and discuss whether you're having a girl or a boy.

Some pregnant women enjoy the attention, while others feel that people are intruding on a personal experience. If you feel uncomfortable, answer questions vaguely or try to change the subject; ask the person about him- or herself instead. Another way of avoiding the unwanted attention is to wear loose clothing that makes your bump look less prominent and attractive to touch.

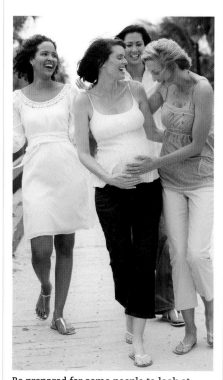

Be prepared for some people to look at, comment on, and want to feel your wonderful bump as it becomes more noticeable. If you're a tactile person by nature, this attention can be easier to handle than if you're not.

AS A MATTER OF FACT

It's not forbidden to eat salt while you're pregnant.

It was once thought that salt increased swelling and the risk of high blood pressure. But your body needs salt to expand your volume of blood and body fluids. Use sea salt (it contains less sodium) and don't have in excess of 6g (0.25oz) a day.

ASK A... DOCTOR

I'm so itchy that I'm scratching to the point of bleeding. What can I do? Most itching in pregnancy, especially on your tummy, is due to stretching of the skin (see p.255), hormonal changes, and heat. Applying moisturizing cream should help.

If you have significant itching, see your midwife or doctor to determine whether you have obstetric cholestasis (see p.473), a serious but rare condition that affects the liver and occurs in about 1 per cent of pregnancies.

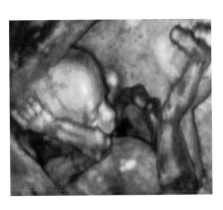

155 days to go...

YOUR BABY TODAY

In this image the whole baby is seen in one view. The legs, held straight, will now be kicking more strongly and, especially if you have had a baby before, you will be increasingly aware of these movements over the next few weeks.

You might want to think about signing up for antenatal classes now as in many areas they get booked up well in advance.

Antenatal classes help to prepare you for the birth of your baby. They usually start in the sixth or seventh month. You'll learn about the signs that you're in labour; breathing and relaxation techniques; pain-relief options; and medical interventions. You'll also be given practical advice on caring for your newborn baby, which can be invaluable if you're a first-time parent.

Depending on where you live, there are various types of classes. These range from free NHS classes run by a midwife at the hospital or clinic, to private classes run by organizations such as the National Childbirth Trust (NCT) (see p.480). You're legally entitled to take time off work to attend classes. Classes are a great way to meet other expectant parents, and by doing so you'll gain an invaluable mutual support system through the rest of your pregnancy and the early weeks of parenting.

By attending antenatal classes with you, your partner can help to prepare for the labour and early weeks of parenting. Classes are also a good way for your partner to meet other dads-to-be. The significant role fathers can play during labour and in the early weeks of parenting is widely acknowledged, and as a result antenatal classes have become much more father-friendly.

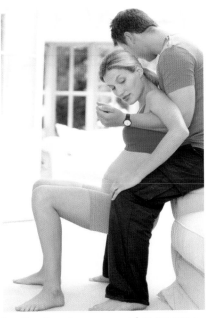

By attending classes, you and your partner can practise and feel more confident about the techniques you'll use in labour.

FOCUS ON... TWINS

Classes for two

As twins are likely to arrive ahead of schedule, you should definitely look into booking antenatal classes now so that you can start them early. Besides, your bump could be very large towards the end, and you may feel less mobile and inclined to go. Because twins sometimes need special care, you should arrange a tour of the Special Care Baby Unit, too.

In some areas, there are special antenatal sessions for those having twins or more, often in the evenings. If your hospital doesn't provide these, a neighbouring hospital might. Ask your midwife.

FIND A CLASSMATE

If you're single, you don't have to go it alone. There's no reason why you can't attend a class with a friend or relative – preferably the person who will be attending the birth. If you'd prefer not to do this, you could find out if there are any classes in your area for single expectant mums. You may feel more comfortable in this environment and you will get the opportunity to meet other women who are in the same position as you.

Don't skip classes just because you're single: they're an invaluable way of learning about pregnancy, labour, and parenting.

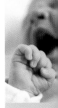

199

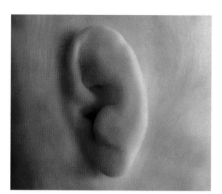

154 days to go...

YOUR BABY TODAY

Like your own ear, your baby's ear is made of soft and flexible cartilage. Although the outer ear is well developed at this stage, inner ear structures will continue to mature throughout your pregnancy.

Is it a boy or a girl? You and your partner may want to start thinking about whether you would like to find out.

The sex of your baby should now be apparent on an ultrasound scan, but you won't have this for a couple of weeks yet (see p.211).

Whether your baby develops into a boy or a girl depends on the presence or absence of a Y chromosome. Males are

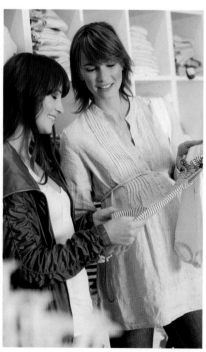

Some pregnant women will want to delay buying a complete set of clothes for the baby until they know the sex, but not everyone wants to settle for either pink or blue.

XY and the Y chromosome instructs the reproductive glands (gonads) to become testes. These then produce testosterone that inhibits the development of the internal female organs and in turn stimulates the normal development of the external male genitalia.

If there is no Y chromosome, the gonad becomes an ovary and the internal genitals are female by default; it's not the ovary that dictates that the female reproductive organs will develop but the lack of testosterone. In the female the uterus is formed first and the vagina lengthens upwards to meet it.

HOSPITAL POLICY

Bear in mind that it might not always be possible to find out the sex of your baby at the 20-week scan. While most units have a written policy to reveal the baby's sex at the 20-week-scan if this information is requested by the parents, some units have a policy of not telling anyone the sex of the baby from scans alone, partly because they cannot be 100 per cent accurate.

If you want to know the policy in your hospital or clinic, ask your midwife or doctor.

ASK A... MUM

Our 20-week scan is fast approaching. I want to know the baby's sex but my partner doesn't. What should we do?
When one person in a relationship wants something that is at odds with what his or her partner wants, tensions can arise.

Like you, I wanted to find out the sex of my baby but my partner didn't. We both explained our reasons: I felt that knowing the sex would better help me prepare for the birth, both emotionally and practically; my partner said he wanted the surprise element of discovering the sex of the baby at the actual birth.

Talk to each other openly and hopefully you'll be able to reach an agreement. Try not to let the issue get out of hand and consider backing down if necessary. It's important that you feel united at this special time.

You may find either one of you doesn't feel as strongly once you start talking. You could agree to find out but not tell anyone else. If you do find out, don't forget the result is not 100 per cent accurate.

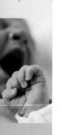

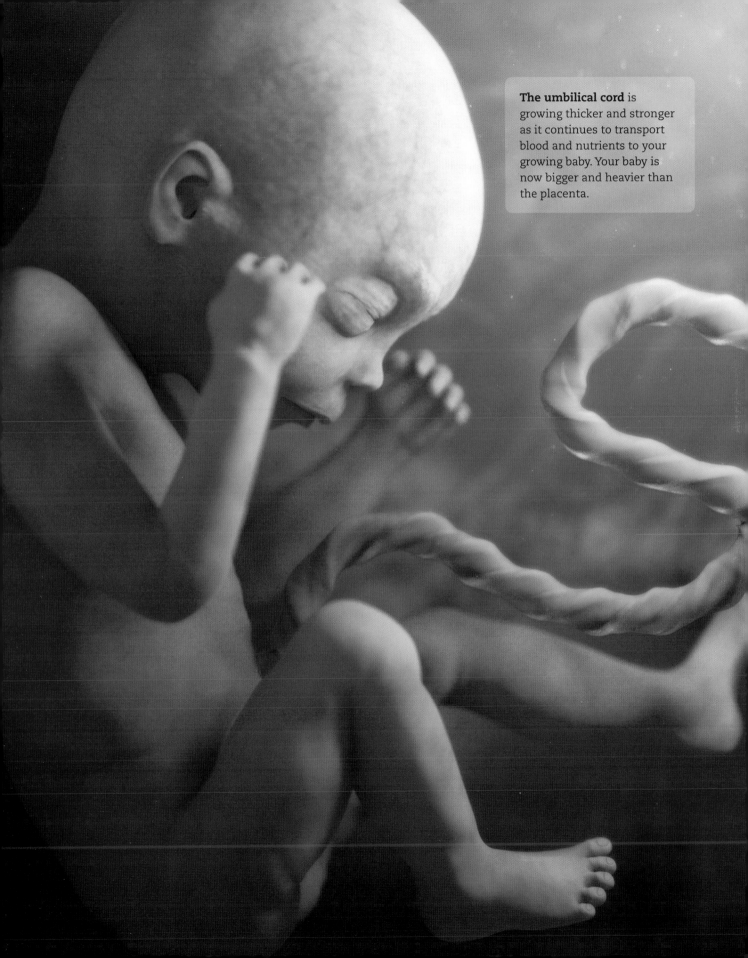

The umbilical cord is growing thicker and stronger as it continues to transport blood and nutrients to your growing baby. Your baby is now bigger and heavier than the placenta.

Your 19th week

YOU'LL PROBABLY FIND YOU'RE BECOMING MORE ATTACHED TO YOUR BABY BY THE DAY

It's easier now to think of your baby as a real person, especially if you see him on another scan around this time. He's almost fully formed and the function of his organs is well advanced. You'll be taking your maternal responsibilities very seriously, but don't let anxieties build up. Talk over any worries you may have with your partner and your midwife; many pregnant women also seek comfort and advice from their own mothers.

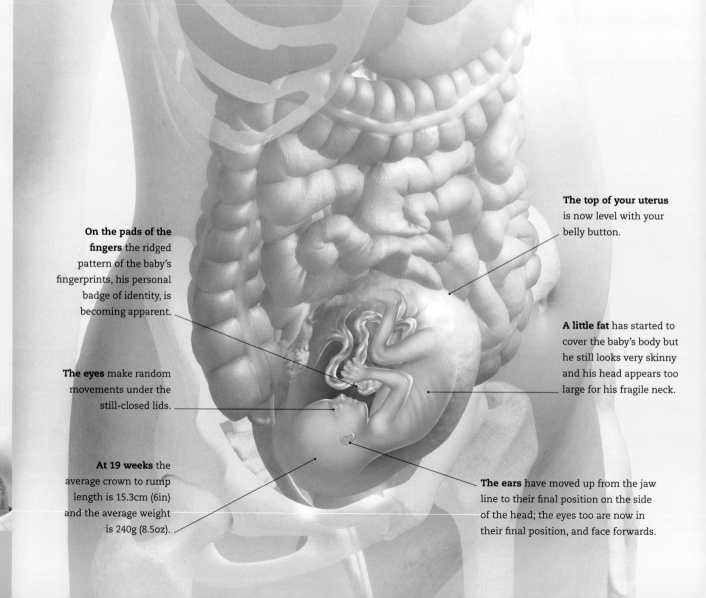

On the pads of the fingers the ridged pattern of the baby's fingerprints, his personal badge of identity, is becoming apparent.

The eyes make random movements under the still-closed lids.

At 19 weeks the average crown to rump length is 15.3cm (6in) and the average weight is 240g (8.5oz).

The top of your uterus is now level with your belly button.

A little fat has started to cover the baby's body but he still looks very skinny and his head appears too large for his fragile neck.

The ears have moved up from the jaw line to their final position on the side of the head; the eyes too are now in their final position, and face forwards.

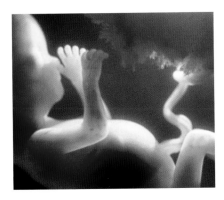

153 days to go...

YOUR BABY TODAY

Anchored to the placenta by the umbilical cord, your baby floats in amniotic fluid. Your uterus provides a warm, protective environment for your baby with lots of room to move in near weightless conditions.

As you approach the halfway mark of your pregnancy, you'll continue to be astounded that there's a baby growing inside you!

The further along the path of pregnancy you are, the more attached and protective you're likely to feel towards your baby. What was once a tiny bundle of cells now looks like an almost fully formed baby – and you will continue to be amazed that you and your partner have made that baby and that this incredible process is happening inside your body.

Once you feel your baby move (see p.213) within the next few weeks, the attachment to him is likely to grow even stronger. While you may have some anxieties at times, try to relax and enjoy your pregnancy – it will be over before you know it.

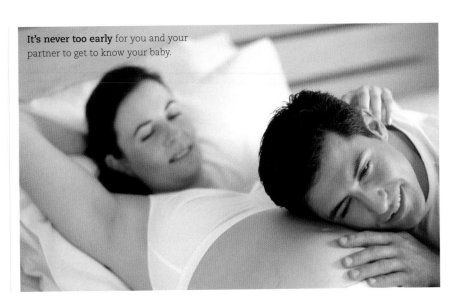

It's never too early for you and your partner to get to know your baby.

ASK A... MIDWIFE

I've got a full-on career and have hardly had any time to think about the baby since I've been pregnant. Will this stop us from bonding?
Even if you work full time while you're pregnant, this doesn't have to have a negative effect on your relationship with your baby. As your baby grows, you will probably find that you start to develop a relationship with your "bump" as you anticipate your baby's movements and perhaps talk to him. Make sure

you plan enough maternity leave before your due date as this gives you time for practical and emotional preparations, as well as time to rest.

There's some evidence to suggest that too much stress in a mother can affect her unborn baby's brain development (see p.187). This highlights the importance of ensuring you have regular opportunities to relax during pregnancy and so, if your work is stressful, maybe this would be a good time to look at your priorities.

FOCUS ON... HEALTH

It's all a blur

Water retention in pregnancy can affect the eyes. Both the lens and cornea can become thicker, and there can be an increase in fluid in the eyeball, causing pressure and blurred vision. This usually resolves itself after the birth. Exercising to keep the fluid moving, and avoiding wearing contact lenses can help. Notify your doctor or midwife if you have vision problems.

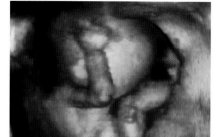

YOU ARE 18 WEEKS AND 2 DAYS

152 days to go...

YOUR BABY TODAY

The sound of your baby's rapidly moving heart muscle can be detected using a simple hand-held listening device – the frequency change it produces is converted into a sound that is easy for you, and your doctor or midwife, to hear.

Your baby's hiccups become stronger and more frequent as pregnancy progresses, and you may be able to feel them now.

Just like your own, your baby's hiccups are short, powerful, jerky contractions of the diaphragm, causing a sudden rush of air that closes the opening between the vocal cords.

Hiccups frequently follow each other in rapid succession and are often followed by gentle limb-stretching movements. No one is certain why babies hiccup. Perhaps it's due to the immaturity of the nerves supplying the diaphragm, or else to your baby's small stomach quickly becoming over-distended.

Your baby's ears and eyes are now in their final position on his face. The ears have moved up from the jaw line and the eyes have moved from the side of the head to lie closer together, looking forward. The eyes move beneath the lids but not yet in a co-ordinated way. He will open them at around 26 weeks.

FOCUS ON... NUTRITION

Not all fat is bad

Many fats are healthy, and should be consumed as part of a heart-healthy diet. The key is to choose healthy fat. For example unsaturated fats, such as those found in olive oil, rapeseed (canola) oil, and in nuts and avocados, are good for you and your baby.

Saturated fats, such as those found in butter and whole milk, and trans fats (chemically altered vegetable oils) found in many processed foods, should be kept to a minimum. Substitute good fats for bad fats in your diet:

■ **When making a salad dressing** or in cooking, choose olive oil or rapeseed (canola) oil. Ready-made salad dressings are often high in saturated fat.

■ **Eat nuts and avocados,** which are full of healthy fats.

■ **Eat white meat** as it is lower in saturated fat than red meat.

Your baby is looking more human and fully formed every day, with well-developed facial features and limbs – and he may even get the hiccups.

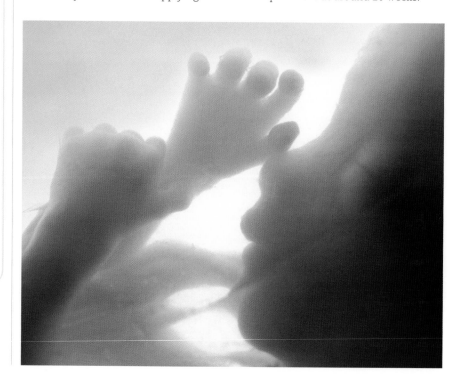

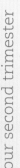
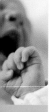

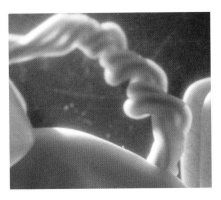

151 days to go...

YOUR BABY TODAY

Coiling is now well established in the umbilical cord. This coiling protects the cord from kinking and from pressing on the umbilical arteries and vein. The coils help to ensure that there is a continuous flow of blood both to the placenta and also back to the baby.

Wanting to protect your baby is a natural maternal instinct and it's likely to have started already.

It's understandable that you want your baby to have the best start in life, but this may lead you to unnecessary anxiety about his health and wellbeing.

You may find yourself worried about things that previously did not bother you. For example, you may use a computer regularly and only now become concerned about the radiation it might produce (see box, right).

Try to relax and keep concerns in perspective; remember that your baby is very resilient and well-protected inside the uterus. If you have concerns about lifestyle issues or how your baby is developing, your midwife can provide information and reassurance.

Meanwhile, you can take good care of yourself by eating well, exercising regularly, and attending all your antenatal appointments.

AS A MATTER OF FACT

There is no significant radiation from a computer that can affect an unborn baby.

There are laws to limit the amount and types of emissions from a computer. For this reason, they aren't harmful during pregnancy.

ASK A... MIDWIFE

What are the risks if I gain too much weight? Pregnant women who overeat tend to have larger babies, which can make the delivery more difficult (the baby is more likely to get stuck during the birth) and increase the likelihood of having a Caesarean section.

Pregnant women who are overweight are also more likely to experience health complications, such as gestational diabetes (see p.473) and pre-eclampsia (see p.474). Their children may be at greater risk of becoming diabetic and being obese in later life.

Most of the research seems to focus on pregnant women who have gained more than 18kg (40lb).

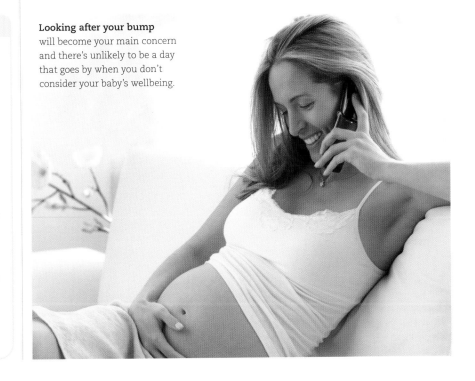

Looking after your bump will become your main concern and there's unlikely to be a day that goes by when you don't consider your baby's wellbeing.

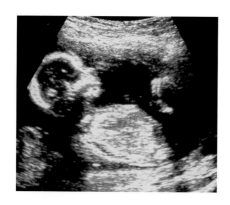

150 days to go...

YOUR BABY TODAY

This is a side view ultrasound scan with the baby's head in the top left. Your baby appears completely human with all fingers and toes fully developed. The skin is now covered with lanugo, fine protective hair.

There's no harm in encouraging your baby to move to increase the likelihood of you feeling his wriggles.

If you're waiting to feel your baby's first movements, be patient. Although it's reassuring to feel him wriggling around, becoming stressed about it won't be good for either of you. Remember, many pregnant women – first-time mums especially – don't feel those first flutterings until 18 to 20 weeks or later (see p.213).

It may be that you have been so busy and active that you have been distracted and not felt your baby's movements. So just stop and relax for a little while; when you're resting the movements will be much more obvious.

Also remember that the baby does not move continuously and there will be periods when the baby is not moving.

There are a few things you can try to stimulate your baby into action – the more he moves, the more chance there is that you'll feel it. It may help to lie down on your side, with your bump supported. Doing this may stimulate your baby to move, as he changes his position to accommodate yours. If all else fails sit down and rest while you have something sweet to eat or drink. This may just do the trick, because babies respond to a rise in their mother's blood sugar.

ASK A... MIDWIFE

I've heard that babies react to sounds with a "startle reflex", so can I prompt my baby to move by playing some loud music?
Your baby cannot hear yet, so playing loud music won't have any effect at this stage.

By about 22 weeks, your baby will be able to hear some sounds (see p.238), by 24–25 weeks he'll be reacting to many different sounds, and sudden noises may prompt a startle response (see p.256).

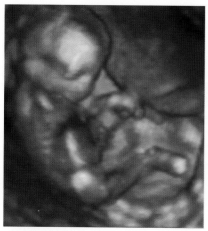

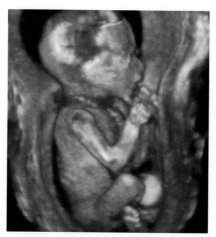

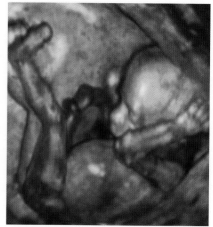

You will probably not be able to feel your baby move yet, but he is incredibly active inside your uterus. Somersaults and stretches are part of his daily routine, as are thumb and toe sucking. Your baby moves when awake and asleep: he has no control over his movements at this stage. Ultrasound scans reveal a huge range of movement in between inactive periods.

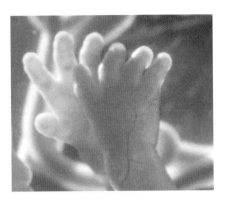

149 days to go...

YOUR BABY TODAY

Your baby's hands – and feet – look quite large at this stage in pregnancy: it is as if your baby needs time to grow into them. The past few weeks have seen rapid changes in the hands and feet and it's now time for the limbs to catch up.

Your baby's fingers and toes are fully developed and their unique prints are beginning to form.

Your baby will be a unique individual and his fingerprints will be proof of this. The ridge patterns in the dermis that will eventually form fingerprints (and "toeprints") are fully developed by this stage of pregnancy. These skin ridges are genetically determined and, as with most developments, are seen about a week earlier in the hands than the feet.

Your baby's sweat glands appeared in his skin in the eighth week, and will continue to increase up to 28 weeks; but they do not function until after birth. The colour of your baby's skin is due to melanin, a pigment produced by "melanocytes", specialized skin cells that have now migrated into the skin. Different skin tones are not due to differing numbers of these cells but due to the amount and shade of pigment that each cell produces. Melanin protects the skin from ultraviolet light which damages DNA.

Although unborn babies produce melanin pigment, they do not achieve their final amount of skin pigment until well into childhood. For this reason it follows that all newborn babies are particularly vulnerable to sunburn. Dark-skinned babies are likely to have a light skin tone when they're born.

AS A MATTER OF FACT

Eating plenty of foods that are rich in vitamin E could reduce the risk of your baby developing allergies, including asthma.

Researchers believe that low levels of vitamin E during pregnancy could adversely affect your baby's lung development or immune system. To boost your intake, improve your diet rather than taking supplements. If you eat more than you need, vitamin E is stored in the body for future use.

ACUPUNCTURE

In acupuncture, certain points on the body associated with energy channels or meridians are stimulated by the insertion of fine needles. The belief is that these conduct vital energy or "chi" around the body. Illness or symptoms are associated with an imbalance of this vital energy.

Acupuncture has been widely and successfully used in pregnancy and regular treatments can help to treat a number of health problems:
■ Pain and nausea – a recent study has shown it to be effective in relieving nausea and vomiting or the potentially more dangerous hyperemesis gravidarum (see p.111).
■ Heartburn (see p.194)
■ Haemorrhoids (see p.468)
■ Stress (see p.187)
■ Carpal tunnel syndrome (see p.471).

Acupuncture has been successful in "turning" breech babies (see p.433), and can also be used during labour to boost energy and relieve pain.

Always use a registered practitioner who is experienced in treating pregnant women.

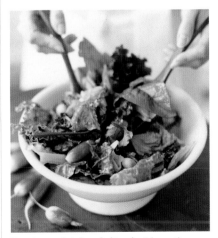

Boost your intake of vitamin E by eating salad leaves, green leafy vegetables, nuts, avocados, eggs, and wheatgerm.

Your 19th week

207

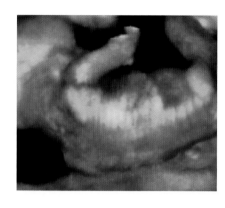

148 days to go...

YOUR BABY TODAY

Your baby appears to be quite thin on early scans. One reason is that fat stores have not yet been laid down underneath the skin, which looks almost transparent. An ultrasound image also highlights the underlying bony skeleton, enhancing this effect.

At around this time you'll have another scan, and your baby will get a thorough health check.

From 18–20 weeks most hospitals offer a detailed ultrasound scan, which is termed an "anomaly" or "anatomy" scan. The scan is used to check the baby's overall development and examine his organs and body systems (see pp.214–5) to check for signs of problems. For most women and their partners, this scan will reassure them that all is progressing well with the pregnancy and the baby's development.

The scan can take some time to perform because of the detailed measurements and investigations taking place. The sonographer can only carry out the checks when the baby is in the correct position – this can be a challenge, given that the baby is likely to be moving around a lot. If the position of your baby makes it difficult to carry out all the checks, you may be asked to walk around for a little while and then return, or even to come back in a week or two for another attempt.

EXERCISING IN WATER

Water is a great environment to work out in during pregnancy: the added support for your bump and extra resistance will enable you to maintain your fitness.

When standing, the water should be just above your waist – too deep and you will not be stable enough and too shallow and you won't get enough support from the water.

You are likely to find aquanatal classes at your local leisure centre, but here are a few simple exercises you can do yourself:

■ **Jogging on the spot:** bring your knees up and push your arms forward and back in a pumping motion. Jog for 3–4 minutes, if possible, but always stop if you feel tired. This exercise has cardiovascular benefits, and will help to tone your legs and arms.

■ **Bicycle exercise:** stand in the water and place a float under each arm. Once you're comfortable, lean back slightly and move your legs in front of you as if you are rotating the pedals on a bicycle. Continue the cycling motion for 3–4 minutes, if possible, but always stop if you feel tired. This exercise will help you to maintain your fitness and help to tone your legs. It's also a good way to strengthen your back and arms.

■ **Arm exercises:** stand with your feet apart and knees slightly bent, then crouch to submerge your shoulders in the water. Lift your arms from your sides to the height of your shoulders and back down again. Pull your arms down in the water towards you and push up as hard as you can (see right). This exercise will help to tone and strengthen the muscles in your arms, back, and abdomen.

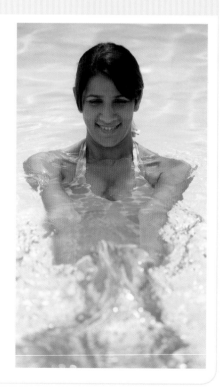

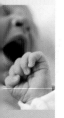

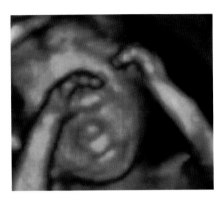

147 days to go...

YOUR BABY TODAY

Your baby has highly flexible joints, enabling her to raise her arms high. This is because her bones are first made of cartilage, which is soft and flexible. Gradually, the cartilage is being replaced by calcium-containing bone.

You'll be getting advice from all quarters, but there's one person you might want to listen to – your mother.

FOCUS ON... YOUR BODY

Taking the strain

There are a number of changes in your body during pregnancy that impact on how you can exercise and how your body moves:

■ **The increased weight** of your baby, placenta, extra blood, enlarged uterus, and breast tissue can cause stress on your body, and most notably on your skeleton.

■ **Postural changes** due to changes in the centre of gravity can increase your chances of developing hip, back, and knee problems.

■ **Relaxin** (see p.197), a pregnancy-related hormone that affects the ligaments, can increase flexibility and result in improper alignment of the spine and pelvis.

Effective and safe exercises are the most efficient way of maintaining and improving your posture and minimizing the stress on your body (see p.196 for a great second trimester workout).

Regular exercise (especially weight bearing exercise such as walking, and using weights – see p.196) generally improves the bone density of your skeleton.

Whether or not you're already close to your mother, being pregnant is likely to affect your relationship with each other. Many women feel naturally closer to their mothers as they go through this significant life event, turning to them for help and reassurance during the course of pregnancy and wanting them to be there in the days and weeks following the birth of the baby.

It's normal for a mother to respond to her daughter being pregnant by being very protective, so do expect a few more phone calls than usual. Your mother is bound to offer lots of advice. Whether or not you take it all on board, do listen – you may just find some of it useful.

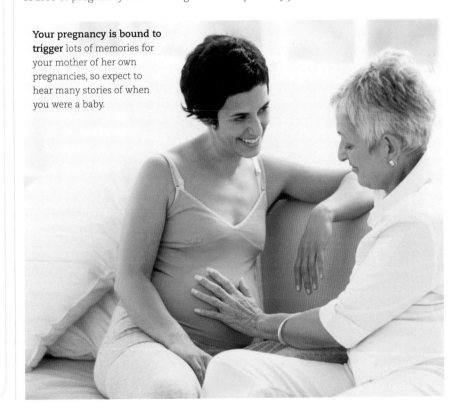

Your pregnancy is bound to trigger lots of memories for your mother of her own pregnancies, so expect to hear many stories of when you were a baby.

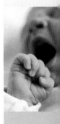

Your 20th week

THOSE BUTTERFLIES IN YOUR STOMACH MAY BE MORE THAN JUST WIND

In the next few days, you might feel your baby's movements for the first time. The little flutter can be such a tiny sensation that many women put it down to wind. But what a wonderful moment when you realize the truth! If you want to find out the sex of your baby, it could be revealed on the ultrasound scan you have this week.

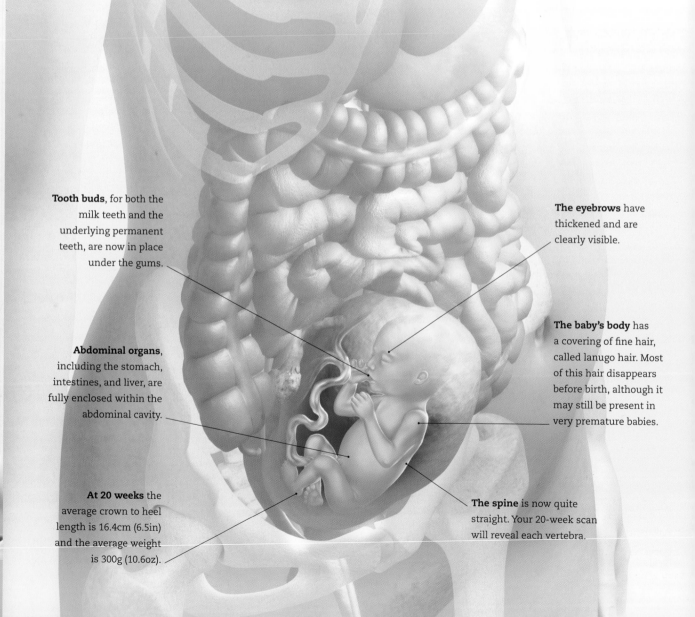

Tooth buds, for both the milk teeth and the underlying permanent teeth, are now in place under the gums.

The eyebrows have thickened and are clearly visible.

Abdominal organs, including the stomach, intestines, and liver, are fully enclosed within the abdominal cavity.

The baby's body has a covering of fine hair, called lanugo hair. Most of this hair disappears before birth, although it may still be present in very premature babies.

At 20 weeks the average crown to heel length is 16.4cm (6.5in) and the average weight is 300g (10.6oz).

The spine is now quite straight. Your 20-week scan will reveal each vertebra.

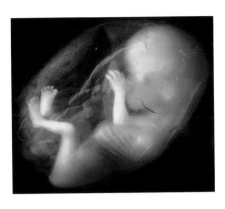

146 days to go...

YOUR BABY TODAY

This image shows the entire baby lying within the amniotic sac. Every finger and toe, and even the lower ribs in the chest, can be seen. Although the head is still quite large, the limbs are much more in proportion with the body.

If you want to know whether you're having a boy or a girl, this is the week you might be able to find out.

You'll have a scan this week and may be given the opportunity to find out the sex of your baby. Identifying the gender is dependent on a number of factors, including the expertise of the sonographer, the quality of the equipment being used, and the position of the baby, particularly the legs, which could obstruct the genitals. Even if all of these factors are favourable and the genitals can be seen, there is an error factor, so the information given is never 100 per cent accurate. You may be able to identify the genitals yourself as you're watching the screen, so if you don't want to know, it's advisable to look away.

If you have an amniocentesis test (see pp.152–3) and want to know the sex of your baby, it can be identified with 100 per cent accuracy.

This 2D scan is a close-up of the baby's profile, showing the bright frontal bone of the forehead, the nose, lips, and chin. The nasal bone appears as a bright area at the top of the bridge of the nose.

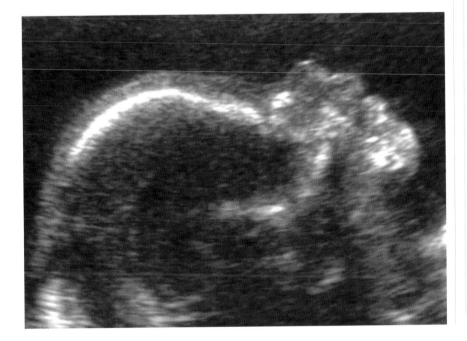

TIME TO THINK ABOUT

Finding out the sex of your baby

Is it a good idea to find out the sex of your baby before he (or she) is born?

Yes...
- Being able to call your baby "he" or "she" rather than "it" or "the baby" may help you and your partner to bond with him or her.
- Knowing the sex means you can choose a name before the big day, although bear in mind that it's not guaranteed to suit him or her.
- Decorating the nursery and buying baby clothes may be simpler.

No...
- Not knowing is a huge motivator during labour and birth for many women, and the excitement of finding out right at the end can help to keep you focused through all the stages of labour and delivery.
- Remember that unless you had an amniocentesis test or CVS test (see pp.152–3), there's no way of knowing your baby's sex for certain. Sonographers can (and do) get it wrong, so don't get too attached just yet to the name you've chosen.

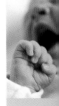

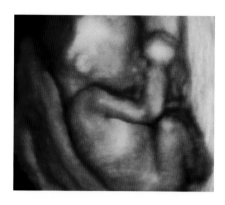

YOU ARE 19 WEEKS AND 2 DAYS

145 days to go...

YOUR BABY TODAY

Your baby is increasingly using her hands and feet to explore her surroundings. All limbs have a full and unobstructed range of movements and the fingertips especially are extremely sensitive. Most of her movements are reflex responses at this stage.

Comfortably floating in her fluid-filled amniotic sac, your baby is made up almost completely of water.

AS A MATTER OF FACT

Pregnant women used to believe that not drinking enough water would make the baby dirty!

While it is important to stay hydrated during pregnancy, the amniotic fluid is not affected by what you drink.

Because water can travel through the skin and the baby is floating in amniotic fluid, her water content is really high, nearly 90 per cent. As your baby's skin thickens and becomes less permeable, and her kidneys better regulate the amount of water lost in the urine, her proportion of water will reduce to 70 per cent at delivery and again to about 60 per cent by the age of 10 as kidney function continues to improve.

Fluids conduct sound waves but the inner ear is still immature and it will be three weeks before a startle response to sounds can be reliably seen on a scan. As both the uterine wall and the ear drums become thinner, she will gradually respond to higher frequencies and quieter sounds.

FOCUS ON... YOUR BABY

Low-lying placenta

Placenta praevia is when the placenta is either partially covering (minor) or completely covering (major) the cervix. In major placenta praevia, the baby cannot be born vaginally. Major placenta praevia poses a high risk of heavy bleeding, either in the later stages of pregnancy or during the actual labour, which is treated as an emergency.

If a low-lying placenta is detected at your 20-week scan, you may be offered another scan at about 34 weeks; the placenta may "move up" as the uterus grows, and by about 34 weeks no longer be low. With major placenta praevia, you may be admitted to hospital for bed rest in late pregnancy.

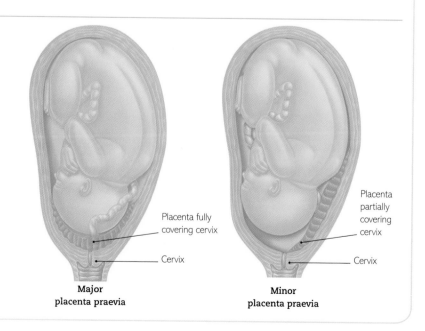

Placenta fully covering cervix

Cervix

Placenta partially covering cervix

Cervix

Major placenta praevia

Minor placenta praevia

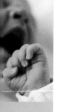

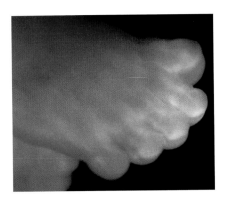

144 days to go...

YOUR BABY TODAY

The toes will wriggle and stretch just as much as the hands and fingers. Your baby is extremely flexible at this time and as likely to bring one or both feet up to her mouth as she is her hands in order to explore them with her sensitive mouth and lips.

Are you feeling your baby kicking? She's letting you know she's definitely in there – a wonderful pregnancy milestone.

At around this time, you're likely to feel that awe-inspiring first kick. While your baby has been moving in your uterus since around the sixth week of gestation, it's only at this stage that she'll make her movements so definitely felt (although some women do feel movements from around 15 to 16 weeks). When exactly you feel that movement can be affected by your body weight, your baby's position, the location of the placenta, and whether it's your first pregnancy.

Experiencing the first sensation of movement, whether it's a feeling of bubbles, butterflies, flipping goldfish, or even a resounding kick, is likely to be an emotionally charged moment. After all, this is the first time your baby has communicated with you, even though she's not aware of what she's doing.

Once you've felt your baby move, you may want her to do so again – just to make sure you didn't imagine it. You may, however, not feel another movement for a few days. A good time to feel the baby moving is when you're relaxed and resting. Your partner may want to place his hand on your tummy to experience those first thumps himself. It won't hurt your baby to play with her, so do gently press on your abdomen when she kicks.

MATERNITY SWIMWEAR

Swimming is fantastic exercise during pregnancy, but you may need to invest in new swimwear as your breasts and abdomen grow.

■ **Comfort and support:** maternity swimsuits have additional support. The costumes are designed to be higher at the back and have more support in the cups. Maternity swimwear is made with stretchy fabric that is comfortable and will give as you grow.

■ **Try a tankini:** this is a two-piece swimsuit that has a vest-style, rather than bra, top. It will flash your bump without revealing too much.

■ **If you're self-conscious** about your bump, wear a sarong. If you prefer to bare your bump to females only, go to women's sessions at your local pool.

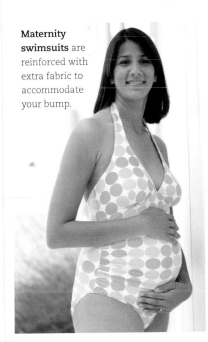

Maternity swimsuits are reinforced with extra fabric to accommodate your bump.

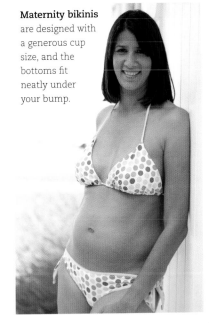

Maternity bikinis are designed with a generous cup size, and the bottoms fit neatly under your bump.

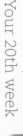

Your 20th week

213

Your 20-week scan

This second-trimester ultrasound, also known as the "anomaly" or "anatomy" scan, looks in detail at how your baby's major organs and body systems have developed, as well as checking the placenta and volume of the amniotic fluid.

YOUR BABY'S CHECKS

What the ultrasound looks at

During this scan, your baby's organs are examined in detail and therefore it can take a little longer to perform than previous scans. For most, the scan provides reassurance that their baby is developing normally. The following areas will be checked.

■ **The brain**, including the fluid-filled spaces inside the brain and the shape of the back of your baby's brain (cerebellum).

■ **The spine**, to check for spina bifida or other problems.

■ **The upper lip**, to check for cleft lip (see p.476).

■ **The heart**, to rule out any major heart malformations. The heartbeat will be checked, too.

■ **The stomach** and diaphragm.

■ **The kidneys and bladder**, making sure that both kidneys are present and there are no blockages or malformations.

■ **The abdominal wall**, to look for a defect, known as gastroschesis.

■ **Your baby's limbs**, to make sure there are no hand or feet malformations, such as club foot.

■ **The umbilical cord**, to check that this has a normal number of blood vessels (see p.113).

What the scan reveals

This scan may be done at 18–20 weeks. By this time, your baby's organs and body systems are well developed and can be seen clearly on an ultrasound scan. The sonographer will look closely at how your baby's major organs and body systems have formed and whether there are any indications of a problem (see box, left). In most cases, the scan will reassure women that their baby is developing normally.

If your baby is found to have a problem, the sonographer will refer you to a fetal medicine expert who will confirm the findings and offer follow-up scans throughout the rest of your pregnancy. He or she will also talk to the hospital paediatrician to ensure that they have enough information to look after your baby at birth.

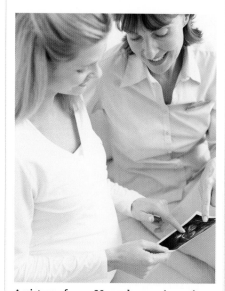

A picture of your 20-week scan shows the incredible detail visible on an ultrasound at this stage of your pregnancy.

Your due date

If you had a dating scan in the first trimester, your dates are unlikely to be changed after a second-trimester scan. This is because dating is most accurate in early pregnancy when all babies essentially grow at the same rate. Later on, individual differences in growth start to appear, making it harder to tell if your baby is just big for dates or if you are further along than thought.

However, if you didn't have a booking scan, the sonographer may change your dates if your baby is 10–14 days smaller or larger than expected. If your dates have been confirmed by a first-trimester scan, such a variation in expected growth may be a sign of a growth problem in your baby (see p.284), although this is rare.

Measuring your baby As your whole baby no longer fits on the screen, the crown–rump length won't be measured. Instead, your baby's size will be calculated by combining a series of measurements in a mathematical formula. The sonographer will measure the width (biparietal diameter) and circumference of your baby's head, the circumference of your baby's tummy (abdominal circumference), and the length of your baby's upper leg bone (femur length). These measurements help to estimate the size of your baby and check that this is within the normal range for this stage of pregnancy.

Placenta and amniotic fluid

The placenta will be examined to ensure that it appears normal and isn't blocking the baby's exit route (the cervix). In early pregnancy, the placenta may be low-lying

During your ultrasound, a picture of your baby is produced when high-frequency sound waves bounce off your baby's organs and tissues and translate into an image on screen. In this image, solid matter, such as bones, are white, while softer tissue appears grey. Areas that contain fluid, such as blood vessels or the stomach, as well as the amniotic fluid, do not respond to the sound waves and therefore appear as black areas on the scan. The sonographer will study these details to assess how your baby is developing in the womb.

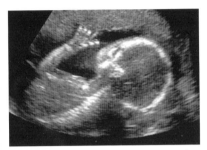

The skull is well developed by now, and features such as the ears are clearly seen.

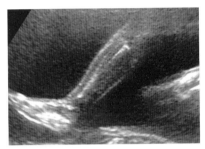

The leg bones are measured to assess how your baby is growing.

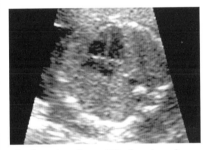

The four chambers of the heart can be identified and certain defects spotted.

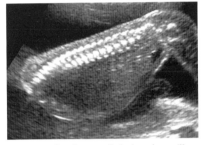

Each vertebra in your baby's spine will be counted to check for spina bifida.

example, because you are over 35 years of age, or you were given a high risk from a previous screening test. Common markers include a bright spot in your baby's heart, seen in about 1–2 per cent of normal babies; extra fluid in your baby's kidneys; short leg or arm bones; thickened neck skin (nuchal fold); and bright (echogenic) fetal intestines.

Some specific abnormalities are linked with a far higher risk of Down's or other chromosomal abnormalities. These include certain kinds of heart defects and other major malformations, such as abnormalities in the bowel.

What happens next If the sonographer detects soft markers, he or she will discuss the findings and may suggest a diagnostic test (see p.152), especially if you already have an increased risk of Down's. However, an earlier all-clear from a diagnostic test means that you can be confident your baby's chromosomes are normal. If an obvious abnormality is seen, and you haven't had a diagnostic test, this will probably be strongly advised. Having information from the scan will help you decide whether you want to proceed with a test. Whatever your decision, any associated abnormalities will be monitored throughout your pregnancy.

(see p.212). This is more common in subsequent pregnancies as the placenta can't attach to the same area twice. In most cases, the placenta moves up and out of the way by the third trimester as the uterus grows. If your placenta is low-lying, your midwife or doctor will arrange a follow-up scan later in pregnancy to check that the placenta has moved up out of the way. If a later scan shows that it has failed to move, a condition known as placenta praevia (see p.473), you will be monitored until the birth.

The amniotic fluid is assessed to check that there isn't too little or too much. If there is too much fluid, it may be possible to drain some using amniocentesis (see p.152) to decrease the risk of later complications such as premature labour (see p.431). Too little fluid can indicate a problem with fetal growth or your baby's renal tract and your baby may need to be monitored.

Markers for Down's syndrome

Ultrasound at this stage is not a reliable way to detect Down's, but it can pick up certain signs known as "soft markers" that may suggest that your baby has an increased risk of Down's. However, many markers are very common and are not usually a cause for alarm unless there are multiple soft markers or you already have an increased risk for Down's, for

Unless your baby is curled up or the legs are closed tight, the sonographer will have a pretty good idea as to whether you're going to have a boy or a girl. Some hospitals have a policy not to reveal the sex, so check this in advance. If you are told which sex your baby is, resist the urge to go out and spend money on all-blue or all-pink décor as sonographers have been known to get it wrong! If you don't want to know the sex, tell the sonographer at the start of the scan.

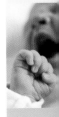

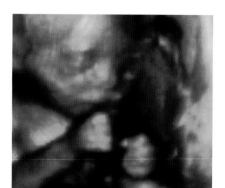

YOU ARE 19 WEEKS AND 4 DAYS

143 days to go...

YOUR BABY TODAY

The appearance of your baby's head is still dominated by a prominent forehead due to the rapidly growing brain. The jaw can seem small but as the toothbuds grow and expand within the jaw, it lengthens and changes proportion.

The foundations are already laid for your baby's teeth – both the milk teeth and the permanent ones that will follow.

Although it's very rare for any teeth to have come through by birth (only a 1 in 3,000 chance), your baby's tooth buds that will form her teeth are already in place within the jawbone.

All of your baby's teeth – both her "milk" teeth and her underlying permanent teeth – start their development beneath the gums while she is developing in your uterus. The milk teeth buds began to develop at eight weeks of pregnancy and by this week all of the buds are formed.

The first milk teeth to harden, as calcium builds up, are the central incisor teeth and the last are the back molars, at around 19 weeks. The crown of each milk tooth does not complete development until after birth and root completion takes until your child is more than three years old.

Buds for the permanent teeth begin to form between the 14th and 20th weeks. These lie deeper than those for the milk teeth and closer to the inner edge of the jaw and gum. They remain dormant until it is time for the milk teeth to be lost.

Your baby's milk teeth will start coming through at around six to eight months and she'll have a complete set of milk teeth by the age of 2½.

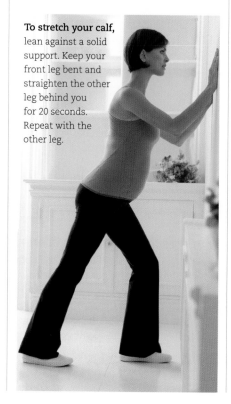

To stretch your calf, lean against a solid support. Keep your front leg bent and straighten the other leg behind you for 20 seconds. Repeat with the other leg.

AS A MATTER OF FACT

Fetal alcohol syndrome leads to serious oral and dental problems in the baby.

Smaller teeth that have weak enamel is just one of the many unfortunate consequences of this condition.

FEELING FLEXIBLE

Stretching and flexibility exercises should be a regular part of your fitness programme at all times, but especially during pregnancy. Being flexible enables your muscles to work more efficiently, alleviates tightness, helps to prevent cramping, and leads to improved balance and posture. Stretching can also help you to feel confident and calm, especially if the exercises are combined with deep breathing.

Flexibility can be maintained or improved during pregnancy by doing a series of exercises that stretch your muscles in a safe and effective way.

■ **Do not stretch further** than feels comfortable or you risk injuring the ligaments and stressing your joints.

■ **Ensure that you're stretching** when the muscles are warm, at the end of a workout or after a warm bath.

During the second and third trimester you should avoid any exercises – stretching or otherwise – that require you to lie on your back for extended periods.

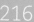

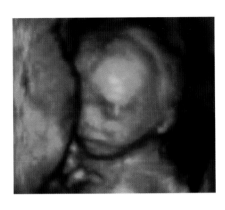

142 days to go...

YOUR BABY TODAY

Your baby often rests against the placenta. This has no effect on the placenta as its surface is protected by the amniotic sac and its composition and blood flow maintain its circulation at all times, leaving your baby free to explore her environment.

As the weeks go by, you'll find that you'll need to rest more and limit the amount of time you are on your feet.

By this stage, you may find it tiring to be on your feet for long periods of time. For one thing, the growing weight of your baby and uterus will lead to discomfort, and potentially to muscle strain. Because your centre of gravity is shifting, too, you may find that you stand awkwardly, putting pressure on your ligaments, which are, themselves, softened due to hormonal changes (see p.197). What's more, prolonged standing can cause blood and other fluids to pool in your legs, which can cause pain and dizziness.

If possible, take short, frequent breaks, so that you can put your feet up. If you do have to stand for long periods, you may find that resting one foot on a stool or box from time to time can help. Make sure your shoes offer good support (see p.257), and consider wearing maternity stockings (see p.225).

It's important not to stand for more than three hours at a time, so if your work involves standing make sure you are given adequate breaks.

ASK A... MIDWIFE

The bigger I get, the more difficult it's becoming to have sex. What should we do? As your pregnancy continues, you will have no choice but to try new sexual positions that will more easily accommodate your growing bump.

You can still use the missionary position but your partner may have to support his weight on his hands instead of lying on you; that way he won't press on your bump. However, you'll find that positioning yourself on top is a better alternative, and as your bump gets bigger you can squat or kneel over your partner. Side-by-side or rear-entry positions are also comfortable during pregnancy. Have fun experimenting to find out what's right for you.

FOCUS ON... YOUR BABY

That's tasty!

The flavours from the foods you eat will be transferred to the amniotic fluid, which is swallowed by your baby in the uterus. Therefore the types of food you eat can influence your baby before her first exposure to solid foods.

Studies show that antenatal and postnatal (through breast milk) exposure to a flavour enhances a baby's enjoyment of it in solid foods. These early flavour experiences may provide the foundation for healthy choices, as well as explain the cultural and ethnic differences in cuisine. So get your baby started on the road to good food choices by making healthy selections now.

Being out and about will make you tired. When you're going out for the day, plan lots of breaks so you can sit and rest.

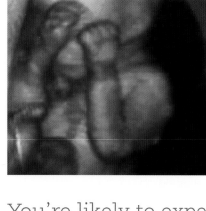

141 days to go...

YOUR BABY TODAY

You will become much more aware of your baby moving as her size and strength increase. You will not be aware of the more gentle movements, or those movements that do not hit the side of the uterus.

You're likely to experience some backache as your baby grows in size and your body continually adapts to accommodate her.

The increasing weight of your developing baby, and the fact that your joints and ligaments soften in pregnancy, can cause backache, but thankfully you don't just have to put up with this pain. There are many simple ways in which you can ease backache or even prevent it (see below).

See your doctor to make sure that the problem and its exact location is properly diagnosed. This way you'll have more chance of stopping it from becoming worse. A common problem, often in later pregnancy, is sciatica (see p.470) – a sharp pain that travels down the back and leg.

see p.470

BANISH BACKACHE

To nip backache in the bud, try the following:
- **Have a warm bath** or use a hot-water bottle on the painful area.
- **Ask your partner** to give you a lovely back rub, or book yourself a massage with an experienced antenatal practitioner.
- **Go to yoga or Pilates classes** to strengthen your back muscles.
- **Watch your posture** (see p.249), and raise your legs when seated.
- **Ensure your car seat** is properly positioned to support your back.

see p.249

FOCUS ON... YOUR HEALTH

Fibroids during pregnancy

In the second trimester, fibroids – benign masses of muscle fibre within the uterine wall, or occasionally attached to it – can become problematic. Increased levels of the hormones oestrogen and progesterone during pregnancy encourage them to grow along with the uterus.

In some circumstances, the rapid growth of a fibroid causes the centre of it to degenerate, leading to severe pain in the uterus and abdomen. When this occurs, the pregnant woman is advised to rest in bed and will be prescribed painkillers, which usually resolves the problem. Fibroids that do not cause discomfort do not require treatment.

Fibroids will not usually affect the developing baby, but if a large fibroid is positioned low down in the uterus or near to the cervix it can prevent the baby from descending into the pelvis, and a Caesarean delivery will be necessary.

Once the baby is born and the uterus shrinks, fibroids also usually shrink to their pre-pregnancy size.

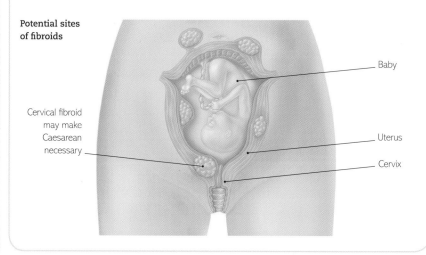

Potential sites of fibroids

Cervical fibroid may make Caesarean necessary

Baby

Uterus

Cervix

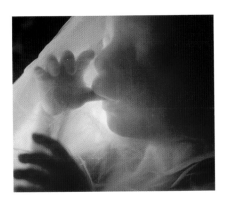

140 days to go...

YOUR BABY TODAY

Although your baby may be sucking her thumb, this is a very complex action that is not fully developed at this stage. For this reason, your baby is as likely to put her fingers or toes in her mouth as her thumb.

Congratulations – you're now halfway through your pregnancy. In around 20 weeks' time, you'll be a mum.

Does it seem like a lifetime, or has it flown by? At least from now on, you really will be counting down. Hopefully, at this halfway point you are feeling fine physically. You're not yet encumbered by a large bump and probably have a reasonable amount of energy. Psychologically, you may still be very emotional, although you will no doubt have got used to any mood swings by now (as will your partner).

At this stage you will start going to antenatal appointments around every four weeks. Remember, your midwife is there to monitor your health and your baby's progress, but also to help, so do get her advice on how to cope with some of the discomforts you might experience as you grow bigger.

AS A MATTER OF FACT

The gestation period for an elephant is an incredible 22 months, making it the longest of any land animal.

In addition to this, the common birth weight for elephants is 120kg (260lb). So, if your pregnancy is already starting to feel long, and your baby a tad heavy, do spare a thought for our large-eared friends!

ASK A... MIDWIFE

I haven't felt my baby move yet. Should I be worried? While you understandably want to feel your baby's movements, there is no cause for concern yet as your recent scan should have shown you that all is well with your baby.

If it's your first baby, you may not notice the early movements as you won't know what to expect. Also, if you're an active person, these slight flutters may be missed. Women with a placenta lying at the front of the uterus may feel movements later, as may larger women as the movement may not be detected through the flesh.

Once you do feel movements, don't become too focused on every one. It's not until around 28 weeks that it becomes important to monitor the pattern. From this stage, the amount your baby moves, as well as the type of movement and when it happens, are relevant as these indicate that the placenta is sustaining the pregnancy and your baby's muscles are developing.

If you're concerned about lack of movement from your baby at any stage, speak to your midwife.

SITTING CORRECTLY

Sit upright on a chair with your legs wide apart and your feet firmly on the floor to align your spine. Make sure your lower back is resting against the chair.

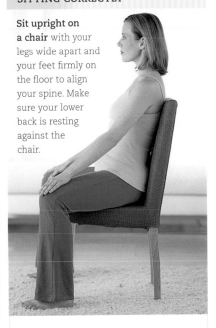

Good posture can help to minimize pregnancy discomforts, including backache (see opposite page). When seated, make sure your lower back is supported by the back of the chair and keep your feet flat on the floor (see above).

Yoga is a great way to learn to hold your body correctly, including how to keep your spine aligned and your lower back supported.

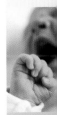

Your 21st week

YOU'RE HALFWAY THROUGH YOUR PREGNANCY ALREADY – IT'S ALL HAPPENING SO FAST

Not all women happily accept their changing body shape, even though they're overjoyed to be pregnant. But bump doesn't have to mean frump. You've got a good excuse to treat yourself to a few attractive maternity clothes or to indulge in some pampering, perhaps by having a gentle massage. Keep up your exercise routine, because you'll feel energized and all the better for it.

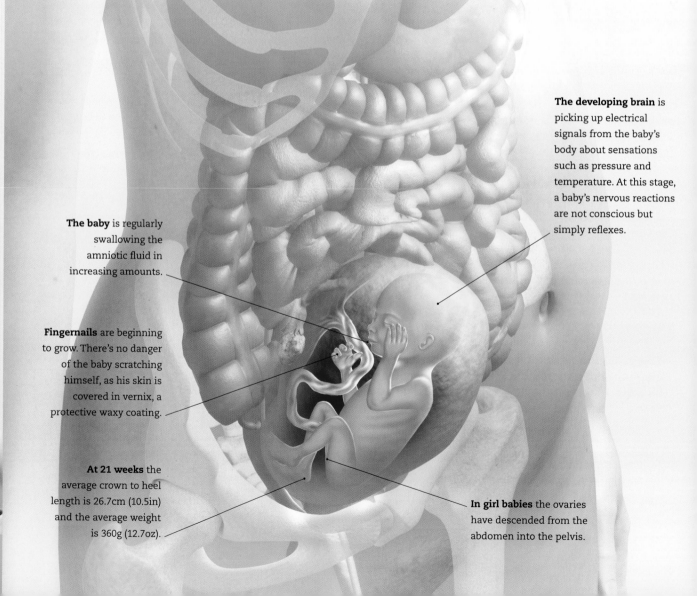

The developing brain is picking up electrical signals from the baby's body about sensations such as pressure and temperature. At this stage, a baby's nervous reactions are not conscious but simply reflexes.

The baby is regularly swallowing the amniotic fluid in increasing amounts.

Fingernails are beginning to grow. There's no danger of the baby scratching himself, as his skin is covered in vernix, a protective waxy coating.

At 21 weeks the average crown to heel length is 26.7cm (10.5in) and the average weight is 360g (12.7oz).

In girl babies the ovaries have descended from the abdomen into the pelvis.

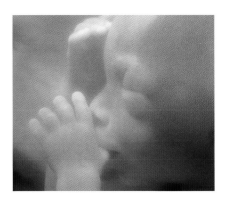

YOU ARE 20 WEEKS AND 1 DAY

139 days to go...

YOUR BABY TODAY

Your baby's movements are still based on a set of reflex actions but this is now beginning to change. As the nerve pathways develop, expand, and mature, your baby gains greater and greater control of his actions.

You're in the second half of your pregnancy and in the months that follow you'll have more regular contact with a midwife.

Your antenatal appointments will become more frequent in the second half of your pregnancy. Even if you are in good health, and your baby has been thoroughly assessed at the 20-week ultrasound scan (see pp.214–5), it can be reassuring to have these regular health checks with the midwife.

The number of appointments you have will differ depending on whether it's your first pregnancy and whether you've had any complications. If it's your first pregnancy, you can expect

around 10 appointments but if you've had a baby before, you may have only seven appointments, unless there are complications. As a general rule you can expect to have antenatal appointments at 25 weeks, 28 weeks, 31 weeks, 34 weeks, 36 weeks, 38 weeks, 40 weeks, and if, your baby is overdue (see p.393), 41 weeks.

If this isn't your first baby and there are no complications, you may not need to attend appointments at weeks 25, 31 and 40. However, you can contact your midwife if you have any concerns.

If you're expecting twins, your antenatal appointments will be more frequent than for a single pregnancy, and will depend on the type of twins you're having: non-identical or identical. If they're identical, the amount of antenatal care will depend on whether they share any of their support system (see p.130).

The wide range of maternity clothes that is now available means you can dress for a multitude of occasions. Look for items that you can also wear after the birth.

FOCUS ON... YOUR BODY

Dressing smartly

With your usual office clothing straining at the seams, you might have to rethink your work wardrobe. The good news is that, unlike in years gone by, there is now a wealth of beautiful maternity clothing available and much at affordable high-street prices. These are often designed as co-ordinated sets, which makes putting them together easy.

Remember that you'll be wearing maternity clothing for a few months, and it's easy to become bored by the same items. If possible, designate a little of your wardrobe budget to buy

yourself one or two items every month. If you're tired of your black elasticated trousers, sleeveless pinafore, and smock dress, buy a pretty new shirt or jacket to jazz them up; you can wear them unbuttoned if necessary.

Don't hesitate to accept hand-me-downs; even if they are not right for your office dress code, wearing them at home will enable you to spend a little more on work clothing. And don't forget your shoes; if you were a stiletto girl before becoming pregnant, you'll need to rethink (see p.257).

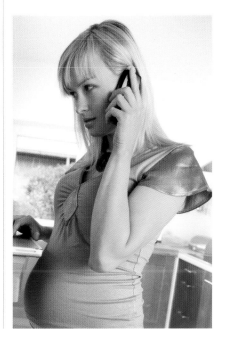

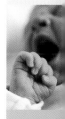

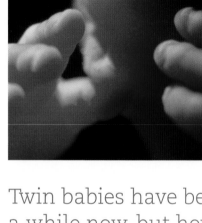

138 days to go...

YOUR BABY TODAY

This close-up of the fingertips shows that the nail beds have formed and the nails are starting to grow. The nails have not yet hardened: this prevents your baby from scratching himself accidentally while he has no control over hand movements.

Twin babies have been sharing a home in the uterus for a while now, but how are they relating to each other?

At 21 weeks, a baby's eyes are still closed, but he'll still be aware of light and dark. Because of this, twins can probably make out their sibling changing position and they're increasingly becoming aware of each other. It's thought that because memory starts developing around now, twin babies may begin to bond at this stage.

As ultrasound scanning has proven, there's plenty of contact between twin babies in the uterus, especially as the amount of space decreases. They have been seen to touch often, kick, and try to grab. Each twin reacts to the other's movements.

They may not act in the same way, with one twin favouring different movements from the other one. For instance, one baby may prefer sucking his thumb, while the other likes clutching his cord. Nor do they necessarily have the same body clock, so they may be active at different times. This proves that, even in the uterus, twin babies are already individuals.

Can my baby feel anything when we have sex? He may be aware of some movements when you have sex and of a change in your heart rate, but he won't be harmed by either. You may find that your baby responds to these sensations by moving a lot while you're having sex, or just afterwards. Some women find this inhibiting, but remember that it doesn't mean the baby is uncomfortable and, of course, he doesn't understand what you're doing! If you have an orgasm, your uterus will feel tight and you may have Braxton-Hicks contractions (see p.410) but, again, this is not harmful to your baby.

Be reassured that your baby is well protected by the pool of amniotic fluid. Also, the cervix is closed by a plug of mucus during pregnancy so no semen can enter the uterus; this helps to guard against infection.

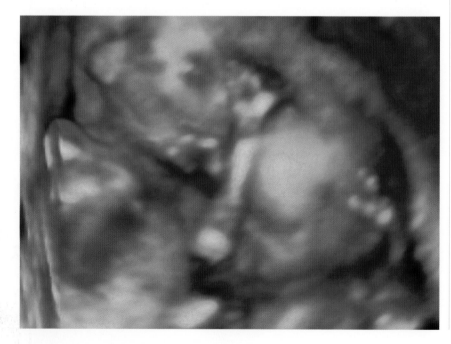

As the pregnancy progresses, contact between your twin babies will increase. As you'll have more ultrasound scans in a twin pregnancy, you'll have plenty of opportunities to see them interacting with each other.

Your second trimester

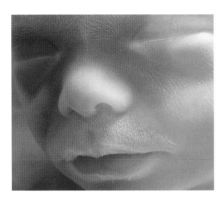

137 days to go...

YOUR BABY TODAY

The eyelids are still fused shut to protect your baby's developing eyes from prying fingers and toes. Deep within the brain, connections are starting to form to link the senses to those areas within the brain that are able to process information.

Part of the fun of not knowing your baby's sex is anticipating what it might be, but be prepared for others to do the same.

If you and your partner decided against finding out the sex of your baby at the 20-week scan, the guessing games will begin and you won't be short of people telling you what they think you're having.

Perhaps your own instinct is the best of all: in one study that asked women to guess the sex of their baby, 71 per cent of the expectant mums surveyed guessed correctly.

THE LOWDOWN

It's definitely a...

If you fancy testing a few old wives' tales on gender, consider these:

- Ask someone to tie a gold ring on to a piece of string and dangle it over your bump to "dowse" for the sex. If it swings from side to side or back and forth, it's a boy; if it spins around in a circular motion, you're having a girl.
- Hairier than usual? Apparently, according to the "old wives", you're more likely to be carrying a boy.
- If your baby's heart rate is faster than 140 beats per minute, you're having a girl (but see p.188!).
- Craving sugar, spice, and all things sweet: girl. Sour or salty foods: boy.

ASK A... MUM

I've found out at the 20-week scan that I'm having my third girl, but I so wanted a boy. How can I pick myself up from this? It can be enormously disappointing to find out that your baby's sex is different from what you wanted, and perhaps even expected. I felt that I'd let my husband down in some way, especially as I knew he wanted a son.

The good news is that by the time our daughter was born, we had both got over the disappointment, and were able to focus on being parents. We always said that if we'd waited until the birth to find out, it would have been hard to come to terms with it at the same time as trying to bond with our newborn baby.

Remember that you haven't met your new daughter yet, and it may be difficult to imagine loving another daughter, but you will do, in time. Try to focus on the fact that she is healthy and that you're having a beautiful baby.

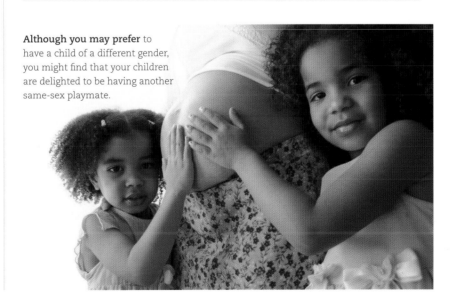

Although you may prefer to have a child of a different gender, you might find that your children are delighted to be having another same-sex playmate.

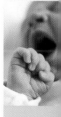

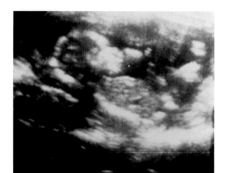

136 days to go...

YOUR BABY TODAY

Shown here is a Doppler ultrasound scan. Your midwife may use a hand-held Doppler ultrasound machine to identify your baby's heartbeat; Doppler scanning can also pick up sudden movements and the whoosh of blood through the placenta.

There are few better ways to relieve those pregnancy aches and pains, and to wind down, than to have a soothing massage.

When you book a massage, make sure you do so with a therapist who is experienced in antenatal massage. Although it's unlikely to occur at this stage, massaging the wrong areas or certain acupressure points can trigger uterine contractions (this can actually make a massage beneficial during labour when you want to speed things up).

Before booking a massage, check with your doctor or midwife that it's okay to have one. It may not be recommended if you've had complications such as high blood pressure or diabetes.

Comfort is crucial and most therapists will position you lying on your side with your head supported by a pillow (see right). Don't hesitate to tell the therapist if you're uncomfortable or if any aspect of the massage hurts. An experienced therapist should check that you're comfortable throughout the massage and stop if you're not.

If you don't want to book a professional massage, you can always call on your partner or a willing friend. It is, however, important that the person who is massaging you is careful and does not attempt to work on the abdominal area.

As well as making a world of difference to those aches and pains and helping you to relax, a massage from your partner is a good way to be intimate with him at times when you might not feel like having sex.

If you don't feel up to having a full massage, a foot, hand, or head massage can be very soothing.

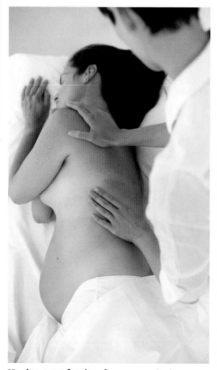

Having a professional massage during pregnancy can be a real treat. Besides feeling blissful, research shows that it eases aches and pains, helps you to sleep, and can reduce stress.

ASK A... MIDWIFE

I can't look in the mirror as I'm feeling so down about my size. Will things get better? You're not alone in battling with your self-image in pregnancy. For some women, their changing body shape can create negative feelings. Eating a healthy diet and taking some exercise helps to prevent excessive weight gain, and exercising will also lift your spirits and improve your sense of wellbeing.

There's no set emotional response to pregnancy, but as well as coming to terms with a momentous life and body change, you are also under the influence of fluctuating hormones, all of which affects your mood and can add to feelings of negativity.

Mild depression in pregnancy is often helped by reassurance and support from your partner, family, or friends. Talking over your fears and concerns may help to relieve your anxieties – you'll probably find that other pregnant women are experiencing the same feelings.

If you are feeling very low and desperate, don't hesitate to consult your midwife or doctor.

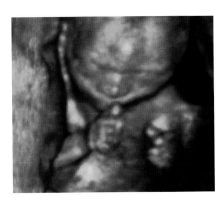

135 days to go...

YOUR BABY TODAY

The skin is less translucent now as your baby is starting to lay down fat stores, which after the birth will help with temperature control and provide an energy reservoir for your baby to call upon when necessary.

Your developing baby is becoming more responsive and aware every day as his nervous system begins to work more effectively.

By this stage, your baby can already detect a number of tastes and in a few weeks he'll start recognizing and responding to sounds. However, the nerve pathways that carry information about pain, temperature, and touch are only just starting to develop at around 20 weeks, and it will be some time before these sensations can be recognized on a conscious level.

Your baby does have reflexes from an early stage – for example, from about 10 weeks he'll close his fingers if they are touched. However, reflexes only require a nerve connection to the spinal cord and do not involve the brain. For information about pain, temperature,

and touch to be recognized, it must travel from your baby's body to his spinal cord and then on to the thalamus, which lies in the centre of the brain. The thalamus then sends signals to the cortex, the outer surface of your baby's brain, where the stimuli can be recognized and also evoke an emotional response. These connections are thought to function after 26 weeks of pregnancy, but it may be several weeks later before their electrical activity can be detected on an electroencephalogram (EEG). Many of these nerves require insulation around them to conduct signals effectively, and these do not develop until much later (see p.300).

ASK A... MUM

This is my second baby – is it worth going to antenatal classes again? I think so. There were three years between my pregnancies and it helped to have a refresher course; I even found that some of the advice had changed in that time. My partner found it helpful, too.

One reason to go is to meet some pregnant mums again; it's always useful to share the experience with others and, as with your first pregnancy, you'll probably find you make some great friends.

WEARING MATERNITY STOCKINGS OR TIGHTS

You probably can't imagine wearing maternity stockings, but they have their uses. They work by promoting circulation and the return of blood back to the heart and may be recommended to prevent vein-related problems, particularly if you suffer from varicose veins (see p.167) or spider veins (see p.134).

They also help to relieve aching feet and mild swelling in the feet, ankles, and legs, as well as fluid retention. They may be particularly helpful

if your work means that you must be on your feet for long periods of time.

Thankfully, an element of fashion has been introduced and many brands are sheer and pretty. There is a variety available: some are thigh- or knee-high (see right) and others cover the whole leg. You'll find lighter stockings for summer wear, when the hot weather can lead to further swelling. You can also buy maternity tights that provide support for your baby and uterus, taking the pressure off your back.

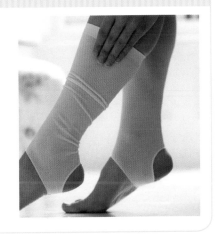

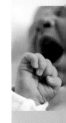

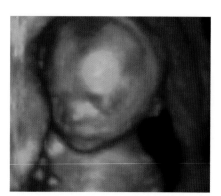

134 days to go...

YOUR BABY TODAY

Your baby is now developing periods of movement and activity and periods of rest and quiet. Soon these periods will become definite cycles of activity, providing something of a daily (and nightly) routine to his movement.

Your baby's reproductive organs are gradually developing and the differences in the genitals are increasingly obvious.

In the absence of high levels of testosterone in a female baby, the reproductive glands become ovaries, which contain six million follicles at this stage, of which about one million will remain at birth. The ovaries have now descended from the abdomen into the pelvis. The testes also undergo a similar descent, but have not yet reached the scrotum. Under the influence of the hormone oestrogen you produce, your baby of either sex may develop breast buds, although these will disappear after birth. Whether your baby is a boy or a girl has very little impact on the pregnancy. Later in pregnancy, there is a slight weight difference, with boys being slightly heavier than girls on average.

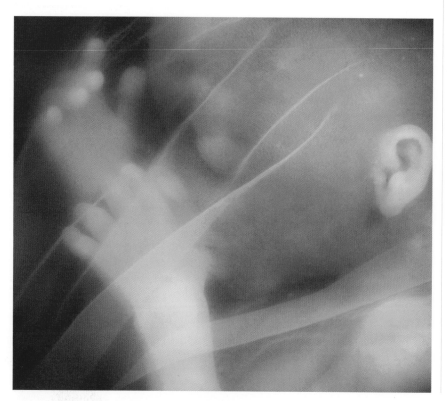

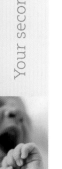

ASK A... MIDWIFE

I fell recently. Could I have harmed my baby? Falling during pregnancy is extremely common, as your increasingly protruding abdomen, softening ligaments and joints, and changing centre of gravity can cause you to lose your balance. The good news is that your baby is safely cocooned in amniotic fluid, which protects and cushions him when you fall. Your injuries would have to be quite severe to cause any harm to your baby.

The best thing you can do is to monitor your baby's movements after a fall. If he's moving as much as normal all should be fine, but if you want reassurance, pay a visit to your midwife. If you do experience any discomfort, or unusual discharge or bleeding from your vagina, seek medical help. If you pass water, this is likely to be urine caused by stress incontinence (see opposite), not amniotic fluid.

The amniotic sac is sometimes referred to as a "bubble" because of its appearance. It may be transparent, but it's tough and extremely difficult to pierce, so your baby is very well protected in this safe environment.

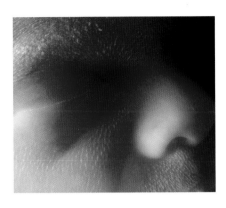

133 days to go...

YOUR BABY TODAY

This image shows just how large the developing eyes are underneath the lids. At birth, your baby's eyes will be large and blue. There are no eyebrows or eyelashes yet, but this will be the first adult type of hair to grow.

Try to find ways to fit in small amounts of energizing exercise every day – you'll feel much better for it.

ASK A... DOCTOR

I seem to have a lot of vaginal discharge. Is this normal? Yes, in the second trimester you may find that you have more discharge than normal. This is usually clear, stringy, or full of mucus and shouldn't smell offensive. If the discharge changes, becoming thick and white, and causes itching, you may have developed thrush, which is common in pregnancy and easily treated (see p.133).

You should see your doctor immediately if the vaginal discharge becomes yellow or greener, or offensive in smell; see your doctor too if you have burning when you urinate, or your external genitals become sore. These are signs that you have an infection that must be treated. Don't ignore any abnormal discharge as, although it won't directly affect your developing baby, an infection can increase the risk of you going in to premature labour.

You may find that you leak urine, especially when you cough, laugh, or run. This is called stress incontinence (see p.471).

Maintaining your exercise routine while you're still working can be challenging. The last thing you may feel like doing is exercising after a day at work, especially as your pregnancy progresses. There are ways of exercising without a visit to the gym; it will just take some thought and planning. For example, every now and then, take the stairs, carefully, instead of the lift, or get off the bus or train at a different stop, so that you walk some of the journey.

If there's a pool near to work, try to fit in an invigorating lunchtime swim. You'll feel much better in the afternoon.

Walk wherever you can, but be prepared: wear comfortable trainers and take your work shoes in a bag with you. Remember to take some water with you when exercising, and keep hydrated throughout the day.

At night before you go to bed, try to fit in some abdominal exercises (see p.250) to strengthen those muscles.

OFFICE WORKOUT

If your job involves sitting down all day, it's even more important to find ways to keep on the move.

■ **Get up from your desk** at least once every hour. Walk to speak to your colleagues instead of phoning or emailing them. Volunteer to fetch drinks for people – this will also make you very popular!

■ **Try this exercise while seated:** straighten your leg out in front of you (see right), keeping your thigh parallel to the floor. Then repeatedly bend and straighten your leg to help your circulation. Follow with flexing and pointing your foot from the ankle. Do each of these exercises at least 10 times with each leg.

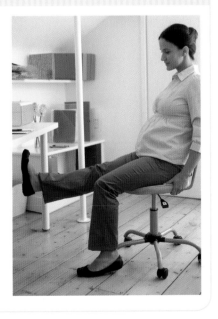

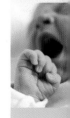

Your 22nd week

DECIDING ON A NAME FOR YOUR BABY CAN BE TRICKY, SO START MAKING THAT LIST

You may not know the sex of your baby but you and your partner can still have fun choosing names. This is a discussion that can run and run. Some couples don't make up their minds until the baby is born. With such matters to preoccupy you, it's probably hard to stay focused at work. Try to pace yourself without letting standards slip. Eating little and often, and drinking lots of water, will help you to stay alert.

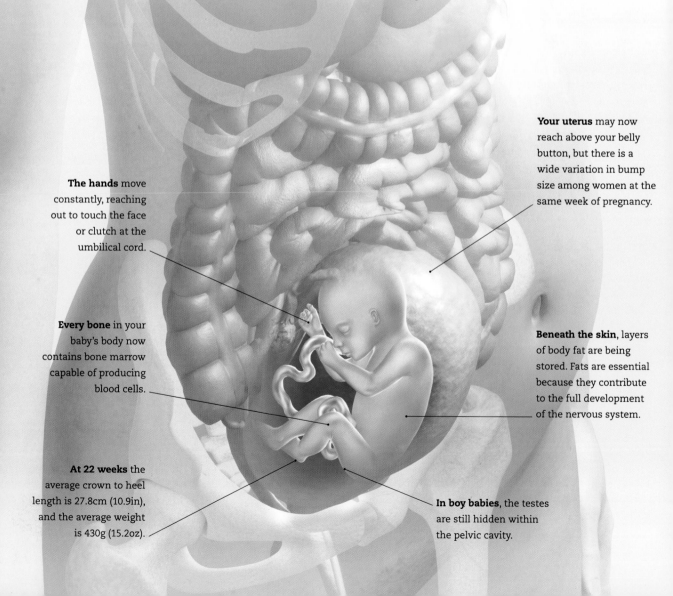

Your uterus may now reach above your belly button, but there is a wide variation in bump size among women at the same week of pregnancy.

The hands move constantly, reaching out to touch the face or clutch at the umbilical cord.

Every bone in your baby's body now contains bone marrow capable of producing blood cells.

Beneath the skin, layers of body fat are being stored. Fats are essential because they contribute to the full development of the nervous system.

At 22 weeks the average crown to heel length is 27.8cm (10.9in), and the average weight is 430g (15.2oz).

In boy babies, the testes are still hidden within the pelvic cavity.

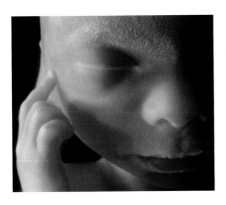

132 days to go...

YOUR BABY TODAY

Fine capillaries carrying blood underneath the skin lend a pinkish tone to your baby. Fat deposits are still sparse so the skin is still quite thin. Within the capillaries red blood cells are carrying oxygen to every part of your baby's body.

If you often walk into a room and forget why you're there, don't be concerned – you've simply developed "pregnancy brain"!

ASK A... MIDWIFE

I've always been a keen walker, but should I cut down on the number of miles now that I'm over halfway through my pregnancy? No, you shouldn't need to, but you might want to take extra precautions. Walking is ideal as it is low-impact exercise that can be maintained throughout pregnancy. In fact, it's a great exercise in the later months because it doesn't jar your knees and ankles.

If you plan to continue lengthy walks and like to walk briskly, try combining this with a slower, more leisurely pace. It's important to control your body temperature so that you don't overheat and feel uncomfortable. To do this, drink plenty of water to avoid dehydration and wear layers that you can take on and off as required.

As your bump grows, you may find hill climbing causes physical instability, as may trekking over uneven terrain, so stick to level paths. If you find yourself getting breathless, take frequent breaks. Do, of course, always make sure you wear good, sturdy footwear, and avoid carrying heavy loads.

Is your mind not feeling quite as sharp these days? Many women find themselves very frustrated by the onset of "pregnancy brain", which makes them so forgetful that they might not remember what they're talking about halfway through a sentence. Your ability to concentrate and pay attention to tasks may also be affected. Doctors are not sure why this

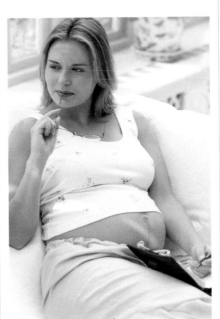

If you're finding you're more forgetful these days, write things down and prioritize so that you aren't overwhelmed with tasks.

happens, but it's likely to be a result of hormonal changes. It may also happen because during pregnancy you're focused internally: you're going through such a major life event, and there are so many changes happening to your body and lifestyle, that you simply pay less attention to other things.

As frustrating as it is, this tendency to forgetfulness is only temporary (although it may last into the first year of motherhood – see below). In the meantime, try making lists at the beginning of each day and tick off tasks as you go. Delegate at home and work when you can and, for once in your life, don't try to multi-task. Focusing on one thing at a time will help you to remember and achieve more.

AS A MATTER OF FACT

"Pregnancy brain" might last until your child's first birthday.

This finding is based on research carried out around the world. After in-depth analysis of the results, the experts concluded that sleep deprivation in the first year of parenting may be a factor.

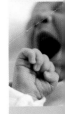

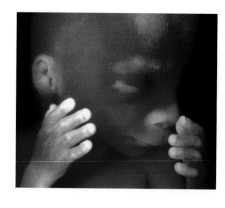

131 days to go...

YOUR BABY TODAY

The next three months are a time of particularly rapid growth for your baby. Cells are dividing, expanding, and maturing in every part of her body. The placenta too is growing and maturing, but this is far less important than your baby's growth from now on.

What's in a name? Well, quite a lot actually, as you'll discover when you start trying to choose one for your baby.

Deciding on a name for your baby is fun but not necessarily an easy task. As well as finding one that you and your partner agree on, it can feel as though everyone has an opinion. Friends may tell you that they have already chosen a name for their baby, so you can't use it! Your family may have traditions that they want upheld, such as passing on a name that has been in the family for generations.

It's a good idea for you and your partner individually to write down a list of names that you like. Then look at each other's list and talk about which ones you do and don't like. If you're lucky, there will be one or more names on both lists that match.

Factors to consider include: does the name sound right with your family name? Does the middle name go well with the first name? What will the initials be? For example, Robert Anthony Taylor will become RAT! Are the meanings of the names important to you? If so, find out what the meaning is of your favourite names – it can be fun to tell your child what her name means when she's older. Is there a short version of the name that you can use informally or, conversely, do you hate names being shortened? If so, avoid those. If you're feeling obliged to use a family name, perhaps make it a middle name.

It's advisable to come up with a few alternative choices, as you may find that the name you have decided upon just doesn't seem to suit your newborn baby when you finally see her.

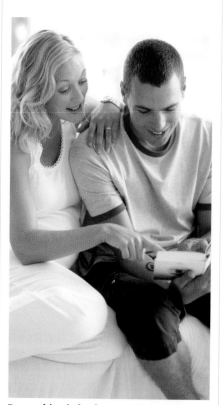

Researching in books or on the internet is a good way to find less popular names, and to discover interesting facts about the origin of names.

POPULAR NAMES

Do you want your child to have an original name, or are you influenced by what's in fashion? Bear in mind that opting for a popular name may mean your child is in a class full of namesakes.

Below is the list of the top 20 most popular girls' and boys' names in the UK in 2012.

Girls' names	Boys' names
1. Emily	1. Oliver
2. Olivia	2. Jack
3. Sophia	3. Charlie
4. Isabella	4. Harry
5. Chloe	5. Oscar
6. Amelia	6. Ethan
7. Jessica	7. Jacob
8. Charlotte	8. Thomas
9. Alice	9. George
10. Lily	10. James
11. Poppy	11. Alfie
12. Lucy	12. Daniel
13. Ava	13. William
14. Evie	14. Henry
15. Isla	15. Joshua
16. Daisy	16. Max
17. Ella	17. Noah
18. Emma	18. Alexander
19. Eva	19. Benjamin
20. Grace	20. Dylan

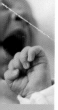

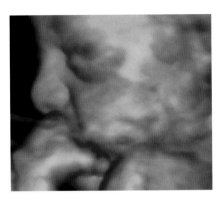

130 days to go...

YOUR BABY TODAY

In this 3D scan the baby's skin looks quite lumpy in parts. This isn't really the case. If the baby suddenly moves during a scan, the image can have difficulty "keeping up" and creates this unusual effect.

As well as using fat for essential growth and development, your baby is now beginning to store it.

Up until this time, your baby has had little opportunity to store fat, because growth has been the most important priority. But now your baby starts to lay down a layer of fat beneath her skin and it becomes less translucent. The placenta is responsible for supplying fats to your baby.

Fat circulates in your bloodstream and within the placenta it is broken down into three free fatty acids, as well as cholesterol, which are passed into your baby's circulation. These fatty acids then recombine to form fats for storage or growth.

Fats are important for adequate nerve and brain development. A layer of fat covers each nerve cell, insulating it from adjacent nerves and improving its connections with other nerve cells.

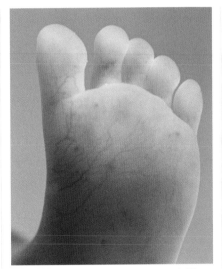

Your baby's veins will become less visible as she gains a layer of fat beneath the skin, making it less transparent than it was in the earlier stages of pregnancy.

Should we tell people the name that we've chosen? I would advise you not to. We told people at first and found it upsetting to find we had so many negative reactions. People freely told us how they had negative associations with the name or that they knew a cat or gerbil called that – a fact that we didn't need to know! Older relatives told us it was "odd" and went on to give us a list of alternatives.

So I would say keep it to yourself until the baby is born and it's all a fait accompli. It takes a bold person to question your choice once your baby has been named.

FOCUS ON... TWINS

Bill and Ben?

Choosing one name can be difficult enough, so if you're expecting twins, start thinking now. If you want to avoid people making jokes at your twins' expense, avoid obvious pairs such as Jack and Jill, and Holly and Ivy. Consider how the names might sound when abbreviated (William and Benjamin, for instance, becomes Bill and Ben).

Finally, it can be worth opting for names of similar length and complexity. For example, young Christopher may be discouraged as he struggles to spell his name, while his twin Jack has no trouble.

AS A MATTER OF FACT

In Hawaii parents often choose names that are associated with beauty.

Some examples of these are: Nohea –"loveliness"; Leia – "child of heaven"; Maka Nani – "beautiful eyes"; Hiwalani – "the attractive one"; Pualani – "heaven's flower"; and Nani, meaning "beautiful, pretty one".

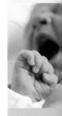

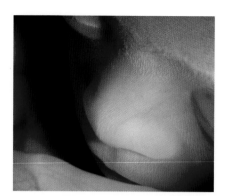

129 days to go...

YOUR BABY TODAY

When looking down on the baby, the nose can look quite wide because the nasal bridge is not yet fully developed. This gives the characteristic "button nose" shape that many babies keep throughout the pregnancy.

Your baby is producing essential red and white blood cells at a rate that is greater than your own.

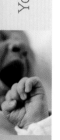

Stem cells in your baby's bone marrow produce red and white blood cells, and platelets – the cells that clump together to form a blood clot. Earlier in pregnancy all of these were produced in the yolk sac (see p.80), then the liver and spleen. Now every bone inside your baby contains red bone marrow capable of producing blood cells. Red blood cells do not last forever and after about 80 days are removed from the baby's circulation. This turnover is higher than your own, where a red blood cell will last for 120 days.

Bilirubin is a breakdown product from red blood cells. It's produced in the liver and removed from your baby's circulation by the placenta. Because your baby's liver takes a few days to efficiently process bilirubin, high levels may lead to jaundice at birth (see p.477). If jaundice does develop after birth then light phototherapy treatment is capable of breaking down bilirubin into a form that can be more easily excreted in your baby's urine.

As a newborn, your baby will be protected against infection by white blood cells and by antibodies from breast milk, especially the colostrum (see p.446). Because of this, breastfed babies are at a lower risk of conditions such as asthma, cow's milk intolerance, and food allergies.

MAKING SENSE OF YOUR ANTENATAL NOTES

As your antenatal appointments are more regular now, it can be useful to get to grips with the medical jargon used in your pregnancy records:

- **Primagravida:** first pregnancy
- **Multigravida:** subsequent pregnancy
- **Hb:** haemoglobin levels
- **BP:** blood pressure

- **Urine tests:** NAD or nil means that no abnormalities have been detected; P or alb means it contains protein; Tr or + indicates a trace of sugar or protein; G stands for glucose; and "other" is anything else.

- **Heart rate:** FHH is fetal heart heard; FHHR is heard and regular; FMF or FMNF – fetal movements felt or not felt.

Your baby's position in the uterus is usually referred to as the presenting part or lie and there are several terms and abbreviations used to describe this. Occiput is the term used for the back of the baby's head.
- **LOL** – left-occipito-lateral. The baby's back and occiput are

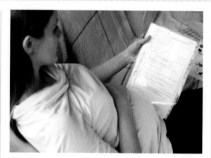

If you're unclear about anything written in your pregnancy records, don't hesitate to ask your midwife to explain.

positioned on the left side of the uterus at right angles to your spine.
- **LOA** – left-occipito-anterior. The back and occiput are nearer to the front of your uterus on the left.
- **LOP** – left-occipito-posterior. The back and occiput are towards your spine on the left side of your uterus.
- **ROL** – right-occipito-lateral. The baby's back and occiput are at right angles to your spine on the right-hand side of your uterus.
- **ROA** – right-occipito-anterior. The back and occiput are towards the front of your uterus on the right-hand side.
- **ROP** – right occipito-posterior. The back and occiput are towards your spine on the right-hand side.

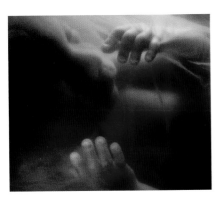

128 days to go...

YOUR BABY TODAY

There is still plenty of room for your baby to move around. Your baby is able to perform complete somersaults and change position several times a day or even several times in a few minutes.

Bumps come in all shapes and sizes and your midwife will keep track of how your baby is growing.

If, like some pregnant women, you are feeling big for this halfway stage, it doesn't necessarily mean that you'll have a big baby. Being large doesn't mean that all your weight is on your bump and from your baby; you may have put on weight on the rest of your body that doesn't affect your baby's size. Women who are carrying twins or triplets do, of course, show earlier and have much larger bumps than those expecting one baby.

The size of your bump is, however, a good indicator of your baby's growth, so it will be measured by your midwife (see pp.284–5). She will measure from a point on your pubic bone in your pelvis to the top, or fundus, of the uterus. This measurement should correlate with the number of weeks you're pregnant, with an accuracy of within 2cm (¾in). So, if you're 28 weeks' pregnant your bump should measure 26–30cm (10¼–11¾in). This symphysis fundal height (SFH) will be written in your notes.

If your bump is found to be significantly larger or smaller than it should be for your dates, you're likely to be referred for an ultrasound scan as this can give a much more accurate measurement of your baby's size.

Remember, though, what you think of as huge and what your midwife and doctor feel is too large can be two very different things! You are used to your body being a certain size and shape and you are much bigger than you used to be, even though to midwives you are a normal and healthy size. This can feel particularly the case if you're someone who has always been slim.

While it's good to spend time with women who are at the same stage of pregnancy as you, try not to make comparisons. Your bump may be bigger than your friend's, but you may end up having a smaller baby.

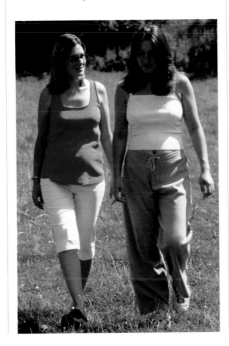

ASK A... NUTRITIONIST

I've been told to rest but will I gain too much weight? It's important that you follow this advice, even though it can be frustrating. Ask your doctor or midwife if you're allowed to do gentle walking or swimming as this will help to keep you fit and burn some calories.

If you're eating a healthy, nutritious diet that includes plenty of fresh fruits and vegetables, complex carbohydrates, and lean protein, you shouldn't gain too much weight.

Never be tempted to diet, or go hungry just because you're less active at the moment. Regular meals and snacks are important. Listen to your body; if you're hungry, it needs fuel.

If full bed rest has been prescribed, light exercise will be out of the question, but make sure you establish at the outset what is and isn't allowed. If you aren't active you are likely to gain some weight, but the aim of bed rest is to ensure that you deliver a healthy baby at full-term, and that's worth a few extra pounds.

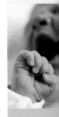

233

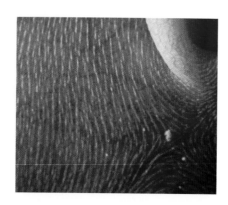

YOU ARE 21 WEEKS AND 6 DAYS

127 days to go...

YOUR BABY TODAY

This is a close-up of the baby's skin just behind the ear. Every part of the skin's surface has small ridges and hollows in a unique pattern. During this week the dermal ridges – the deeper layers of skin – start to mature, giving rise to finger- and toeprints.

Your baby has been filtering amniotic fluid and storing the waste as a substance called meconium.

At the end of this week, your baby's anal sphincter muscle is fully functional. This should prevent any small particles of meconium being passed into the amniotic fluid. Meconium is first produced at 12 weeks. It is the rather greenish/black first poo that nine out of 10 newborn babies pass in the first 24 hours.

Meconium is formed mainly from cells discarded from the lining of the gut as it lengthens and expands, and the waste of any nutrients which have been absorbed from the swallowed amniotic fluid. It is continuously produced, slowly moving down the gut to enter the large bowel (colon) by 16 weeks. Meconium is sterile as there are no organisms inside the gut and no bowel gas is produced.

AS A MATTER OF FACT

The unborn baby will move her hand to her mouth and even suck her thumb.

Research has shown that the baby may even open her mouth in anticipation. Anything that the hands encounter is firmly grasped and this grip is strong enough to support the whole of the baby's body weight.

KEEP TONED

Effective strength training during pregnancy, using free weights (see right) or a machine at your gym, will help your body to cope with the demands of pregnancy. Being stronger will help you to carry the increase in body weight and also help you to recover after the baby is born. Having more toned limbs will help you look and feel better, too.

Like all aspects of exercise during pregnancy, there are guidelines that should be followed:
■ **If you've been doing regular weight training,** continue with your programme, but do not increase the weight loads or repetitions.
■ **If you're new to using weights,** begin with very light ones and few repetitions and build up slowly. Do not increase the weight load until you are confident that you are able to cope with the increase.
■ **Take a deep breath** to start and breathe out as you lift the weight.
■ **Free weights,** rather than machines, are safer to use during pregnancy. If you're using a machine, make sure a trainer has shown you how to use it correctly.

■ **If you find standing up while doing strength training too tiring,** sit on a chair to lift your weights (see below).

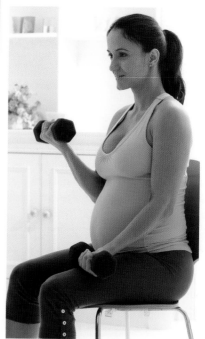

If you're sitting and using weights, keep your back straight and relax your shoulders. When standing, make sure that you have your legs hip-width apart and your knees slightly bent.

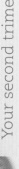

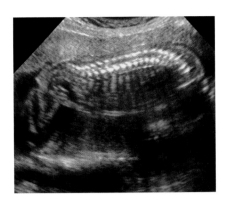

YOU ARE 22 WEEKS EXACTLY

126 days to go...

YOUR BABY TODAY

The vertebrae that make up your baby's spinal column encircle and protect the spinal cord. The vertebrae are seen here on an ultrasound scan, forming a long chain (white areas) that narrows at the base of the spine and ends with a slight outward curve.

Maintaining a professional manner at work will set the standard for how colleagues treat you during pregnancy.

Chances are that everyone in your office will be aware that you are expecting a baby by this stage, even if you haven't told them personally. Good news does have a habit of travelling fast, and you may have that pregnancy "glow" that makes your condition pretty clear – as well as a fairly prominent bump.

If word of your pregnancy is getting round the office, it might be best to tell your boss now. It's only a couple of weeks until you have to tell him or her officially anyway (see pp.348–9), and it's better and more professional if the news comes directly from you.

You may need to adapt your working day a little, but play it carefully. Try to keep up with your work, and act professionally. Your colleagues are, hopefully, thrilled that you're pregnant, but try not to expect special favours or extra attention.

While being pregnant isn't an illness, do take adequate breaks to recharge your batteries, or work flexible hours, if that's on offer, so that you can avoid travelling at the busiest times.

Try to go for a short walk in your lunch hour for fresh air and to get some gentle exercise. Drink plenty of water to keep you hydrated and alert, and eat little and often to keep your energy levels high.

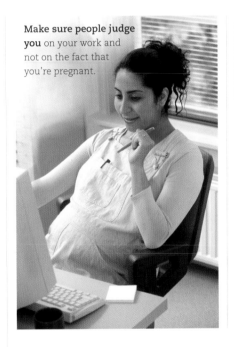

Make sure people judge you on your work and not on the fact that you're pregnant.

FOCUS ON... HEALTH

Vaginal bleeding

If you have any vaginal bleeding, always see your doctor or midwife. Growths on your cervix, or some inflammation, can produce light bleeding from time to time.

Heavy bleeding in the second trimester may suggest a problem with your placenta, such as placenta praevia (see p.212). Similarly, the placenta may pull away from the wall of the uterus, causing some bleeding, or, very rarely, uterine rupture can occur, usually only in women who have had a Caesarean section in the past.

ASK A... MIDWIFE

My manager said I can't have time off to attend antenatal classes. What should I do? You're legally entitled to paid time off to attend antenatal appointments as required by a registered medical practitioner, midwife, or health visitor. You must show a certificate issued by one of the above professionals to confirm you are pregnant, together with proof of the appointment. Antenatal appointments also include childbirth preparation or relaxation classes.

If your employer is refusing to allow you time off, talk it through with him or her. If this doesn't help, seek advice from your human resources department or another senior member of staff, or contact your trade union if you have one.

Your 22nd week

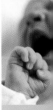

235

Your 23rd week

YOU COULD BE FEELING A LITTLE OFF-BALANCE, BOTH PHYSICALLY AND EMOTIONALLY

Being pregnant can have all kinds of unexpected effects. There will probably be days when you just don't feel in control of your emotions and they get the better of you, making you cry for no reason. Or your body feels clumsy and unco-ordinated, and you keep walking into the furniture. Just chat to some other mums-to-be and you'll find that these side-effects are all a normal part of the pregnancy experience!

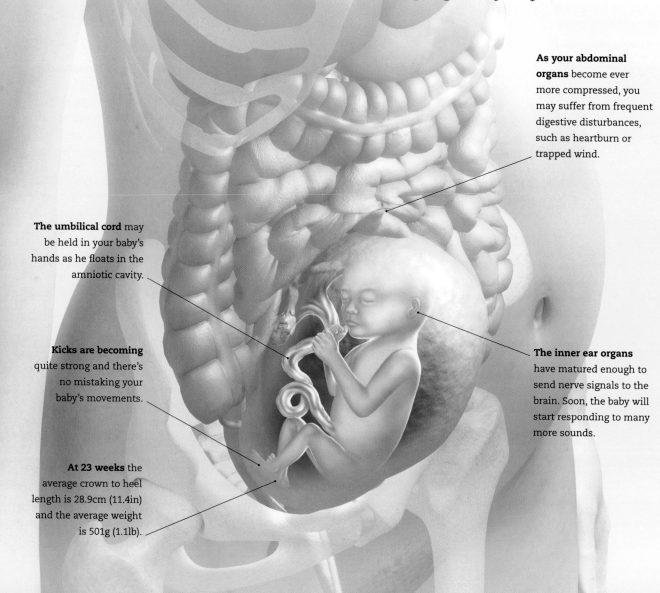

As your abdominal organs become ever more compressed, you may suffer from frequent digestive disturbances, such as heartburn or trapped wind.

The umbilical cord may be held in your baby's hands as he floats in the amniotic cavity.

Kicks are becoming quite strong and there's no mistaking your baby's movements.

At 23 weeks the average crown to heel length is 28.9cm (11.4in) and the average weight is 501g (1.1lb).

The inner ear organs have matured enough to send nerve signals to the brain. Soon, the baby will start responding to many more sounds.

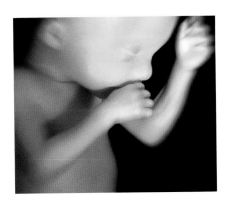

125 days to go...

YOUR BABY TODAY

This is a landmark week for your baby's senses: hearing and balance, both controlled by the inner ear, start to mature now. As this image shows, the ears are still not in their final position at the side of the head.

If your emotions are all over the place, try having a good cry, preferably on someone's shoulder. You'll feel a whole lot better.

It's normal to feel a bit up and down emotionally. The best way to cope is to give yourself some time out and the low points will soon pass. If you find yourself crying at an advert yet again, try to see the funny side! Sharing this fact with someone else may also help, especially a pregnant friend or new mum – she more than anyone else will be able to relate to how you're feeling and reassure you.

The good news is you don't need to worry about your baby – he won't be affected by your occasional mood swings. However, it might not be good for him if you get too stressed as this causes your body to produce more cortisol, a hormone which can have adverse effects on your baby (see p.187). So, when you're feeling stressed, make adequate time to relax and take care of yourself, for your baby's sake.

ASK A... DOCTOR

I think I may have food poisoning. Will this harm my baby? Some food-borne pathogens, such as salmonella, campylobacter, and E. coli will not directly harm your baby but can make you very unwell, causing profuse vomiting and diarrhoea that could lead to extreme dehydration. It's important to keep up your fluid intake both to flush out the offending pathogens, and to ensure you're sufficiently hydrated. If the vomiting is so serious that you can't keep any fluid down, ask for an emergency appointment with your doctor.

Infection with listeria bacteria is the most serious as it can infect the baby and may cause a miscarriage or premature labour. It is, therefore, essential that you contact your doctor if you believe that you've eaten a contaminated food (see p.17), so that the relevant checks can be carried out and treatment given, if necessary.

Always take special care when choosing food and follow hygiene rules when preparing it. Avoid eating foods commonly associated with food poisoning (see p.17).

FOCUS ON... TWINS

Maternity matters

If you're having twins, now is the time to discuss your maternity leave with your employers. In the UK, most women expecting multiples take maternity leave from around 29 weeks, unless they still feel up to carrying on or they're advised to finish earlier for health reasons.

You may also want to take off as much time as possible after the babies are born, and your partner will want to take the maximum amount of paternity leave (see p.349). Aside from help from family and friends, which will be essential, consider what you can afford in terms of additional childcare.

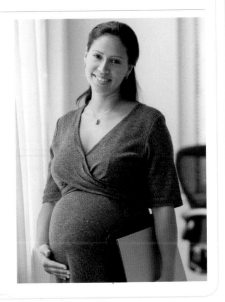

237

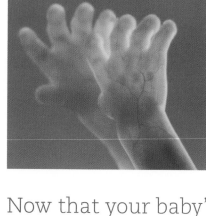

124 days to go...

YOUR BABY TODAY

The hands and fingers are clearly visible and the nail beds have been laid down. The baby's fingers will close if the palm of his hand is touched. The tips of the two bones in the forearm, the radius and the ulna, can just be seen in the lower part of this image.

Now that your baby's ears are sufficiently well developed to process sounds, his hearing will gradually improve.

Your baby's external ears have been developed for some time but for him to hear, the internal ear structures also need to mature. In the middle ear, three bones – the malleus ("hammer"), incus ("anvil"), and stapes ("stirrup") – conduct sound into the inner ear. These bones are formed initially from soft cartilage and embedded within connective tissue. The bones begin to harden and the connective tissue gradually dissolves. This allows the ear drum to vibrate on to the hammer, which passes the movement on to the anvil, and then the stirrup. The vibrations are then passed to the cochlea, a cavity of the inner ear, where they are translated into nerve impulses to be sent to the brain.

At 22 weeks, your baby's inner ear has matured adequately for sound to be processed into neural signals to the brain. The first part of the cochlea to develop is responsible for receiving lower sound frequencies. As your baby develops, he will gradually be able to recognize and respond to higher sound frequencies. Over the next three weeks, your baby's responsiveness to sounds will gradually increase. At first the responses are slow and sluggish, but by 25 weeks he will react to a range of sounds by moving around.

As well as being responsible for your baby's hearing, the inner ear also controls his balance. Small fibres within three semicircular canals of the inner ear are able to sense acceleration in any direction, providing the sense of motion and balance. Floating in the amniotic fluid is similar to weightlessness and, although your baby is very active, he has no sense yet of moving up and down.

AS A MATTER OF FACT

Men are faster than women at changing nappies.

Research shows that the average time a woman takes is 2 minutes and 5 seconds, whereas the average man takes 1 minute and 36 seconds! So that's a job for him, then.

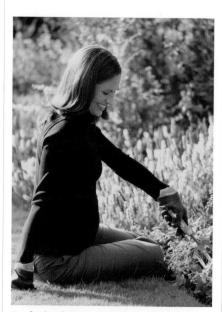

Gardening is great exercise and will also ensure you get some fresh air. Make sure you wear gloves as the soil may contain toxoplasmosis parasites (see pp.25 and 86).

RARING TO GO

If, like many pregnant women at this stage, you feel incredibly energized, make the most of it. Here are some ways to direct that energy:

■ **Get some exercise,** including doing some gardening (see left).
■ **Organize your paperwork** and get your finances in order.
■ **Clear out any clothes** that you know you won't wear again.
■ **Learn to knit** or, if you already can, get going on some baby clothes.
■ **Make time to see all the friends** you haven't been in touch with for a while – you may not feel up to socializing in later months.

However good you're feeling, always make time to relax and recharge your batteries.

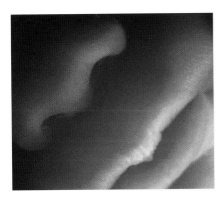

123 days to go...

YOUR BABY TODAY

The baby's mouth and nose are well developed. The nervous and muscular systems are now mature enough for the baby to suck in amniotic fluid, which the kidneys slowly process. Waste is eliminated via the placenta.

During your pregnancy you'll probably make some new friends, but you may find that some old friendships are affected.

One thing you may not have anticipated before you were pregnant is how your friendships might change. It's normal to be drawn to other women who are pregnant or who have recently had a baby, and common to make friends at antenatal classes (see p.199). It's natural to want to surround yourself with people who are going through or who have been through the same experience as you, not least because you will have so many questions they can answer. You might also feel closer to female relatives, especially your mother (see p.209).

You may find that friends who are not pregnant or who don't have children may not be as interested in all the details of your pregnancy. It may be difficult for them to comprehend how all-encompassing pregnancy and then having a child is; it may be literally all you can think about. If these are friendships you value, make an effort to have some "non-pregnancy" chats. It will be good for you not to be 100 per cent focused on the pregnancy.

If you find you drift apart from these friends for a while, don't worry. Good friends will always remain just that, whether or not your lives temporarily go in different directions.

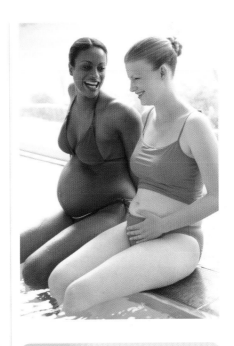

By spending time with women who are also expecting a baby, you can share the ups and downs of your pregnancy experiences. It can also be fun to do activities together, such as going swimming or to aquanatal classes.

Your 23rd week

ASK A... DOCTOR

My fingers are tingling and I've been told I have carpal tunnel syndrome. What is it? This condition occurs when swollen tissues in the wrist compress the nerves and cause pins and needles and numbness in your fingers. There may also be difficulty grasping and a weakness in the hands. In pregnancy, it's caused by an increase in blood volume and fluid, especially in the second and third trimesters. There are ways to reduce the symptoms, such as circling and stretching exercises to improve circulation and increase wrist mobility. Your midwife will be able to demonstrate these exercises. Wearing wrist splints and elevating your hands on a pillow at night can also help.

Carpal tunnel syndrome disappears after the birth, once there is no longer excess fluid.

AS A MATTER OF FACT

The number of women over 40 becoming pregnant continues to increase.

According to the UK Office for National Statistics, the conception rate for the over 40s rose from 9.4 pregnancies per 1,000 women in 2000 to 13.9 pregnancies per 1,000 women in 2011. The most common age for pregnancy is between 25 and 29.

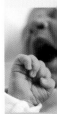

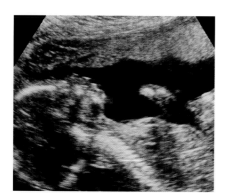

122 days to go...

YOUR BABY TODAY

Seeing your baby on a 3D or 4D scan gives you a better view, but most of the information that enables doctors to plan your care comes from looking inside your baby using 2D ultrasound, which provides the clearest images of internal structures.

Now that he can hear, your amazing baby is starting to develop the ability to remember things, too.

As your baby's nervous system develops, and especially once his sense of hearing evolves, he has the opportunity to learn and remember from experience. How this process develops is not fully understood, but experts believe that the first signs of learning coincide with the unborn baby's ability to hear, at around this mid-stage of pregnancy.

In later months, more sound will reach your baby as the walls of the uterus become thinner. Although babies have been seen to be startled by a noise at this stage, they seem to learn not to react to the sound if it is repeated again and again, gradually adapting to it as it's repeated over time, and eventually ignoring it.

This simple test demonstrates that a fetus can adapt to a repeated stimulus. If, however, the sound pattern is not repeated for some time, your baby will have forgotten it and become startled by it if it occurs again.

Retaining a memory for events is a much more complex function and relies on pathways in the grey matter of the brain. It will be weeks before learning and memory are linked in the last stages of your pregnancy.

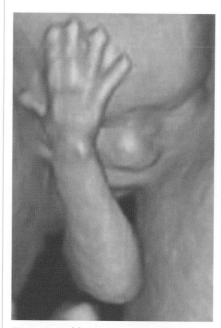

3D scans enable you to see your baby's face and features, such as the hands, in incredible detail. As these images are so real, they often improve the feeling of bonding a mother has for her baby.

Your second trimester

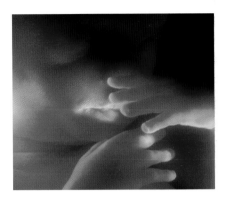

121 days to go...

YOUR BABY TODAY

Extremely fine hairs called lanugo hairs cover your baby's entire skin surface. These are constantly shed and replaced but, during the final few weeks of pregnancy, will be replaced by thicker, permanent hairs. Lanugo cells help to insulate the skin.

The occasional dizzy spell is common in pregnancy and not a sign that anything is wrong.

As your body works hard to nourish your baby, you may find yourself feeling dizzy from time to time. It's common to feel dizzy when you stand up suddenly; this is because, although your blood supply has increased during pregnancy, getting up quickly causes the blood to rush into your legs. This reduces the supply of blood to your brain, making you feel light-headed.

Dizziness can also be a symptom of anaemia. Although you produce more red blood cells in pregnancy than before, your volume of blood also increases. This means that proportionally there are fewer red blood cells and your blood count will drop.

You may also become short of iron and, if this is the case, you will be prescribed iron tablets. As well as dizziness, symptoms of anaemia include tiredness and shortness of breath. Low blood-sugar levels (see p.92) can also cause dizziness and can be prevented by eating snacks regularly.

If you're feeling dizzy, although it's likely to be due to the physiological changes in pregnancy, inform your midwife so you can be examined and any relevant blood tests taken. If you feel dizzy when you're out and about, or if you need a seat on a bus or train, always tell someone – the majority of people will be understanding.

AS A MATTER OF FACT

Not all pregnant women toe the good health line.

We're constantly bombarded by healthy eating messages so pregnant women are well informed about eating well. But in a recent UK research study, 5 per cent of women were found not to be including any calcium-rich foods (see p.16) in their diet at all. Only 4 per cent were trying to eat more omega-3 foods (see p.169).

If you can't face crowds, see one friend at a time in a home environment. Be selective and prioritize those people who really matter to you, rather than trying to fit everyone in.

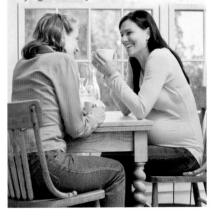

ASK A... MUM

I don't feel up to socializing but should I force myself to go out?
I remember that feeling well! When you're pregnant, it's normal to feel like battening down the hatches sometimes because you're too tired to socialize. It's worth, however, trying to make the most of your leisure time before the baby arrives. You may not feel like getting out and about, but once you do you'll probably be glad you made the effort and it will help you to maintain friendships.

I chose my activities carefully, opting for early evening or weekend meet-ups, and went to cafés rather than bars. I also had friends round for lunch and dinner but asked everyone to bring a course. I realized I might not get to the cinema or theatre for a while once the baby was born, so planned lots of great trips. You can always go to weekend matinées if you're too tired in the evening. When I was really too tired to go out, I'd catch up with a friend on the phone.

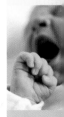

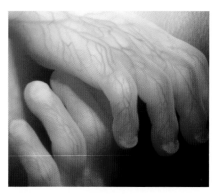

120 days to go...

YOUR BABY TODAY

Your baby's nervous system and muscular co-ordination are now much more developed. He has a grasping reflex – when his palm is touched his fingers will close – and he is able to suck his thumb purposefully, rather than through random movements.

When clumsiness strikes, something as simple as walking in a straight line may prove difficult!

If you find that you're often bumping into things and tripping over, it sounds as though you've been hit by clumsiness, a common side-effect of being pregnant.

Clumsiness in pregnancy has physical causes: the hormone relaxin causes your joints to loosen, your centre of gravity changes as your abdomen expands, and your extra weight shifts you off balance. There are, however, also emotional reasons: if you're pre-occupied by being pregnant, your concentration is bound to slip now and then, making you less likely to notice potential hazards in your path.

The good news is that your usual grace will return once you're no longer pregnant, but until that time it's important to avoid situations that might put you at risk of injury. So wear flat shoes rather than heels, avoid wet or slippery surfaces, and take care on steep staircases. Tape down the edges of loose rugs, and keep the stairs and hallways clear of things that might trip you up.

Be particularly careful when you're lifting something as it's very easy to lose your balance if you're leaning forward. Take care, too, getting into and out of the bath or shower, as these are notorious hotspots for pregnancy-related injuries.

It's worth noting that normal clumsiness in pregnancy is not accompanied by visual disturbances, headaches, or dizziness, so if you have any of these symptoms, you should see your doctor.

TIME TO THINK ABOUT

Preparing your home

If your partner's nesting instinct has kicked in, make the most of it by working out what needs doing around your home.

■ **Decorate the room** your baby will eventually sleep in once you move him out of your bedroom.
■ **Take the opportunity** to have a sort-out and take any unwanted clutter to the tip or charity shop.
■ **Make storage space** by putting up some extra shelves and cupboards where you can. Work out where you'll store large items, such as the pram.

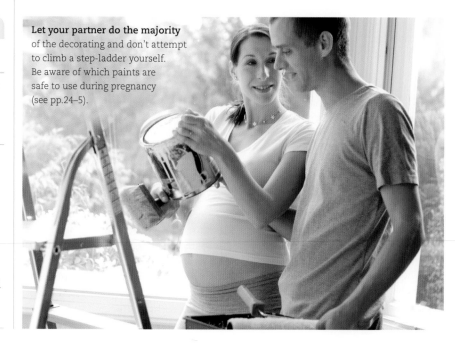

Let your partner do the majority of the decorating and don't attempt to climb a step-ladder yourself. Be aware of which paints are safe to use during pregnancy (see pp.24–5).

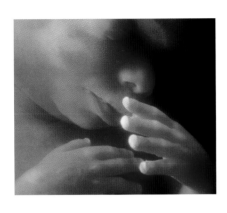

119 days to go...

YOUR BABY TODAY

External appearances are deceptive: although your baby seems very well developed, it's still early in the pregnancy – the state of the cervix and progesterone produced by the placenta both play a part in ensuring that labour does not start for some months yet.

You may be surprised by the strength of feeling you have for your baby, and this maternal instinct will grow stronger each day.

Do you feel as though you're a mum yet? Whether or not you're a maternal person, you'll already have started, instinctively, the process of becoming a mother. You may be taking better care of yourself, eating better, and making lifestyle changes, not necessarily to benefit your own health but for your baby. You're likely to find yourself being very protective and nurturing towards your bump, wanting the best for your baby, and being worried about anything happening to him. It's nothing to worry about if you don't feel this strong bond: all women are different and it may not be until you're holding and caring for your baby that you experience strong maternal feelings.

Your partner may not have this strong parental instinct, but the more you involve him in the pregnancy, the greater the chance of him getting close to his unborn child. By reading in books or on the internet about how the baby is developing at every stage, and attending some or all of the antenatal appointments with you, he will be able to picture the baby and follow his progress as closely as possible.

You'll find that your baby occupies your thoughts a lot of the time. Being pregnant makes most women act selflessly in the best interests of their baby.

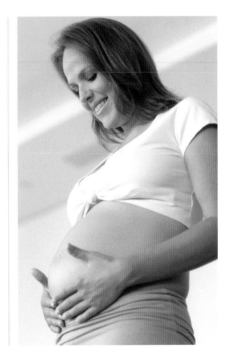

FOCUS ON... RELATIONSHIPS

What's that, Mum?

If you have a toddler already, she will undoubtedly be curious about why you have suddenly got so fat! Keep things simple, along the lines of "Mummy is growing you a baby sister or brother, but she/he won't be here just yet." Over the coming weeks, explain in more detail what having a new baby means.

There's no need to tell your toddler how the baby got there, or to keep reminding her about it. Just answer her questions when she asks, without showing too much preoccupation with the matter.

ASK A... DOCTOR

I've got flu. Will this harm my baby? No, your baby should be fine but because your immune system is compromised during pregnancy, your symptoms might last longer than usual. Drink plenty of fluid to stay hydrated, and eat several small meals a day to maintain your energy levels. Call your doctor if you don't improve after 24–48 hours, or your temperature exceeds 101°F (38°C).

Very few pregnant women do experience complications, but if you feel very unwell, and, in particular, you experience problems breathing, see your doctor immediately. Ask the pharmacist's advice before taking any over-the-counter medication.

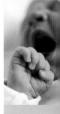

Your 24th week

YOUR BABY'S BODY SYSTEMS ARE BECOMING MORE AND MORE EFFICIENT

A baby getting prepared for independent life needs all the help you can give her. Keep up your good habits by nourishing the two of you with healthy food; and make sure your own body is in peak physical condition to support your pregnancy. Some minor discomforts, such as feeling too hot, leg cramps, and piles may be plaguing you. These annoying problems are only temporary and will disappear once your baby is born.

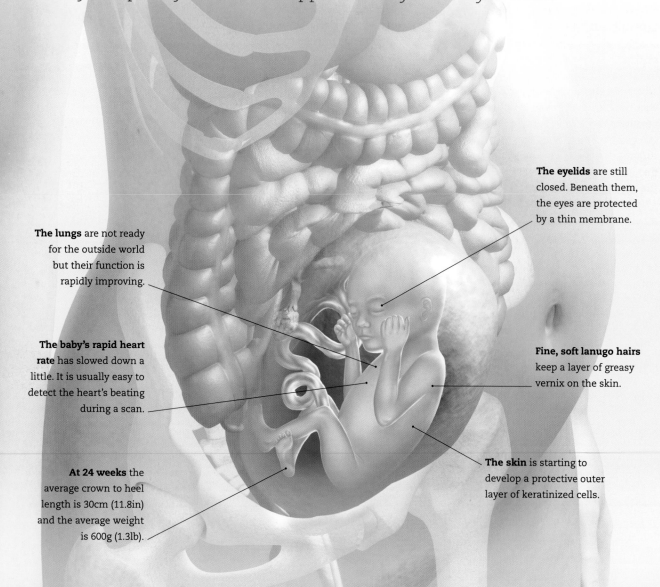

The eyelids are still closed. Beneath them, the eyes are protected by a thin membrane.

The lungs are not ready for the outside world but their function is rapidly improving.

The baby's rapid heart rate has slowed down a little. It is usually easy to detect the heart's beating during a scan.

Fine, soft lanugo hairs keep a layer of greasy vernix on the skin.

The skin is starting to develop a protective outer layer of keratinized cells.

At 24 weeks the average crown to heel length is 30cm (11.8in) and the average weight is 600g (1.3lb).

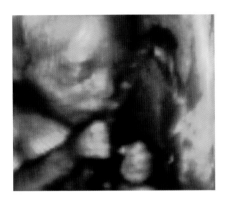

118 days to go...

YOUR BABY TODAY

There is no light in the womb, but 3D ultrasound is designed to produce highlights and shadows to give the same effect as if you shone a torch into the womb. Now your baby may be holding her hands flexed into a fist.

From this point onwards, your baby is considered "viable" and would receive life-saving treatment were she born early.

Week 24 is considered the legal age of viability for your baby, and therefore an important pregnancy milestone. Like many women, you may feel relieved to get past this point.

If you went into labour and delivered your baby before this week, she would be unlikely to survive and you would be considered to have had a miscarriage. After 24 weeks, the doctors have a legal duty to do everything they can to save the baby. Babies born after 24 weeks receive special care and are resuscitated, if necessary. The more advanced you are in your pregnancy before you deliver, the less likely it is that your baby will face the problems associated with being born prematurely.

Incredible scientific and technological advancements have meant a huge increase in the survival of premature babies, with health complications kept to a minimum.

AS A MATTER OF FACT

The world's youngest surviving premature baby was born in Florida at just 21 weeks and six days.

The baby weighed only 283g (10oz) and measured 9.5cm (3.75in). Her feet were the size of an adult's fingernail. It was the first time a baby born before 23 weeks had survived and led to calls for the legal age of viability to be lowered.

SPECIAL CARE BABY UNITS

Babies who are born prematurely, or newborns who are sick, will receive specialist round-the-clock care in a special care baby unit (SCBU) (see pp.452–3). The earlier the baby is born, the more chance there is of complications, such as infections, occurring. If your baby is born several weeks prematurely, she may need to be cared for in a neonatal intensive care unit (NICU) – this may not be in the hospital where your baby was born.

Your baby may be put in an incubator with monitors attached and receive oxygen through a special ventilator. Some of the equipment looks very frightening, but remember it is there to help your baby stay warm and nourished and improve her health.

The staff will readily explain what is going on, and they will be keen for you to be involved as closely as possible in your baby's care and encourage bonding.

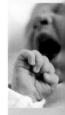

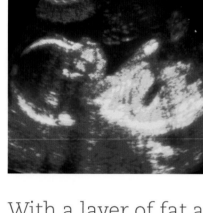

YOU ARE 23 WEEKS AND 2 DAYS

117 days to go...

YOUR BABY TODAY

You will probably be aware of your baby's movements by now: the number of movements and their nature will vary during the day and night and you may notice that they start to form into a particular pattern or respond to your own activity.

With a layer of fat and a tough layer of cells, your baby's skin is now becoming more resilient.

Your baby's skin is continuing to develop and has now started to "keratinize". Keratin is the substance that transforms the skin's outer layer into a protective layer of dead cells. Hair and nails also form from keratin.

The outer keratinized layer of skin cells, plus a layer of fat laid down between the skin cells, gives the skin a waterproof covering. This process of keratanization reduces the amount of water your baby loses into the amniotic fluid. Each new skin cell, made in the deepest part of the skin, matures as it gradually moves up towards the surface and, now keratinized, becomes part of the outer protective layer before it is eventually shed. The cycle takes approximately 30 days.

The thickest layers of keratinized cells are on the palms of the hands and the soles of the feet. The keratinizing process has only just begun. As the fat layer is very thin at this stage, your baby's skin will still appear translucent, but less so than it did in earlier weeks.

At this stage of pregnancy, your baby still has plenty of room to manoeuvre inside the uterus, and although you're likely to be feeling lots of movements by now this will only be a fraction of the total. This is because the only movements you'll feel are those that cause your baby to kick or bump into the wall of your uterus. You will be unaware of many of the finer movements that are performed close to the baby's body as they won't make any contact with your uterus.

COPING WITH LEG CRAMPS

Getting painful spasms in the leg muscles is common in pregnancy, particularly at night. You may find that you wake up due to the sudden and severe localized pain in your legs or feet. This is thought to be due to the pressure of the uterus on the pelvic nerves.

Some experts believe that cramp during pregnancy may be caused by a lack of calcium or salt or an excess of phosphorus, but these theories are as yet unproven.

When you get a spasm, relieve it by flexing your foot or leg (see far right), and gently massaging the affected area. The cramp should resolve itself once you are out of bed and using the muscle. However, if the pain doesn't recede and there is any reddening or swelling in the leg, you should seek medical advice urgently to eliminate the possibility of a clot (see p.186), as this can be dangerous.

To reduce the incidence of cramp or its severity, drink lots of water to prevent dehydration and regularly do leg stretches (see right) and ankle exercises, circling your heel and wiggling your toes.

Doing gentle exercise, such as walking or swimming, can also help, as can regularly massaging the calf muscle to improve circulation.

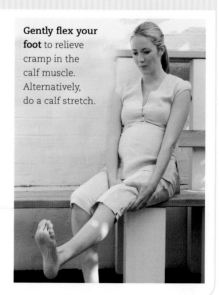

Gently flex your foot to relieve cramp in the calf muscle. Alternatively, do a calf stretch.

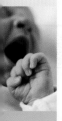

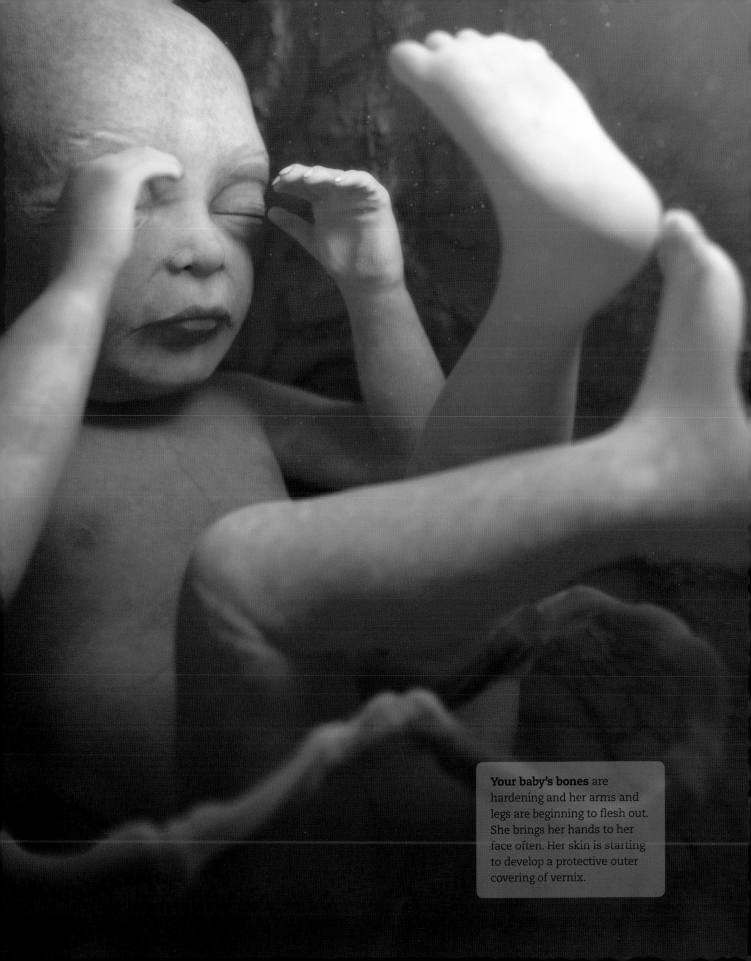

Your baby's bones are hardening and her arms and legs are beginning to flesh out. She brings her hands to her face often. Her skin is starting to develop a protective outer covering of vernix.

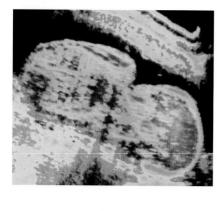

116 days to go...

YOUR BABY TODAY

Ultrasound uses sound waves of a very high frequency, well beyond the audible range of the human ear, so your baby's hearing will be completely unaffected by the sound waves transmitted during these scans that check her growth and development.

Are you feeling hot? Being pregnant can sometimes feel as though you have your own personal radiator strapped to you.

You may find that you're much hotter and sweating more than normal during pregnancy. This is because you're carrying more weight than usual and you have more blood pumping around your body.

If you're pregnant during the summer, this can be difficult to bear, so find ways to stay cool (see p.324). If you're pregnant in the winter, you may find yourself walking down the street in a light jumper while other people are all bundled up in coats and scarves. You might get into debates with your partner if he wants the heating on and you want the windows open!

Make sure you drink enough fluid throughout the day. You might find that the increased sweat causes a rash in the creases under your breasts or in your groin, so wash frequently and make sure that you dry these areas well.

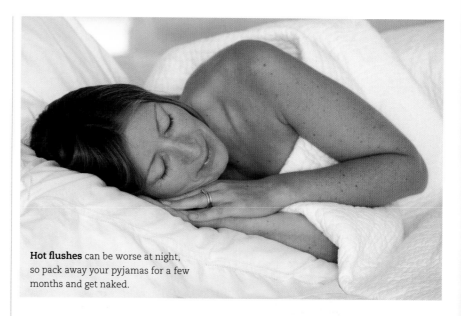

Hot flushes can be worse at night, so pack away your pyjamas for a few months and get naked.

AS A MATTER OF FACT

It's common to dream that you give birth to an older baby, who is born walking and talking!

This is thought to reflect a mother-to-be's insecurities about caring for a tiny, helpless baby. The older the baby, the more self-sufficient she appears.

ASK A... MIDWIFE

I keep having really strange and vivid dreams. Is this normal in pregnancy? Yes, when you're pregnant, it's common to dream more and to remember your dreams. Experts attribute the vividness of these dreams to all the emotional and physical changes a pregnant woman is going through.

The vivid dreams may be a way for your unconscious to deal with all the hopes and fears you may have about your unborn baby and impending motherhood.

The increase is also believed to be due to hormonal changes: increased levels of oestrogen are thought to cause longer periods of REM (rapid eye movement) sleep – the phase of sleep in which we are most likely to dream.

If your dreams are disturbing, try writing them down to get them off your mind.

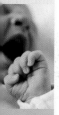

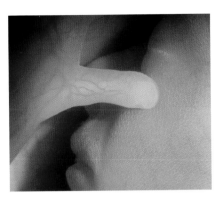

YOU ARE 23 WEEKS AND 4 DAYS

115 days to go...

YOUR BABY TODAY

The joints and bones of the hand are still very soft, although the cartilage skeleton is now gradually being replaced by bone. This image shows well the numerous capillaries supplying blood to the hands, right down to the fingertips.

Over the next few weeks, your baby will take on more of the appearance of a newborn.

Your baby's eyelids and eyebrows are well developed by this week of pregnancy, but the eyelids remain fused. The cells that are destined to become your baby's fingernails were present at 10 weeks, and the cells for the toenails were present four weeks later.

Now, at 23 weeks, the nails are just beginning to make an appearance at the base of the nail bed. The nails will grow continuously throughout life,

but it will be several weeks before they have reached the tips of the fingers and then the toes.

Your baby's skin is developing quickly and often appears wrinkled at this stage; it is as if the baby has yet to grow into it. Your baby is now covered in extremely fine and short hairs, known as "lanugo". This layer of hair will be almost completely lost before birth. The hairs help to trap vernix on to the surface of the skin; this is the white,

greasy layer that you often see in patches on a baby's skin at birth. It collects in the skin folds and creases and helps to protect the baby's skin not only from the water content of the amniotic fluid, but also the waste products within it.

As your pregnancy advances, your baby's kidney function is improving and the amniotic fluid produced becomes increasingly similar to urine in its composition.

PREGNANCY POSTURE

Your posture will naturally change as a result of pregnancy; this is due to the extra weight you're carrying and the softening of your joints.

Prior to pregnancy, your centre of gravity was directly over your hips; during later pregnancy it shifts forwards to your enlarged abdomen. This dramatic shift in your centre of gravity increases the curve of your lower spine, and can result in lower back pain (see p.218). The weight you gain during pregnancy can also put a strain on the back.

Exercises can help to balance your body and alleviate the muscular aches associated with changes in your posture (see right for one example).

It's important to adapt to these postural changes in pregnancy:
■ **Do abdominal exercises** (see p.250), to strengthen the core muscles, as well as back stretches. These help to maintain good posture and avoid back pain later in pregnancy.
■ **Be aware of** the way you're walking and standing: pull your shoulders down and back, do not arch your lower back and keep your pelvis in a neutral position.
■ **Avoid balancing anything** on your hip, as this can affect your hip and back alignment.
■ **Don't hold a phone between** your head and shoulder as this can result in neck pain.

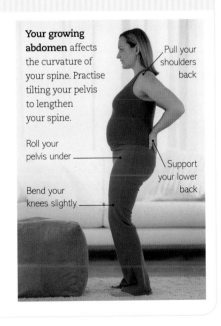

Your growing abdomen affects the curvature of your spine. Practise tilting your pelvis to lengthen your spine.

Pull your shoulders back

Roll your pelvis under

Support your lower back

Bend your knees slightly

Your 24th week

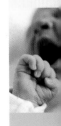

249

Abdominal exercises

Strong abdominal muscles are beneficial during pregnancy as they will help you carry the weight of your baby and assist you during labour and birth.

Abdominal exercises done while lying on your back aren't recommended after the first trimester. The reason for this is that when you lie on your back, your enlarged uterus presses on one of your major blood vessels, reducing the amount of blood pumped around the body and causing dizziness. However, you can strengthen the oblique abdominal muscles without lying on your back by using gravity and your body to strengthen and tone the torso. In pregnancy, you can tone your abdomen with exercises where you adopt an all-fours position or an upright sitting position. Aim to do the exercises below three to four times a week.

Benefits of abdominal exercises

Strong abdominal muscles enable your body to work more efficiently in labour. They also help support the weight of the baby, which takes pressure off the spine, reducing the likelihood of backache. In addition, keeping your abdominal muscles strong means that you're less likely to get a condition called *diastasis recti*, in which the abdominal wall muscles separate, often following childbirth. This makes it harder to regain your figure and fitness.

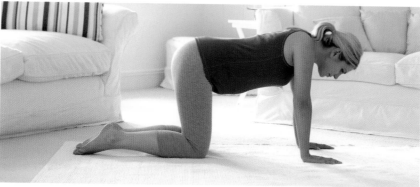

The sling Get down on all fours with your hands on the floor, feet and knees apart, and arms straight. Keep your back flat in a neutral position, taking care not to arch your back. Imagine the abdominal muscles as a sling holding your baby. Take a deep breath, then slowly pull your abdominal muscles (the sling) in towards your back, pulling the baby closer to you, and gently release, returning to the starting position. Repeat around 20 times, or as feels comfortable. Breathe properly during the exercise, breathing in to start and breathing out as you pull in your tummy.

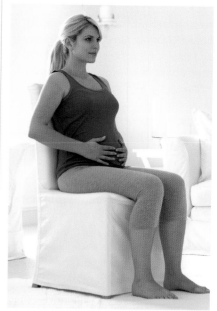

The abdominal pull This can be done anywhere and at any time. It's advisable to start by doing the exercise sitting in an upright chair with your shoulders relaxed away from your ears and your back straight. Make sure your lower back is well supported, if necessary using a pillow. Put your hands around your tummy below your navel. Breathe in slowly and at the same time gently pull in your abdominal muscles for two seconds and then release on the exhalation. Repeat the exercise 10 times. Take a short break, then start again.

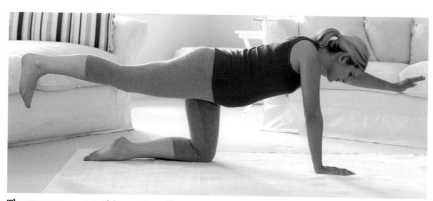

The superman pose This exercise will strengthen your core muscles, keeping your abdomen and back strong, and helping to prevent lower back pain. It also stretches your leg and arm muscles. Start from an all-fours position. Keeping your back in a neutral position, lift your left arm in front of you and your right leg up behind you. Be careful not to arch your back or lift your leg higher than the hips. Hold for a count of five and slowly lower. Then repeat with your right arm and left leg. Do around 10 repetitions for each arm and leg, or as many as feel comfortable.

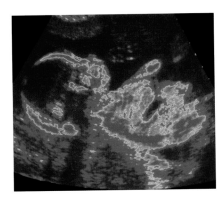

114 days to go...

YOUR BABY TODAY

In this coloured 2D ultrasound scan the baby is lying face upwards. It is now increasingly difficult to show the whole baby using this type of ultrasound as it only shows a thin slice at any one time. Here, only the upper part of the baby can be seen.

Practising yoga in pregnancy can be hugely beneficial, both physically and emotionally.

As well as strengthening and toning muscles, yoga aims to bring about a greater awareness of your breathing. Learning to control your breathing is a great way to relax during pregnancy and an invaluable way to prepare to breathe through the contractions when you're in labour.

Standing poses in yoga focus on achieving core stability, thereby strengthening the back and abdominal muscles. This is beneficial during pregnancy when the additional weight you're carrying can affect your balance and cause unsteadiness. Calm sitting poses that concentrate on aligning your spine help you to focus on steadying your breathing and centring yourself. If you feel unsteady doing yoga poses, you can simply lean against a wall.

Pilates is also a good exercise to do in pregnancy as it heightens your bodily awareness, giving you greater control of – and confidence in – your body. Pilates also incorporates pelvic floor exercises (see p.69).

Whatever classes you're doing, it's important to find an accredited instructor who is experienced in teaching pregnant women. There are now many specialist pregnancy yoga and Pilates classes.

AS A MATTER OF FACT

Practising yoga in pregnancy is safe and it may reduce the risk of pregnancy complications.

A recent study found that pregnant women who practised yoga had a reduced risk of developing pregnancy-induced high blood pressure and of going into premature labour.

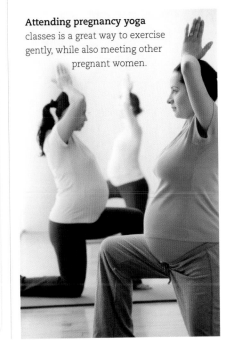

Attending pregnancy yoga classes is a great way to exercise gently, while also meeting other pregnant women.

ASK A... DOCTOR

Why are piles common in pregnancy? Piles (haemorrhoids) are, like varicose veins (see p.167), dilated veins, but they occur around your anus. The weight of your baby pushes down on your back passage, restricting blood flow and causing the veins to dilate.

Piles can be itchy and sore, and may cause a throbbing sensation. The discomfort can be relieved with cold packs and creams containing lubricants to help the passage of stools, and/or local anaesthetics to relieve soreness. Piles can bleed – you may notice bright red blood on the paper after you pass a stool.

If you have piles, it is important to try not to get constipated (see p.468) as this means you have to strain and push to pass your stools, which increases the pressure on the piles and makes them worse. Ensure that you drink lots of water and eat sufficient fibre.

If your piles are becoming very problematic and uncomfortable, seek your doctor's advice.

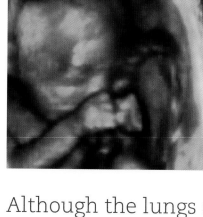

113 days to go...

YOUR BABY TODAY

Your baby is now making regular deep breathing movements. These have been present for some weeks, but not in a sustained and co-ordinated fashion. These breathing movements are critical for the development and expansion of your baby's lungs.

Although the lungs are the last of your baby's organs to be fully functional, they are undergoing rapid development now.

ASK A... MIDWIFE

Is it true that playing music to my unborn baby will enhance her development? Some research into this claim finds that playing music to an unborn baby will lead to a shorter labour and easier birth, and to the newborn baby crying less, being more relaxed, and, overall, being in better health. At the moment, there doesn't seem to be any significant research to suggest that babies who listen to music in the uterus are more intelligent, or develop at a greater speed.

The jury is still out on these findings, but there is anecdotal evidence from pregnant women that their babies move to the rhythm of music. It makes sense that as you relax to gentle music or are invigorated by livelier music, your baby will respond in kind. Many mums say that music played frequently during pregnancy seems to be familiar to their newborns, and soothes them.

So whether your baby is simply experiencing the benefits of your happy state as you listen, or responding to the rhythm, playing music is a good idea.

At this stage, your baby's lungs are starting to mature, as the barrier between the bloodstream and what will become air-containing sacs gradually starts to thin. The thinner this barrier, the more easily oxygen and carbon dioxide will transfer into and out of the baby's bloodstream.

The lungs remain filled with fluid during your pregnancy and when your baby practises breathing, the fluid moves out of her lungs into the amniotic fluid.

At 23 weeks, cells begin to line the smallest branches within the lung and start to produce surfactant, a substance that greatly assists lung function. This substance enables the smallest air sacs to remain open when the newborn baby breathes in and out so that gas transfer can continually take place. Without it, the tiny air sacs would collapse after each breath and it would take much more effort to move air in and out of the lungs. The cells that produce surfactant are not, however, fully functional yet.

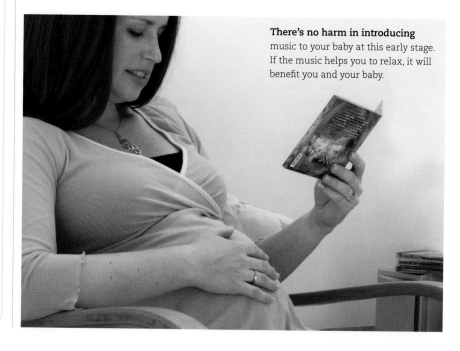

There's no harm in introducing music to your baby at this early stage. If the music helps you to relax, it will benefit you and your baby.

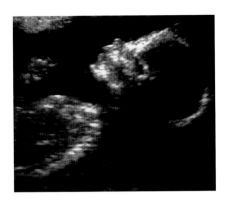

112 days to go...

YOUR BABY TODAY

As your pregnancy advances your baby's skeleton starts to harden, reflecting more of the ultrasound beam and casting black shadows. In this scan, the forehead casts a shadow, and it is no longer allowing the brain beneath to be easily seen.

Even though you're well settled into your pregnancy, ensure you maintain all those healthy lifestyle habits you've established.

You've been pregnant for almost six months and are, hopefully, feeling great in yourself. Don't, however, let this make you complacent. Even though your baby is well developed by this stage, it's important to maximize her health, and your own, by continuing to eat well and taking care of yourself. Changes, such as not smoking or drinking alcohol, will probably be part of your normal lifestyle now as opposed to something that you have to think about and work hard at.

If you have not managed to change your lifestyle to become more healthy, then it is never too late to start. Any changes you make now will benefit both you and your baby.

While you'll need to adapt your exercise routine, if you have one, in these later stages, ensure you continue to be active and, ideally, do something physical every day, even if it's just a 20-minute stroll. Also keep up your daily pelvic floor exercises (see p.69) – once the baby is born, you'll be thankful you did.

(see p.69)

AS A MATTER OF FACT

A correctly worn seat belt reduces the risk of injury to the unborn baby by 70 per cent.

In recent research, over half of pregnant women did not wear their seat belt correctly, positioning it too high across the abdomen and putting the torso strap behind them rather than over the shoulder.

FOCUS ON... DADS

Hello, it's Daddy

Don't be afraid to talk to your baby. To begin with, she will recognize lower-pitched sounds, such as deep male voices, more than higher-pitched sounds, like your partner's voice. This is good for you as it means that there is plenty of time for your baby to get to know your voice before she is born.

After birth, your baby will recognize your voice and this will have a calming effect when she is distressed. So tell her about your day and even read to her – it all helps to create a bond.

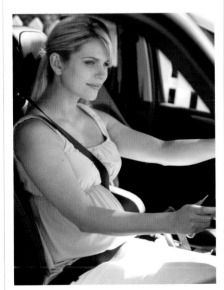

For maximum safety and comfort, wear the seat belt positioned between your breasts and under your bump.

HOW TO WEAR A SEAT BELT

It may feel cumbersome to wear a seat belt while you're pregnant, but it is essential, and a legal requirement. The good news is it's possible to buckle up comfortably.

■ **Fasten the belt** over your shoulder, as normal, and between your breasts (see left).

■ **Position the lower part** of the belt below your bump, and flat over your hips (see left).

If an emergency stop is necessary, be reassured that your baby is very safely cushioned by the amniotic fluid that surrounds her and your strong uterine muscles.

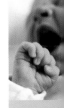

Your 25th week

IT'S THE END OF THE SECOND TRIMESTER, SO YOU MIGHT WANT TO START LOOKING AHEAD

The rest of your pregnancy will pass before you know it. Make sure you have all the practicalities in hand, such as deciding what date to stop work, and you might want to give some thought to the birth. Meanwhile, friends and family will no doubt be monitoring your growing bump with interest. Try to be patient if they bombard you with advice and don't listen to too many "tall tales" about pregnancy and childbirth.

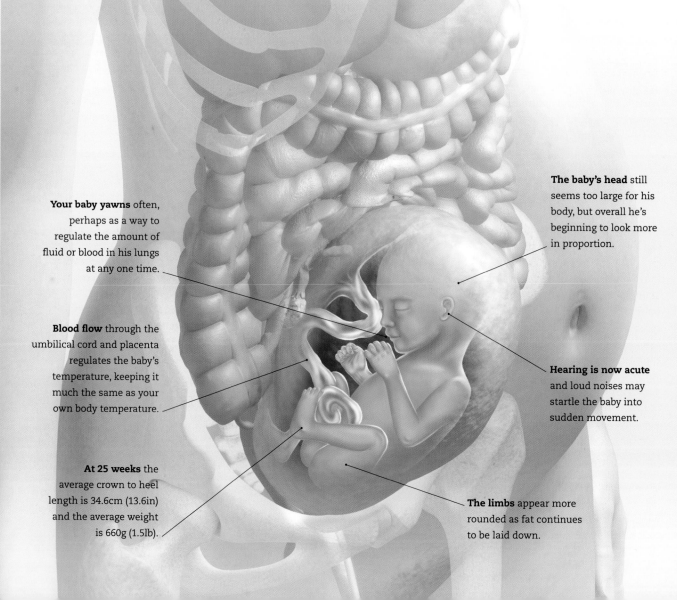

Your baby yawns often, perhaps as a way to regulate the amount of fluid or blood in his lungs at any one time.

Blood flow through the umbilical cord and placenta regulates the baby's temperature, keeping it much the same as your own body temperature.

At 25 weeks the average crown to heel length is 34.6cm (13.6in) and the average weight is 660g (1.5lb).

The baby's head still seems too large for his body, but overall he's beginning to look more in proportion.

Hearing is now acute and loud noises may startle the baby into sudden movement.

The limbs appear more rounded as fat continues to be laid down.

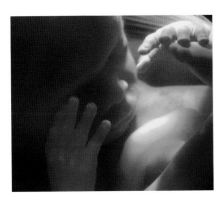

111 days to go...

YOUR BABY TODAY

From this week, brown fat is laid down in your baby's neck, chest, and back to be used after birth to produce heat and energy. At the moment he has no control over his temperature, which is efficiently maintained at a perfect level by the placenta.

This week you're legally obliged to inform your employer of the date you want to start your maternity leave.

At least 15 weeks before your due date, when you are 25 weeks pregnant, you must tell your employer when you want to start your maternity leave. You can stop work and start your leave any time from 29 weeks of pregnancy, but you can opt to work later into your pregnancy. If you work until the end, but take days off due to a pregnancy-related problem or illness in the last four weeks, your employers can insist you start your maternity leave. This only applies in the last four weeks; up until then, time off would be considered sick leave. If you have your baby earlier than your planned leaving date, maternity leave starts from the day your baby is born.

FOCUS ON... YOUR BODY

Stretchy skin

You may have developed stretch marks due to your skin stretching rapidly as you gain pregnancy weight. Initially, these marks are pinky/red and can be itchy. After pregnancy, stretch marks fade to a lighter, silvery colour and become less obvious. They generally occur on the breasts, tummy, hips, and thighs, and affect the majority of pregnant women.

Stretch marks can be genetic and are more likely to occur the older you are because older skin is less elastic. Moisturizing the skin won't prevent stretch marks but it may help to keep it smooth. A combination of exercising and eating healthily can minimize the rate at which you gain weight and "stretch".

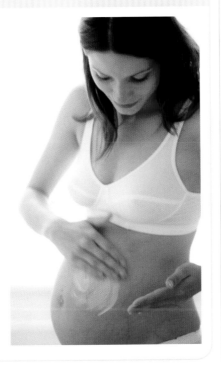

ASK A... MIDWIFE

My midwife measured me and said I seem small for dates. What does this mean? It means your baby appears to be small for your stage of pregnancy, but it doesn't necessarily mean there's a problem. You'll be given a scan for an accurate measurement and so that your baby's development can be thoroughly checked.

Sometimes slow growth is due to a condition called intra-uterine growth restriction (IUGR). It can be due to a problem with the baby or the placenta, affecting the amount of oxygen and nutrients reaching the baby. Pre-eclampsia (see p.474) can cause IUGR, as can smoking, drinking alcohol, and taking recreational drugs.

AS A MATTER OF FACT

You will get Statutory Maternity Pay if by week 25 you've worked for your company for 26 weeks.

This is paid at 90 per cent of your weekly earnings for the first six weeks of your maternity leave (see pp.348–9).

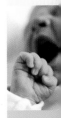

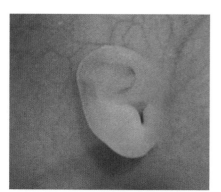

110 days to go...

YOUR BABY TODAY

In the uterus, your baby's ears not only have fluid around them but also inside. This is part of the reason that he can only hear certain lower sound frequencies. Yawning may be a way to unblock the ears, and from now on your baby spends a lot of time yawning.

If you're feeling tired, you're not alone. Your developing baby has been yawning for some weeks now.

All babies are known to yawn in the uterus, although the reason why they do this remains unclear. Yawning is often accompanied by shrugging of the shoulders or stretching, exactly as you would do when tired. Unborn babies have even been seen to rub their eyes!

Your baby first started yawning at around 15 weeks and has gradually yawned more and more frequently. The precise function of yawning for the baby remains in doubt and there are several hypotheses. Whilst it's difficult to imagine that an unborn baby is actually tired, it has been found that babies who are anaemic yawn much more frequently than others. Another theory is that yawning may help the unborn baby to regulate the amount of fluid or blood flow he has within his lungs. Or yawning may simply be a primitive reflex, a remnant from an earlier evolutionary stage, with no current function.

Whatever the reason for yawning, the early stage at which this develops in the unborn baby, and the fact that all mammals are known to yawn in the uterus, does suggest that it plays an important, though unknown, role in fetal development.

AS A MATTER OF FACT

Women aged over 40 are more than twice as likely to have left-handed babies.

This is according to a Canadian study and may be related to the fact that older women are more likely to experience complications in pregnancy and have more arduous deliveries. Several studies show a correlation between left-handedness and birth stress.

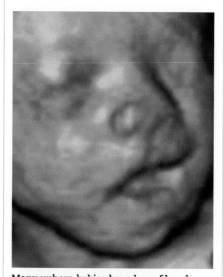

Many unborn babies have been filmed yawning on 4D scans, which give a very close-up view of fetal behaviour.

Listen to Mummy

Your developing baby's ears are structurally complete, and studies show that he can hear clearly now. Your breathing and heartbeat and the gurgles of your digestive system provide a constant background rhythm, but he's also aware of other sounds.

Talking to your baby will help you to bond: research indicates that newborns recognize – and turn towards – the sound of their mother's voice in preference to other female voices. To begin with he'll hear deeper voices more clearly, but later he'll register higher-pitched sounds. He will, of course, become more familiar with his mother's voice, partly because this is what he will hear most often and also because her body is a good conductor of sound and vibration.

You may have noticed that sudden noises make your baby startle. In one study, ultrasound scans of fetuses showed that they had a "blink-startle" response to loud noises from around 24 weeks.

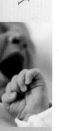

109 days to go...

YOUR BABY TODAY

Here the baby is lying with an arm up to the face and the face lying on the placenta. The eyes are shut at this time and it will be a couple of weeks before they start to open. The hand is held in the most relaxed position, with the fingers slightly curled.

Your body is working hard to grow your baby, so take care of it by enjoying some pampering.

Think of your pregnancy as a time to focus on yourself and your body; once your baby is born, the majority of your focus will be on babycare.

If you have the time and money, treat yourself to a day at a spa. Most do special packages for pregnant women. Spending time at a spa, where you can go for a gentle swim, have some pampering treatments, and enjoy being in a tranquil environment, is a great way to relax and unwind. If a spa day is out of the question, create your own at home. Run a bath, add some relaxing essential oils (see p.163 for a list of those that are safe to use in pregnancy), light some candles, and relax. If you don't want to be disturbed, let your partner know and turn off the phone.

Pregnancy massage (see p.224), either from a professional or your partner, can be very therapeutic, both physically and emotionally. Another great treatment to have at this stage is a pedicure; you'll increasingly be unable to see your toes, let alone reach them, so it's a treat for someone else to take care of them for you.

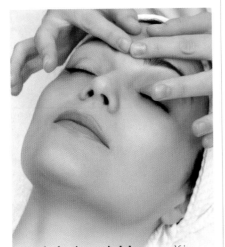

Now is the time to indulge yourself in a little pampering. When booking beauty treatments, always make it known that you're pregnant.

ASK A... DOCTOR

I haven't felt my baby move for four hours. Should I be worried? Contact your midwife and explain your baby's usual pattern of movements. She can examine you and provide reassurance.

If you're not familiar with your baby's movements, lie down – he is more likely to sleep when you're active. Try encouraging him to move around (see p.206).

ON YOUR FEET

You may now find it more of a struggle to be on your feet, especially for long periods of time. Weight gain, changes in your centre of gravity (particularly during the second and third trimesters), and hormones can cause foot pain and swelling (see pp.225 and 466). The pregnancy hormones that relax your joints ready for childbirth can also work to loosen the ligaments in your feet and hips, which can cause some discomfort.

To minimize foot discomfort:
■ **Wear sports shoes** that have a good arch support to help to reduce strain on your spine. They may also prevent a condition called plantar fasciitis – this is where the large ligament that connects the heel to the ball of the foot becomes inflamed.
■ **Avoid wearing high-heeled shoes.** As well as being uncomfortable, they may make you unsteady on your feet and cause you to fall.
■ **Ensure that your shoes fit** correctly and invest in new ones if not. Some pregnant women's feet expand by a size, and never return to their normal size after pregnancy.
■ **Take regular exercise,** and avoid standing for long periods. Take regular breaks if your job involves standing.

257

108 days to go...

YOUR BABY TODAY

This 3D scan shows the baby thumb sucking. The 3D technique uses several routine 2D images, linked together to give the 3D effect. In a 4D scan, a series of 3D images are shown in quick succession to give almost real-time movements: the 4th dimension is time.

A natural temperature-regulating mechanism within the uterus means your baby never gets cold.

The temperature inside the uterus is between a third and half a degree higher than yours. Because your body temperature is so closely controlled, your baby never becomes cold so never needs to shiver. He has started to lay down a special form of brown fat, particularly around the neck, chest, and back. After birth, metabolism of this fat produces both energy and heat. In the womb, however, the baby cannot use this fat to raise his temperature. Some temperature control occurs as heat is lost from the baby's skin into the amniotic fluid through the uterine wall and then into your body tissues. However, the regulation of temperature is predominantly achieved by means of the blood flow to the placenta. The large surface area of the placenta allows it to act as a heat exchange, keeping the temperature of the blood leaving the baby in the umbilical arteries constant with that of the oxygenated blood returning to the baby through the umbilical vein.

After birth, babies lose heat quickly. They are still unable to shiver and cannot maintain their temperature, cooling rapidly if they're not wrapped up warmly or held skin-to-skin shortly after the birth.

SENSIBLE SNACKING

In addition to eating three meals a day, you may find you need to snack throughout the day, too. There's nothing wrong with that as long as you're choosing the right foods, and not reaching for the biscuits and crisps all the time. These tempting foods might satisfy a hunger pang, but the lack of nutrients and empty calories mean they won't serve you any real purpose. Healthy snacking can be accomplished with a bit of planning before you go shopping:

■ **Dried fruits** should be a mainstay of your snacking, since they can easily be stored and carried. Enjoy a wide variety of dried fruits, as the more variety you consume, the more likely you are to obtain the nutrients you need. Try dried apricots, raisins, cranberries, cherries, and peaches.

■ **Lightly salted mixed nuts** will satisfy any salt craving you may have in a healthy way.

■ **Opt for pretzels, oatcakes,** or crackers, rather than crisps.

■ **Fresh fruit** is a convenient and nutrient-rich snack; always carry one or two pieces with you when you're out and about, and make fruit salads that you can keep in the fridge. Keep frozen fruit on hand, and along with some vanilla yogurt, you can whip up a smoothie in no time at all.

■ **Frozen yogurt and low-fat ice cream** both make good snacks and desserts. Stock up on a variety of low-fat yogurt brands.

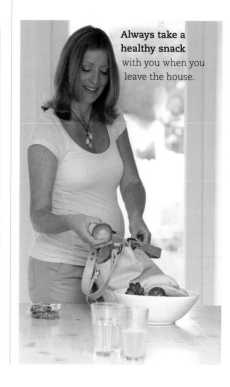

Always take a healthy snack with you when you leave the house.

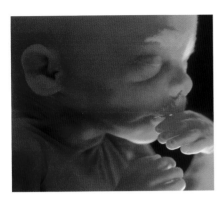

107 days to go...

YOUR BABY TODAY

Here the skin looks almost loose around the neck as the baby has turned his head slightly. This is normal at this stage: the lack of fat beneath the skin and the need to grow rapidly can make your baby appear as if he needs time to "grow into" his own skin.

Some meals may be followed by an uncomfortable bout of indigestion, but you can take steps to prevent and relieve this.

ASK A... NUTRITIONIST

What natural remedies could I try for my digestive problems?
Peppermint in its fresh or dried herbal form is most definitely beneficial for treating a wide range of symptoms, the most important of which are digestive problems. Try drinking tea (see right) or sucking on peppermint sweets, especially if you've eaten a big meal.

Peppermint contains menthol, which has been shown in studies to be an effective digestive muscle relaxant and an effective remedy for wind, nausea, and indigestion. It has a "carminative" effect, meaning that it works specifically on the digestive system.

The intensity of your symptoms can be relieved by eating raw garlic or taking a garlic capsule every day. A garlic supplement that is rich in the active ingredient allicin will be more effective.

Other herbal teas that may ease heartburn are cardamom, camomile, lemon balm, orange peel, and meadowsweet. To aid digestion, try drinking a teaspoon of cider vinegar in warm water 20 minutes before a meal.

While you may be enjoying your food, you could be paying the price with indigestion. The pregnancy hormone progesterone relaxes the muscles in the whole of the digestive tract. This slows digestion and the

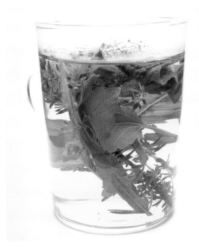

sphincters, or rings of muscles, at each end of the stomach become less effective. This can cause heartburn and indigestion as acidic juices from the stomach leak back into the oesophagus. In addition, as your pregnancy progresses, your growing baby is squashing your stomach so that you have a smaller space to digest food.

To relieve indigestion, eat little and often, eat slowly, don't eat late at night, and cut down on fatty or spicy foods. You could also try natural remedies, such as peppermint (see left). Rather than lie flat, prop yourself up with pillows. Check with your pharmacist before taking over-the-counter remedies.

Make your own peppermint tea by steeping fresh or dried leaves in hot water. Drink the tea after you've eaten for the best results.

FOCUS ON... DADS

Organizing paternity leave

Depending on how long you've worked for your company and their company policy, you may be entitled to paternity leave and pay (see p.349). Speak to your human resources department now to find out your rights and whether your company offers additional perks. You may also be entitled to unpaid parental leave. To maximize the time you can take off once the baby is born, work out how much holiday you have left and consider saving up days.

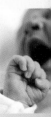

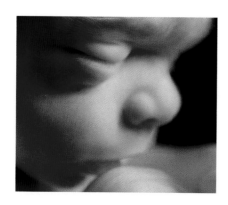

106 days to go...

YOUR BABY TODAY

The nose is well defined and as well as regularly swallowing the amniotic fluid your baby is breathing it in and out through each nostril. Just as adults do, your baby will tend to favour breathing more through one nostril than the other.

The proportions of your baby's body are becoming much closer to those of a newborn baby.

Up until the third month, your baby's head accounted for almost half of his overall length. Now his head, trunk, and legs account for a third each. At birth your baby's head will still be large in proportion compared to an adult's, but it will be just a quarter of his overall length.

Still very skinny, your baby is now starting to fill out more as fat stores continue to be laid down. Until about 14 weeks, most babies are approximately the same size and

weight. After this point, genetic and especially environmental forces increasingly come into play, influencing how quickly your baby can grow and whether his full growth potential is eventually reached.

Because different babies increasingly vary in size as the pregnancy progresses, ultrasound dating becomes less accurate at determining the number of weeks you are into your pregnancy. The best time to date the pregnancy is between 11 and 14 weeks, by simply

measuring the baby from the top of his head to his bottom (the crown–rump length, see p.138). The 20-week scan (see pp.214–15) also dates the pregnancy very accurately from the head and abdominal circumferences and the bone measurement in the leg.

If your first scan is at this late stage, it is only possible to estimate roughly the stage of pregnancy and age of the baby. It is never appropriate to change your due date if an earlier, more accurate scan has been performed.

IT'S ALL IN THE BUMP

The general story goes that if you're carrying your baby low, you're having a boy, if you're carrying high, then you're having a girl. The truth is, the way you carry is probably determined by the tone of your abdominal and uterine muscles as well as the position of your baby.

According to those "old wives", there are other physical clues: if you've gained weight on your face and it's round and full, you're having a girl. If your right breast is larger than your left, it's a boy – and if your partner gains weight, you're "definitely" having a girl!

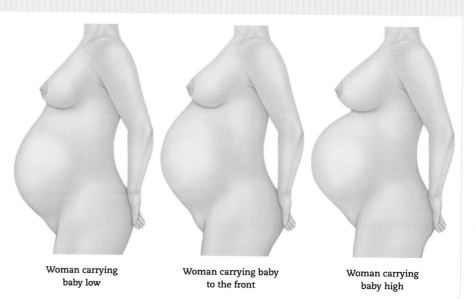

Woman carrying baby low

Woman carrying baby to the front

Woman carrying baby high

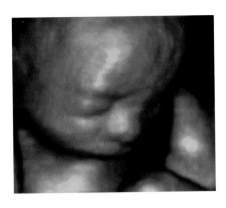

105 days to go...

YOUR BABY TODAY

Here the baby's head is looking down towards the chest. The right arm is bent at the elbow to lie across the neck, the left arm is only just visible as it is partly in shadow, and finally the tip of a knee can be seen tucked up just below the right forearm.

You can expect to be subjected to a few unwelcome birth stories, whether you want to hear them or not!

Birth partners

The benefits of having a supportive birth partner are indisputable, so it's worth thinking about it now.

■ **Research shows that** women who receive continuous emotional and physical encouragement during labour are less likely to need pain relief or medical intervention, such as an epidural (see pp.404–5), an assisted delivery (see pp.436–7), or a Caesarean (see pp.438–9), and should experience a shorter labour.

■ **Women who feel their birth partner** was supportive are more likely to view their birth in a positive light, and to take to motherhood and breastfeeding easily, and are less prone to postnatal depression.

■ **Your birth partner** doesn't have to be the baby's father (although he may be there as well); in fact, studies indicate that a woman may do the job better. A close female friend who's had her own children could be ideal; your mum is another option.

■ **You could consider** hiring a doula (see right).

It appears to be a rite of passage for some women to describe the birth of their babies in minute detail, literally giving an hour-by-hour account. For these women, it appears to be part of the recovery process and they like nothing better than a new audience, and, especially, a woman who is pregnant for the first time. So you'll no doubt find yourself on the receiving end of a few birth horror stories – sometimes from complete strangers!

These women may feel it's their duty to "warn" you about the "reality" of childbirth, and what you should and shouldn't do – for example, "definitely

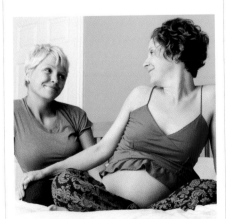

Having a close female friend or relative with you during labour, even if it's only at home in the early stages, may prove to be a great help to you and your partner.

have an epidural, otherwise the pain is horrendous". Remember that every woman's experience is different and stay focused on your own birth plan. Childbirth is undoubtedly difficult for some women, while others have straightforward deliveries, without complications. Tell the story-teller you'd rather not hear the gory details but promise to book a date for a joint debrief once your baby is born!

The prospect of giving birth and then looking after a newborn can be daunting. For some mums, hiring a doula is the perfect way to ensure a gentle progression from pregnancy to motherhood.

Doulas are women who "mother the mother" by providing emotional and physical (but non-medical) support before, during, and after childbirth. Widespread research shows that the presence of a doula can help you have a shorter, easier birth, making it less likely that you'll need pain relief or medical intervention (including an epidural or Caesarean). To find out more about hiring a doula, contact Doula UK (see p.480).

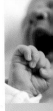

Welcome to your third trimester

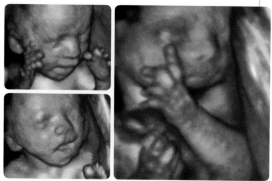

A new person emerges Your baby is close to being a fully functioning individual. His major organs are almost ready to work in the outside world, but he would need medical help should he be born now.

Monitoring growth By measuring your growing abdomen, your baby's rate of growth is assessed and any concerns addressed with further tests.

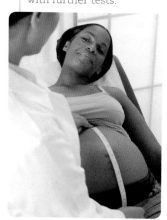

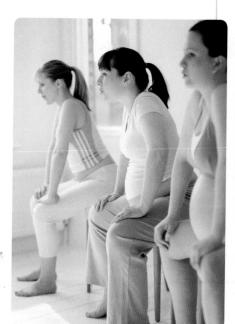

Sleeping comfortably You need to take the weight off your bump, but relaxing is easier said than done. Use lots of pillows to cushion you when you rest in bed.

From weeks 26 to 40, your baby will probably grow by about 2.7kg (6lb) and 15cm (6in).

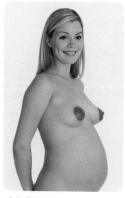
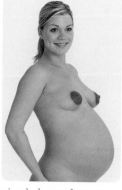

Third trimester Your growing baby pushes out your lower ribs and fills up most of the space in the uterus. **Ready for birth** Your bump is huge and you're tired and breathless, but excited, too.

A new brother or sister Include older children as you prepare for your new baby. They can help you to choose clothes and think about names.

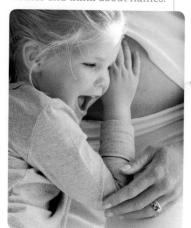

Preparing for labour Attending antenatal classes and exercise sessions will help you to prepare both mentally and physically for the approaching labour and birth, and to feel confident about how you'll cope.

You're on the home straight now and your thoughts turn increasingly to the birth of your baby.

33	34	35	36	37	38	39	40

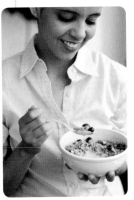

Fibre fit An adequate fibre intake is especially important in late pregnancy when a sluggish digestion makes constipation more likely.

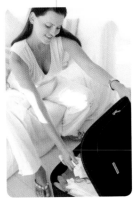

Ready to go Delivery date is on the horizon. If you're planning a hospital birth, pack your bags in good time. Start gathering up essential items.

Nearing the end As you reach the end of your pregnancy, you'll marvel at the size of your bump.

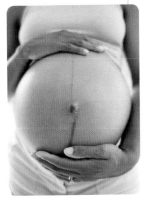

38 weeks It's a tight fit now for your baby, so he hasn't much room to turn and kick. You should still feel him moving, though – so it's important to be aware of any change in activity.

Facts and figures By week 38, the placenta's role is nearly over and it starts to age.

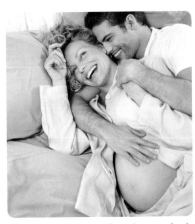

Bringing on labour If you've reached 40 weeks with no sign of labour, you may be starting to think about ways to trigger its onset – making love is one of several methods to try.

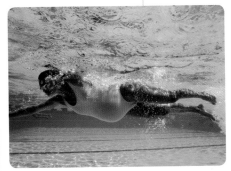

Taking the weight It's worth continuing with swimming for as long as you feel able, as the water supports all your additional weight, bringing welcome relief.

Facts and figures By 33 weeks, your baby is rapidly putting down fat deposits and is starting to look more like a newborn baby.

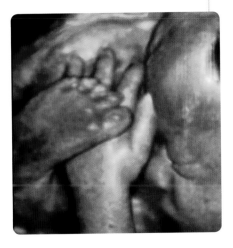

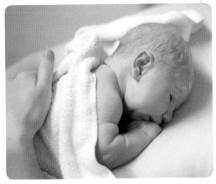

Hello, baby Here at last, and worth all the waiting. Immediate skin-to-skin contact has significant benefits for your baby.

Your 26th week

YOU'VE REACHED THE THIRD AND FINAL TRIMESTER AND WILL BE HEAVILY PREGNANT BY NOW

You're on the last lap and, although your bump is probably big, you've still got a lot more expanding to do. Your baby will be moving about quite vigorously and may even respond to loud noises and music. Nerve cells in her brain are beginning to join up and her co-ordination is improving. Keep your own brain stimulated by attending antenatal classes for fun, company, and information.

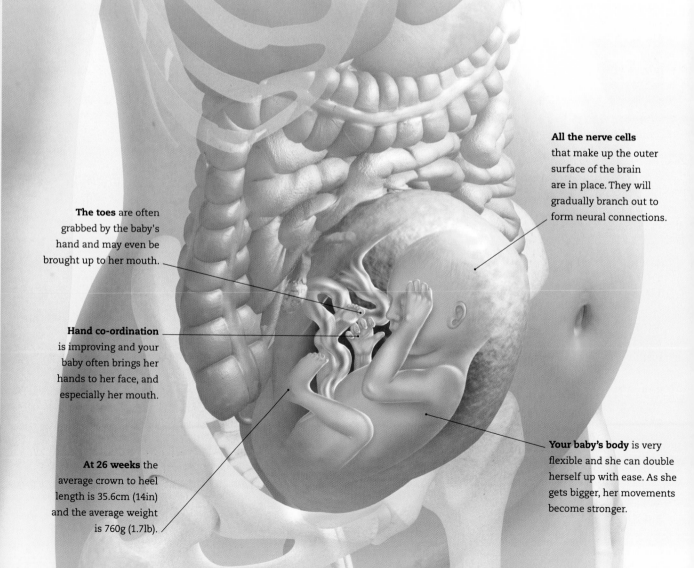

All the nerve cells that make up the outer surface of the brain are in place. They will gradually branch out to form neural connections.

The toes are often grabbed by the baby's hand and may even be brought up to her mouth.

Hand co-ordination is improving and your baby often brings her hands to her face, and especially her mouth.

At 26 weeks the average crown to heel length is 35.6cm (14in) and the average weight is 760g (1.7lb).

Your baby's body is very flexible and she can double herself up with ease. As she gets bigger, her movements become stronger.

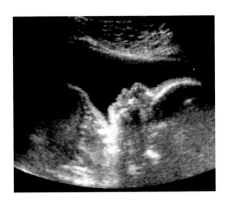

104 days to go...

YOUR BABY TODAY

Here the baby is looking directly upwards. The profile is nicely detailed with the nose, lips, and chin clearly outlined. The neck is still short so, as this image shows, the head is still held quite close to the chest.

Your antenatal classes will give you a chance to learn about labour, birth, and life with a newborn, and make new friends.

If you booked them earlier in your pregnancy (see p.199), you may be starting antenatal classes (also called parentcraft classes) about now. Classes may be held in the hospital where you have chosen to give birth, or they can be run by the National Childbirth Trust (NCT), or privately by midwives. The aim of the classes is to inform you about pregnancy, labour, and the first few weeks after the birth. For example, you may be taught relaxation or breathing techniques, or be told about the different types of pain relief on offer. You'll also be given advice on what to buy for the baby and on topics that are relevant after the birth, such as breastfeeding, sleeping, and nappy changing.

It's common to feel excited about the classes and keen to learn about what's going to happen and to meet other people going through the same experience. But antenatal classes are not just about gathering information, they're also about meeting others, which is difficult for some people. However, as you're all parents-to-be, you're likely to find things to talk about. Just talking with others about your symptoms or worries can help, especially if they're going through the same emotions as you. It can be reassuring to know that you're not the only person to feel a certain way.

If you do make friends in your antenatal class, this support group can also be very helpful after you all have your babies.

FOCUS ON... YOUR BODY

Rib pain

As the uterus expands, the rib cage is pushed outwards to make room for it, and this can lead to rib pain or discomfort. This is not inevitable, but it is more likely if you have a smaller than average body frame or you're carrying twins or more. It can be made worse if your baby kicks a lot or if she spends a lot of time in the breech position as her head will push against your diaphragm and rib cage.

Sitting down may make the pain worse since being seated compresses your internal organs more. If you have a sedentary job, get up and move around as often as you can, and if you're forced to sit for long periods, keep adjusting your position until you find one that's comfortable.

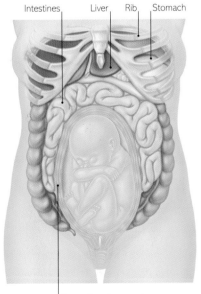

Intestines   Liver   Rib   Stomach

Expanding uterus reduces space for stomach and intestines

ASK A... DOCTOR

I think I have a vaginal infection. Will this harm my baby? A vaginal infection is very unlikely to harm your baby since the mucus plug around the cervix stops infection reaching her. You may find the symptoms of an infection – itching, irritation, and a discharge with an unpleasant odour – uncomfortable. Your doctor will prescribe medication to clear it up.

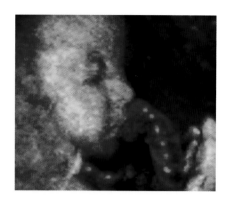

103 days to go...

YOUR BABY TODAY

This image shows the baby in profile, this time in 3D. The coils of the umbilical cord are just seen in the background passing behind the baby's head. The eyelids can be seen, still firmly closed. Fat stores are now giving the face a much more rounded contour.

Two tiny glands control your baby's growth and development now, and give her the ability to face up to life's stresses later.

Relative to body size, your baby's adrenal glands are 20 times larger than your own. The adrenal glands are roughly triangular in shape, with their base wrapped over the top of each kidney. They have an outer layer, or cortex, which releases steroid hormones such as cortisol, and an inner layer, or medulla. Adrenaline and the related hormone noradrenaline are secreted from the medulla in response to stress.

Adrenaline prepares the body for a "fight or flight" response, increasing the availability of glucose, speeding up the heart rate, and maintaining or raising blood pressure. These are vital adaptive responses for your baby that will help to maintain a stable environment

within the uterus and prepare her for the stresses of life later on in the outside world.

It is the outer cortex, however, that needs to work hard, producing many hormones that help to co-ordinate your baby's growth and development. The cortex produces three types of hormones: mineralocorticoids that

regulate salt balance; glucocorticoids that help to control the availability of sugars, fat, and amino acids in the bloodstream; and androgens, male-type sex hormones, such as testosterone. It is the cortex that accounts for the large size of your baby's adrenal glands. After birth, in the first couple of weeks, the adrenal glands rapidly reduce in size.

ASK A... DOCTOR

I've noticed lumps in both my breasts. Should I be worried?
Breast lumps can be normal in pregnancy, especially in the third trimester as the breasts get ready for breastfeeding. These lumps are generally soft and may move around; they may also be tender. However, breast lumps should never be ignored, so always see your doctor who will be able to confirm that they are pregnancy related.

FOCUS ON... TWINS

How identical are identical twins?

Twins from the same egg have the same DNA. In a way, they're natural clones, so you might expect them to

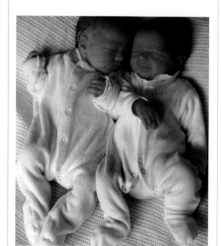

be identical in every way. They will certainly look very alike, and have the same hair colour, eye colour, and skin colour. They will also have the same blood group and tissue type.

However, the environment isn't the same for each baby, even pre-birth. Small differences in blood flow, and in location in the uterus, can have far-reaching effects.

■ **There may be recognizable differences** in the weight, height, and head shape of identical twins.
■ **Each twin** has unique fingerprints and iris patterns.
■ **Identical twins** can have different personalities too, partly because of subtle dissimilarities in their very early environment.

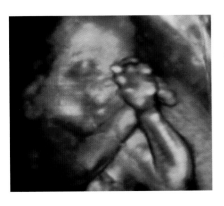

102 days to go...

YOUR BABY TODAY

This baby has her hands held up in front of her face. In the top right-hand corner, the curved inner lining of the uterus can be seen. Shadows in the image give the impression of hair but ultrasound is not detailed enough to show hair – even if there was any to see at this stage.

Attending antenatal classes together is a good way for your partner to stay closely involved with your pregnancy.

Not all dads-to-be are keen on going to antenatal classes. They might not feel the classes apply to them, and may fear that they will be asked to do exercises that they find embarrassing.

If your partner is reluctant, discuss it with him, pointing out what the classes are for and why you feel that you need his support. You could explain that you want him to be informed about labour so that he is not anxious in the delivery room. He might find it useful to chat to male friends who attended classes when they were expectant dads.

Classes may include some sessions with men and women together and others where the women attend on their own, for example to practise breathing techniques, while the men have a separate session where they can share any concerns. If time off work is an issue for your partner, ask for a list of what topics will be covered each week and pick those sessions that you think are the most relevant for him. If your partner is well informed, he'll feel more involved in the pregnancy and more confident in helping you during labour and birth.

What you learn at antenatal classes may bring you closer. Try to stay in touch with each other at home, spending time relaxing together and feeling your baby moving.

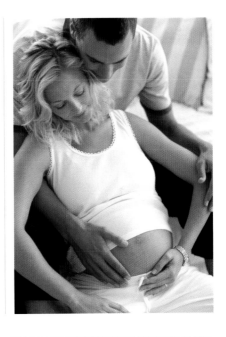

TIME TO THINK ABOUT

Maternity rights

To qualify for maternity and paternity benefits and leave:

■ **Obtain a MATB1** form from your doctor or midwife after week 20 (they won't give it to you before this time). Fill it in and give it to your employer.

■ **Tell your employer** your expected week of delivery and the date you plan to start your maternity leave.

■ **Your partner** should also inform his employer in order to qualify for paternity leave (see p.349).

FOCUS ON... RELATIONSHIPS

Anticipating changes in your relationship

It might seem obvious, but once your baby is born your relationship won't just be about you and your partner any more. Suddenly there is a tiny new person around, who wakes during the night and who has her own needs. By necessity, after your baby is born you and your partner will pay less attention to each other. There may also be less physical intimacy between the two of you, not least because you both will be very tired.

It's best to talk about, and acknowledge, these issues before the birth. This way, you and your partner will better accept that these factors are a normal part of making the life change from coupledom to being a family.

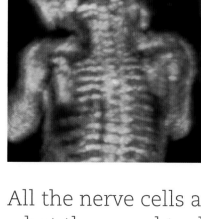

101 days to go...

YOUR BABY TODAY

This 3D image shows the back of the baby, taken using a scanner setting that enhances the reflections from the skeleton. The back of the spine, ribs, and shoulder blades are clear. This technique has opened up many new possibilities for visualizing your baby's development.

All the nerve cells are now on the surface of your baby's brain; what they need to do next is make connections with each other.

Your baby's brain is so complex that it needs the entire length of your pregnancy not only to grow, but also to mature. It is continually forming new connections and sensory pathways.

The nerves that make up the brain's grey matter started in the centre of the brain on the outer surface of the lateral ventricles (there is one ventricle in each hemisphere of the brain). The lateral ventricles contain the part of the brain known as the choroid plexus, a loose, seaweed-like structure that produces the fluid that bathes your baby's brain and spinal cord. Constantly circulating around the brain, this fluid protects and buffers the brain from the harder structure of the bones of the surrounding skull.

The gradual, wave-like, outward movement of nerve cells in the grey matter, which started more than 12 weeks ago, is now complete. Coming to rest close to the brain's surface, these cells need to mature, branching out to make multiple connections, or "synapses", with other nerve cells.

The surface of your baby's brain is very smooth at this stage but as the cortex matures, beginning to form six clear layers, it takes on its familiar wrinkled appearance.

FOCUS ON... YOUR BUMP

Your bump: to show or not to show?

Whether you want to clothe your bump in figure-hugging fabrics and proudly show it off, or choose looser styles that may fit you for longer and obscure just how pregnant you are, is a personal choice.

■ **If you're happy to show your bump,** you may feel comfortable in stretchy fabrics that can expand as your tummy does. The downside to wearing tight clothing is that your skin may be sensitive to anything snug-fitting. Tight tops will also bring attention to your breasts.

■ **If you feel more comfortable** not showing the profile of your bump, choose baggier clothes, such as tunics, smocks, and overshirts. These may be more comfortable and will cloak your bump for longer.

■ **If you want to bare your bump,** do so when the weather is warm enough. One advantage is you may find you can wear some pre-pregnancy tops.

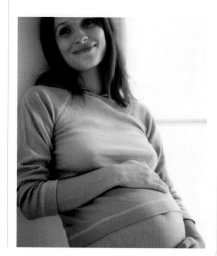

ASK A... MIDWIFE

I'm getting quite big – should I adapt my swimming style?
You may find that in these final couple of months, you need to change your swimming style to one that is more comfortable; many women opt for breaststroke, which can also help to get the baby in to an optimum position (see p.329).

If you don't feel up to swimming lengths, just relax in the pool instead. Being in the water will relieve pressure on your abdomen and help to ease lower back pain.

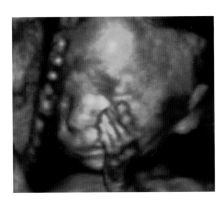

100 days to go...

YOUR BABY TODAY

With fingers held up to the cheek, eyes closed, and the ear just visible in the background, this image shows a very peaceful baby. To the left, the umbilical cord is visible on its way to the placenta, seen further left still.

It will be some years before you'll know your child's personality, but even in the uterus she has some likes and dislikes.

As your baby continues to grow you may find yourself wondering what she is going to be like: easy-going or demanding? Funny or serious? Happy playing alone or sociable? Boisterous or quiet? You may believe that babies are born with their personalities already developed, or that they are born with a personality that is further shaped and developed as they grow. The nature versus nurture debate rages on and, in all likelihood, it's a combination of the two: some aspects of your child's personality may already be decided before birth, some may be developed later in childhood, or even adulthood.

You may already have noticed that your baby has certain likes or dislikes, for example she may kick or move in response to loud music or to a certain genre of music, though it's difficult to tell whether the increased movements mean your baby is enjoying it or not.

Your baby is very stimulated inside the uterus. By this third trimester, she can feel vibrations, and hear not just sounds from inside your body, such as your heartbeat, but also sounds from outside, such as people talking. Your baby is aware of when you're moving or are still and you may have noticed a pattern of movements from her, not least that she "communicates" more when you're resting.

As part of her activity, she will continue practising for life after the birth, with breathing movements and swallowing – and she may even suck her thumb.

BUYING FOR YOUR BABY

Preparing for your baby's arrival doesn't have to break the bank.
What your baby needs:
■ **Milk:** breast milk is free (and best for your baby). For bottle-feeding, you'll need bottles, teats, formula, and a sterilizing system.
■ **Nappies:** you'll need to decide between disposables, reusables, or a combination of the two (see p.291). Whichever type you choose, you'll also need to use nappy wipes.
■ **Somewhere to sleep:** she can sleep in a cot from birth if you don't want to buy a crib or a Moses basket. Even if you buy a second-hand cot, always buy a new mattress.

■ **Lots of babygros**: don't buy too many newborn size.
■ **Transport:** a buggy (with a lie-option until your baby can sit up), or a sling or backpack in which to carry your baby.
■ **Car seat**: this is a legal requirement for car travel. Don't buy second hand.
What your baby can live without:
■ **Changing station:** a mat (or towel) on the floor is cheaper and safer.
■ **Bottle warmer:** heat in a jug instead.
■ **Designer wardrobe.**
■ **Travel cot:** borrow one if necessary.
Save money by shopping online. Scour second-hand shops and car-boot sales. Swap clothes and toys with friends, family members, and other parents.

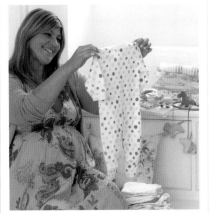

Babies soon outgrow babygros and get little wear out of them so you may be offered some from friends. You can cut the feet off the babygros if they're too tight.

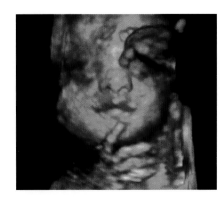

99 days to go...

YOUR BABY TODAY

A 3D scan can be coloured in different ways. This image demonstrates that by this stage your baby's lip shape is clearly defined. The lips are the most sensitive part of the entire body and your baby's hands are often held up towards them.

Your baby can make co-ordinated movements with her hands and feet, make a fist, and grab hold of her toes.

Your baby's hand co-ordination dramatically improves now and she constantly brings her hands up to her face, particularly her mouth. The face, and especially the lips, are extremely sensitive, and this heightened sensitivity provides strong positive feedback as your baby successfully co-ordinates smooth, purposeful movements between hand (and foot) and mouth.

There is still plenty of room in the uterus for all sorts of movements and your baby is extremely flexible. It is quite easy for her to adopt a doubled-up position, with her feet up by her mouth or even on top of her head, and to do full somersaults.

Your baby's bones are hardening from the centre out so their outer edges are still formed of soft cartilage.

FOCUS ON... YOUR BABY

Birth weight

A woman's weight gain during pregnancy influences her baby's birth weight, which in turn influences the future health of the baby. Birth weights that are too high or too low have been associated with an increased chance of health problems in the baby's future. Thus, pregnancy is a balancing act, in which women need to take in enough, but not too many, calories and gain the right amount of weight (see p.99).

Health experts are increasingly concerned about the fact that fetal over-nutrition is resulting in high birth weight. Being overweight, or putting on excessive amounts of weight during pregnancy, increases the chances of gestational diabetes in the mother (see p.473), a Caesarean delivery, complications during delivery, large newborns, and childhood obesity. If a child is obese, there's an increased risk of a lifetime of being overweight or obese, which increases the chances of diabetes, high blood pressure, cancer, and heart disease.

ASK A... MIDWIFE

Why do I get so hot when I'm exercising? During pregnancy, your core body temperature rises due to the effects of the hormone progesterone, your increased weight, and the greater demands on your body. Exercise generates heat and raises your core temperature even further, which is why you're likely to feel extra hot when you exercise during pregnancy.

You'll also sweat more easily while you are pregnant. This is because pregnancy-related hormones cause dilation of blood vessels and thus blood flow to your skin (this explains the rosy "glow" some women get), allowing your body to lose heat through the skin more readily. This means that, although you

get hotter while you're exercising, you'll cool down more quickly than usual. When you're exercising, always remember to:

■ **Drink water** before, during, and after a workout.
■ **Wear suitable clothing** that will allow your skin to breathe.
■ **Avoid exercising** when conditions are hot and humid.

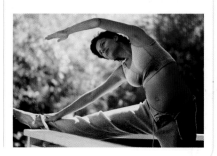

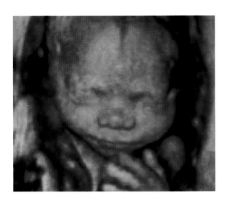

YOU ARE 26 WEEKS EXACTLY

98 days to go...

YOUR BABY TODAY

The space between the two frontal bones of the forehead (the dark line) has now nearly closed. The bones on the left and right sides come to lie very close to each other with a small gap to allow for further growth of the head and brain.

Dreaming is a natural and healthy part of your sleep cycle, but at this stage of pregnancy unsettling dreams can be common.

Vivid dreams are common among women in the third trimester. You may, in fact, not be dreaming more than usual, but difficulty in finding a comfortable sleeping position and waking often to go to the loo may mean that you remember your dreams more than usual (you normally would not wake during the dreaming phase of your sleep cycle, so often do not recall your dreams in the morning).

It is common to dream about babies and small children in distress or danger. It is not uncommon for women to feel anxious about such dreams, but you should know that they are in no way insights into what is in store for you. Dreaming is a way of filtering any negative emotions so that you do not have to experience them at first hand. Rest assured that, although disturbing, these dreams will help you to cope with your natural concern for your baby's welfare.

GOING ON A HOSPITAL TOUR

As part of the build-up to your baby's birth, you may be offered a tour of the hospital. Not only will you be able to see first hand where you're likely to deliver your baby, and what the wards are like, but you can also work out the practical details, such as parking, admission procedures, what you'll need to bring, and what facilities there are, such as cafés and shops for visiting friends and family.

Ultimately, a hospital tour offers you a reassuring chance for you and your partner to prepare yourself mentally for the big day and what will follow your baby's birth.

Use the opportunity as a fact-finding mission. Ask how the hospital uses birth plans (see p.303), and when and why they might have to be adapted. Ask how many other mums there will be on the ward, and, if you wish, how you can arrange a private room. There is usually a fee for this. Find out what support you'll have in the first 24 hours. Most hospitals now expect the mother to keep the baby with her during the night. Ask about visiting hours, and the number of visitors you can have at any one time. You could also ask how many babies are born at the hospital each year, and how many of these are born by Caesarean (emergency or otherwise). Request information about who might be delivering your baby, how long the staff shifts are, and what is done to provide continuity of care during labour and birth.

Are there birthing pools or baths available? Do they have TENS machines or any other form of pain relief you may be considering? What support is there for breastfeeding, and are there breast pumps available?

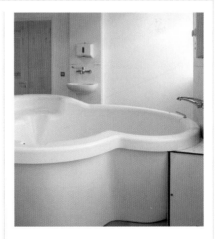

Finally, although you probably won't need to use it, you may wish to see the special care baby unit (SCBU) (see pp.452–3). If your baby needs this sort of care, it can help to have seen the equipment and gained a basic understanding of what it's used for.

Your 27th week

YOU MAY FIND IT DIFFICULT TO SLEEP DUE TO YOUR BABY'S ACTIVITIES

Space is now getting tight in your uterus. The baby is likely to give you a few sharp jabs with his feet and fists as he stretches and turns. However uncomfortable the kicks may be, you'll find them a welcome reassurance that the baby is thriving. Relax in bed or in the bath and watch your bump – you'll be amazed and amused at how it pops up and down and moves around.

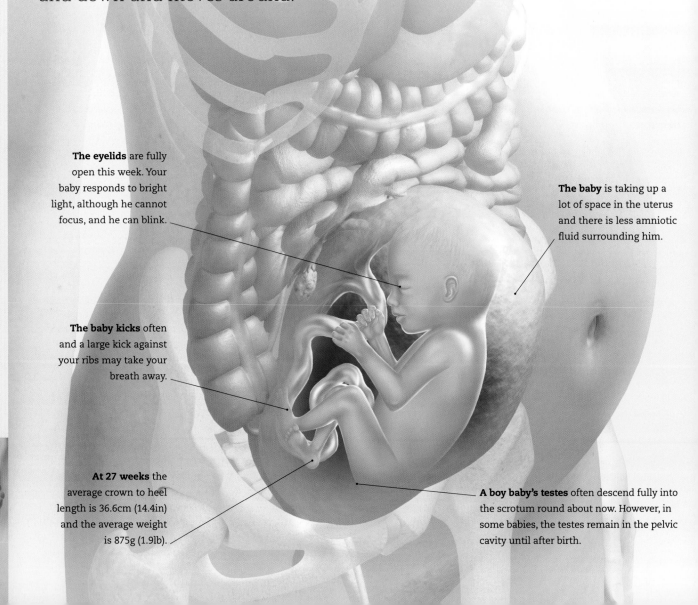

The eyelids are fully open this week. Your baby responds to bright light, although he cannot focus, and he can blink.

The baby is taking up a lot of space in the uterus and there is less amniotic fluid surrounding him.

The baby kicks often and a large kick against your ribs may take your breath away.

At 27 weeks the average crown to heel length is 36.6cm (14.4in) and the average weight is 875g (1.9lb).

A boy baby's testes often descend fully into the scrotum round about now. However, in some babies, the testes remain in the pelvic cavity until after birth.

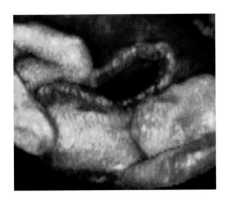

97 days to go...

YOUR BABY TODAY

The coiling umbilical cord is very clearly seen in this image. The umbilical cord grows as your baby grows and will be about the same length as your baby at this stage of your pregnancy: about 36.6cm (14.4in).

When you settle down for a nap it can be frustrating if your baby starts exercising, but take this as a sign that all is well.

You may have noticed that your baby is more active at some times than at others, often when you're trying to relax or sleep! This is likely to be because when you're busy or distracted, you're less aware of your baby moving because you're not paying him as much attention as at other times. The moment you stop and sit down to put your feet up or go to bed will be the time your baby starts to do his somersaults.

Remember that, like newborns, babies still in the uterus spend a lot of time sleeping, so there will be periods when you don't feel your baby being very active – it's fine for him not to be moving all the time. Every baby has a different cycle of waking and sleeping, and there are no rules as to when your baby should be kicking and when he should be still.

If you're familiar with your baby's pattern of movements and are concerned that you haven't felt him move, try lying down on your side and relaxing or playing music to see if your baby responds. If, however, you're concerned, then see your doctor or midwife, who will be able to examine you and listen for the baby's heartbeat.

Some women count their baby's kicks using a chart, noting down when they feel the baby move. Kick charts are not often used now, unless recommended by a doctor or midwife, as they are thought to cause unnecessary concern. Babies have an individual pattern of movements, and it is this, rather than the number of kicks, that's important.

ASK A... MUM

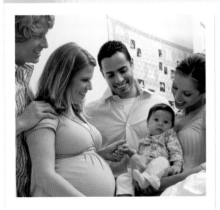

I've never looked after a baby and I don't even know how to put a nappy on one! What can I do?

You're not alone: I had never been around babies much and was full of questions. How do nappies work? What do babies do all day? What if I drop my baby? Luckily a friend had a three-month-old who we "borrowed". As you'll soon realize, there are plenty of weary mums and dads out there, and almost certainly someone among your family and friends will be only too happy to take a break. But before you remove the baby from his comfort zone, spend time with him and his parent(s). Feed him and change nappies under his mother's watchful eye. If she's confident that you're up to the job, offer to take charge, perhaps just for a few hours at first.

If all goes well, you could build up to a day – or even overnight. It'll work wonders for your confidence and eliminate any fears you have about babycare. When it comes to looking after your newborn, you'll have some idea of what to expect and feel more sure about what you're doing.

AS A MATTER OF FACT

During pregnancy your total volume of blood is 50 per cent higher than normal.

The amount of blood pumped with each heartbeat increases by about 40 per cent and you make around 20 per cent more red blood cells than normal.

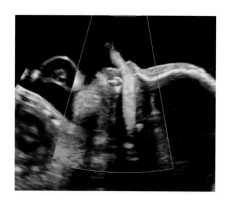

96 days to go...

YOUR BABY TODAY

This coloured ultrasound shows the baby breathing the amniotic fluid (red, flowing towards the ultrasound beam) in and out. The baby is breathing a stream of fluid out through the nostrils and, at the same time, a smaller amount through the mouth.

As the development of your baby's eyes and sense of sight continues, he reaches another milestone: the eyelids open.

Although your baby's eyelids formed at nine weeks of pregnancy, they have remained fused together until this week. Your baby is not in complete darkness, however, because as the uterus grows its wall thins allowing in increasing amounts of light. Now, your baby's eyes have reached a stage of development where they can open.

Even with the eyelids open, the delicate structures of the eyeballs are protected by a fine membrane that will completely disappear during the final month of pregnancy.

It's too early for your baby to respond to light in a fully co-ordinated way, but he may turn towards very strong lights or, if startled by a sudden loud noise, he will often respond with a blink, just as children and adults do.

The retina has just started to be lined by light-receptive rods and cones. The cones are responsible for colour vision and develop later than the more numerous rods. The rods transmit an image in black and white and are used for night-time vision and for peripheral vision. Connections form between the retina and the optic nerve, which then transmits the information it receives to be decoded in the visual cortex at the back of the brain.

Your baby will often bring his hands up to his face. However, because his limb movements are now so well co-ordinated, he won't touch his eyes.

ASK A... MIDWIFE

I've got inverted nipples. Will I be able to breastfeed? Babies breastfeed rather than "nipple feed" and if your baby latches on to your breast correctly (see p.448), inverted nipples shouldn't cause difficulties. About 10 per cent of women have flat or inverted nipples. The best way to find out whether you can breastfeed is simply to try once your baby is born. There are various techniques that may help: consult your midwife if you're having problems or contact a breastfeeding counsellor through your local NCT or the La Leche League (see p.480).

FOCUS ON... TWINS

Growth of twins in the last trimester

In these last three months, you're likely to get very big. As you'd expect, the more babies inside, the greater the challenge for your body to provide enough space as well as the perfect conditions for growth. You'll probably be advised to gain just under 0.5kg (1lb) a week for the first half of your pregnancy and slightly more each week in the second half.

From around 28–29 weeks, the growth of twins and other multiples slows down compared with that of singletons. But they still move and kick as much as possible, cushioned by amniotic fluid, which continues to increase in volume until 36 weeks.

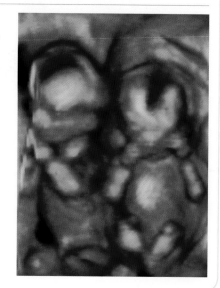

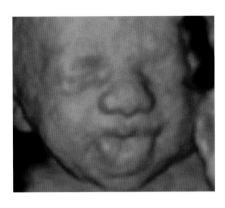

95 days to go...

YOUR BABY TODAY

Your baby sticks his tongue out often especially before or after a particularly large gulp of amniotic fluid. Fluid doesn't enter the lungs but is swallowed into the stomach. Your baby would be completely unaware of the ultrasound scan, so is not reacting to the scanner.

It's a natural instinct that parents are fiercely protective of their children, and not unusual for this to start well before the birth.

You may be feeling very protective of your bump and baby. The bump almost acts as a beacon to other people, making them aware that you're pregnant. It's not unusual to feel quite vulnerable, for example in a jostling crowd or when you're out shopping. When this happens, make it clear to people that you're pregnant and, hopefully, they'll give you more space and give up their seat, if necessary.

When you're driving, you may find you're doing so even more carefully than normal, or becoming a very nervous or critical passenger. You may become more irritated than usual by people who you feel are driving without concern for your safety.

This protective instinct is a natural part of becoming a mother. It's the desire to protect and nurture your child, even before yourself. Rest assured, though, that your baby is in the safest possible environment inside your uterus. Your body is providing your baby with warmth, food, and oxygen. The baby is cushioned and protected by the amniotic fluid in which he floats, and this acts as a buffer to any shoving or bumping by crowds of people.

ASK A... DOCTOR

Why am I being told I need a glucose tolerance test? In pregnancy some women develop a form of diabetes known as gestational diabetes (see p.473), which disappears when the baby is born. It may be suspected if you have signs such as tiredness and thirst and is confirmed by testing urine for glucose. If it's found, you'll be advised to have an oral glucose tolerance test (OGTT) between 24 and 28 weeks. This test is also advised if you have a BMI over 35, a close relative with diabetes, or had diabetes in a previous pregnancy.

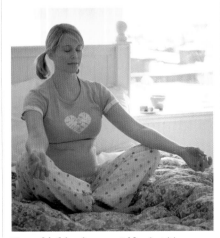

Hypnobirthing is a great idea but it's important that you are taught the various relaxation and visualization techniques and practise them regularly during pregnancy.

THE LOWDOWN

Hypnobirthing

The idea of hypnobirthing – giving birth in such a relaxed state that you barely feel pain – sounds too good to be true. But the research extolling its benefits is impressive. Several studies have shown that self-hypnosis helps women to feel less anxious about labour and birth. They also tend to require minimal pain relief and medical intervention: many women succeed in giving birth at home.

■ You learn a series of self-hypnosis, relaxation, visualization, and breathing techniques, which over time become second nature, enabling you to approach childbirth in a calm, positive frame of mind.

■ **By practising hypnobirthing,** you should feel in control of your body and able to manage the pain during labour and delivery.

■ **The key is to practise frequently,** and a supportive birth partner is invaluable for helping you perfect the techniques, and use them in labour.

■ **Ask your midwife** to recommend a course near you or contact your local NCT (see p.480).

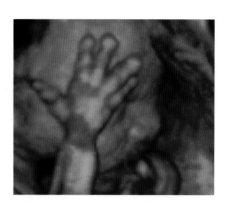

YOU ARE 26 WEEKS AND 4 DAYS

94 days to go...

YOUR BABY TODAY

On this 3D image each finger is held outstretched. Holding the fingers in this way for any length of time is tiring so most of the time the hands are held with the wrists slightly flexed and the fingers bent, ready to grasp any object that floats into reach.

Your baby's reproductive organs are now in place; a boy's testes have descended and a girl's ovaries have all their follicles.

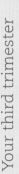

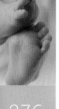

ASK A... MUM

Is it normal to argue all the time when we should be happily looking forward to our baby's arrival? Expecting a baby puts pressure on even the strongest of relationships. Concerns about having a healthy baby and adjusting to parenthood were at the heart of most of our arguments. And when we started to talk about it, we found we had conflicting opinions about big child-rearing issues. I was sensitive, irritable, and moody, and often snapped when I didn't mean to.

We sat down and talked calmly and agreed not to "sweat the small stuff", avoiding areas of contention, and compromising when it didn't really matter. In the throes of a disagreement, I'd stop and think: I love this man, we're having a baby together, is this really important in the long run? We also made time to do positive things together that we had enjoyed before I was pregnant, and tried to find opportunities to laugh, to reduce stress, and to put things into perspective. By the time the baby arrived, we were both much more relaxed.

If your baby is a boy, it's at about this time that the testes complete their descent into the scrotum. This is often associated with a small amount of fluid around each testis called a "hydrocele". This fluid will disappear naturally either before or after birth.

The cremaster muscle, part of the spermatic cord, is able to raise the testes back into the groin. This helps to regulate the temperature within the testes after birth, relaxing when cooling is needed. If your baby is slightly cool when he is examined, the cremaster muscle retracts the testes, giving the impression of undescended testes in your newborn baby.

Temperature control is not required in the uterus and the testes slowly move down into the scrotum. It is by no means unusual for one testis (or both) not to have descended at birth. Your doctor will check for this as part of the routine baby development check and confirm that both testes can be brought down into the scrotum.

Unlike the ovary, which already contains all of the egg-producing follicles that it will ever make, the testes do not start to make sperm until puberty.

Differences in the speed of growth and weight gain become more apparent now, and boys tend to be slightly heavier than girls at birth.

WEIGHT GAIN IN THE THIRD TRIMESTER

In your third trimester gaining weight steadily is important. If you were a healthy weight before your pregnancy, you can expect to gain about 0.5kg (1lb) a week up to week 35 or 36, and not much thereafter. Keep in mind that the largest contributing factor to your overall weight gain will be your baby, followed by extra fat, which you will need to sustain your pregnancy and when breastfeeding. Your midwife will monitor your weight gain to ensure it's healthy.

Weight gain chart

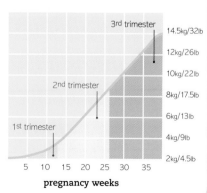

3rd trimester — 14.5kg/32lb
12kg/26lb
10kg/22lb
8kg/17.5lb
2nd trimester — 6kg/13lb
4kg/9lb
1st trimester — 2kg/4.5lb

5   10   15   20   25   30   35
pregnancy weeks

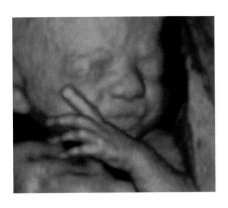

93 days to go...

YOUR BABY TODAY

This week, some babies open their eyes for the first time but this is a brief event, difficult to capture on ultrasound, so you may not see it on a scan. Some light is reaching your baby but he hasn't developed a sleep–wake cycle that corresponds in any way with day and night.

As each day passes, your baby is getting bigger and bigger and you will be more conscious of his body and movement.

As wonderful as it is to feel your baby move inside you, sometimes it can be uncomfortable. As your baby grows there is less and less room for him to move around, especially as he kicks or stretches against the walls of your uterus. These movements can vary from gentle paddling motions to feeling as though the baby has hiccups. Sometimes the baby will kick hard; if it's under the ribs it can take your breath away and leave you feeling quite sore. The kicking can also wake you when you're sleeping, and many women say that their babies are more active at night. If you're sitting or lying in a position that the baby doesn't like – for example, if you spend too much time on one side – your baby may well kick until you move.

Although sometimes these movements can be uncomfortable or take you by surprise, most of the time they're just a gentle reminder of your growing baby and, as such, are something to look forward to feeling.

ASK A... DOCTOR

If I went into labour now, would my baby survive? Until relatively recently, babies born before 28 weeks' gestation often did not survive. Today, with medical advances in special care baby units, babies of 22 weeks' gestation have survived outside the uterus, although this is still very rare. The guideline – and legal requirement – for most hospitals is that 24 weeks is the earliest point at which they will resuscitate a baby, unless the newborn shows clear signs of life.

Extremely premature babies have an increased risk of disability, even with the best medical care, and often the delivery itself can put an enormous strain on the baby. Very experienced doctors, midwives, and nurses are involved in the care of extremely premature babies.

If possible, the delivery should take place in a hospital with a dedicated special care baby unit (SCBU) (see pp.452–3). If this isn't possible, babies are often transferred to a specialist centre when they are stable enough to be moved. Very premature babies take a long time to "catch up" and meet developmental milestones. Each day and week of pregnancy is a milestone, and the nearer to full term (37–42 weeks) you deliver, the better it is for your baby.

FOCUS ON... SAFETY

Buying bedding

Use the right bedding and follow safe sleeping guidelines (see p.444).

■ **Based on your baby wearing a nappy, vest, and babygro,** you'll need to cover him with a sheet and one to two lightweight blankets (a folded blanket counts as two) if the room is 16–20°C (61–68°F). If the room is warmer, he'll only need a sheet; if colder, add more blankets. An ideal room temperature is 18°C (64.5°F).

■ **If your baby sleeps in a Moses basket or carry cot,** buy sheets designed specifically for these.

■ **If using a sleeping bag,** ensure it's lightweight, the correct size, and doesn't have a hood.

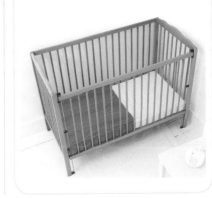

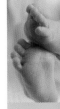

277

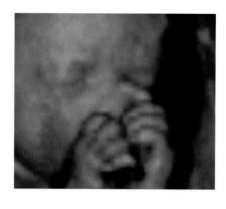

92 days to go...

YOUR BABY TODAY

At this stage, thumb sucking is becoming much more co-ordinated as the sensitive lips and fingers meet. On scans most babies look as if they enjoy it, and there's no doubt that it provides important sensory feedback and perhaps reassurance to your developing baby.

The thought of being off work in the last months of pregnancy is tempting, but it will give you less time off with your baby.

As long as you're feeling in good health, try to work into the last month of your pregnancy. It can be particularly frustrating if you finish two months before, only to find that your baby is born later than expected. Working as late as possible may also allow you to spend some time with your replacement. If you're finding work tiring, try to adapt your working day and avoid travelling in the rush hour, if possible. Whenever you start your leave, colleagues may hold a party and want to buy gifts for your newborn. If you're asked what you want, suggest gift vouchers as these will allow you to purchase some of the more expensive baby equipment, and prevent duplication of gifts. Many shops also offer gift lists for babies, which are a good way to choose the items you want.

BACK PAIN IN THE THIRD TRIMESTER

One of the most common pregnancy complaints, back pain is generally a reaction to your increased weight and the laxity of the joints that are an integral part of pregnancy. There are some ways to alleviate this, and anecdotal evidence suggests that women who exercise are far less likely to suffer from extreme back pain than those who don't.

It is best to try to avoid back pain by exercising your abdominal muscles, which will give your back support, and keep your legs and arms strong too. See page 250 for an effective abdominal workout.

Carrying does not end when you have had your baby. You will have a car seat, baby bag, and perhaps shopping to carry, as well as your newborn. So it's best to keep your muscles strong throughout your pregnancy to prepare for this. Here are five top tips to avoid back pain in the third trimester:

■ **Stay strong:** strength training for all parts of your body (see p.196) will help you to cope with the increased weight you gain during pregnancy.
■ **Support:** invest in a support belt that will give your back a break from bearing the load of your bump. It will also support your sagging stomach and may relieve discomfort in your legs. This can be particularly useful if you're carrying twins or more.
■ **Sleep:** while sleeping, place a pillow between your legs to ease the stress on your back. Buy or borrow a shaped pillow that gives your belly and back support at the same time.
■ **Stretch:** flexibility will help your back to relax and avoid your muscles getting too tense.
■ **Sit:** keep your back supported by the back of a chair (see p.219). Use a pillow to increase the support in your lower back, if necessary. If you work at a desk, make sure your chair adequately supports your back.

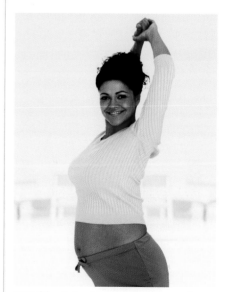

Stretching helps to prevent your muscles from tightening, so you feel less tense and more relaxed. Put on some comfortable clothes and stretch as often as you can, and always stretch before and after exercise.

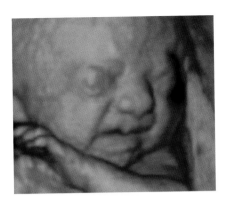

91 days to go...

YOUR BABY TODAY

This baby looks quite cross. Your baby often makes strange and funny faces in the uterus. It's as if he is practising every type of facial expression in preparation for after the birth when these will be one of the tools he uses to communicate his needs and emotions.

As you soak in a relaxing bath, it's an amazing sight to look at your baby moving and stretching your belly.

Your belly is a marvellous thing. It's already changed so much over the last 27 weeks and will continue to grow until you give birth.

Inside that bump your growing baby is moving around. When your baby is kicking and turning around, take the time to look down, and you may be able to see him move or even see the imprint of a foot as it kicks you.

While you're having a bath is a good time to watch your belly – you may find that your baby is more active around this time because you're relaxed – and you can take time out to observe his movements. Keep your partner involved when your baby is active by encouraging him to touch your bump.

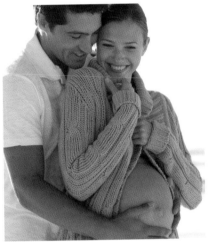

Watching your baby move is wonderful. You may even miss your ever-expanding and active bump once you're no longer pregnant.

ASK A... MIDWIFE

My tummy measurement has been the same for three weeks. Why isn't my baby growing? From 24 to 36–37 weeks of pregnancy, your abdomen can be measured to establish the height of the top of the uterus, which indicates how the baby is growing. In early pregnancy, this type of measurement doesn't give an indication of fetal growth.

When a midwife measures your abdomen, there is an element of subjectivity depending on the technique he or she uses. So if you've been measured by different midwives the results may be difficult to compare. However, even with the same person measuring you, the estimation of your baby's growth may still not be 100 per cent accurate. If there are any concerns, you will probably be referred to a consultant to decide whether you need to have further investigations, such as a scan.

FOCUS ON... DADS

Are you tired too?

Being pregnant is more tiring than most women anticipate. In the third trimester, your partner's bladder is under pressure and this can cause her to wake during the night to go to the loo. The size of the bump starts to become uncomfortable, and it can be difficult for her to find a relaxing sleeping position. The other changes she's going through, from shifting internal organs through to altered hormone levels, can contribute to her restlessness. And if she's having troubling sleeping, you are likely to be disturbed too. The end result is that both of you feel constantly tired.

Unfortunately there is no answer. Going to bed earlier can help, but having some time to relax together before bed is just as important. The bottom line is that disrupted sleeping patterns will now become part of the norm for both of you. There is no quick fix to this problem, but it may help to cut back your social life in the evenings.

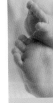

Your 28th week

EVEN BEFORE BIRTH, YOUR BABY IS ESTABLISHING A PATTERN OF BEHAVIOUR

Your baby is beginning to have regular sleep–wake cycles and her breathing, yawning, and swallowing are taking on a more definite pattern. However, your own life may seem less rhythmical. You may find things are slightly different at work and, perhaps, be seeing less of some friends because you don't always feel up to socializing. Don't become isolated, though – if nothing else, stay in touch by phone, email, and social media.

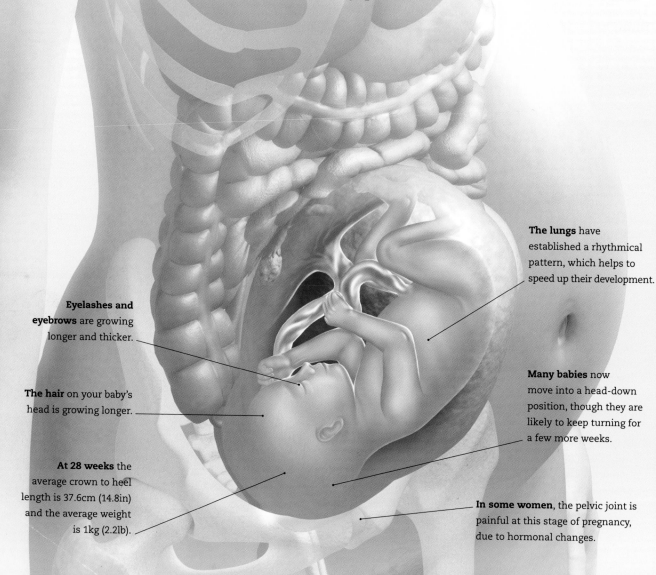

The lungs have established a rhythmical pattern, which helps to speed up their development.

Eyelashes and eyebrows are growing longer and thicker.

The hair on your baby's head is growing longer.

Many babies now move into a head-down position, though they are likely to keep turning for a few more weeks.

At 28 weeks the average crown to heel length is 37.6cm (14.8in) and the average weight is 1kg (2.2lb).

In some women, the pelvic joint is painful at this stage of pregnancy, due to hormonal changes.

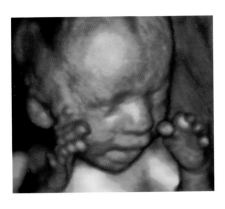

90 days to go...

YOUR BABY TODAY

On a scan the space between the frontal bones of the forehead appears as a dark line on the soft spot at the top of your baby's head. This is not a line on the skin: instead where there is no underlying bone, more of the ultrasound beam passes through rather than being reflected.

Do all you can to stay involved with medium- and long-term plans at work so that you continue to feel part of the team.

The difficulty of balancing

motherhood and a career can crop up even while you're still pregnant. Depending on your career, you may find yourself excluded from long-term planning discussions as colleagues assume that you won't be around, or won't come back after your maternity leave. Some colleagues may simply treat you differently just because you're pregnant, assuming you can no longer do your job in the same way. You may feel left out of future planning, or feel that your opinions are disregarded as you will not be there to implement them. This can be compounded by the fact that it can be difficult to motivate yourself if you know you won't be there to see a project through to the end.

No one can be certain of being in a job in six months' or a year's time, but you have the advantage of knowing how much longer you're going to work and you may even have a reasonable idea of when you're intending to return to work. Continue to do your job and make it clear by your actions that you want to provide input on all projects, even though you may not be there to see them through to the end. If at this point in time you're intending to return to work after the baby is born, make this clear to any colleagues who may doubt your long-term commitment.

You can also help to plan for your maternity leave by, perhaps, dividing up your workload or helping to search for a replacement to cover your role. Being organized now will make the countdown to going on maternity leave much easier in the coming weeks.

ASK A... MUM

Should we buy a baby bath or can the baby use our bath? I thought a baby bath was an optional extra, but having bought one found it really useful. A huge advantage is that you can use it in any room (though if the room doesn't have a water supply, you'll need to transport water).

I was a bit apprehensive the first few times we bathed the baby, then experienced parents told me even they found it tricky to hold a wriggling baby safely in a bath of water. Using a smaller baby bath is less daunting and helps you to develop confidence. However, a baby outgrows a baby bath by around six months and, once not in use, the bath can take up a lot of storage space (unless you can recycle

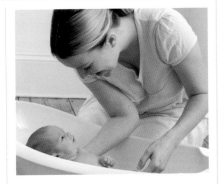

it to a pregnant friend). Many parents choose a bath seat designed for newborns in the family bath. Alternatively, enjoy a bath together, although you must keep the water tepid for the baby and you may find this too cold for you.

AS A MATTER OF FACT

As your uterus grows, your diaphragm is compressed with the result that you may find it difficult to breathe deeply.

In fact, you're actually taking in more air. It's important not to fight the natural tendency to hollow your back. This opens up your rib cage to let in more air, and also helps to balance the excess weight of your bump.

281

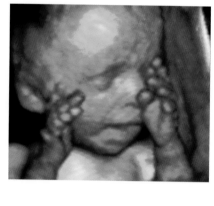

89 days to go...

YOUR BABY TODAY

Your baby may be looking happy today. Babies smile and grimace, wrinkle their foreheads, and stick their tongues out. Many of these behaviours are only becoming more apparent now as 3D ultrasound has provided a unique opportunity for their study.

Your baby has developed a sleep–wake cycle very similar to the one she will have in the days and weeks after birth.

Your baby's yawns have, until this point, occurred only occasionally as a single event, but they are now becoming more repetitive, with several yawns following one another. Your baby's swallowing reflexes were developed at 25 weeks but still need time to become much better co-ordinated.

The baby's breathing movements are vital for the normal development of the lung tissue. Your baby does not breathe amniotic fluid into her lungs. The lungs are filled with fluid produced by the lung tissue itself, and as breathing movements are practised, small amounts are expelled. With each breath, the diaphragm pushes down, and the chest wall moves in as the larynx relaxes, allowing fluid to escape. Only a tiny proportion (0.5 per cent) of the fluid in the lung escapes with each breath. This compares to a fifth (20 per cent) of the air in the lungs moving in and out with each breathing movement.

Your baby has been breathing for some weeks, but the pattern up until now has been somewhat random. Now, the baby's breathing patterns start to reflect her better developed sleep–wake cycle, and becomes more rhythmical.

FOCUS ON... NUTRITION

Burning calories

During pregnancy your body will store fat – mainly in the hips, thighs and abdomen – to ensure there is enough energy for your baby to grow. Usually, the body relies on glucose for energy but in mid and late pregnancy, hormonal and metabolic changes facilitate the use of fat as an energy source. If you exercise regularly without topping up your calories, you could be reducing the amount of stored fat. In addition, doing cardiovascular and weight-bearing exercise regularly tends to increase your metabolic rate slightly; therefore even when you're not exercising, your body will burn more calories.

It's important that you do exercise regularly during pregnancy but you need to make sure that you're taking in enough calories to meet the demands of your growing baby and your body. A simple guideline is that during the third trimester you should be taking in an extra 200 calories a day, with an extra 150 calories on the days that you exercise.

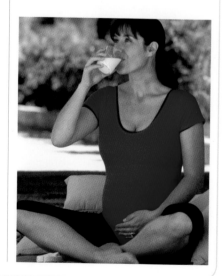

TIME TO THINK ABOUT

Antenatal care

You should have an appointment this week and at 31 and 34 weeks.

At each one, your blood pressure will be measured, and your urine tested for protein. The midwife will also check the size of your baby by measuring the height of your uterus, and she will listen to any concerns and offer you advice.

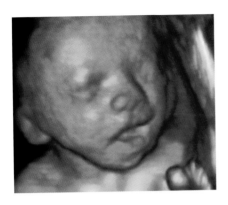

88 days to go...

YOUR BABY TODAY

This baby is at the end of a yawn. Your baby is yawning in a more co-ordinated way now with one yawn often following another. It may look as if this image shows the fingertips in the bottom right but in fact it is a foot, brought nearly up to the mouth.

Pregnancy is a subject about which everybody has an opinion they want to share with you, whether you like it or not.

Although you may have become very proud and protective of your bump, it can be extremely irritating if other people become over-protective of you. You may find that everyone has an opinion on your pregnancy, and what you should and should not be doing to stay healthy. Some women find all the attention comforting, but others find it frustrating or suffocating. If you're someone who finds all the advice difficult to handle, try to remember that people mean well.

Of course, it's your body, and you'll do what is best for you and your baby. If it's all getting too much, then try talking to the main offenders, often a partner, mother, or mother-in-law. Explain that you're trying your best and that you're aware of what you should and shouldn't do while you're pregnant and are following the advice of your doctors and midwives. Politely thank them for their input and reassure them that you're taking good care of yourself and your baby.

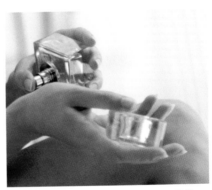

Choose the perfume you put on carefully as you may find that some scents, even one you're used to wearing, make you feel nauseous or light-headed during pregnancy.

On smelling good

Are you wafting through pregnancy feeling fresh as a daisy? It's rarely discussed, but being pregnant may make you feel less fragrant than usual, not least because you will sweat more than before – although it's unlikely that anyone else will have noticed. An increase in vaginal discharge is also nothing to worry about, but if it smells offensive or is yellowish or greenish in colour, you could have an infection so see your doctor. To stay smelling sweet:

■ **Shower or bath regularly** and apply deodorant every time. Take handy wipes with you to stay fresh all day.
■ **Use body sprays** and lotions if your usual fragrance doesn't smell "right": they tend to be lighter and are less likely to cause headaches.
■ **Avoid wearing tight clothing:** wear loose clothes in natural fabrics, which absorb sweat and allow your skin to breathe.
■ **Wear cotton underwear,** and change it more often, if necessary.
■ **Use disposable panty liners,** if needed, to stay feeling fresh.

FOCUS ON... YOUR HEALTH

Blood pressure checks

About a quarter of first-time mums develop high blood pressure in pregnancy. High blood pressure can be an indication of pre-eclampsia (along with protein in the urine). Pre-eclampsia (see p.474) can affect the liver and kidneys and, if untreated, lead to eclampsia, a serious condition that causes convulsions. If you have pre-eclampsia, your midwife will closely monitor your blood pressure. Medication will be offered until you are far enough into your pregnancy for it to be induced or to have a Caesarean.

Assessing fetal growth and wellbeing

As well as monitoring your own health and wellbeing throughout your pregnancy, the midwife will also assess how your baby is growing and will refer you for further tests if she has any concerns about your baby's wellbeing.

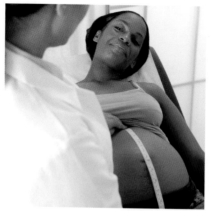

Measuring your abdomen helps the midwife to monitor your baby's growth.

Measuring your baby

In a low-risk pregnancy, the abdomen is measured at antenatal visits to assess the baby's growth. The measurement in centimetres from the top of your pubic bone to the top of your uterus (the fundus) should be about the same as the number of weeks you are pregnant, with an allowance of up to 2cm either way. For example, if you are 26 weeks' pregnant, you should measure between 24 and 28cm. Your fundal height can be measured between 24 and 36–37 weeks, as once your baby "drops" into the pelvis in late pregnancy, the measurement may not reflect her true size. If there is a variation of 3cm or more, your doctor will arrange for an ultrasound to check your baby's growth (see below) and the amount of amniotic fluid. If the scan indicates a problem, the doctor will arrange for scans every two weeks as analyzing growth patterns over time gives a more accurate assessment of whether your baby's growth is normal.

In certain cases, for example if a woman is obese, in twin pregnancies, and where there are large uterine fibroids, the only accurate way to assess growth is by ultrasound.

UNDERSTANDING RESULTS

Growth charts

If your midwife or doctor has any concerns about your baby's growth later in pregnancy, he or she may arrange for scans to be done over a period of time so that your baby's growth can be plotted on a chart and monitored. Individual measurements will be taken of the head, abdomen, and limbs. Measurements of the head and abdomen are most important as an unequal growth pattern in these areas may indicate a particular problem.

The three lines on the graphs here represent the normal range for growth. The red line in the centre, referred to as the 50th percentile, shows an average pattern of growth. The pink lines above and below, the 90th and the 10th percentiles, show the top and bottom ranges of normal growth. As the head and abdominal circumferences are measured over time and plotted on a graph, a pattern of growth becomes clear. Here, the head is growing normally, but growth has slowed in the abdomen, possibly due to a placental problem that in itself may be caused by a condition in the mother. For example, conditions such as high blood pressure (see p.283) or diabetes (see p.473) can affect placental blood flow. If the blood flow to the baby is restricted, this can result in the oxygen and nutrients carried in the blood being diverted to the baby's most vital organs, the brain and heart, rather than to the abdominal organs, which results in unequal growth patterns in the head and abdomen.

Head circumference

cm
36
32
28
24
20
16
12
8

14 18 22 26 30 34 38 42
Weeks of gestation

Abdominal circumference

cm
36
32
28
24
20
16
12
8

14 18 22 26 30 34 38 42
Weeks of gestation

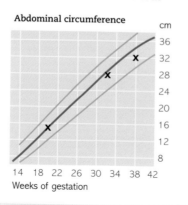

Measuring growth with ultrasound in late pregnancy

By late pregnancy, the length of your baby can no longer fit on the screen and so her size will be calculated by combining several measurements in a mathematical formula, as is done at the 20-week scan (see p.214). Measurements taken include the width of the head (biparietal diameter), circumference of the head, and the abdominal circumference, which are plotted on a graph over a period of time (see box, opposite). The length of the upper leg bone (femur length) may also be measured. If your baby is smaller than the 10th percentile or has a small abdomen, you may have more tests to assess her wellbeing (see below). A measurement above the 90th percentile can be a sign of gestational diabetes (see p.473) and will need investigating. Also, if your baby is at the larger end of the scale, your doctor or midwife may recommend a Caesarean delivery.

Your baby's wellbeing

If there are concerns over your baby's growth, you may be referred for fetal heart rate monitoring and/or biophysical profile testing, which observe how your baby responds to stimuli and if there are signs of fetal distress. If you have a known condition that can affect your baby's growth (see box, opposite), your doctor may arrange for you to have one or both of the above tests once or twice a week after about 32 weeks' gestation as a matter of routine, whether or not there are concerns about your baby's growth. Some hospitals also perform special scans, known as Doppler scans (see box, right) to assess placental blood flow.

Fetal heart rate monitoring This uses a cardiotocograph (CTG) reading (see p.418) to assess your baby's wellbeing. Two monitors are placed on your abdomen: one monitors uterine contractions while the other listens to

Doppler scans

A Doppler scan is a specialized scan that analyzes blood flow through the placenta. If the placenta is functioning well, the blood flows easily. If there is a problem in the placenta, it is resistant to the blood flow and the baby's heart has to work harder to pump blood. In extreme cases, there are periods between your baby's heartbeats of no blood flow or reversed blood flow through the umbilical cord. In this case, an early delivery may be suggested unless you're very premature.

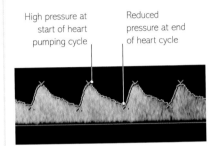

High pressure at start of heart pumping cycle

Reduced pressure at end of heart cycle

High pressure at start of heart pumping cycle

Very low pressure at end of heart cycle

A normal Doppler reading shows the continuous blood flow to the baby via the placenta. At the beginning of a heart cycle, the pressure is high; it then reduces at the end of the cycle, but doesn't ever stop.

An abnormal reading indicates that there is resistance to blood flow in the placenta, resulting in very little or no flow at the end of the cycle. The baby may not receive sufficient oxygen, which can affect growth.

your baby's heart rate, and the results are plotted on a graph. The heart rate speeds up in response to contractions and fetal movements. The test result is thought to be "reassuring" if the heart accelerates twice over 20–30 minutes, and there are no large decelerations. About 10–20 per cent of babies have a test with less than two accelerations. This doesn't necessarily mean there is a problem: your baby may just have been asleep, and the test may be repeated.

A biophysical profile (BPP) If, after monitoring the heart rate of your baby, your doctor has concerns, a BPP may be carried out. A BPP combines the results of a CTG reading with a scan to evaluate four factors: the volume of amniotic fluid, fetal movement, fetal muscle tone and posture, and fetal breathing. Two points are given for each part of the test, so a "reassuring" BPP result would be eight points.

I've heard about "kick counts". Should I be doing these?

Kick counts – counting how many times your baby kicks over a period of time – used to be advised to check that your baby was doing well. However, more recently, women have been encouraged to be aware of their baby's individual pattern of movement rather than the amount of kicks, as this is thought to be a more reliable indicator of how your baby is doing. If you think there is a change in the pattern of movement, call your midwife or doctor at once.

Can my baby move too much?

The more movement the better, even if this keeps you up at night or causes discomfort. An active fetus is not a sign that you'll have a restless baby or hyperactive child.

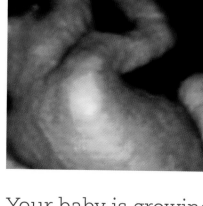

YOU ARE 27 WEEKS AND 4 DAYS

87 days to go...

YOUR BABY TODAY

This baby's back is turned and she's facing away from the ultrasound scanner. The skin is much less transparent than before as your baby is constantly laying down fat stores beneath it. This fat accounts, in part, for much of your baby's weight gain from now on.

Your baby is growing eyebrows and eyelashes – and hair on her head – and making good use of all the space in your uterus.

Your baby's eyes are now open, and both the eyebrows and the eyelashes have grown. The hair on your baby's head continues to get longer.

It's quite likely that your baby is making use of all the space available and may well be in a breech position (bottom down), at least some of the time. This is the case in a third of pregnancies at this stage but your baby's position is unlikely to stablize until after 36 or 37 weeks.

Because the shape of your uterus naturally favours a head-down position, only 3 to 4 per cent of babies remain in the breech position after 37 weeks. It may be quite difficult for you (and your midwife) to tell the position of your baby at this stage. For example, just because the feet kick you in one particular place doesn't tell you much about your baby's position. She is very flexible and a scan might show that she is doubled up with her feet on her head.

BLOOD TESTS

Some time between 26 and 30 weeks your blood will be tested to check you aren't anaemic. If you're found to be anaemic you may be prescribed iron tablets. Because of an increase in the fluid content of your blood, your haemoglobin count is likely to fall later on in your pregnancy, so it's worth addressing this now. Iron tablets can cause digestive problems, such as constipation or diarrhoea, so if this happens to you, ask if your prescription can be changed. The liquid medications available over the counter are kinder on the digestive system than tablets, so ask your doctor if one is suitable for you.

The same blood sample will be used to re-check your blood group and rhesus status. As a result, you may be offered an anti-D injection (see p.123) at about 28 and 34 weeks, with another scheduled for after the birth, if your baby is rhesus positive.

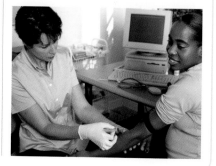

FOCUS ON... YOUR HEALTH

Pelvic girdle pain

You know you've got pelvic girdle pain – or PGP – when sneezing hurts, you're waddling like an old woman, and turning over in bed is a major task (see p.470). Formerly known as SPD, or symphysis pubis dysfunction, PGP affects one in five pregnant women. It's caused by hormonal changes that change the way the pelvic joint functions and it can be extremely painful. Try the following if you have PGP:

- Keep your legs together when getting in and out of bed or the car (place a plastic bag on the seat to help you swivel).
- Sleep on your side with a pillow between your legs.
- Wear comfortable shoes.
- Avoid doing tasks that hurt, such as housework or pushing a supermarket trolley.
- Relax in warm water.
- Ask your doctor for a support belt or an elasticated tubular bandage to hug the lower pelvis.
- Get some therapy: studies show that physiotherapy and acupuncture may help.

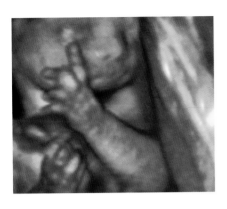

86 days to go...

YOUR BABY TODAY

A finger is held close to the eye in this image. The eyes are shut for most of the time but also a simple reflex action will prevent a stray finger (or toe) from touching the eye. Furthermore, the fingernails are still well away from the fingertips at this time.

Deciding to go it alone is never an easy option, but with the right support, you can look forward happily to your baby's birth.

It's reassuring to know that many women have babies on their own and do not find life an endless struggle. Although it would be wrong to pretend that parenting alone is as easy as it is when you share the care, with additional support it is possible. Even if you are in a relationship, you may feel you are going it alone at times. You may have very strong reasons why you want a baby, for example your increasing age, and this determination will give you strength and focus.

It is helpful for all pregnant women to find someone to talk to and confide in. This could be your mother or a close friend or relative. As you are making far-reaching decisions about your future, it's important that you have support, accurate information, and time to think things through without fear, panic, or pressure from others. Finding somebody you really trust and whom you know can give you support when you need it – especially in labour and in the first days and weeks with your baby – may help to relieve any pressure you are under. It will also enable you to think more calmly and clearly about your situation and make plans.

It's worth, even at this early stage, starting to think about who you would like to ask to be your birth partner: this is a big decision that should not be rushed.

BUILDING UP A SUPPORT NETWORK

It's important for all pregnant women to have emotional and practical support, and this is especially true if you're single.
- **Attend all your antenatal appointments** and build up a relationship with your midwife; she is an invaluable source of information.
- **Book yourself in for antenatal classes.** If you're single, you may find that daytime courses are less populated by "couples"; this gives you a chance to build up a network of female friends. Also try to go to classes, such as yoga and aquarobics.
- **Give plenty of thought** to choosing your birth partner: a trusted friend, or perhaps your own mother, who is likely to be thrilled to be asked to share this experience with you.
- **Don't be too proud to accept offers of help** from friends and family – most will genuinely want to be involved now and after the birth.

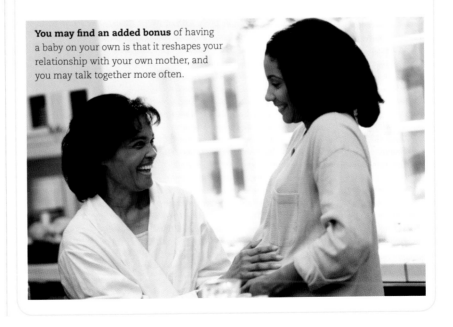

You may find an added bonus of having a baby on your own is that it reshapes your relationship with your own mother, and you may talk together more often.

85 days to go...

YOUR BABY TODAY

Although ultrasound cannot show it, there is now some hair on your baby's head and her eyelashes and eyebrows have grown. The pattern and colour of hair growth has a significant impact on the overall look of your baby but this is not apparent on a scan.

While women who are pregnant in the summer may find it hard to stay cool, being pregnant in the winter is also challenging.

Most women are understandably reluctant to buy a winter coat that will see them through pregnancy and may well never be worn again. The good news is that you probably won't need one at all! You're likely to feel very warm towards the end of your pregnancy, and may find it more comfortable to wear plenty of layered knits rather than one warm coat or jacket. Layers can also be easily discarded if you become overheated while you're travelling.

You can also probably hijack some of your partner's wardrobe, and borrow a coat or jacket that will fasten over your bump if you're planning to be outside for extended periods. Alternatively, go to a local charity shop – you may well find a larger coat or jacket for a bargain price that will last the few weeks of your pregnancy.

Another thing to consider is wearing your own coat unfastened, with a long scarf hanging down to fill the gap.

Think about purchasing a large shawl or wrap, which will see you through the winter months, and keep you and your baby warm after the birth. Shawls and wraps are ideal for keeping you warm when your baby is in a sling, and also for unexpected breastfeeding sessions outdoors.

You'll need to take extra care in the winter, when you're in icy conditions. Make sure you wear sensible flat shoes when you're out and about to reduce the risk of slipping over.

ASK A... NUTRITIONIST

My midwife has told me I'm anaemic. Can I improve my iron levels through my diet? All pregnant women should be offered screening for anaemia, which is done early in pregnancy (at the first appointment), and again between 26 and 30 weeks (see p.286). Generally, an iron-rich diet is advised in pregnancy and this is enough to prevent or improve anaemia. Eat plenty of lean red meat, beans, dried fruits, dark green vegetables, fortified cereals, and bread. Try including a vitamin C-enriched food or drink in your diet, as vitamin C helps the body to absorb iron more efficiently. Vegetarians need to eat plenty of eggs, pulses, beans, and nuts to boost iron supplies.

Taking iron tablets may be recommended depending on how low your iron levels have become.

FOCUS ON... TWINS

Practical adjustments

If you're having two or more babies, you'll need to consider making some adjustments to your living space. To reduce the risk of cot death, it's best for babies to sleep in the same room as their parents for the first six months but you don't need two cots. You can put both your newborn babies to sleep in one cot (see p.335), but this isn't recommended after they're three months old.

It's a legal requirement for each baby to have an individual car seat if you plan to drive them anywhere, including home from the hospital.

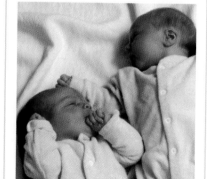

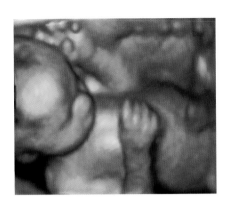

84 days to go...

YOUR BABY TODAY

The amniotic fluid is approaching its maximum amount at this time and your baby will have plenty of space in which to move. Here the baby is looking down towards the umbilical cord. Your baby is still likely to change position several times a day.

If you're the first among your friends to have a baby, be prepared for friendships to evolve and change.

Some friendships change as you go through different life stages. You'll probably have had different groups of friends through school, college, and different jobs, with one or two close friends throughout. Friendships often develop with people when you're at a similar stage in your lives. This means that during your pregnancy and when you have young children you may feel most comfortable with other women in similar situations. You'll meet new friends at antenatal classes or postnatal groups, or in situations such as toddler swimming or music classes.

As you make new friends, you may find your old relationships begin to change. Friends without children may find it difficult to understand your new role as a mother, and the intense love that you have for your child, and you may start to drift apart. Of course this is not always the case; some friendships are unchanging, irrespective of whether your lives go along different paths.

ASK A... MIDWIFE

I've seen a second-hand car seat advertised. Is there any reason why I shouldn't buy it? Don't use a second-hand car seat unless you can be absolutely certain of its history as it may have been in an accident or damaged.

Car safety experts suggest that if you must use a second-hand car seat, only accept one from a family member or friend when you're absolutely sure of its history and if the original instructions for the seat are still available. They strongly discourage purchasing a car seat for your baby through a second-hand shop or classified advertisements, or on the internet.

FOCUS ON... NUTRITION

Choosing organic

Eating organic food is one way to eat more healthily during pregnancy. Organic fruit and vegetables are grown without any chemical pesticides or fertilizers. Organic meat, poultry, eggs, and dairy products come from animals that are not given growth hormones or antibiotics. For these reasons, organic foods are free from pesticide residues, additives, and preservatives. They are also usually higher in nutrients. Organic farming also promotes the use of environmentally friendly practices. Most additives are safe during pregnancy, but eating organic is a second step that can add to a healthy foundation of food choices.

The downside of eating organic food is that it tends to cost more than regular groceries. Given the price of food, many families cannot afford the extra that goes with eating organic. If you can't afford organic foods, eating whole foods in their least processed, most natural form, and plenty of fresh fruit and vegetables is the next best thing, and is still a very healthy diet.

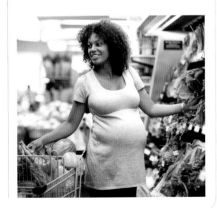

Your 29th week

USE THIS THIRD TRIMESTER TO GET ORGANIZED BEFORE YOUR BABY IS BORN

You may feel a little bored and back-achey at this stage of pregnancy, but there are plenty of positive ways to take your mind off things. For example, you could start to make enquiries about breastfeeding classes, plan your maternity leave, and draw up shopping lists of baby essentials, such as nappies, a changing mat, babygros, bibs, and muslin cloths, and perhaps buy a couple of items each week.

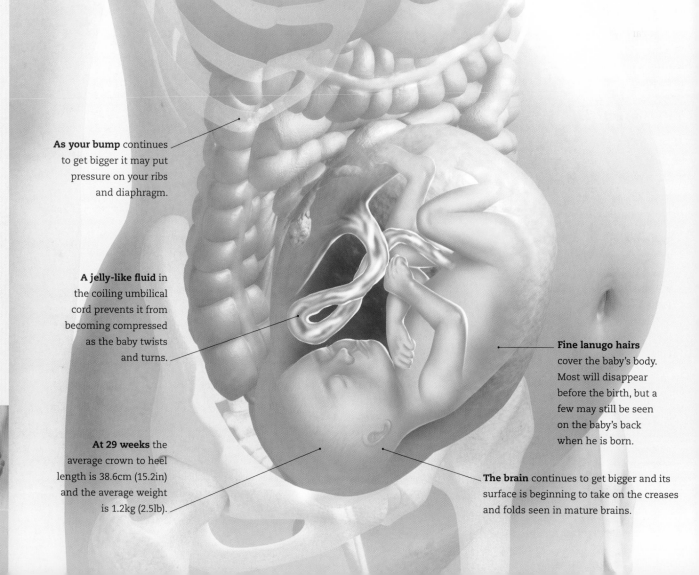

As your bump continues to get bigger it may put pressure on your ribs and diaphragm.

A jelly-like fluid in the coiling umbilical cord prevents it from becoming compressed as the baby twists and turns.

At 29 weeks the average crown to heel length is 38.6cm (15.2in) and the average weight is 1.2kg (2.5lb).

Fine lanugo hairs cover the baby's body. Most will disappear before the birth, but a few may still be seen on the baby's back when he is born.

The brain continues to get bigger and its surface is beginning to take on the creases and folds seen in mature brains.

Your third trimester

290

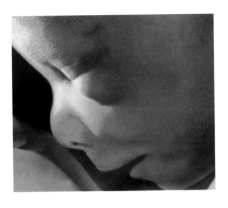

83 days to go...

YOUR BABY TODAY

This week is something of a landmark in your baby's development. Although a baby born at this stage would still need help with breathing, the lungs have matured to an extent that survival chances outside the womb are significantly better than earlier in the pregnancy.

It's never too early to start thinking about the financial implications of maternity leave, and whether to return to work.

When you're on maternity leave, it may be the first occasion that you haven't worked for a long time. This change can be quite daunting, even though you know you'll soon be busy looking after a baby. Depending on your contract, you'll be entitled to varying amounts of pay during your maternity leave. If you've worked for your employer for at least 26 weeks (full or part-time) by the 15th week before your baby is due, you'll be entitled to statutory maternity pay (SMP), an allowance set by the Government which can be paid for up to 39 weeks (see pp.348–9). You're then entitled to a further three months of unpaid leave. This means that you could be off work for up to a year and still be able to return to your job. Some companies are more generous than others, offering a percentage of your salary during your maternity leave. Going on maternity leave may cause a significant drop in your income. You should talk to your partner about how much money will be coming in and going out and how you will manage a change in your finances.

Even though it's a long way in the future, you might also start thinking about plans for working after the baby is born. You may think that you have no real option financially and have to return full time, but explore the possibilities of working more flexibly, or working part time, or from home one or two days a week. You may also want to start thinking about your childcare options (see p.332).

CHOOSING NAPPIES

Should you opt for disposables (use once, then throw away) or reusables (wash, dry, and use again)?

■ **Disposable nappies** are slim fitting, super absorbent, and will keep your baby dry, even overnight. However, they cost more (by some estimates, up to £1,000 per child by the time you start potty training) and there's the landfill factor to consider. Eco-friendly nappies, however, are now available – they use no polluting bleaching agents and fewer chemicals are used to produce them.

■ **Reusables** cost less – although the initial investment is greater. They also provide a softer landing for toddlers who topple over. However, all that soaking, washing, and drying could get you down (plus there is an environmental impact). You may opt to use a nappy-laundering service each week (at a cost). Reusables need changing more often than disposables. They are slightly more difficult to put on and take off, but modern reusables are fastened with Velcro, not pins.

■ **Using a combination** of reusable nappies and disposable nappies can work well: buy the occasional pack of disposables for when you're out and about or if you leave your baby with a babysitter, but opt for reusables the rest of the time.

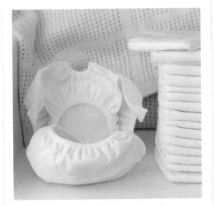

Reusable nappies (left) cost less than disposables as they can be used over and over but washing and drying them is labour-intensive. **Disposable nappies (right)** are easy to use but more expensive.

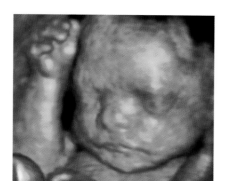

82 days to go...

YOUR BABY TODAY

This image shows a typical chin-on-the-chest position with an arm held up to the side of the face. A knee is just visible on the left with a loop of umbilical cord next to it. Your baby is now likely to be in a head-down position but there's still time to change.

The coiled umbilical cord connects your baby to the placenta, his life-support system until birth.

Most umbilical cords finally grow to be about the same length as the baby (although there are exceptions), reaching a final length of 50–60cm (20–23.5in). The umbilical cord has up to 40 turns along its length and these turns are seven times more likely to twist to the left than the right. The coiling pattern was in place nine weeks after conception, with more coils at the baby's end than the placental end; this may be a response to your baby's movements. The cord contains three blood vessels: two arteries taking deoxygenated blood and waste from your baby to the placenta and one vein carrying oxygen-rich blood from the placenta to the baby. The cord diameter is usually less than 2cm (¾in) and the blood vessels are embedded in and protected by a layer of jelly. The watery composition of the jelly, together with the cord's coiling pattern, prevents compression of the cord.

After the birth, your midwife will check the number of vessels in the cord as in 1 per cent of pregnancies the cord contains only one umbilical artery.

ASK A... DOCTOR

If my baby is a low birthweight, will he have health problems?
A low birthweight is less than 2.5kg (5½lb) and although the majority of small babies thrive, some do have difficulties. Most low birthweight babies are small because they are premature. There are many ways you can reduce the risk of your baby being a low birthweight: eating adequate amounts of healthy food to gain the right amount of weight (see p.99), not smoking or drinking alcohol, reducing stress, and keeping all antenatal appointments so that your health – and your baby – can be monitored.

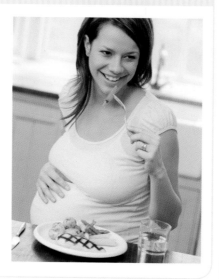

FOCUS ON... YOUR BODY

Restless legs

Some pregnant women experience restless legs syndrome (RLS), whereby they have an irresistible urge to move their legs. It most commonly happens while resting, so can be very disruptive to sleep. The exact cause isn't known but it may be related to an imbalance of a brain chemical called dopamine. The level of dopamine can be affected by a lack of iron. Restless legs syndrome will pass once you're no longer pregnant. To minimize the effects of restless legs syndrome:
■ **Ensure your diet** includes an adequate intake of iron (see p.154).
■ **If you're in bed** when you get restless legs, don't lie there and suffer: get out of bed and fill a bowl with cold water and soak your feet until they feel freezing cold. When you get back in to bed, try raising your feet on a pile of pillows.
■ **Avoid stimulants** such as caffeine, and before bed try to eat something that contains tryptophan (see p.177) – the amino acid that encourages sleep and relaxation. Also avoid exercising close to your bedtime.

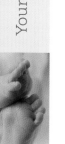

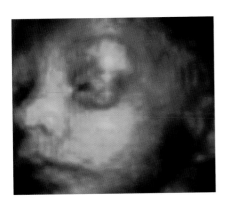

81 days to go...

YOUR BABY TODAY

This image offers the first view of the eye opening. The lids have separated and the dark pupil can be seen. There is no true reflection of colour on ultrasound so the white of the eye is coloured the same as the eyelids and face. The "eyebrows" are in fact shadow.

If you're starting to feel that you've been eclipsed by your bump, it's time to do something just for you.

Like many pregnant women, you may feel that you've disappeared behind your bump; that the essence of who you are has been lost in the guise of "pregnant woman". People may no longer ask about how you're feeling, or what's going on in your life. Instead of "How are you?", they might ask, "Is everything OK with the baby?"

It can be difficult for people, and even for you, to remember that you still exist in a role that is separate from pregnant woman or mother. If during your pregnancy you are feeling very frustrated by this, consider doing something just for you, maybe some pampering or a dinner for two, to make you feel special again.

FOCUS ON... NUTRITION

Grazing through the day

You need to eat plenty of good-quality protein to encourage your baby's growth and keep you in glowing good health, so try to eat either eggs, cheese, lean meats, fish, pulses, or wholegrains at every meal. Add to that lots of fruits and vegetables, nuts, seeds, and some unrefined carbohydrates (see p.92).

Break the food down into a plan of five to seven small meals and snacks each day. If you usually have soup and a sandwich for lunch, try a vegetable soup mid-morning, and have the sandwich later; prepare snacks such as raw vegetables, cheese, nuts, and fruit and graze on them through the afternoon. Perhaps have a bowl of porridge early evening, followed by fruit later.

There are no "rules" about when food needs to be eaten, so eat these "mini-meals" when you're hungry. So long as you get the nutrients you need and don't overeat, you can graze as often as you like.

ASK A... DOCTOR

I have a sharp pain in my lower back and leg. What causes this?
This sounds like sciatica, a sharp pain that travels down the back and leg when the sciatic nerve – the longest nerve in the body – is trapped in a joint in the lower back. This is not related to your pregnancy, although it can get worse in pregnancy. For lower back pain, warm baths and a warm compress can help, as can gentle massage by an experienced practitioner. Exercise such as yoga or aquanatal classes can help to strengthen back muscles, but check with your doctor before embarking on a new exercise regime. Watch your posture (see p.249) and wear comfortable, supportive shoes.

If you have sciatica, ask your doctor or midwife to refer you to a physiotherapist. You'll be shown exercises to help relieve the pain and minimize the risk of it recurring.

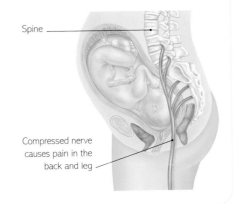

Spine

Compressed nerve causes pain in the back and leg

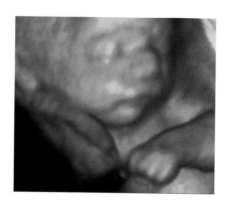

80 days to go...

YOUR BABY TODAY

The sleep–wake cycle is now more established, however just because your baby is moving you cannot assume that he is awake. He spends little time fully active with his eyes open, so many of the movements you are feeling are happening while he is asleep.

Your baby's growth depends on many factors and its rate varies through the course of your pregnancy.

The growth of your baby relies on a steady stream of nutrients. Most nutrients are transferred unaltered across the placenta, but some substances are made by the placenta itself and a few are produced from scratch by your baby. These include the hormone thyroxine, the production of which depends on iodine from the mother crossing the placenta. Thyroxine has several functions and its level needs to be controlled very precisely. The placenta forms a near-perfect barrier to thyroxine, enabling you and your baby to adjust thyroxine levels independently of each other.

In the early stages of pregnancy, genetic factors largely determined the size of your baby, but by now environmental factors are becoming more important. Overall, your baby's final birthweight is determined about 40 per cent by genetic factors and 60 per cent by environmental factors. Your baby grows at a steady rate from 24 weeks until the last 2–3 weeks, when growth continues but more slowly. (If you're expecting twins, your babies grow as if alone in the uterus up until 28 weeks but from this point there is a reduction in their growth rate.) Your baby's internal organs account for much of his current growth.

The liver and brain, in particular, continue to enlarge and muscle mass increases. Later, fat will be deposited under the skin, rounding out your baby's contours.

AS A MATTER OF FACT

The incidence of identical twins has been stable for some years.

Identical twins represent about a third of all twin pregnancies, regardless of race, maternal age, or geography.

FOCUS ON... TWINS

Buying for your twins

The clothes you buy for your twins should be easy to put on and take off, and, of course, machine washable. You'll probably be given outfits as presents, so just buy the basics.

For each baby, you're likely to need at least:
- Six vests
- Six babygros
- Two jackets
- One or two hats (sunhat for summer)
- Several muslin cloths and bibs.

Keep in mind when choosing nappies that twins are often smaller on arrival than a single baby, and you may therefore get through a wide range of sizes in the first few months.

It's advisable to buy a good-quality double buggy, as it will be used for quite a while. When choosing a buggy, a side-by-side model is preferable to a tandem buggy, so that your babies can see each other and communicate as they grow older.

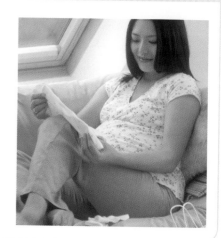

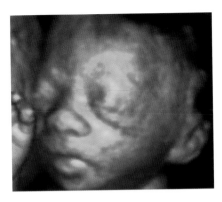

79 days to go...

YOUR BABY TODAY

Although many babies look similar on 3D ultrasound, particularly strong features, such as the ears, lips, or nose, may be distinctive. From now on these features will become more and more individualized and recognizable.

Breastfeeding may be natural but it can be tricky to get started, so try to attend a class or two now while you have the time.

There is a lot of pressure on women to breastfeed: breastfeeding has health benefits for both you and your baby and it helps with bonding. People may already be asking you whether you intend to breastfeed or not, and it's reasonable that you don't yet know the answer. After all, you haven't tried!

Most women want to try breast-feeding, but some feel uncomfortable with the thought of doing it, especially in public. You should be able to find breastfeeding support in your local area; there will a counsellor in the hospital and your local NCT will know of support groups. In some areas you can attend classes during pregnancy, which will explain the benefits of breastfeeding and aspects such as positioning the baby so that you're both comfortable and the baby is latched on (see p.449).

The expectation of breastfeeding is that, because it's natural, it's easy. The reality is that until you get the hang of it, it can be a little more difficult. Ask your midwife to show you how to position the baby. Most importantly, keep an open mind and try it. Once breastfeeding is established, it's beneficial to your baby's health, great for your figure, and a wonderful way to be close to your baby.

THE LOWDOWN

On leakages

Some pregnant women experience some leakage of breast milk, perhaps when their breasts are massaged or sexually stimulated, and sometimes for no apparent reason. Some discharge in pregnancy does mean that things are working properly, but women who don't experience this symptom are perfectly able to produce and provide milk for their baby.

FOCUS ON... NUTRITION

Cultured foods

Naturally cultured and fermented foods – such as some yogurts, vegetable pickles, sauerkraut, and miso (a Japanese paste, often used in soups) – contain enzymes and bacteria that help your body to digest food, and build up friendly bacteria in the intestines. If your digestion is sluggish and you're finding constipation a problem, try increasing the amounts that you eat of these foods.

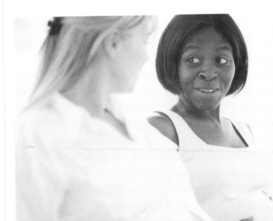

Talk to pregnant friends about breastfeeding now, and you can support each other once you start feeding your babies. Also get your partner involved: research shows that partners who are aware of the benefits of breastfeeding are more likely to be supportive.

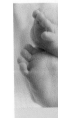

78 days to go...

YOUR BABY TODAY

Your baby's external features are fully formed but inside there is still a great deal of activity as many of the organs are continuing to mature. Even after pregnancy further development occurs, especially of the brain and lungs.

Back pain is not an inevitable part of being pregnant: there are lots of things you can do to help prevent and relieve it.

Yoga and other stretching exercises are great during pregnancy, as they strengthen key ligaments while relaxing areas that are tight and painful. Although it may seem easier to rest when you experience pain (especially back pain), and to avoid exercise, gentle stretching and movement often decreases muscle spasm and improves the function of the spine, resulting in less pain. Exercise also boosts energy levels and contributes to an easier labour, delivery, and post-natal recovery. Try stretching and relaxation techniques as a first resort for back pain.

If the pain is severe, ask your partner to massage the area with 3–4 drops of lavender oil in a tablespoon of grapeseed oil, which will encourage healing of strained muscles. If the area feels inflamed and painful, try placing a cold pack on the affected area for 5–10 minutes, several times a day.

I'm bored with being pregnant! How will I get through the next couple of months? I felt the same at about six months but found the last three months went quite fast just because more was happening. Along with more antenatal visits and classes, there was planning when to start maternity leave, then finishing work, then getting the nursery ready, and buying things for the baby. And I made an effort to see all my girlfriends – it all made the time pass quickly.

FOCUS ON... YOUR BODY

Minimizing strain on your back

Your growing bump shifts your centre of gravity to the front of your body. As the baby strains your abdominal muscles, and pregnancy hormones soften your ligaments, your abdominals give less support to your spine, which can result in back pain. Lifting and bending can exacerbate back pain, so try these strategies to help avoid added strain.

■ **To lift something from the floor,** stand close to the object with one foot in front of the other. Bend your knees, then straighten them, so that you use your thigh muscles to lift. Avoid locking your knees: always bend from the waist with your knees bent. If you need to pick something up, consider sitting, kneeling, or squatting to reach it to avoid putting your lower back under stress.

■ **If you have to move a heavy object** (try to avoid this if you possibly can), push it rather than pull it: that way, your legs, not your back, take the strain.

■ **To get into and out of a car,** or bed, keep your hips, pelvis, and back aligned in the same direction. To get out of bed, roll on to your side, and use your arms to push yourself up.

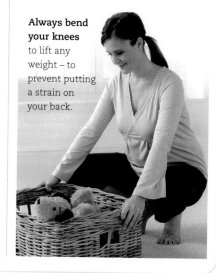

Always bend your knees to lift any weight – to prevent putting a strain on your back.

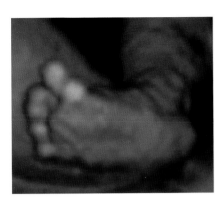

77 days to go...

YOUR BABY TODAY

This close-up shows how the baby's foot looks now. Your baby will easily put his feet on top of his head one minute only to bring them down the next, so just because your baby is kicking you at one end it doesn't mean the head is at the other.

Pregnancy can be a time of information overload, and sometimes it's difficult to know which sources are reliable.

In today's society women are simply overloaded with information about pregnancy, from newspapers, magazines, books, and the internet. Photographs of glamorous pregnant celebrities, who look as if they don't have a care in the world, abound in the media. Two sources on the same topic can offer conflicting opinions. Although the internet can be a wonderful source of useful information, it has drawbacks: you don't know who has written an article on a website, it may not have been written by a health professional, and some recommendations may even contradict standard medical advice.

This means that constantly scouring the internet and reading everything you find can be confusing and scary.

Articles telling you that you risk the health and wellbeing of your baby by doing something can make you feel inadequate. Keep telling yourself that women have been having children for centuries without the aid of the internet! If reading lots of information makes you feel empowered and better able to make informed choices, then read away, but if it makes you feel confused then don't. A sensible course might be to pick just one reliable book or information source to read instead.

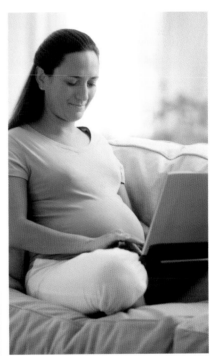

Use the internet to gather information about your pregnancy, using reputable health sites. However, if too much information makes you anxious or stressed, take your midwife's advice.

ASK A... MIDWIFE

I plan to bottlefeed. What do I need to buy in advance? You'll need plastic bottles (teats are included), a sterilizing unit or kit (see p.449), which often has everything you need, and your preferred formula. Each comes in a range of options, so you need to decide what works best for you.

As you get to know your newborn baby, you may have to change the type of teat and/or formula, so it's not advisable to buy too many before the birth.

FOCUS ON... NUTRITION

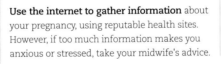

Immunity-boosting blueberries

According to an American study, blueberries topped a list of more than 40 fruits in terms of antioxidant activity. They are also a source of fibre, which is great during pregnancy, especially if – like many women – you suffer from constipation. Blueberries also contain nutrients that can prevent or repair damage to the body's cells. This may strengthen the body's immune system and your ability to fight infections.

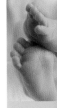

Your 30th week

YOU'RE GETTING TIRED MORE EASILY BUT THAT PROBABLY WON'T STOP YOUR NESTING PLANS

The nest-building instinct often kicks in as a woman approaches her due date. You may be overwhelmed with the urge to clean and decorate, but although it's natural to want a perfect home for your baby don't wear yourself out. Work, travelling, and a constant round of antenatal appointments are probably all much more of an effort these days. If you need to keep stopping to rest, listen to your body and do just that.

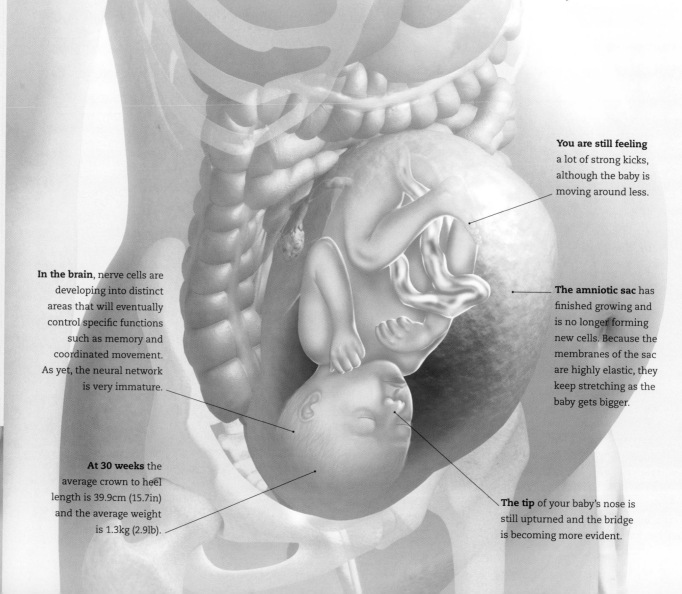

You are still feeling a lot of strong kicks, although the baby is moving around less.

In the brain, nerve cells are developing into distinct areas that will eventually control specific functions such as memory and coordinated movement. As yet, the neural network is very immature.

The amniotic sac has finished growing and is no longer forming new cells. Because the membranes of the sac are highly elastic, they keep stretching as the baby gets bigger.

At 30 weeks the average crown to heel length is 39.9cm (15.7in) and the average weight is 1.3kg (2.9lb).

The tip of your baby's nose is still upturned and the bridge is becoming more evident.

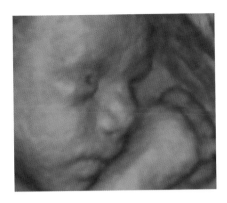

76 days to go...

YOUR BABY TODAY

The image shows the eyes are open once more for a brief look around. It's not completely dark within the uterus and the more advanced your pregnancy, the more light can penetrate inside. Your baby will gradually be assimilating this information.

Be prepared to spend more time in waiting rooms from now on, as your care providers ask to see you more often.

It's important to remember that your pregnancy is a natural, healthy process, but with more regular antenatal appointments, and a lot of time spent sitting in a waiting room at the hospital or midwives' clinic or your doctor's surgery, surrounded by people with various illnesses, you may start to feel that you have a medical problem. Even though you're visiting the hospital so often, you are fit and well; you just also happen to be pregnant.

At every antenatal appointment you will be asked for a urine sample, which is checked for protein. If you find it's getting increasingly difficult to catch your sample in the tiny, fiddly bottle you're given, don't worry. Only a small amount of urine is needed, so if you can't see anything just start to urinate and then move the bottle underneath the flow to catch some. Urine is sterile (unless you have a urinary tract infection) so don't worry about getting some on your hands – just wash them thoroughly afterwards.

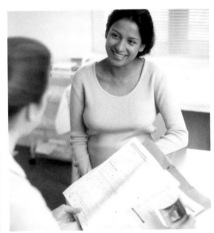

Regular appointments with your midwife take time out of your day, but they offer reassurance that all is well with your baby.

ASK A... DOCTOR

We know our baby has Down's syndrome. How can we prepare ourselves? Knowing now will give you time to come to terms with the fact that your baby will have Down's syndrome. You won't need any special equipment or toys when your baby is born, but you will need emotional support, so turn to the people now who you think will best give you this.

Contact the Down's Syndrome Association (see p.480) for information and support, including getting in touch with parents of children with Down's syndrome through your local support group.

THE LOWDOWN

Freebirthing

Giving birth without any medical assistance from a midwife or doctor might seem a little crazy, but a small minority of women believe that so-called freebirthing is the ultimate way to welcome their baby into the world. Some mums-to-be plan an unassisted home birth after having a negative experience during a previous labour; others want their birth to be "natural", "private", and devoid of medical intervention.

■ **Freebirthing is not against the law,** but it is radical. It's also potentially very risky, because an apparently textbook delivery can swiftly turn into a medical emergency that can only be resolved by trained medical professionals. Complications such as the baby needing oxygen can and do happen.

■ **Some women have an unplanned DIY delivery** – usually because of a short labour – and in these instances the mothers and babies are usually fine. But actually choosing to go it alone is definitely not something that should be considered lightly.

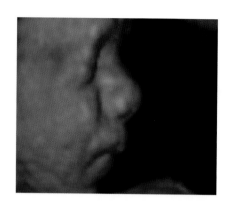

75 days to go...

YOUR BABY TODAY

Now the bridge of the nose is more apparent than earlier in the pregnancy. The tip of the nose can still look slightly upturned at this stage adding to the "button nose" appearance. As the face lengthens, the tip of the nose does move downwards slightly.

Your baby's nerve cells are developing, but they are still not mature enough for her to feel pain, temperature, or touch.

Electrical activity can now be detected in the increasingly convoluted folds of grey matter, the part of your baby's brain that controls the higher functions, such as memory and consciousness, as well as muscle control and sensory perceptions, such as seeing and hearing.

The neurons of the cortex – the outer layer of grey matter – have started to develop into six distinct layers with separate functions, a process that will be completed in about five weeks, although further maturing will be needed. Your baby is born with almost a full complement of neurons, but there is further growth in early childhood.

For nerves to function effectively and signals to pass along them faster, they need insulating. In a process known as myelination, the nerves are insulated with myelin sheaths of fat. Although all of the components of the nervous system are present from an early stage of development, the peripheral sensory and motor nerves, spinal cord, and brain need the entire pregnancy to develop and function as a unit.

The nerves of the brain and spinal cord carry the sensations of pain, temperature, and touch. However, the process of myelination is ongoing and will not be complete until the final few weeks of pregnancy, so your baby does not register or recognize pain, temperature, and touch at this stage.

ASK A... MIDWIFE

The reality of having to give birth is hitting me now! How can I avoid getting too anxious? A little way into your third trimester, the reality of childbirth may sink in. You may be experiencing some pregnancy discomforts, including Braxton Hicks' contractions (see p.410), which give an indication of what is to come.

First of all, remember that the calmer and more relaxed you are, the easier your birth will be. Try to use a little positive visualization – your baby coming out easily in a "whoosh" of fluid, and contractions being "positive pain" to bring your baby into the world. Remember that your baby will be fine, however long she takes to arrive, and that your pain and discomfort are all controllable. In other words, even if you decide on a natural birth now, you can get help and relief when you need it.

Try to relax and enjoy the last months of your pregnancy. Treat yourself to a massage, and keep yourself busy – perhaps undertaking a creative project for your new baby. Above all, don't worry. Think about childbirth as welcoming your baby into the world, and focus on this rather than any concerns.

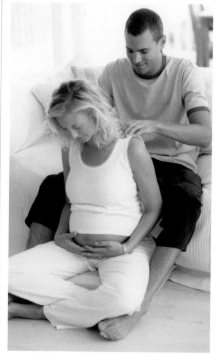

A massage is soothing and relaxing and can be very welcome attention as you wind down towards the birth of your baby.

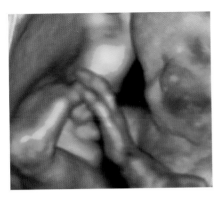

74 days to go...

YOUR BABY TODAY

Your baby often grasps one hand with the other or, as this image shows, grasps a foot. This helps with important sensory feedback to the brain as the nerves within the brain start to mature and become insulated along their length to carry signals more effectively.

Start getting your baby's room ready now, while you still have the energy for shopping and helping with decorating.

It's recommended that your baby sleeps in the same room as you for the first six months, but many parents-to-be still like to prepare the baby's bedroom. This room can still be used for the baby's clothes and any newborn gifts you're given. You might also want to breastfeed, and set up a nappy-changing area in there.

The NCT often holds sales of second-hand baby equipment, and this can be a good opportunity to purchase some of the bigger items at a reduced price. If you buy a second-hand Moses basket or cot, it's recommended that you buy

a new mattress. Hand-me down clothes, sheets, and towels are another way to save money. If this is not your first baby you may find that you have more or less everything you need, apart from disposables, such as nappies (unless you are using washable nappies – see p.291).

Although it's good to be prepared (and sometimes babies do arrive early), remember you won't be trapped in your house forever more so you don't need to prepare as if for a siege. If you don't have something you need or you run out, you can always go and get it after your baby is born.

If you don't know the sex of your baby, opt for a neutral colour scheme for your baby's room. If you do know, then you can decorate accordingly.

Do I need a pram/travel system/buggy? Most parents-to-be are unsure about the type of pram they'll need for their baby and, as there are a number of options and types available, this can make choosing the right item difficult. You will need to buy some type of travel equipment for your baby and what you choose will vary depending on your circumstances.

If you're mainly a car driver, you may want to consider a car seat that attaches to a pram, or a car seat and separate travel cot. If you intend to walk a lot, you may find a lightweight pushchair or buggy more suitable than a pram. Keep in mind how long your baby will be in the buggy: it must be comfortable, have a lie-flat option for the first six months, and adjustable seat options as your baby grows. The buggy must also be weatherproof.

If you do a lot of "around town" travel, you might consider a lightweight option in addition to your main system. It's worth having a look around in shops and online to compare different models and get the best price.

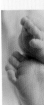

Planning for your birth

As your due date approaches, you may start to think in greater detail about how you would like to manage your labour and birth. Being informed will help you to feel more confident about the choices you make.

Your choices for birth

When planning the type of birth experience you would like to have, you'll need to consider a number of factors. One of the most important decisions is where you would like to give birth. You may also want to think about the details of your birth, such as which positions you would like to adopt during the birth, and what sort of pain relief you might choose to use (see pp.396–407).

It's important to be flexible. You may have preferences as to the type of birth you want, but accepting that your choice may be limited or advised against because of a pre-existing medical problem, or because a problem arises in labour, will help you to prepare mentally and to curb disappointment if events don't go to plan. It is generally accepted that the care of healthy women in labour who have had a straightforward pregnancy should be undertaken by midwives, with advice and support from doctors, with transfer to doctors only sought if a medical opinion is needed.

The place of birth Earlier in pregnancy, you'll probably have thought about where you would like to give birth and discussed the options with your midwife or doctor. Although you may have already stated a preference, it's important to know that you can review your choice and change your mind towards the end of pregnancy.

Where you give birth may be influenced by factors such as whether you've had complications in pregnancy, for example gestational diabetes (see p.473) or high blood pressure (see p.283), that would make a hospital birth preferable. On the other hand, if your pregnancy has been straightforward and you have become more informed about labour and birth over the course of your pregnancy, your confidence may have grown and you may decide to opt for a home birth in familiar surroundings, or to investigate midwife-run birthing units in your area.

Sometime in the third trimester you may have a hospital tour, which gives you a chance to see the labour and postnatal wards in the local hospital, and to ask questions about hospital policies and what facilities are available. Ask your midwife for details of tours.

An active labour In antenatal classes, you'll learn a range of techniques to help you cope with pain during labour. Most methods centre around breathing and relaxation techniques that help you to focus during labour and birth and don't inhibit movement. Maintaining mobility and an upright position during labour is thought to help you cope with

NEW PROCEDURES

Stem cell collection

The collection of stem cells, which are found in the umbilical cord, is a relatively new private service. Stem cells develop into many different types of cell in the body and can be used to treat diseases such as leukaemia by replacing diseased cells (see p.310). Stem cells are collected from the umbilical cord immediately after birth and sent to a laboratory where they are frozen and stored, acting as health insurance for the baby in future life. If you want to have this done, you must make arrangements with a private company and check that the hospital has procedures to allow the collection to be carried out.

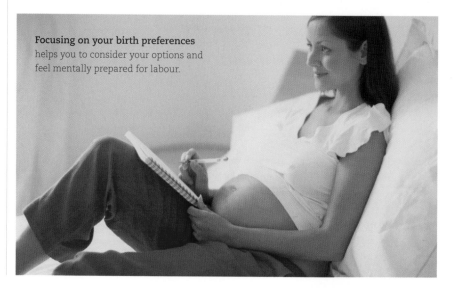

Focusing on your birth preferences helps you to consider your options and feel mentally prepared for labour.

contractions and to use gravity to help push your baby down the birth canal.

If you want an active birth, this may influence how you feel about the type of pain relief you want to use (see below) and about monitoring in labour. For example, continuous monitoring (see p.418) can limit your movement. If the staff at the hospital want to monitor your baby continuously, talk to the midwives about how you can maintain some mobility; for example by sitting on a birthing ball, or adopting an all-fours position on the bed or on a mattress on the floor.

Your pain relief options Factors that may influence the type of pain relief you would like include how active you want to be (see above); what effect different drugs may have on how you experience labour; and how drugs can affect the baby.

Natural methods, such as breathing techniques, labouring in water, and TENS (see p.399), and some medical pain-relief options, such as gas and air and pethidine,

or similar opiate-based injections (see pp.402–3), allow an active birth. However, drugs such as pethidine easily cross the placenta and can affect the baby's breathing at birth. Regional anaesthetics, such as epidurals (see p.404), limit movement and can mean that you will have a decreased urge to push.

Making a birth plan

Writing your preferences in a birth plan helps you to consolidate your thoughts and to pass this information on to your midwife. Or your midwife may discuss a birth plan with you. A birth plan is useful, too, for your birthing partner, who may need to advocate on your behalf in labour. Birth plans also allow you to state any special needs, such as the help you will need if you have a disability.

Make your birth plan straightforward and accessible. Working with your carers as a team will help you to cope best with labour and to feel that you're involved in decision making, whatever the outcome.

THINKING ABOUT THE BIRTH

Questions to consider

When planning where and how you ideally want to give birth, you need to consider both what you would prefer and what the hospital or birthing unit can offer. The following questions may act as helpful prompts.

Questions to ask yourself
■ Who would you like to have with you during the labour and birth?
■ Do you want an active labour?
■ What pain relief do you want?
■ If you have an assisted birth, would you prefer ventouse or forceps?
■ Do you want your partner to be present if you have a Caesarean?
■ Do you want the third stage of labour to be managed naturally or assisted with drugs?
■ How do you want to feed your baby?

■ Are you happy for your baby to have a vitamin K injection (see p.442)?

Questions to ask the hospital
■ What is the policy on induction? Will the hospital monitor your baby before labour if you don't want to be induced?
■ Will the choice of pain relief and the place of birth change if you're induced?
■ Are there birthing pool facilities?
■ Will you be able to bring in aids such as aromatherapy oils or music?
■ How much privacy will you have?
■ Can you have a female doctor?
■ Will your baby remain with you throughout your stay in hospital?
■ Does the hospital have facilities for sick babies, or are babies transferred?
■ Can you go home when you feel ready, or is there a set discharge time?

WHO'S WHO

Birth ideologies

In the mid-20th century, labour and childbirth in the West became highly medicalized. In reaction, several childbirth philosophies emerged that focused on empowering women and viewed childbirth as a natural rather than a medical experience. Many of these approaches are integral to the way childbirth is managed today.

Dr Grantley Dick-Read, a British obstetrician, linked labour pain to fear when he was working during the 1950s. He promoted breathing and relaxation to help cope with pain, and his methods are now commonplace.

Dr Ferdinand Lamaze was inspired by the Russian scientist Dr Pavlov, who trained dogs to have a set response to stimulus. In the 1950s, Lamaze extended this idea to childbirth, believing that women could be trained to respond positively to labour pain.

Sheila Kitzinger, a well-known birth practitioner who became prominent in the 1960s, believes in a woman's right to choose how to give birth.

Frederick Leboyer, a French obstetrician, came to prominence in the 1970s with his book *Birth without Violence*. He focuses on the baby, believing that a traumatic birth could impact negatively later in life. He promotes "gentle birthing" where the baby is immersed in warm water after birth and has skin-to-skin contact.

Michel Odent, a birth practitioner, advocates active birthing, believing that women act on instincts in labour. His birthing centre in Pithiviers, France, has the lowest national rates of intervention.

Janet Balaskas founded the Active Birth Movement in 1981. At her Active Birth Centre in London, she teaches relaxation, breathing, and yoga.

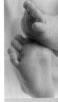

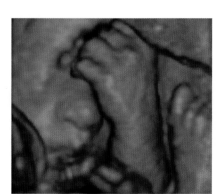

73 days to go...

YOUR BABY TODAY

In this image a hand is held up to the forehead and, to the right, part of a foot can be seen. The groove between the nose and the upper lip is visible and the nose has the characteristic "button" shape. It looks cramped in there but there is still room to move.

Your baby is cushioned in a sac of amniotic fluid, which surrounds her until your waters break and you go into labour.

As your uterus has enlarged throughout your pregnancy, the amniotic sac has expanded to accommodate both your baby and the amniotic fluid. From now on, however, the sac will grow by simply stretching rather than forming new cells.

The amniotic sac is formed from two distinct layers or membranes, an inner "amnion" and outer "chorion". The chorion originally had a blood supply of its own, but this has now been lost. The thinner amnion is able to slide over the chorion as your baby pushes against it. Neither layer contains nerve cells: this explains why it's not painful when your membranes rupture or "waters break".

Combined, the layers are only 0.5mm thick. Collagen fibres in each layer allow for a great deal of stretch – this is vital in these final months to avoid early rupture of the membranes. Indeed, the membranes may be so resistant to rupture that they don't break until the final stages of your labour (see p.411).

As well as holding in the amniotic fluid and providing a barrier to possible infection through the cervix, the membranes contain substances that form prostaglandins. Prostaglandins play an important part in the initiation of labour. This is one of the reasons why labour often starts when the membranes have ruptured.

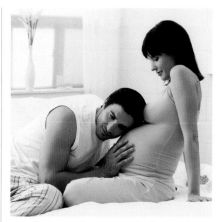

Your baby may have several episodes of hiccuping in a day, or only one or two – you will both be able to feel these as a series of light, rhythmic movements.

AS A MATTER OF FACT

The only reliable way to discover the sex of your baby is to have a diagnostic test (see pp.152–3), such as amniocentesis or chorionic villus sampling.

Even ultrasound can be wrong. And despite the common belief that the size and shape of your bump indicates the baby's gender, these are in fact determined by your muscle tone, your baby's position, and the amount of weight you've gained.

FOCUS ON... DADS

Kicks and hiccups

By now, it's possible to see and feel your baby moving, often with kicks and punches. This may happen more often in the evenings, when your partner finally gets to sit down and relax. Watching your baby's movements can be a great way to bond with her, and with your partner.

Your baby will respond to your voice, to music, and may even jump at unexpected noises (see p.256);

it's impossible to say whether this is because these noises are enjoyed or because they're irritating.

Your baby will also hiccup sometimes (see p.204) and you have a better chance of feeling her moving while she's hiccuping than during any other form of movement. This is because hiccups occur over prolonged periods of time, while kicks and punches can be fairly random.

72 days to go...

YOUR BABY TODAY

The lip shape and groove between the nose and upper lip are particularly well shown here. If you or your partner has a prominent groove, or philtrum, above the upper lip, your baby may too, or she may inherit characteristics that are somewhere in between.

Regardless of your size – and that of your baby – nature won't let her grow too large for you to be able to give birth.

Your body shape isn't an indication of whether you'll have an easy birth. The size of your hips is not always a good indication of the size of your pelvis so having slender hips doesn't mean you'll have a difficult birth, and having larger "child-bearing" hips doesn't mean you'll have an easier birth.

What is known is that, although how big your child will be is determined genetically, women have an extra influence on the size of their babies while they are in the uterus. So, even if your child ends up growing to 1.80m (6ft) tall, if you're small you'll limit how big she gets in the uterus. This makes sense – if you're small, you wouldn't be able to deliver a hefty 5.5kg (12lb) baby, so your body limits the baby's size at delivery. Your baby will then catch up on her expected growth after the birth.

There's a condition called cephalo-pelvic disproportion in which the baby is too big or the pelvis is too small for the baby to engage. An MRI scan will be performed to get exact measurements.

ASK A... MIDWIFE

Do twins run out of room to turn around in the womb? It does tend to be the case that, in the third trimester, twins find a position and settle there at an earlier stage of pregnancy than if there was just one baby. Generally, with twin pregnancies, there seems to be a lot less movement in presentation from about 32–34 weeks. How your twins are likely to be delivered depends largely on the direction that the twin who is lowest in the pelvis is facing. If this twin is head down, then a vaginal delivery should be possible and the second twin may be able to be gently coaxed to turn head down.

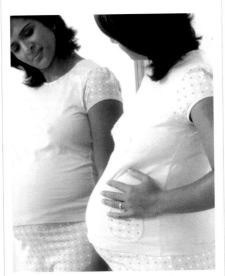

As you marvel at the size of your bump, you may be concerned about how you'll ever deliver your baby. But don't worry – nature is on your side.

TIME TO THINK ABOUT

A support network

After giving birth, your body will spring back into shape overnight; you'll be bursting with energy and raring to go. That's one scenario! The other – more realistic – possibility is that you'll find yourself struggling to get breastfeeding established and to clean your teeth before teatime. If you don't like living in a mess, act now to prevent resentment (and the washing) building up in a few months' time.

- Talk to your partner now about how you're going to split the chores once you're parents.
- Your "job" will be to nurture your newborn, so you'll need domestic backup, if possible, particularly during the first few weeks. Recruit helpers (family and friends; or pay professionals if need be). Delegate so that you won't have to think about shopping, cooking, or cleaning.
- New parents need their own space, so it's never too early to organize some babysitters for a few weeks after the birth. If you're breastfeeding, you'll need to express your milk.

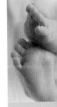

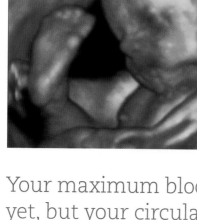

71 days to go...

YOUR BABY TODAY

Increasingly sounds enter the womb and your baby will respond to some of the loudest. The fluid all around her can have quite an effect on the sounds that your baby can hear: the effect is similar to how you might feel when you swim with your head under water.

Your maximum blood volume won't be reached for a few weeks yet, but your circulation is working harder than ever at this stage.

Your blood volume is likely to be about 5 litres (8.25 pints) between weeks 25 and 35 – an increase of about 25 per cent. This increased blood volume means that your heart is pumping harder and faster. Your blood vessels are as relaxed as they can be by this stage of pregnancy, and will not stretch any further to accommodate this extra blood flow. You may notice that you sweat more, and that your skin feels hotter (this is the rosy glow that many women experience).

In addition to this extra blood, there is also a lot more fluid circulating around your body. This makes all your body tissues thicker. It's common and normal for your face, fingers, and ankles to be puffy or swollen (see pp.466–7). However, since puffiness is also a sign of pre-eclampsia (see p.474), it's important for your doctor or midwife to check this out.

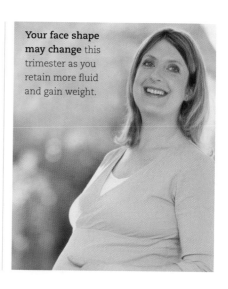

Your face shape may change this trimester as you retain more fluid and gain weight.

ASK A... MIDWIFE

I've noticed that I get short of breath very easily. Should I be concerned? No, when you're pregnant, your lungs have to work much harder to meet your body's increased oxygen needs. To help you take in more air, your ribs spread sideways and your lung capacity increases dramatically. This can make you feel breathless, particularly from mid-pregnancy.

In the last three months of pregnancy, most women find they get breathless even during mild exertion, which happens as the expanding uterus pushes up against the lungs. However, being breathless can also be a sign of anaemia (see p.472), which may need to be treated. Your breathing may start to get easier when your baby engages (moves down into your pelvis ready to be born) (see p.361).

FOCUS ON... TWINS

Exercising safely

If you're pregnant with twins, it's recommended that you don't do any vigorous or aerobic exercise in the third trimester. The last three months are particularly tiring so you probably won't feel up to doing much anyway. You'll also get bigger sooner than someone who is having a single baby, and your size may preclude you from doing certain activities.

If you do want to be active, go for a gentle walk or swim, or to an antenatal yoga or Pilates class. If you want to do anything more vigorous than this in the third trimester, first check with your antenatal carers.

Your doctor and midwife will be monitoring your babies' progress and they may advise on your level of activity if there is any slowdown in the babies' growth and development.

Whatever activity you're doing, always follow the guidelines for safe exercising (see p.18).

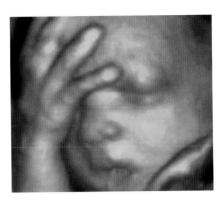

70 days to go...

YOUR BABY TODAY

Does your baby start to feel tired? Certainly on some scans it can look as if she is. In fact, your baby actually spends most of the time in a state of sleep rather than full wakefulness: it seems that during pregnancy your baby does need to spend most of the time asleep.

You probably won't want to stop working just yet, but you may need to make some adjustments if you're feeling very tired.

Later on in the third trimester you may begin to feel more tired than usual. The strain on your body may begin to show itself – you may find yourself uncomfortable and easily fatigued. Things that never bothered you previously, such as standing for long periods of time or walking a lot, may get increasingly difficult. For example, your journey to and from work may tire you much more than it did previously. If that is the case, find out whether you can alter your hours to avoid travelling at the busiest times of the day and, if you find yourself travelling in the rush hours, don't be shy about asking someone to give up their seat for you. If there is a room in which you can rest at work, you may be able to take a short nap in the middle of the day or early afternoon, which might help to alleviate your tiredness a little.

You may want to discuss with your employer ways to make your job less physically demanding, or ask for help, for example if you need to carry heavy files or your job involves walking long distances. With a few adjustments you should be able to keep going until the start of your maternity leave, but above all, listen to your body: if you're tired, rest; if your feet and legs hurt, sit down.

USING A BIRTHING POOL

Labouring and giving birth in water can not only relieve much of the pain, discomfort, and stress of childbirth, it can also induce relaxation and reduce blood pressure. Research shows that warm water on the lower back (the area of the spinal cord that receives the nerves from the lower abdominal region) can reduce labour pain, while the level of endorphins, or natural painkillers, rises in the same environment. Whether you choose a birthing pool or a warm bath, water is a great way to deal with contractions.

If you give birth in water, your baby's umbilical cord will continue to provide her with the oxygen she needs, but she will have to be brought to the surface quickly to encourage her to breathe on her own.

You will be able to arrange to hire a pool for your own home, or may be allowed to use one in some hospitals (see p.343). Make sure you include these details on your birth plan (see p.303). Using a birthing pool will not be recommended if your birth is considered to be high risk.

FOCUS ON... TWINS

Caesarean birth

Over half of all twins are delivered by Caesarean (see pp.438–9). Many of these are elective: the decision is made in advance, and the mother doesn't go into labour. A Caesarean is major surgery, but for the babies it's often the best way to arrive and a small price to pay for the mother.

Vaginal birth can be complicated for twins, especially the second twin who goes through two lots of uterine contractions. It's considered to be high-risk if the babies are premature.

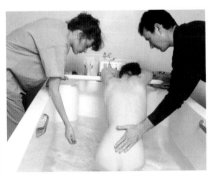

It's relatively easy to hire a birthing pool if you're planning a home birth, and you can check the availability of a pool at your hospital when you tour the facility.

Your 31st week

EVEN IF YOU HAVE A BIRTH PLAN IN MIND, BE PREPARED TO BE FLEXIBLE

You may have firm thoughts about what you consider to be the ideal birth experience. However, keep an open mind because many factors can influence where and how your baby is born. There's nothing unusual in a woman changing her mind, even after her labour has actually started. Your healthcare team will expect you to ask a lot of questions about childbirth, so take advantage of their experience and expertise.

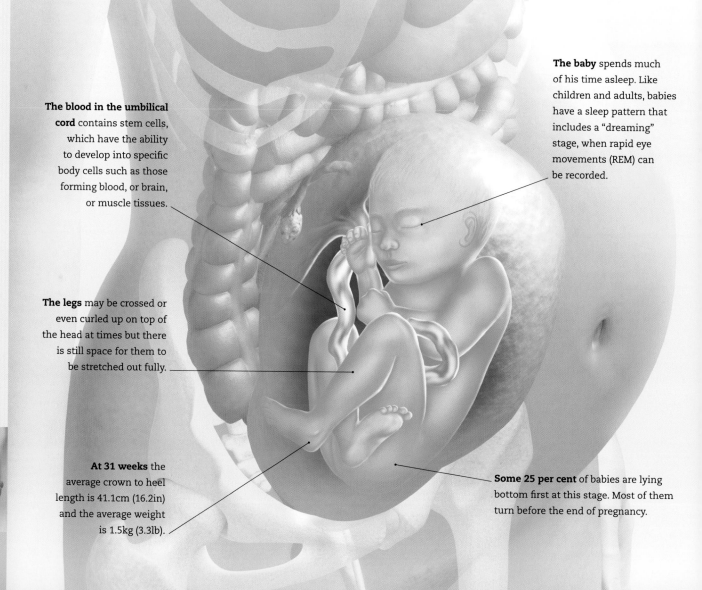

The blood in the umbilical cord contains stem cells, which have the ability to develop into specific body cells such as those forming blood, or brain, or muscle tissues.

The baby spends much of his time asleep. Like children and adults, babies have a sleep pattern that includes a "dreaming" stage, when rapid eye movements (REM) can be recorded.

The legs may be crossed or even curled up on top of the head at times but there is still space for them to be stretched out fully.

At 31 weeks the average crown to heel length is 41.1cm (16.2in) and the average weight is 1.5kg (3.3lb).

Some 25 per cent of babies are lying bottom first at this stage. Most of them turn before the end of pregnancy.

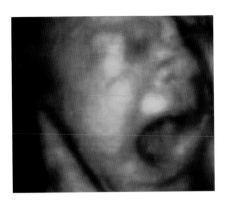

YOU ARE 30 WEEKS AND 1 DAY

69 days to go...

YOUR BABY TODAY

From this point in the pregnancy your baby will yawn just as often as during the first few weeks after birth. Exactly why babies yawn before birth remains unknown, but seeing your baby yawn on a scan is quite likely to make you yawn as well.

It's well worth giving some thought to where your baby is going to sleep before you actually bring him home from the hospital.

It's recommended that your baby sleeps in a cot or crib in your bedroom for the first six months. See the box below, if you're considering co-sleeping. With your baby in your bedroom, you'll be close by when he cries in the night and able to attend to him easily. This is especially useful if you're breastfeeding.

Remember that babies are not necessarily quiet sleepers: they may wriggle, grunt, and move around and these noises may disturb you or your partner. If your partner has to go to work the following day this extra disturbance may affect him. It will

affect you, too, but you may have a chance to "catch up" on some sleep, or at least rest, when your baby naps. You should do what is best for all three of you, even if that means your partner spends some nights in the spare room. Some new parents find that they are so exhausted by life with a newborn that they sleep, regardless of whether their baby is snuffling or not.

If the baby is in his own room you may worry that you may not hear him cry, but you will if you use a baby monitor. When he does cry, yet again at 3am, be aware that a short trip along the landing can seem like a mile.

SHOULD YOU CO-SLEEP?

You may want to put your baby into your bed with you, especially if you're breastfeeding. This is not recommended before a baby is three months old, if he was born prematurely, if he weighed less than 2.5kg (5.5lb at birth), or if you or your partner smoke, have drunk alcohol, taken sedating medication, or are extremely tired. If you put your baby in your bed to sleep when he's older, be reassured that you and your partner are highly unlikely to roll over on to him.

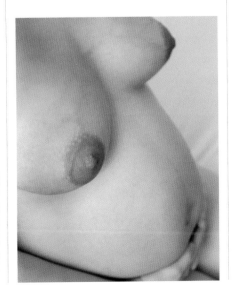

FOCUS ON... YOUR BODY

Breast changes

In the third trimester, your breasts will begin to prepare themselves for feeding your baby, and you may experience some discomfort and changes that you had not anticipated. Your breasts will become fuller, and may actually feel very heavy; your areolas (the area around your nipples) will become darker, and you may feel lumps and bumps in your breasts, as the first milk, colostrum, begins to be produced. This may leak out a little (see p.295).

The small glands on the surface of your areolas (known as Montgomery's tubercles) will also become raised bumps. You may have darkened veins along your breasts, due to their increased blood supply. Your breasts may also feel more tender and sensitive than usual, especially if touched.

Your breasts will change in preparation for breastfeeding, whether you intend to breastfeed your baby or not. They become fuller and heavier, the areolas (dark areas around the nipples) become darker and the veins under the skin more obvious.

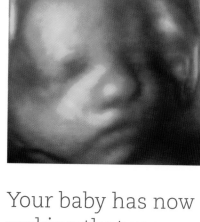

68 days to go...

YOUR BABY TODAY

You will be aware of times when your baby is especially active and times when he is more quiet. There is still a lot of space for your baby to move within the uterus but it is likely that there will be a favourite spot that receives more kicks than any other.

Your baby has now developed a clear rhythm of sleeping and waking that may mimic your own or be personal to him.

Exactly when and how your baby develops a cycle of sleeping and waking before birth remains a bit of a mystery. It's not known whether your own rhythms influence your baby's sleep–wake cycle or whether your baby develops his own internal clock. Indeed, such a clock might be triggered in response to the small amount of light that is able to penetrate through the uterus during the last few weeks of pregnancy. It's apparent from brain scans, however, that by this stage of pregnancy, your baby does have very separate periods of activity.

There is a clear cycle, alternating between periods of quiet rest, sleep with rapid eye movements (REM), wakefulness with activity but no eye movement, and wakefulness with lots of activity and eye movements. During this sleep–wake cycle, the baby's actions become more co-ordinated as periods of activity are linked to rhythmical breathing and increased heart rate, and eye movements.

By this stage of pregnancy, electrical activity in your baby's brain shows patterns reflecting periods of sleep or wakefulness. An EEG of your baby's brain would show that the quietest period, deep sleep, takes up almost half of the time. The next most common state is REM sleep (the sleep stage during which children and adults dream). This is a time of great electrical activity within your baby's brain. During REM sleep the baby may be quiet or making lots of movements, so it's not possible to tell whether your baby is truly awake at this time or if he's dreaming. Paradoxically, the least electrical activity happens when your baby is most awake – in fact less than 10 per cent of your baby's time is spent truly awake at this stage.

STEM CELL COLLECTION

The blood in your baby's umbilical cord contains "cord blood", which is rich in stem cells. These cells are the building blocks of organ tissue, blood, and the immune system. Some parents save these cells and store them (in a private facility at a cost) in the event that their child or another family member needs their healing benefits (see p.302).

Studies have found that they are very effective in the treatment of more than 70 diseases including juvenile arthritis, cancers, heart disease, and brain injury.

Stem cells are widely used, but there is significant evidence to show that using cells from the cord blood of a sibling or other family member is more effective than using cells from an unrelated donor, or bone marrow from relatives.

Cord blood can be pricey to store. The NHS keeps a cord blood bank in which donated blood is stored, and this is used to treat patients who need it most. This means that your baby's cord blood may have been used before your baby, or one of his siblings, needed it.

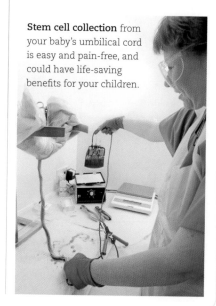

Stem cell collection from your baby's umbilical cord is easy and pain-free, and could have life-saving benefits for your children.

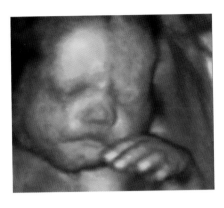

67 days to go...

YOUR BABY TODAY

It can come as quite a surprise to see that your baby will be increasingly pulling all sorts of expressions. Here the baby has his mouth turned down but the next minute will be yawning, grimacing, or peacefully sleeping.

Natural birth has many advocates, but the best birth is one that delivers your baby safely with minimum trauma for both of you.

Many women want a natural delivery, with no pain relief or other medical intervention. Giving birth naturally is for some reason perceived as the "best" way, and to do otherwise means that you somehow "failed" at childbirth. This pressure means that women can feel guilty or even depressed if they needed pain relief or a Caesarean section, for example.

Bear in mind that some women have higher pain thresholds and can get through labour with simple breathing or relaxation techniques, while others need more help. Pain is subjective, no one else can feel your pain; if it is too much for you, then ask for help. Your options (see pp.402–7) will be explained to you by the midwife.

Childbirth is hard work, but the experience should not be so painful that it scars you. Being pain-free may mean that you have a more enjoyable, even empowering, labour experience. The medical team is on the labour ward to help you, and will be called only when necessary either for your wellbeing and safety or that of your baby.

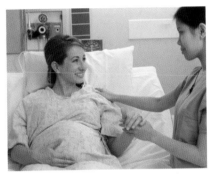

Having a natural birth is high on the list of many women's priorities, but it's worth preparing mentally for medical intervention, in case it becomes necessary.

ASK A PANEL ABOUT... NATURAL BIRTH

I want a natural birth but everyone says I'll change my mind once I'm in labour. Are they right?

Mum: Nothing can prepare you for the discomfort of labour, and I found my carefully laid plans were unrealistic and impractical when the pain kicked in. No matter how well prepared you are, you may change your mind during labour, and it's worth being prepared for that. I did feel a bit disappointed that I couldn't manage without pain relief. It helps if you focus on what's important – delivering a healthy baby. If you achieve this aim, you've succeeded, no matter what happens along the way. I would say to stick it out for as long as you can, but you'll be doing yourself and your baby no favours if you both become exhausted and distressed.

Midwife: Many women are shocked by the intensity of the birth experience, and soon forget about their idealistic birth plan. It's better for all involved that you allow for contingency plans, and keep an open mind. Pain relief (see pp.396–407) and interventions are designed to make the experience better for you and your baby, and will not be offered unless they're necessary, or you feel that you can't do without them. Some women get through labour naturally; others need some help. A lot of women do change their mind about "going natural", and there is nothing wrong with that. A mum who has her pain under control will find that the delivery is much quicker, and she'll have much more energy for her new arrival.

Twins

Just a few weeks to go. By now, you're probably quite large and, of course, excited at the imminent arrival of your twins, or more. However, you may also be concerned about how you will manage during and after the birth.

Getting ready for the birth

Although multiple pregnancies and births are more likely to have complications, they are now safer than ever as advances in antenatal and postnatal care have dramatically improved the outlook for premature babies – the main concern with multiples (see below).

You can prepare for the birth by getting plenty of rest. Putting your feet up, or even having a lie-down during the day, helps to improve the blood flow to the placenta, which in turn helps your babies to grow. Practising pelvic floor exercises (see p.69) is important with a multiple pregnancy as your pelvic floor muscles are under an additional strain.

Bonding with twins

Often, expectant mums of twins or more worry about how they will bond with more than one baby. It's true that bonding can be harder with twins, and even more so with higher multiples. After all, it's hard to fall in love with more than one person at a time, especially when you're exhausted caring for two babies or more. Being aware of this and arranging extra help for after the birth may ease your anxiety. Also, accept additional offers of help that allow you to rest or spend time with one twin. If someone offers to take the twins out, you might consider one twin going and the other spending time with you.

TWINS

How your babies lie in the uterus

In the final weeks, your babies will take up their positions for the birth. The most common position is with both babies lying vertically. With 75 per cent of twins, the first is head down (cephalic); the second twin may be head down or breech, or one twin may lie across the uterus (transverse). You may suspect their position from the kicks, but only a scan confirms this.

A Caesarean will be recommended if you have triplets or more, or your first twin is breech or transverse (25 per cent of cases). A vaginal delivery is most likely if both twins are head down. If the first is head down and the second is transverse or breech, there are different opinions as to the best type of delivery, which you can discuss with your obstetrician.

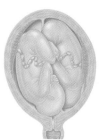 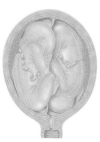 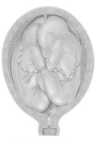 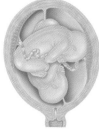

Both babies head down (cephalic)	**One baby head down, and one breech**	**Both babies in a breech position**	**One baby head down and one transverse**

A shorter pregnancy Twins or more usually arrive earlier than singletons. Space in the womb is one factor. In addition, with multiple pregnancies the placenta becomes less efficient towards the end of pregnancy. As a result, the ideal length of pregnancy is shorter: for twins, 37 weeks is considered full term, for triplets, the average pregnancy is about 34 weeks, and for quadruplets, pregnancy lasts around 32 weeks. The average birth weight for each twin is 2.5kg (5lb 8oz) at full term.

You may deliver even earlier than this, as nearly 50 per cent of twins are born prematurely. However, nowadays expert care for premature babies means that over 80 per cent of babies weighing less than 1kg (2lb 3oz) at birth, some born as early as 23 weeks, survive.

Preparing for more than one

Even if your twins are identical they're individuals, and relating to them as separate people will help their development and your relationship with them. Even in pregnancy, some expectant mums notice how different their babies are from their different movement patterns in the womb.

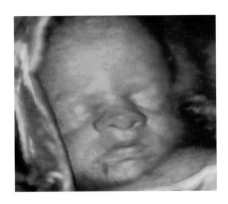

66 days to go...

YOUR BABY TODAY

In this 3D scan the baby's arm is held up next to the face. This type of scan shows external features but also looks inside the baby in 3D so you may see some parts of your baby "through" an arm or leg. Here, the baby's ear can be seen through the arm.

In the uterus and in the first months of his life, your baby relies on your immunity to various infections.

Your baby does not have the ability to produce antibodies (which would attack you) in the uterus: he relies completely on you to protect him from infection, not only in the uterus but also after birth. Protection after birth is possible because antibodies from your immune system cross over the placenta into your baby's bloodstream, while you're pregnant. If you have immunity to a disease such as measles, mumps, polio, and many other severe infections, your baby will carry your antibodies to these conditions. Childhood immunizations provide immunity to many severe infections.

Owing to a large outbreak of whooping cough cases in 2013, a recommendation was introduced that pregnant women between 28 and 38 weeks be vaccinated against this. The immunity your baby acquires from your antibodies is lost with time, so from two months he will require a programme of immunizations.

FOCUS ON... YOUR BODY

There have been numerous studies over the past few years involving women exercising while they're pregnant. The bottom line is that exercise performed effectively and safely, at a moderate intensity and in healthy women, is beneficial.

As well as being good for your health and making you feel more energized, exercising will get you into great shape for labour and childbirth, which is, in effect, a workout!

Here are the myths:

■ **Exercising will harm my baby if I move too much.** Your baby is protected by amniotic fluid and nourished by the placenta. By keeping within safe exercising guidelines (see p.18), and not doing any high-impact sports or activities where you are at risk of falling or injuries, you are not putting your baby at risk.

■ **Exercise will use up some of the nutrients my baby needs.** Your baby's growth will be monitored at antenatal appointments, so you and your midwife will be able to tell whether your baby is growing at a usual rate or whether you should increase your calorie intake. If you're concerned, increase your calorie intake on the days that you exercise.

■ **Doing tummy exercises will harm the baby.** You can do abdominal exercises but you should not do them lying on your back in the second and third trimesters. The risk of lying on your back is that your enlarged uterus can press down on the vena cava (the large blood vessel that returns blood to your heart). This causes your blood pressure to fall and compromises the oxygen flow to the baby. The first sign of a problem will be feeling dizzy: if you roll on to your left side, any symptoms

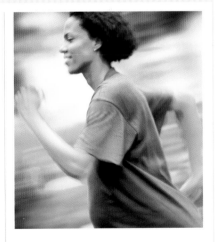

should disappear. Don't hesitate to consult your midwife if you're concerned. The abdominal exercises that are shown on page 250 give you some great ways of doing safe abdominal exercises that do not put you or your baby at risk.

65 days to go...

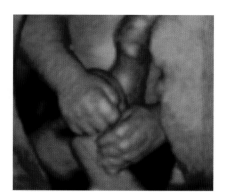

YOUR BABY TODAY

Here the hands are holding the umbilical cord as it arises from what will become the tummy button, or umbilicus. The umbilical coils and its covering of firm, clear jelly protect the cord from kinking and prying fingers.

If you want a home birth atmosphere with additional support, consider having your baby in a birthing unit.

Birthing units are run by midwives and the emphasis is on a natural birth. They can be situated next to a hospital maternity unit or on a separate site. Some hospitals have a birthing unit facility in the maternity unit. As the majority of women give birth without needing medical intervention, these units provide a good alternative to a more medicalized hospital environment. The environment in a birthing unit tends to be more relaxed and flexible than a hospital environment. You'll have continuous support from midwives and may even be attended by the same midwife throughout your labour and birth. Furthermore, the midwives in these units are very experienced at handling a birth without medical intervention. All of these factors therefore increase your chances of having a straightforward birth. To be eligible to give birth in such a facility, you would need to have had an uncomplicated pregnancy and be unlikely to require specialized medical care or monitoring in labour and birth. If complications did occur, you would be transferred to the nearest maternity unit, although this is rare.

ASK A... MIDWIFE

I'm having a home birth. Can my older children, aged four and six, be present at the birth? There is nothing more wonderful or miraculous than the birth of a baby, and it's natural to want your older children to be present and witness it for themselves. However, do consider this carefully before you give them the go-ahead. For one thing, even the easiest of labours are painful, and young children will be distressed to see mum in pain. What's more, they may be slightly daunted to see their new sibling emerging from your body, probably covered with various substances. Having said that, many kids handle the experience well if they know what to expect, so outline everything, and explain that any cries, shrieks, or swearing on your behalf are necessary to help get the baby out. You could also mention that you may cry or even vomit, just so they are prepared. Let them know to expect some blood, and that baby will be attached to a (rather gruesome!) cord. If they're squeamish, get them to position themselves by your head, or bring them in immediately after.

HOME IS WHERE THE HEART IS

The prospect of sleeping in your own bed and being looked after by people who love you are reason enough to opt for a home birth. It's natural to feel less inhibited at home, and you may be more inclined to move around more and for longer, be as vocal as you like, use gravity, and try different birthing positions, all of which can make labour and delivery shorter and easier. Your midwife will explain what's involved, so seek her advice. On the big day be flexible: you may want to head for hospital.

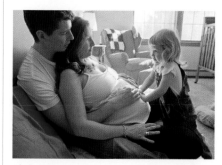

It's important to prepare an older child for the arrival of a new brother or sister. Involve her as much as possible in your pregnancy: allow her to touch your expanding tummy, encourage her to talk to the baby, and take her with you for antenatal visits.

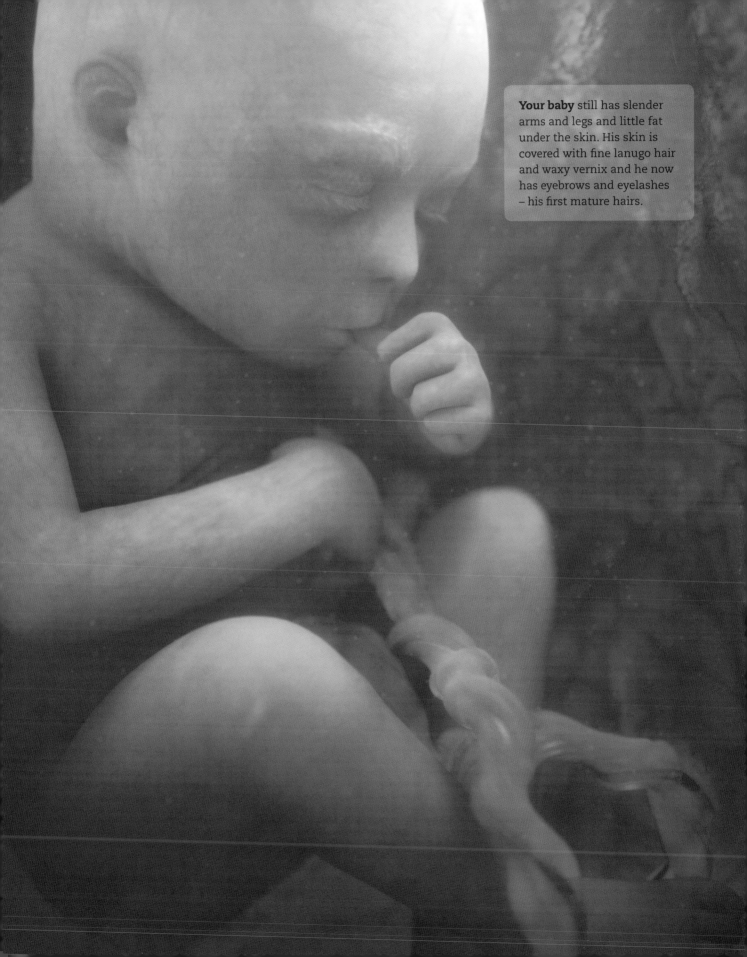

Your baby still has slender arms and legs and little fat under the skin. His skin is covered with fine lanugo hair and waxy vernix and he now has eyebrows and eyelashes – his first mature hairs.

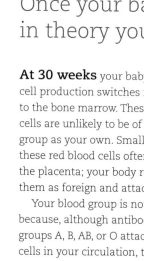

64 days to go...

YOR BABY TODAY

Here the baby is resting on the placenta, seen at the right-hand side of the image, with the umbilical cord just below the baby's chin. The eyes are closed and this image was taken at a time when the baby was at his quietest, during deep sleep.

Once your baby's production of red blood cells is in full swing, in theory your immune system could begin to harm your baby.

At 30 weeks your baby's red blood cell production switches from the liver to the bone marrow. These red blood cells are unlikely to be of the same blood group as your own. Small numbers of these red blood cells often leak across the placenta; your body recognizes them as foreign and attacks them.

Your blood group is not important because, although antibodies to blood groups A, B, AB, or O attack your baby's cells in your circulation, they are too large to cross the placenta and attack your baby. Therefore differences in ABO blood groups do not matter. However, everyone is also rhesus positive (85 per cent) or negative (15 per cent). If you are rhesus negative (see p.123) and

your partner is rhesus positive, your baby may also be rhesus positive.

Rhesus negative women produce antibodies to rhesus positive blood cells; these are smaller than ABO antibodies and can cross the placenta. Once they do, large numbers of antibodies can attack your baby's blood cells, leading to anaemia. First pregnancies are rarely affected. In a second pregnancy a rhesus negative woman is given one or two injections of the rhesus antibody "anti-D" in the third trimester (see p.123). Anti-D is in a form that is too large to cross the placenta. This mops up any of your baby's blood cells in your circulation, preventing your immune system from attacking your baby.

AMNIOTIC FLUID

Your baby excretes and reabsorbs about 0.5 litre (18fl oz) of urine daily, and the amniotic fluid reaches a peak volume of about 1 litre (35fl oz) at 33 weeks. After this time the volume starts to decline and can be as little as 100–200ml (3.5–7fl oz) in an overdue pregnancy (see p.393).

Low levels of amniotic fluid, known as oligohydramnios (see p.473), can be a sign of a growth-restricted baby or a baby with kidney problems.

Excessive amniotic fluid, known as polyhydramnios (see p.473), may be seen in twin or triplet pregnancies, and is also associated with physical abnormalities in the baby or diabetes in the mother.

After 40 weeks, the fluid level needs to be checked regularly to ensure that there is not too steep a decline in fluid levels. If the overdue baby is thought to be at risk, an induction (see p.432) will be recommended.

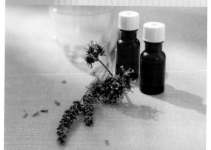

FOCUS ON... YOUR HEALTH

A good night's sleep

Insomnia is a common problem during pregnancy and can lead to fatigue, feelings of stress and anxiety, and irritability.

■ **The herbal teas** valerian and passiflora are both safe during pregnancy, and can be drunk before bed to relax and encourage sleep.

■ **Essential oils** of lavender and Roman camomile can be added to the bath, or dropped on to your pillow, to calm and relax.

■ **The homeopathic remedies** Passiflora 6C, Coffea cruda 6C, and Nux vomica 6C are all good for sleep problems, and can be taken before bed and if you wake up during the night.

■ **Bach flower remedies** (see p.372) can relieve stress and aid sleep.

63 days to go...

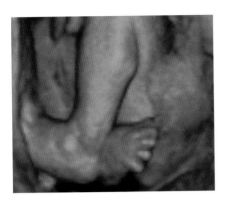

YOUR BABY TODAY

One leg is shown here crossed over the other. Your baby can still stretch her legs out fully and even curl up in such a way that the feet can rest on top of the head. However, she'll often be seen with her legs in this crossed position.

Epidural is a common form of pain-relief during labour and may be an option for you if you have a low pain threshold.

Many women have decided that they want a pain-free delivery with an epidural (see pp.404–5) even before they go into labour. It's worth knowing, however, that labour has to be well established before you can have an epidural, so you'll still experience some painful contractions. Epidurals generally work well, but sometimes the block isn't complete or is more effective on one side than the other. Some women decide to have an epidural because they know they're unlikely to cope well with labour pain. Many women start off saying that they don't want an epidural and change their minds halfway through – if it's your first pregnancy, you can't possibly know how you'll feel.

An elective Caesarean (see pp.438–9) is one that is planned and generally performed for medical reasons – for example, because of a low-lying placenta (see p.212) – and not simply because a woman wants to have one. Having a Caesarean is major abdominal surgery and in most circumstances it is safer to have a vaginal delivery. Recovery after a Caesarean usually takes longer than after a vaginal birth, so one is only performed if necessary.

THE LOWDOWN

Tokophobia

This condition is an intense fear or dread of childbirth. There are two types: primary tokophobia pre-dates pregnancy and can start as early as adolescence; secondary tokophobia is associated with an earlier traumatic experience in childbirth. This fear can manifest itself as nightmares, intense anxiety, or panic attacks.

If you have tokophobia, your midwife will refer you to a consultant obstetrician who deals in mental health issues, or you may be referred directly to a psychologist to discuss your fears. Some experts believe that hypnotherapy can help to tackle any subconscious fears of childbirth. An elective Caesarean (see pp.438–9) may be recommended if your fear of having a natural birth cannot be overcome.

FOCUS ON... RELATIONSHIPS

Comfortable lovemaking

You may need to experiment to find lovemaking positions that are comfortable. Most women find that the missionary position becomes increasingly uncomfortable as your partner presses on your bump. You may find being on top is enjoyable and does not put pressure on your tummy. Lying in the spoons position, with your partner behind you, can also be pleasurable. Other positions that don't restrict your pleasure and are comfortable include sitting together, kneeling while your partner enters from behind, and lying side by side with your legs entwined.

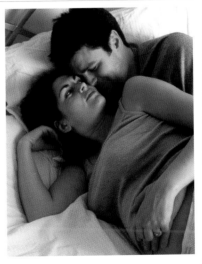

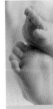

Your 32nd week

The baby won't have settled into her final birth position just yet, but an assessment of how she's lying will be made at every routine check-up. There's still room in the uterus for your baby to exercise her limbs and she's getting much stronger and more active. You'll know all about it! As your bump gets bigger, it may become more difficult to be very active and to get comfortable when you're sitting or lying down.

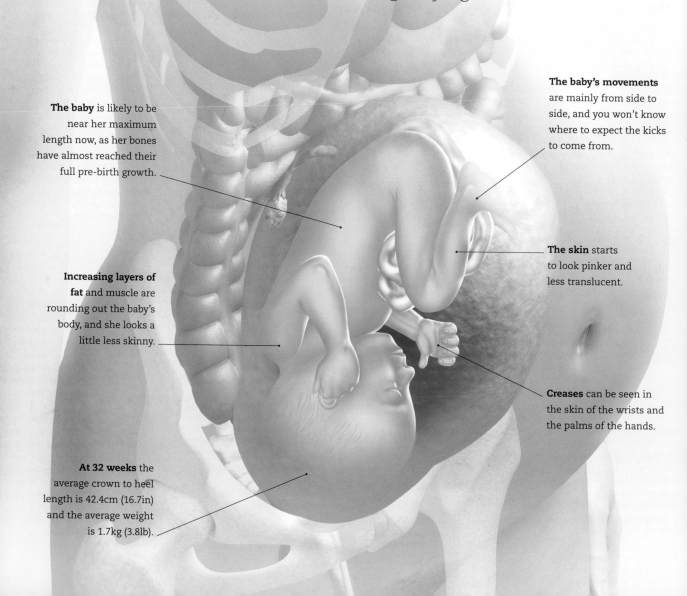

The baby is likely to be near her maximum length now, as her bones have almost reached their full pre-birth growth.

The baby's movements are mainly from side to side, and you won't know where to expect the kicks to come from.

Increasing layers of fat and muscle are rounding out the baby's body, and she looks a little less skinny.

The skin starts to look pinker and less translucent.

Creases can be seen in the skin of the wrists and the palms of the hands.

At 32 weeks the average crown to heel length is 42.4cm (16.7in) and the average weight is 1.7kg (3.8lb).

Your third trimester

318

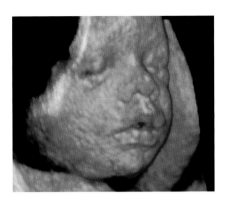

62 days to go...

YOUR BABY TODAY

The amount of amniotic fluid within the uterus reaches its maximum over the next two weeks but will then start to reduce gradually. Measurements of the four deepest pockets of amniotic fluid can add up to 15–20cm (6–8in), allowing space for your baby to move.

If you listen to music while you're pregnant, your baby will be tuning in, too – and it might just benefit her.

You might have noticed that your baby becomes more active when you're listening to music. It's been noted that unborn babies move and even breathe in time to music, and there have been claims that by exposing your baby to certain types of music, you can enhance her brain development.

One study, relating to a "Baby Mozart" brain-enhancing product, claimed that the structure of, say, a particular Mozart arrangement, stimulated brain development to a greater extent than other genres, and even other classical composers. This theory has, however,

been debunked. Some research found that college-aged students who listened to classical music showed a brief and temporary improvement in spatial intelligence. However, the same research was not tested in children or babies. The research has not been repeated and the results are open to several different interpretations.

Whether or not it enhances your baby's intelligence, listening to classical music can relax you, which is always a good thing during pregnancy. And if you gently sway to the music, your baby may enjoy being "rocked" to sleep.

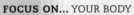
FOCUS ON... YOUR BODY

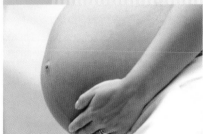

Protruding navel

You may be surprised to find that by now your perfectly formed navel is protruding. This is caused by the pressure of your rapidly expanding uterus, which presses against your abdomen and literally pops your belly button out.

Some women find their protruding navel unsightly, and choose to wear skirts or trousers with a high waistband to cover it; you can also invest in a belly band (see p.179), which keeps it all tucked in.

A protruding navel is a normal consequence of pregnancy and it will return to normal a few months after delivery. However, you may find that, like other parts of your body, your navel sags a little more than it used to.

ASK A... MIDWIFE

What exactly is an "active birth"?
Having an "active birth" – staying mobile during the first stage of labour and remaining upright, squatting, kneeling, or on all-fours during the second stage – can make labour and delivery easier and less painful. Working with gravity helps your pelvis to open and encourages the baby's head to press on your cervix, helping it to dilate. To get active:
■ **Practise squatting (see p.424):** it takes time to learn to do it, but it's an effective way to speed labour up. When squatting, make sure you

have sufficient support – from your partner, for example.
■ **Relax by kneeling** with a birth ball or beanbag.
■ **Use a birthing pool** if you want to relax in water for a while.
■ **If you need a drip,** because you've been induced (see p.432), ask for one with a long tube that will leave you free to move around a little.
■ **Choose a mobile epidural,** which should enable you to stay active.
■ **If lying down** makes your contractions stop, get up and start moving again.

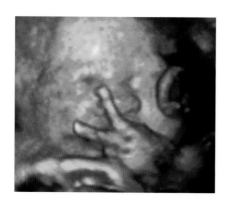

YOU ARE 31 WEEKS AND 2 DAYS

61 days to go...

YOUR BABY TODAY

Your baby's hand co-ordination continues to improve as her brain is better able to make sense of the feedback it receives. The eyes will often open but only for short periods at a time, reducing the chance of a stray finger coming too close.

By this stage, your baby is the length she'll be at birth, but she's still very thin and needs to gain fat and muscle.

At this stage of pregnancy, your baby's muscle mass and fat are continuing to increase. Her skin is now thicker and less translucent, and begins to look pink rather than red as the underlying blood vessels are overlaid with more flesh. Growth hormone is being produced by your baby's pituitary gland but before she's actually born this does not influence her growth. Instead insulin and insulin-like growth factors are key. As your baby's skeleton is now close to its final size, her overall length is established. Your baby is still, however, very skinny.

A sonographer can make a good estimate of your baby's weight from an ultrasound scan but her final birthweight will very much depend on when she is born. She'll continue to grow throughout the pregnancy, although in the last few weeks growth is mainly due to fat deposits rather than to muscle mass.

If you're trying to guess how heavy your baby will be at birth, the latest research indicates that the size of your baby has a lot to do with "imprinted" genes. These are genes that are marked as having come from the father, which promote the baby's growth, or the mother, which are growth limiting and attempt to preserve her resources.

FOCUS ON... TWINS

Dressing your babies

Twins look adorable when they're dressed alike, so you may be buying – and certainly will be given – lots of sets of matching clothing. But it's much easier to tell identical twins apart when they're dressed differently. It also helps everyone relate to them as individuals, which is good for their development.

Also keep practicalities in mind: every time one of your twins gets dirty, are you going to change them both? You may find it pays to be flexible: if there are only two clean babygros, then that is what they'll have to wear, regardless of style or colour match.

Newborns don't care what they wear, but if you get in the habit of dressing them the same, they may become conscious of it in the toddler years and get distressed if they're wearing something different.

How you dress your babies is your decision, but you could:

■ **Dress your babies in matching outfits but different colours,** or the same colours but different styles.
■ **Only dress them identically on the odd occasion,** for instance for a family photograph or special occasion.
■ **Give any identical outfits you receive to one twin.** The next batch of identical outfits goes to the other twin.

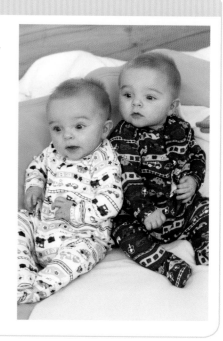

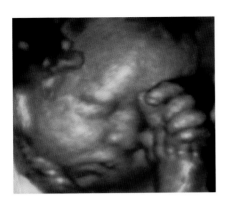

60 days to go...

YOUR BABY TODAY

Here the umbilical cord is seen lying over the baby's shoulder. This is very common; in fact at some time every baby will have the umbilical cord lying close, especially during the next few weeks while the baby frequently changes position.

Jolts and jostles are all part of being pregnant – and your baby probably won't even notice them.

ASK A... MUM

I'm finding it increasingly hard to focus at work. How can I best get through the next few weeks?

As your baby – and you – get bigger, you may find that you have less energy and your concentration span decreases accordingly. This is normal, but it can pose problems if you have a job to do! First of all, take regular breaks, putting your feet up or closing your eyes for a few minutes to rest. Make sure you drink enough, as dehydration can affect your performance. Similarly, eating healthy snacks, little and often, can keep you from flagging. Iron-rich foods, such as dried fruit, are particularly important: low iron levels can make you tire easily.

Carry a small notebook with you, and jot down anything that you need to remember, no matter how trivial. This can help to overcome lapses of memory, and keep you focused on what needs to be done. It may also help to start your day with a "to-do" list, and tick your way down it in order of priority. Finally, try to get enough sleep, which will give you at least half a chance of feeling refreshed the next morning.

Your bump is getting larger and larger. As you walk you may notice that your bump also appears to move, swaying from side to side with each step. It can be difficult to remember that you're so much bigger than you used to be. You may find yourself trying to squeeze through tight spaces, or between tables and chairs in a restaurant that previously you would have fit through and now find yourself a

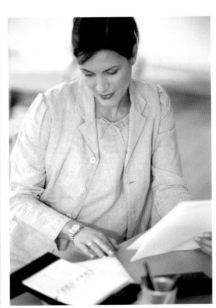

To help you focus at work keep a notebook handy and jot down everything: what to do today, what to say when you make a call, and what you need to cover in a letter or e-mail.

bit stuck! Even if you find that your bump is getting bumped around occasionally this really is nothing at all to worry about: your baby is safe, protected by the pool of amniotic fluid that acts as a cushion against the odd jolt. Soon enough you will be back to your normal shape, or nearly your normal shape, and it can be odd to think back to having to compensate for a bump.

FOCUS ON... YOUR HEALTH

Heart palpitations

Having a run of fast heartbeats, or missing a beat occasionally – or simply being acutely aware of your heartbeat – is defined as heart palpitations (see p.469). It's common to have these in late pregnancy. They are usually nothing to worry about and are simply the result of changes to your blood circulation, coupled with a large abdominal bump, although unnecessary stresses and anxieties can play a part as well.

If, however, palpitations are accompanied by chest pain or breathlessness, or if you think they are occurring more frequently, mention this to your midwife.

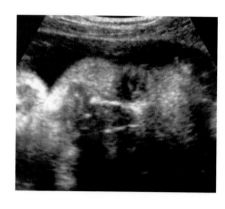

YOU ARE 31 WEEKS AND 4 DAYS

59 days to go...

YOUR BABY TODAY

Measurements around the head, abdomen, and thigh bones are used from the ultrasound image to estimate the weight of your baby. Interestingly, on average, boys are now starting to be slightly heavier than girls.

As your baby puts on muscle and its tone improves, she begins to be capable of more complex and stronger movements.

Your baby's muscle tone takes some time to develop fully. By this week of your pregnancy, head control is improving and in the legs muscle tone now allows for smoother and more complex movements. For once, the arms and hands lag behind the legs and feet in development, taking another three weeks to achieve the same level of tone and movement.

In the last few weeks the familiar "fetal position" is increasingly seen on scans: this is not only due to lack of space, but also because your baby's flexor muscles (those that bend the elbows, hips, and knees) have a better tone than her extensor muscles (the muscles that extend the arms and legs) in each limb.

You will also be aware that your baby is moving more now than at any other time. You only feel the movements that hit the lining of your uterus, but there will be many more small movements of which you are completely unaware. Movements inside the uterus are important: they help your baby's co-ordination, strengthen her bones, and increase muscle mass. The number of muscle cells increases up until 38 weeks. From this point on, individual muscle cells lengthen and expand in response to exercise, further increasing muscle mass and strength.

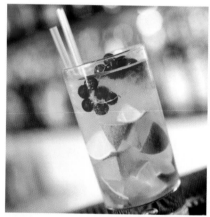

There is no need to feel left out when all around you are partying: enjoy fresh fruit juices over ice, topped with soda, tonic water, or ginger ale to add a little fizz.

NON-ALCOHOLIC DRINKS

Here are some ideas for delicious non-alcoholic drinks:
- Cranberry juice/orange juice/lemon juice/ginger ale
- Grapefruit juice/cranberry juice/soda or tonic water
- Sparkling apple juice/dash of angostura bitters/sugar to taste
- Orange juice/bitter lemon
- Lemon juice/pineapple juice/orange juice/grenadine/soda
- Diced lemon/diced lime/diced orange/ginger ale/sugar to taste
- Apple juice/pear juice/ginger ale.

ASK A... MIDWIFE

Will having an orgasm cause me to go into labour? In a pregnancy without problems, an orgasm will not cause premature labour (see p.431), and at full term orgasm will only cause the onset of labour if it's going to happen anyway. If you have had any signs of premature labour you'll be advised to avoid sexual intercourse. This is because the hormone oxytocin increases during sexual arousal, and oxytocin causes the muscles of the uterus to contract. Orgasm may increase Braxton Hicks' contractions (see p.410). You should also avoid sexual intercourse If your waters have broken, due to the risk of infection.

If you've gone past your due date and your body is ready to go into labour, sexual intercourse may help things to start for two reasons: prostaglandins in semen help the cervix soften at this stage of pregnancy, and the contractions stimulated by orgasm are more likely to develop into early labour contractions.

Your third trimester

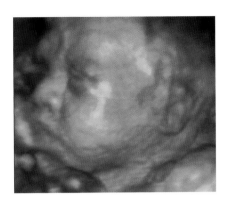

58 days to go...

YOUR BABY TODAY

This image shows a furrowed brow and an open-eyed expression. Just as the muscle tone in the limbs is strengthening, so the muscles of the face are being used and tested. This can produce some unusual expressions that do not necessarily reflect your baby's emotions.

How your baby is positioned can affect your delivery, but there is plenty of time at this stage for things to change.

Each time you are examined at an antenatal appointment your midwife will assess your baby's lie and presentation (see p.336). About 15 per cent of babies are breech at 32 weeks, but only about three or four per cent are breech by full term. This is because there is plenty of room for the baby to turn around. After about the 35th or 36th week, the baby is unlikely to change position as there is less room for large manoeuvres. Your midwife can give you advice on helping to reposition your baby (see p.329) or may suggest an external cephalic version (ECV) (see pp.364 and 433), a procedure to try to turn the baby. If your baby is breech, your midwife may recommend that you have an extra ultrasound scan at about 37–38 weeks of pregnancy to check the baby's position. It may be difficult for your midwife to be completely sure, on examination alone, whether she is feeling the baby's bottom or head.

FOCUS ON... DADS

Getting the balance right

Much of later pregnancy involves your partner doing less than normal. This may range from doing less exercise to not doing household chores. It may be challenging for your partner to realize that she's not able to do things as easily as before and, to a certain extent, is less independent.

You can be a great help to her in the final weeks of pregnancy, but be aware that there's a fine line between being supportive and being over-protective. Deep down you may want to turn into "superman" and do everything, but it might frustrate your partner if you become too over-protective. Try to take the lead from her and give her help as and when she needs it, as well as space to do her own thing.

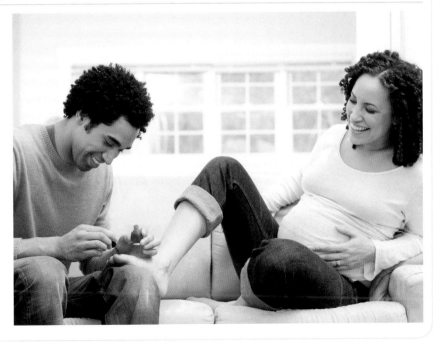

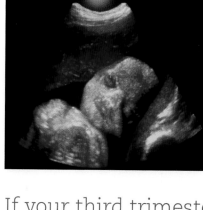

57 days to go...

YOUR BABY TODAY

You can see from this image just how much amniotic fluid is around your baby at this time. Ultrasound displays the fluid as black on the screen. Sometimes there will be speckles within the fluid: these represent skin and hair cells that are shed as your baby grows.

If your third trimester coincides with the summer months, staying cool and comfortable can be a real challenge.

When the weather is hot, your baby makes you sweltering! Keep yourself hydrated by drinking lots of cool water. Consider carrying a spray bottle of water (keep it in the fridge overnight so that it's nice and cold next day) to spritz you when you're too hot.

Opt for sleeveless clothing that is made of natural fabrics, such as linen and cotton, which will help to keep the air circulating. If you want to keep some or all of your arms covered, wear short-sleeved jackets or cotton cardigans. Wear a sun-hat and sunglasses, especially if you're in direct sunlight for any length of time.

Opt for flip-flops or low-heeled sandals to let your feet breathe – these can also be a good option if your feet are swollen (see pp.466–7).

FOCUS ON... YOUR BABY

Listening to your baby's heartbeat

From the very earliest stages of pregnancy, your baby's heart will be beating, and there can be nothing more uplifting and reassuring than hearing this for yourself. Your midwife can use a variety of instruments to hear your baby's heartbeat, including a Pinard stethoscope and a Doppler monitor, which uses ultrasound technology (see right). A baby's heart beats between 120 and 160 times per minute (with slight variations) – quite a few more than your own heartbeat, which is normally under 100. The sole purpose of listening to the heartbeat is to ensure that it falls within a normal range, and to reassure mums-to-be that all is well. If there's

an unusual rhythm or the heartbeat speeds or slows unexpectedly, your doctor or midwife can arrange for tests to confirm that all is well. Some women feel that hearing their baby's heartbeat helps the bonding process in advance of the birth.

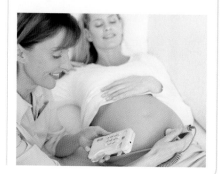

THE LOWDOWN

First hours and days

To help you prepare for what will follow the birth of your baby, here are a few interesting facts you might like to know:

■ **You may shake all over** just after giving birth and don't be concerned if you vomit; this is quite normal and nothing to worry about.

■ **Newborn babies don't always master breastfeeding** (see pp.448–9) straightaway. Just like you, they need to practise.

■ **Afterpains** (the clamping sensation in your uterus when your baby suckles) can hurt almost as much as contractions.

■ **The first time you urinate** and defecate after giving birth can be uncomfortable.

■ **You may feel very vulnerable,** and in need of your own mum, in the first few days of parenthood.

■ **Lochia (after-birth bleeding)** can be a challenge at first, even if you're using larger-sized sanitary towels.

■ **Bonding with a newborn doesn't always happen** immediately for all mothers, but it's worth the wait.

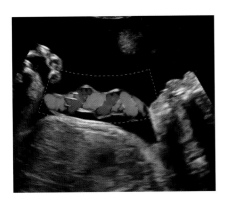

56 days to go...

YOUR BABY TODAY

The blood flow in the umbilical cord is highlighted in this image. The colours show the direction of flow. The smaller umbilical arteries that carry blood towards the placenta are seen in blue as they wrap around the more central umbilical vein (coloured red).

The best way to make sure you get enough sleep is to find ways to slow down mentally and relax.

You may find that you're having difficulty sleeping, partly because your bump makes it uncomfortable to lie down in certain positions, but also because you have lots to think about at the moment. Try to take some time out with your partner each evening relaxing and bonding together with your bump. Even spending 10 minutes doing nothing except focusing on yourself, your body, your partner, and your baby can be invigorating and rejuvenating.

Get yourself in a comfortable position, and try to focus inwards on your body, turning your mind away from all your external worries. First focus on slowing down your breathing. Then turn your thoughts to a place and a time when you felt relaxed and happy – for example, when you were on holiday, walking on the beach. Next focus on clenching and then relaxing each set of muscles in turn, or imagine a ball of heat passing slowly through your limbs and body making them feel warm, heavy, and relaxed.

You might like to involve your partner: perhaps he could sit with you with his hands or head on your bump and try to adjust his breathing so it's in sync with yours. Just lying next to your partner, even without talking, can relax you and bring you close together.

DRESSING FOR EXERCISE

In this last trimester, dressing appropriately for exercise can make all the difference to your activities and the way that you feel.

During pregnancy it is possible to look good in your workout clothes, while still supporting your bump and your breasts. Ensure you wear the correct size clothes – trying to squeeze into a size you outgrew three months ago will be uncomfortable and restricting.

There are some great pregnancy exercise ranges on the market, which are cut well and have ample room for your bump. If, however, you'd rather

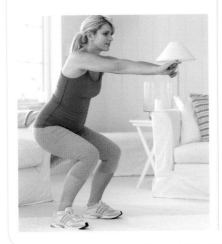

cover up while you're exercising, just wear a large T-shirt and baggy tracksuit bottoms or loose-fitting shorts. Wear whatever makes you feel confident and comfortable.

There are some good support belts available, which may make your cardiovascular exercise that much more comfortable. If you're carrying twins or more this will be even more of a welcome addition to your workout wardrobe. Most of the support belts are made from elasticized fabric with Velcro fastenings that can be adjusted to suit your bump size. Alternatively, wind a crepe bandage around your pelvic region – just under your bump – to support its weight.

Your breasts will need additional support by this stage of pregnancy, but especially when you're exercising. A well-fitting sports bra is vital for any activity as the delicate breast tissue can weaken due to the increased pressure of your larger and heavier breasts. If your breasts are very large, and you feel they're unsupported by just wearing a sports bra, try wearing it on top of your usual bra.

Your 33rd week

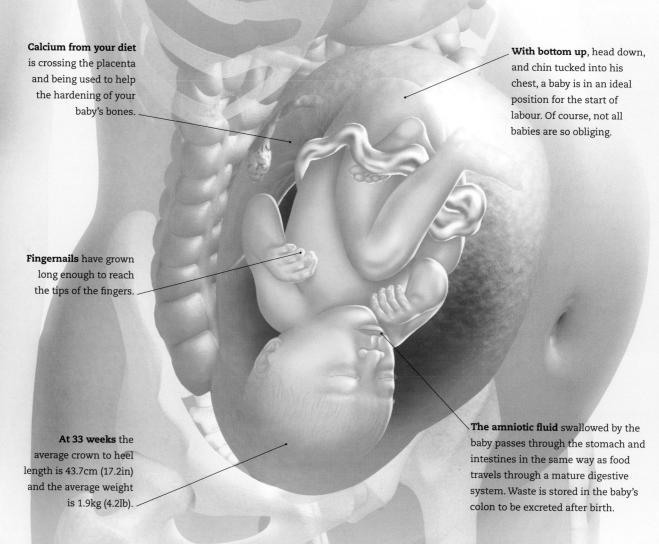

IT'S HARD TO IMAGINE HOW LIFE WILL BE WITH A NEW BABY

All prospective mums, and not just first-timers, find it difficult to envisage the future after the arrival of the baby. The imaginings, dreams, and hopes of the last few months are about to become realities – which may be very different from what you expect. You may find that it helps to concentrate on practical matters, such as the birth celebrations and future childcare. You could make plans for recovering your pre-pregnancy figure. The bump won't be with you forever, even if it feels like it!

Calcium from your diet is crossing the placenta and being used to help the hardening of your baby's bones.

With bottom up, head down, and chin tucked into his chest, a baby is in an ideal position for the start of labour. Of course, not all babies are so obliging.

Fingernails have grown long enough to reach the tips of the fingers.

At 33 weeks the average crown to heel length is 43.7cm (17.2in) and the average weight is 1.9kg (4.2lb).

The amniotic fluid swallowed by the baby passes through the stomach and intestines in the same way as food travels through a mature digestive system. Waste is stored in the baby's colon to be excreted after birth.

Your third trimester

326

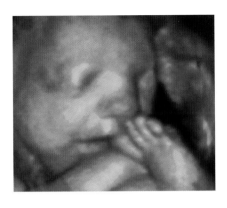

55 days to go...

YOUR BABY TODAY

In this image the hands are folded over beneath the chin and there's a foot up by the mouth and nose. It can look as if your baby is quite a contortionist but because he is still quite skinny, the joints allow for a great deal of flexibility.

If you feel you have little control over your own body, it's natural to think your figure will never be normal again – but it will!

At this stage of the third trimester, you'll still be gaining 0.5–1kg (1–2lb) per week but weight gain tends to slow down in the last few weeks of pregnancy. By now, your tummy will have stretched and your belly button may have popped out – this can be quite protruding and may be seen through your clothes (see p.319). In your second trimester you may have developed a linea nigra, a dark line of pigmentation down the centre of your abdomen (see p.170).

Like most women you are probably happy and excited about having a baby but a little concerned about getting your figure back after the birth. Some women get quite upset at the thought that their stomachs may not return to their previous shape, and this is completely normal. Rest assured that with a bit of hard work and exercise and the continuation of your healthy pregnancy diet after the birth, your figure can return to its pre-pregnancy state and your belly button should pop back to its normal shape of its own accord. The key is to remember it will take a bit of time: it did, after all, take nine months to gain the weight.

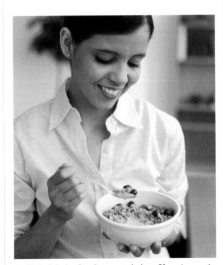

A diet rich in foods containing fibre is good for health at any time of life but especially during these three months as it helps to prevent the common problem of constipation. Snack on wholegrain breads and cereals.

ASK A... MIDWIFE

I want to work right up to the birth – is that allowed? Yes, you can do this, but you may need a doctor's medical certificate to confirm that you are fit to do so. Think carefully before making this decision. Late pregnancy can be extremely tiring and, if your job is mentally and/or physically taxing, it may be better to begin your leave before your due date. You will also need time to prepare for the arrival of your baby.

FOCUS ON... NUTRITION

Fabulous fibre

Fibre is very important in the third trimester, since it will help your digestive system work more efficiently. Dietary fibre – the indigestible part of plant foods – is the best natural way to keep the bowels regular. Most pregnant women who eat a diet based on wholegrains, fruits, and vegetables, are likely to be getting enough fibre.

Pregnant women should aim for 25g (1oz) of fibre daily. To give a sense of what it takes to achieve this, there are around 3g in a medium avocado or banana, or a serving of broccoli, blueberries, brown rice, or beans. Eating three or four servings of fruit a day, vegetables with your meals, and eating wholegrain breads and brown rice will provide plenty.

Fibre makes you feel fuller sooner and for longer, and can help to prevent over-eating and excess weight gain. It also contributes to the management of diabetes, lowers cholesterol, and decreases the risk of heart disease.

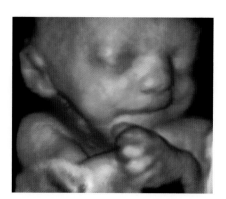

YOU ARE 32 WEEKS AND 2 DAYS

54 days to go...

YOUR BABY TODAY

During this week your baby's fingernails have become fully developed and now approach the tips of the fingers. Bathed in amniotic fluid, the nails are kept very soft: it's only after birth that your baby might tend to scratch and need to wear mittens.

Every 40 minutes, your baby swallows enough amniotic fluid to fill his stomach, before emptying it back into the amniotic sac.

Your baby is swallowing and recycling almost half a litre (18fl oz) of amniotic fluid each day. As well as providing him with nutrients, especially proteins, this fluid is important for the healthy development of the gut. Your baby's sense of taste is thought to have developed to such an extent now that if you have eaten spiced food he can distinguish this in the fluid he drinks.

Amniotic fluid does not enter the lungs but travels down the oesophagus into the stomach where it is stored for a short time. At this stage, the stomach fills every 40 minutes, but, from 35 weeks, as the stomach enlarges, this rate slows down to every 80 minutes. Muscle contractions move the fluid in waves into the small and then large bowel. As it travels along the bowel, water is reabsorbed so that only waste material or "meconium", enters the colon, the final section of the large bowel. This meconium accumulates in the large bowel, which is completely full by the time your baby is born. Babies don't usually pass meconium before the birth but do so soon after. Meconium consists mainly of skin cells, lanugo hairs, and vernix. It has a greenish colour due to the presence of bilirubin, a breakdown product from red blood cells.

FOCUS ON... THE BIRTH

False alarms

In the next few weeks, as you and your partner await your baby's arrival, you may experience one or two false alarms, especially if it's your first baby. A false alarm can come at any time of the day or night and it won't respect important meetings or deadlines.

It can help if you – as well as your partner – familiarize yourself with all the signs that indicate labour may be starting (see pp. 409–11). If, however, you're ever in doubt, do contact your midwife to ascertain that labour has not started, rather than assuming that this is the case. She will be very experienced in dealing with false alarms and won't mind you contacting her.

ITCHY SKIN

Having itchy skin on your bump is common: as the skin there stretches and thins, it can become dry. You could try using a moisturizing lotion to soothe this.

If, however, you have severe itching on your abdomen, or on the palms of your hands or soles of your feet, see your doctor. This itching can be a sign of obstetric cholestasis (see p.473), a rare pregnancy condition involving the liver, which causes bile salts to enter the bloodstream, making the skin (especially on the hands and feet) itchy, although there is no rash. The condition may also cause a vitamin K deficiency. Vitamin K helps the blood to clot, so a deficiency increases the risk of bleeding for both mother and baby. Medication to bind the bile salts and vitamin K supplements are effective treatments. Some studies suggest early induction of labour (at around 37 weeks) helps to avoid complications. The condition resolves after delivery, usually without any long-term liver damage.

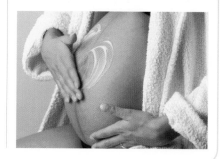

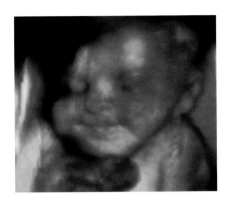

53 days to go...

YOUR BABY TODAY

Your baby's position in the uterus is influenced by your own posture. Gravity has some effect on your baby, so whether you are standing or sitting, and which side you lie down on affects the way your baby's back is turned and which side he rolls onto.

As your abdomen grows, it's normal to feel you want to support your bump when you're walking around.

You've probably had to change the way that you exercise by now due to your growing abdomen. You may well have had to replace jogging on the treadmill, for example, with going for long, brisk (or not so brisk!) walks. If you find that even walking makes your tummy and pelvis sore or uncomfortable, you may find you naturally hold up your bump with your hands to try to give it some extra support and to give your pelvis and back a break. Some women say it feels as if the baby "might fall out".

You might want to invest in a pregnancy support band; made of stretchy fabric, this useful item supports the bump and can help to prevent lower back pain.

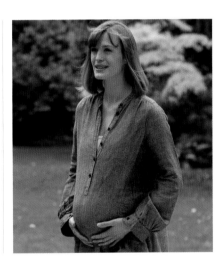

Walking at a comfortable pace when you are heavily pregnant will cause your bump to shift around and your instinct may be to support your baby with your hands.

BUYING A BABY MONITOR

Baby monitors first appeared in the UK in the early 1980s and today there is a huge range of different models on the market, so choosing one can be daunting. Although monitors vary, they have the same basic components – a minimum of two units: one to transmit your baby's sounds, and one that stays with you so that you can hear if your baby is crying or fussing.

Additional features include: a moving lights-sound display, low power and out-of-range warnings, the option to use mains or batteries, a talk-back function, and a temperature sensor. Some have a night light function. With all these features available, your choice largely depends on your personal preferences and your budget.

FOCUS ON... YOUR BABY

Repositioning your baby

Your movements during late pregnancy can affect the position of your baby. Ideally, he'll lie head down, facing your back, with his chin tucked into his chest. You can encourage this optimum fetal position by:
■ **Spending time on all fours,** wiggling your hips from side to side; or arch your back, then drop your spine down.
■ **Sitting with your knees lower than your pelvis,** and your body tilted slightly forwards.
■ **Kneeling on the floor,** leaning over a beanbag, cushions, or birth ball.
■ **Sitting on a birth ball,** with your legs positioned slightly apart and knees lower than your hips, then rocking your pelvis.
■ **Assuming the tailor pose:** sit on the floor with your back straight and the soles of your feet together. Let your knees fall to the side and rest your elbows on your inner thighs.
■ **Swimming:** breaststroke helps to open the pelvis.

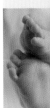

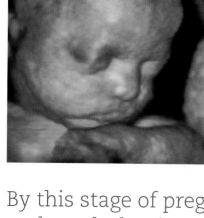

52 days to go...

YOUR BABY TODAY

This image shows that the bridge of your baby's nose is now more fully formed. The face is taking on a more rounded shape and some babies may look quite chubby from now on. Shadows around the top and sides of the head will increasingly give the illusion of hair.

By this stage of pregnancy, your baby's fingernails have grown and reach the tips of his fingers.

By now, your baby's fingernails have reached the tips of the fingers. The fingernails first appeared at 23 weeks, and as the development of the arms is consistently ahead of the legs, the toenails started to develop four weeks later. The future nail begins at the tip of each finger or toe, where a nail fold is formed. At the base of this nail fold, the cells start to harden into nail, in a process known as keratinization. The nails grow from new cells formed in the soft nail bed. It takes nine weeks for the nails to reach the fingertips and it will be a further four weeks before the toenails reach the tips of the toes.

The nail is actually all the same colour, but the white part of the nail appears white because it does not have the nail bed, with its rich blood supply, beneath it to give the illusion of colour. Since the nails already reach the fingertips, it probably won't be long after the birth before your baby's nails need trimming – they are very fine and soft and you may find it easier to trim them by nibbling them away rather than trying to cut them. Or cut them with baby nail scissors while your baby is asleep and not wriggling around.

FOCUS ON... YOUR BODY

Yoga is excellent exercise for the mind and body while you're pregnant, and may be a cornerstone of your birth preparations if you choose to take active birth classes (see p.333). An instructor will tailor a routine for your body and the stage of your pregnancy. The individual stretches shown below are ideal for opening up the pelvis and strengthening the legs. By practising them while you're pregnant, you'll be able to use them more effectively and confidently during labour. When you're practising squatting, it may help if your partner supports you from behind.

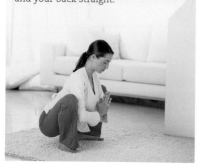

Get into a squatting position. Squat only if you find it easy to hold this position with your heels on the floor and your back straight.

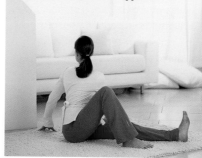

Sit with your left leg stretched out in front of you and right leg bent. Gently twist your body, placing your hands on the floor for additional support.

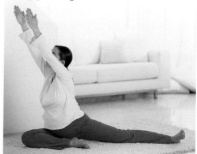

Sit with one leg stretched out behind you, and the other tucked beneath your bump. Stretch upwards, breathing deeply throughout.

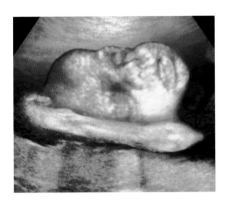

51 days to go...

YOUR BABY TODAY

In this image of the baby lying on his side, the arm is positioned beneath the head and is partly outside of the 3D view, allowing structures within the arm to be seen. Part of the bones in the elbow and forearm show here as bright reflections.

To get used to the fact that your newborn will arrive very soon, start focusing on life after the birth.

Friends and family might now begin talking about what will happen after the birth and what it will be like for you to have a baby.

If this is your first baby, you probably can't really envisage what it will be like to be a mum, and even if you have had a baby before you've never had a second or third and so don't know what it will be like to have another one. Of course you know that life will carry on, but it can be difficult to see past the labour to the realities of life with a newborn. As ever, keep talking to those close to you about how you feel, be it excited or scared and unprepared (usually all three in rapid succession). Talk about what you think or hope it will be like after the baby is born, for example when are grandparents and other key people going to visit, and whether you would like a christening or naming party – or perhaps neither of these. This may help you to get used to the idea that not only are you pregnant but there is a baby coming.

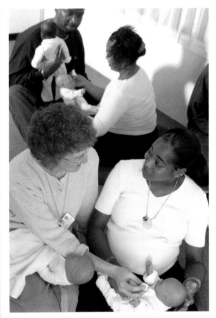

Antenatal classes are a wonderful opportunity to swap ideas and information with a group of people in the same position as you. Long-term friendships can be made here.

ASK A... MIDWIFE

How will I benefit from going to antenatal classes? You'll get the opportunity to share information, ideas, fears, and concerns about childbirth in a comfortable environment, and to discuss and decide upon issues that will affect the way you choose to give birth. You'll also meet other parents-to-be. Often friendships formed at classes continue after the birth as you support each other in your new parenting role. In most classes, you'll be given advice about:

■ **Tried-and-tested labour techniques,** such as breathing through the pain, massage, suitable sustenance, and some positive visualization exercises

■ **Pain-relief options** and a range of natural alternatives (see pp.396–407)

■ **How to present** (and preserve) your birth plan (see p.303)

■ **The practical and emotional support** a birth partner can offer

■ **The items required** for a hospital or home birth (see pp.341 and 358).

You'll be advised on how to prepare yourself for the birth, what to expect in the first few days, and how to encourage healing afterwards, as well as being given tips on looking after a newborn, including nappy-changing, bathing, and establishing breastfeeding.

AS A MATTER OF FACT

In a first birth, the cervix dilates by about 0.5cm every hour, compared to 1.5cm every hour for subsequent babies.

First-time mums push for around an hour, compared with about half an hour for a second baby.

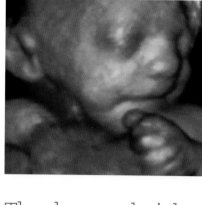

YOU ARE 32 WEEKS AND 6 DAYS

50 days to go...

YOUR BABY TODAY

This image may show the start of a smile. Your baby will often be smiling, sticking his tongue out, and pulling all sorts of faces. He may also still be experiencing hiccups, which may be something that you are now becoming aware of.

The days and nights fly by with a newborn, so it's a good idea to start thinking about childcare well before you need it.

It may seem impossible to believe that you should be considering childcare before your baby is even born, but it can be useful to think through the options while you have the time. There are two main types of childcare: in and out of your home. In the first case, you can have a live-in or live-out nanny or mother's help, an au pair (which may be acceptable if you work from home, for example, and can supervise), or perhaps a family member or friend who is prepared to come to your house to look after your baby. If you choose outside childcare, there are a number of options including nurseries, daycare centres, workplace crèches, childminders, and

even relatives in their own homes. Before you set your heart on one particular type of care, it's a good idea to investigate the costs and the availability in your area. You may wish to pay a visit to some of the nurseries or other facilities near to you, just to get a feel for what's on offer, and establish now what you do and don't want. Secondly, remember that good-quality childcare facilities and carers are usually in demand, and, even if you aren't entirely sure when you will be going back to work, it's probably a good idea to put your baby's name (or surname, at least!) down for a few, to give you options when the time comes.

CALCIUM INTAKE

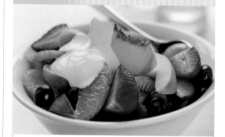

Your baby's skeleton began forming at the end of the first trimester, but the majority of your calcium is transferred to the baby from your body in the third trimester. This happens regardless of your calcium intake. If a mother-to-be's diet is low in calcium, it will be taken from the reservoir in her bones, which can affect her bone density.

The recommended amount of calcium in pregnancy is 800mg daily. Calcium needs to be accompanied by vitamin D in order to be absorbed by the body.

Dairy products are a rich source of calcium, and some, such as margarine and low-fat spreads, are often fortified with vitamin D. Vegetarian sources of calcium include tofu, leafy green vegetables, dried fruit, seeds, and nuts.

FOCUS ON... DADS

Being at the birth

Many dads-to-be are anxious about being with their partners during labour and birth. This is often because they will be witnessing their partner experience one of the most intense things a woman can ever do and they may be unsure of how to help.

There are plenty of ways in which you can support your partner during labour: being aware of her wishes, speaking for her if she is unable to,

and repeating what midwives and doctors have said if she didn't hear clearly; passing her a drink; rubbing her back; holding a flannel to her face; switching music on or off; being encouraging and reassuring her.

Attending antenatal classes can be useful (see p.331). You will learn more about labour and birth, and how to support your partner physically and emotionally.

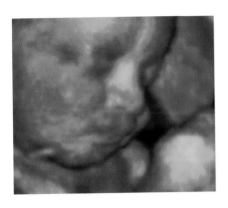

49 days to go...

YOUR BABY TODAY

Soon your baby will be approaching a time when the lungs can fully support him after birth. At 33 weeks though, most babies would still need some help with breathing if born this early. You baby will be regularly practising breathing movements inside.

Choosing who will be present at the birth with you is a big decision, so start thinking about it in good time.

You can choose whoever you like to be your birth partner, though the labour ward staff might object if you have a team of people! If you do want more than one partner, get approval ahead of the birth and put this in your birth plan (see pp.181 and 303). You may want to ask your mum, sister, or close friend in addition to your partner. You might also find that your partner is unable to be there, for example if he is unavoidably going to be out of the country. If you're comfortable with it and feel that you will benefit from someone else being there, then ask away. You can put who you want to be

your birth partner or partners on your birth plan. Of course, if you're going to ask someone else apart from or in addition to your partner to be present, discuss it with him first. He might not be so thrilled at the idea of your mum being present, but explain why you would like her there. Remember that this is a special occasion for him as well and he may have his own preferences for who is or is not present at the birth.

Now might also be a good time to discuss things like whether you want a video made of the birth, but you may prefer your partner to be supporting you, rather than handling the camera!

(see pp.181 and 303)

TIME TO THINK ABOUT

Active birth classes

The aim of active birth classes is to make women feel good about their bodies and give them the confidence that they have the mental and physical reserves to have a successful birth experience. Classes are generally suitable regardless of fitness level, flexibility, and your stage of pregnancy.

■ **Active birth classes** promote the benefits of yoga and exercise as both physical and mental preparation for childbirth.
■ **Yoga strengthens the body,** improves posture and circulation, and teaches how to use relaxation and breathing techniques to relieve stress.
■ **Like antenatal classes,** active birth classes allow you to meet other parents-to-be and share their pregnancy experiences.
■ **The downside of active birth classes** is that not all NHS trusts run them and finding classes can be difficult. They can get booked up quickly and can be quite expensive. Ask your midwife if she has details of any local active birth classes.

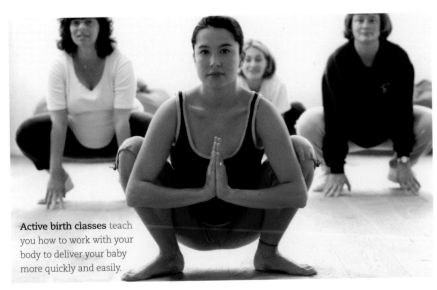

Active birth classes teach you how to work with your body to deliver your baby more quickly and easily.

Your 34th week

YOUR BABY IS ALMOST FULLY EQUIPPED FOR THE OUTSIDE WORLD

If your baby was born this week, she'd still need some help with breathing and feeding. But it's reassuring to know that basically she's in pretty good shape for survival. However, you are unlikely to go into labour this early. Now is your chance to start practising the relaxation and pain-relieving exercises that you've been learning at your antenatal classes. The more familiar you are with the techniques, the more they will help you during labour.

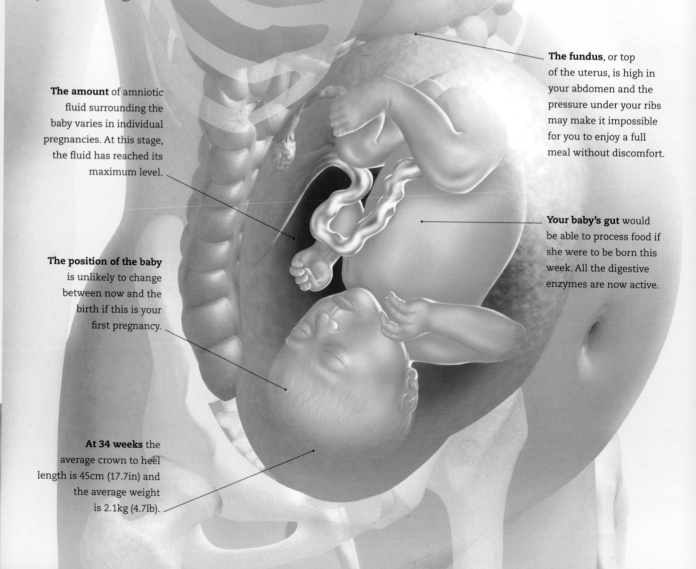

The amount of amniotic fluid surrounding the baby varies in individual pregnancies. At this stage, the fluid has reached its maximum level.

The position of the baby is unlikely to change between now and the birth if this is your first pregnancy.

At 34 weeks the average crown to heel length is 45cm (17.7in) and the average weight is 2.1kg (4.7lb).

The fundus, or top of the uterus, is high in your abdomen and the pressure under your ribs may make it impossible for you to enjoy a full meal without discomfort.

Your baby's gut would be able to process food if she were to be born this week. All the digestive enzymes are now active.

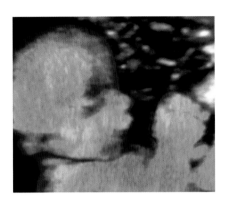

48 days to go...

YOUR BABY TODAY

Your baby may well be head down by this stage. The head is the heaviest part and gravity plus the shape of your womb favours a head-down position. Ask your midwife or doctor at the next clinic visit if she can determine the position for you.

Premature labour is highly likely in a twin pregnancy, so your antenatal carers will be on alert and monitoring you closely.

There are still six weeks to go until the due date for a single pregnancy, but if you're expecting twins they may arrive any time from now. Thirty-seven weeks is considered full term for twins, and about half are born before this date. Women expecting twins are at higher risk of high blood pressure, pre-eclampsia, placental insufficiency, gestational diabetes, and premature labour. That said, many women do go on to deliver twins naturally and many consultants will allow you to continue to 40 weeks, after which time an induction is offered.

If the babies are in any position other than "head down", or the placenta is in an awkward position, such as near the neck of the uterus, a Caesarean may be recommended. Some consultants prefer to deliver twins by Caesarean

because the second twin may run into difficulties during the delivery, particularly if she is not head down. Premature babies are more at risk of complications than those who go to full-term. A Caesarean delivery ensures the babies are delivered quickly without having to go through hours of potentially stressful labour.

If your babies share a placenta or a sac, induction or a Caesarean will be suggested at 34–37 weeks, possibly because one baby is not growing as well as the other (see p.130).

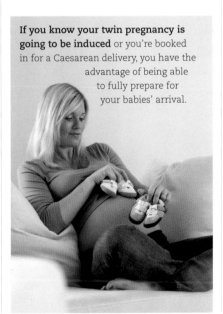

If you know your twin pregnancy is going to be induced or you're booked in for a Caesarean delivery, you have the advantage of being able to fully prepare for your babies' arrival.

AS A MATTER OF FACT

The average birth weight of twins is 2.5kg (5lb 8oz).

This is compared to 3.5kg (7lb 8oz) for singleton babies. It's not unusual for there to be a difference in birth weight between the babies. The average weight of a triplet is 1.8kg (4lb) and of a quadruplet 1.4kg (3lb).

ASK A... DOCTOR

I'm having my twins in a couple of weeks. Can they sleep in the same cot? Having shared the same tight space in the uterus for many months, it seems natural to allow twin newborns to sleep together and, in fact, research indicates that it may have some benefits. Not only has it been found to be safe for twins of roughly the same size to sleep together until three months of age, but one study found that putting newborn twins in the same cot helped to regulate their body temperature and their sleep cycles.

They can be placed side by side, or head to head. Ideally each should have her own set of covers, to avoid overheating. Like single babies, twins should be put to sleep in the safe sleeping position, on their backs (see p.444).

You can purchase a double cot, which will last until your twins are old enough to move to a bed, but many experts believe that twins should be given their own sleeping space from three months, so that they can be given individual attention and the opportunity to develop their own sleep patterns.

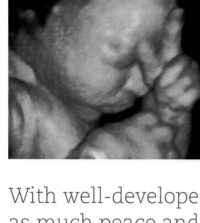

47 days to go...

YOUR BABY TODAY

Shadows give the impression of hair on the eyebrows and eyelashes on this 3D image. Because this baby was lying head down, the view of the top part of the head is lost in the shadows caused by the mother's pelvis.

With well-developed hearing, your baby may not be getting as much peace and quiet as she would like in the uterus.

Although some quieter high-pitched sounds don't penetrate the uterus, it is not quite as peaceful for your baby as you might think. There will be a constant background noise produced by your heart beating, your breathing, and your stomach rumbling. The uterus and amniotic fluid will prevent many quieter sounds from reaching your baby, but voices do penetrate quite easily. Your baby has already learnt to adapt to repetitive sounds but is now acquiring a memory for familiar noises. The most familiar sound is, of course, your voice. Your baby will startle and turn towards loud or unfamiliar sounds and these will also cause her heart rate to increase.

FOCUS ON... YOUR BABY

Lie and presentation

Your baby's lie and presentation will be assessed by your midwife at every antenatal appointment.

Your baby's "lie" means which way round she is lying, vertically or horizontally – a horizontal lie is known as transverse. The "presentation" refers to which part of the baby is nearest the pelvis, and would come out first.

The most common presentation is head down, bottom up, called a cephalic presentation (see right). Breech presentation (see far right) is when the baby is bottom or feet down with the head upwards. A footling breech means that the baby is head up, with one leg and foot extended downwards while the other is tucked in. In an anterior presentation, your baby's head is down and faces your back. In a posterior presentation, your baby's head faces your tummy, which can prolong labour and may increase the chances of an assisted delivery. (See also p.388)

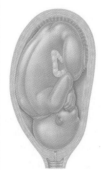 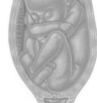

Cephalic presentation   **Breech presentation**

ASK A... MIDWIFE

What is perineal massage and how do I do it? Spending just five minutes a day massaging your perineum (the area between the vagina and anus) with oil could reduce your risk of tearing or having an episiotomy (see p.427) during the birth. It also means you're less likely to experience pain in that sensitive spot postnatally – even after an episiotomy.

Here's how to do it:

■ Wash your hands. Apply a pure cold-pressed oil, such as olive oil, to your perineum and your thumbs, then slide both thumbs about an inch inside the vagina. Gently stretch the vagina until you feel a slight stinging sensation.

■ When you feel that sensation, hold the pressure steady until you no longer feel the stinging. Then gently massage the lower half of the vagina with your thumbs. With your thumbs hooked in the vagina, pull forwards to stretch the skin as you massage.

■ Not sure you're doing the first part properly? Insert your fingers into the corners of your mouth and pull your mouth open to the sides for a similar "burning" sensation.

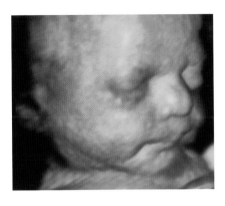

46 days to go...

YOUR BABY TODAY

At this stage it is simply no longer possible to see the whole baby on a scan. The ultrasound scan cannot step far enough back to include the whole baby in a single view. Instead it is necessary to move the probe around, to examine one area at a time.

Most women want to wait as long as possible to start maternity leave, but you must make the decision that is right for you.

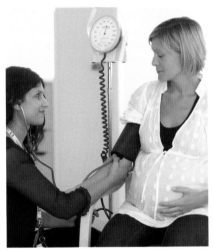

Your blood pressure will be monitored regularly at this stage as a high reading can be a sign of pre-eclampsia (see p.474).

There is generally no risk in working up to the final month of your pregnancy. Like many women you may decide to work up to around 37 weeks, but, by this week you are highly likely to find it increasingly tiring. If you are feeling exhausted and think you want to start your leave sooner, speak to your manager without delay. Hopefully, he or she will be understanding, although legally a manager can insist that you give the full 28 days notice before you start your maternity leave (see pp.348–9). Be aware that if you're struggling to cope with the discomforts of late pregnancy and decide to take sick leave during the last four weeks, your employer can also insist that you start your maternity leave early, from the time of your sick leave.

Another desirable option is to work flexi-time, so that you can travel at a less busy time and, if it's possible with your type of employment, work from home sometimes to cut out some of the commuting.

FOCUS ON... YOUR HEALTH

Essential checks

Some of the regular tests you will have in the third trimester are designed to check for pre-eclampsia (see p.474). A combination of high (or rising) blood pressure and protein in your urine can be an indication of pre-eclampsia; another sign of this condition is extreme swelling, particularly of the face and/or ankles.

ASK A... MIDWIFE

Will I have to give back my maternity pay if I decide not to return to work? This is a little bit complicated, and it's worth getting some legal advice.

In a nutshell, if you do not wish to return to work after your maternity leave, you must resign, and you must give the notice required by your contract. So, if you have an eight-week notice period, you must resign eight weeks before the end of your maternity leave. You can string this out a little by including unused holiday allowances.

If you don't give your notice until the date you are due to return to work, you'll theoretically be obliged to work out your notice period.

In terms of maternity pay, it's really up to your employer. You do not need to return SMP (statutory maternity pay) if you resign. If you did, however, receive maternity pay beyond this, you'll need to look at your contract. In most cases, you are legally obliged to repay contractually agreed maternity payments; however, many employers will not request this.

You are also entitled to be paid for outstanding holiday that has accrued during your maternity leave, which may reduce the sum you need to repay a little.

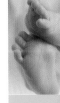

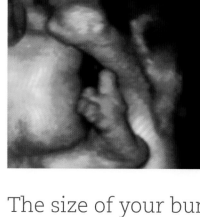

45 days to go...

YOUR BABY TODAY

A foot is shown here with the toes spread out. Not all of the movements that you feel will be due to kicks; some movements will be shrugs or punches and some will come from the bottom or head as it touches the sides of the uterus.

The size of your bump will increasingly be due to the baby alone as the amniotic fluid now reduces slightly each week.

The amount of amniotic fluid that surrounds and protects your baby is now at its maximum and the placenta has almost completed its growth.

Amniotic fluid is essential for your baby's lung development, gut maturation, protein requirements, and temperature control. Adequate fluid also allows your baby to move easily since she is in an almost weightless state. There is about 1 litre (35fl oz) of fluid around your baby. The range, however, is quite wide and "normal" can be anywhere from 300ml to 2 litres (11–70fl oz). Sometimes there is too little fluid surrounding the baby, a condition called oligohydramnios (see p.473), or too much fluid, called polyhydramnios (see p.473). In this situation you would be closely monitored and premature delivery might be necessary.

It's not surprising that the size of your uterus may not reflect the size of your baby as there can be so much variation in the quantity of fluid.

As the amount of amniotic fluid reduces in late pregnancy, your baby is not as well cushioned and her movements may become more obvious, although you should bear in mind that increasingly, as she grows, she has less space in which to move around.

AS A MATTER OF FACT

One of the most common concerns for women in late pregnancy is that their waters will break in public.

The reality is that the amniotic fluid is unlikely to gush out. It is much more likely to trickle out because in a head-down position, the baby will press down on the cervix and prevent the liquid from escaping. If it does happen in public, don't worry – you won't be short of people to help you.

FOCUS ON... DADS

What's in your hospital bag?

Once your partner's labour begins, your attention will need to be focused on helping her both practically and emotionally. So as well as helping your partner prepare her maternity bag (see p.358) in advance, it's a good idea to prepare a bag of your own.

Understandably, dads are not always well supported in delivery units, and certainly don't get fed. You'll also find that you're at the hospital for several hours.

Consider packing the following:
- Snacks
- Drinks
- A pillow
- Something to read or play
- A reasonable amount of change to pay for car parking and to buy tea, coffee, and soft drinks if they're in vending machines
- A list of phone numbers, or enter them into your mobile phone now
- A camera.

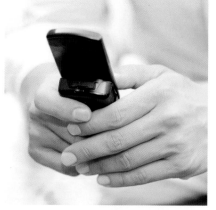

Text messaging is an effective way to inform some family and friends about the birth. Make sure you've entered all the numbers into your phone before the big day.

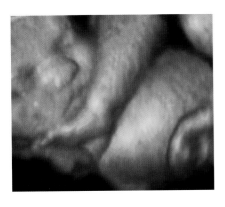

44 days to go...

YOUR BABY TODAY

At this stage your baby may lie transversely (see p.336) across your uterus as here, but such a position becomes increasingly less likely as the pregnancy advances. The more babies you have had the more likely it is that the shape of your uterus allows this lie.

You may be learning breathing and relaxation techniques at antenatal classes, but practise them at home, too.

When you are tense and frightened, pain can feel much worse, so teaching yourself to relax and stay calm can help. With around six weeks to go, you still have plenty of time to try out some of the breathing and relaxation techniques that will help you during labour. It's true that practice makes perfect and it can take some time to train your mind to relax at will, especially if you are in pain.

Spend a short period of time as often as you can, every day if possible, practising your breathing – close your eyes and slow your breathing down, breathing in through your nose and out through your mouth. As you breathe in, imagine your breath entering your body and relaxing you and as you exhale you

breathe out any pain or tension. You might want to involve your partner by asking him to breathe with you or count your breathing, a slow count to three or five for every inhale and exhale.

Some women like to practise using the techniques while pinching their arm temporarily to simulate a contraction – although of course it won't mimic the pain exactly! Practising these techniques in a calm, relaxed manner in late pregnancy will help you to use them effectively on the big day.

A banana is a fabulous fruit to eat before exercising because it gives you a slow and steady release of energy.

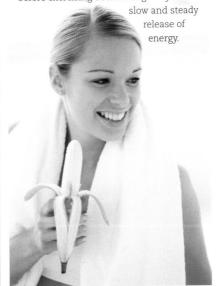

AS A MATTER OF FACT

You're more likely to get a seat on public transport in Japan due to the "manners squadron"!

If you find that no one gives up their seat for you on public transport, you're not alone. In Japan, however, the "manners squadron" mission is to patrol trains and make sure that any seats are vacated by the young and offered to those who need them.

FOCUS ON... NUTRITION

Fuel for fitness

Demand for nutrients is higher when you're exercising and even higher when you're pregnant. This is not the time to reach for low-nutrient, high-calorie snacks; ensure you make careful choices when it comes to the nutrients you put into your body.

You should be eating a snack before you exercise, consisting of a complex carbohydrate and a protein. You should also eat frequent small meals and snacks if you are feeling hungry. It's fine to snack throughout the day.

Some healthy snack ideas are as follows:
- Half a bagel spread with two teaspoons of peanut butter
- An apple or banana and a handful of raw almonds
- A pear with two slices of Cheddar cheese
- Carrot, celery, and cucumber sticks and/or breadsticks dipped into two tablespoons of hummus
- Cottage cheese or cream cheese spread on two Ryvitas (or other crackers) or wholemeal toast.

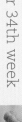

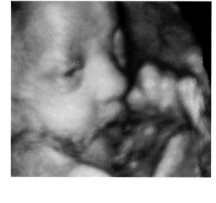

43 days to go...

YOUR BABY TODAY

Your baby is now capable of producing all of the enzymes that will process food within the digestive tract. If born early, your baby could now feed normally although some will still require help as they need to fine-tune the co-ordination of their suckling reflexes.

Your baby is naturally nourished inside the uterus and her own digestive tract is now functioning well.

Eighty per cent of your baby's energy needs are met by carbohydrates, mainly in the form of glucose, and almost 20 per cent from protein. Fat is not used as an energy source but it is used for growth. All mineral, vitamin, and calcium needs are met from your own reserves and your diet. Two possible exceptions are iron and folate, a water-soluble vitamin

that occurs naturally in foods; folic acid is the synthetic version. Folate does not easily cross the placenta to reach and nourish your baby. Your own iron stores may already be low if you eat little or no red meat or if this pregnancy has followed on quickly from your last one. Your baby needs iron (and folate) to make red blood cells and because only a small percentage of iron in your diet

is absorbed, iron supplementation is often recommended at this stage.

While all of your baby's gut structures were present by 20 weeks, it is not until this stage that all the enzymes needed for digestion are activated and the absorptive surface of the gut is established to a degree that would enable your baby to feed if she were born now.

GETTING UP FROM LYING DOWN

After you've exercised on the floor, or have been resting in bed, you may find it a struggle to get up from lying down. This simple manoeuvre can put a strain on your abdominal muscles, which are stretched, and it isn't helped by your altered centre of gravity. The technique shown below was

originally devised by yoga teachers to help you get up safely from a lying down position.

As with any strenuous manoeuvres at this stage of pregnancy, always take your time and remember to breathe slowly and deeply throughout.

Step one: With your knees bent, roll on to your right side bringing the knee beneath you up to waist level. Keep your right hand aligned with your bent knee.

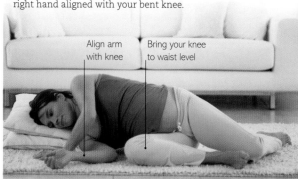

Align arm with knee

Bring your knee to waist level

Step two: Shift your weight on to your left hand and knee. Position your right knee under your right hip and your right hand under your shoulder and come up slowly on all fours.

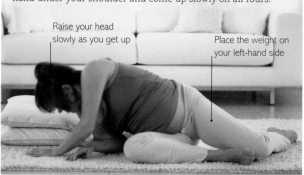

Raise your head slowly as you get up

Place the weight on your left-hand side

42 days to go...

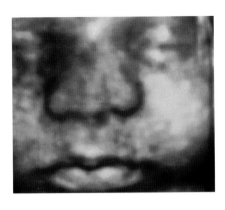

YOUR BABY TODAY

This close-up of the baby's face clearly shows the lip shape and slightly separated eyelids. The slight shadowing seen to the left of the image is from the wall of the uterus, which at this stage of the pregnancy will always be very close to your baby.

If you've made the decision to have a home birth, you'll need to ensure you're fully prepared in good time.

ASK A... MIDWIFE

What additional things do I need to think about if I'm having a home birth? Have all the items you need for labour and birth gathered in the place you intend to deliver, and organize your items separately from the baby's items.

As well as practical items, such as clothing, toiletries, and sanitary pads, you may also want to have to hand music, phone numbers, and a camera. It's a good idea to have a well-stocked fridge so make a list of nutritious foods to stock up on before your due date. This will help you during labour and in the first week of parenthood. Your baby will need nappies, cotton wool, vests, clothing, sheets, and blankets.

If you have other children, you may need to make arrangements for them to be cared for.

Even though you're planning to have your baby at home, there are circumstances in which you may need to be transferred to hospital. This can happen before, during, or after labour and so, even though you may not wish to contemplate this outcome, have an emergency bag packed (see p.358) just in case.

Women had their babies at home for generations; it was only in the 20th century that women began to have hospital births. If you're considering a home birth, remember that the majority of pregnancies and deliveries are normal and do not need any medical intervention.

Be reassured that if you have decided to have a home birth and then change your mind, for example if you decide you want an epidural, or your midwife advises you that the baby needs help, you will be transferred to hospital.

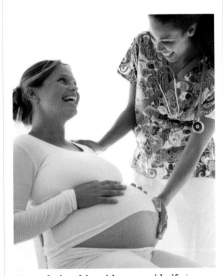

Your relationship with your midwife is even more important if you're giving birth at home as she will be your sole medical support.

Group B strep test

Around 20–30 per cent of pregnant women carry the strep B bacteria in the vagina or rectal area. Known as GBS (group B streptococcus), it is usually harmless in adults, but can cause a rare and serious infection in newborn babies if untreated.

■ **There is no routine screening policy in the UK,** but some hospitals screen for GBS at 34–37 weeks of pregnancy. If the result is positive, antibiotic treatment can be given during labour that will reduce the risk of the baby becoming infected. Some hospitals don't screen but if the bacteria is detected in a urine test or a swab is taken for another reason and is positive, antibiotic treatment may given in labour.
■ **The test is very straightforward** and involves taking a swab of the area around your vagina and rectum.
■ **If GBS is detected,** and treatment given as soon as labour starts, there is little risk to the baby.
■ **It is possible to be infected with GBS** in a second pregnancy, even if you didn't have it first time round.

Your 35th week

TRY TO STAY ACTIVE, EVEN THOUGH YOU MAY BE WADDLING BY NOW

Taking exercise is probably the last thing you want to do, but it's worth the effort. The more you move, the more energy you will gain. Gentle exercise will also help to relieve some of the aches and twinges of late pregnancy. The baby's movements may change as he has less room to move around. Instead of kicks, he may be shuffling around. He's busy, though, practising for the outside world, teaching himself to suckle and focus his vision.

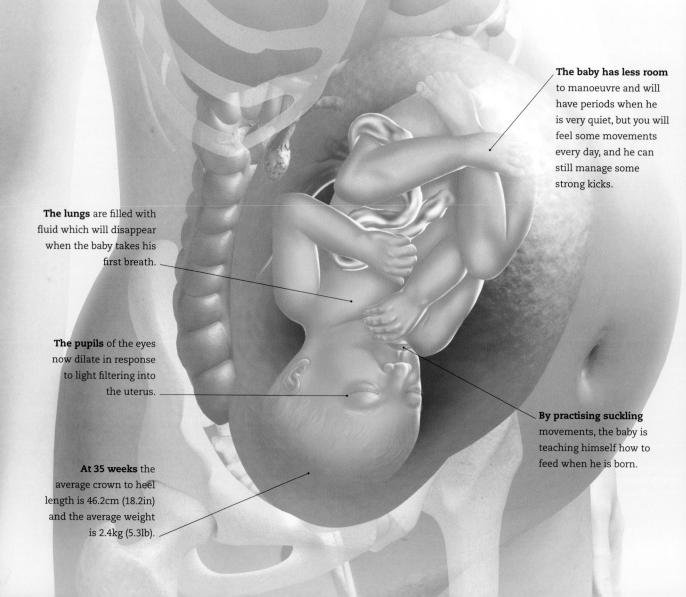

The baby has less room to manoeuvre and will have periods when he is very quiet, but you will feel some movements every day, and he can still manage some strong kicks.

The lungs are filled with fluid which will disappear when the baby takes his first breath.

The pupils of the eyes now dilate in response to light filtering into the uterus.

By practising suckling movements, the baby is teaching himself how to feed when he is born.

At 35 weeks the average crown to heel length is 46.2cm (18.2in) and the average weight is 2.4kg (5.3lb).

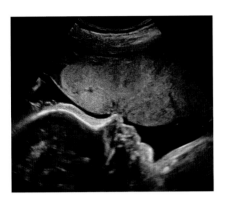

41 days to go...

YOUR BABY TODAY

This profile of the baby shows the tip of the nose touching the placenta. Your placenta will not be growing any more and now thins slightly. Within, the placenta continues to mature and it remains a highly efficient means of supplying your baby's energy needs.

As your size begins to have an impact on your daily activities, you'll find that a few practical adjustments are necessary.

Your posture will change as your bump continues to grow. To compensate for the heavy weight you're carrying, you might find that you lean back slightly, especially when you're walking downhill. You might also waddle when you walk as you shift your weight from side to side. In a few weeks' time, when the baby begins to engage into the pelvis (see p.361), you may find that you waddle even more.

It's normal at this late stage of pregnancy to move more slowly than normal. You may find yourself struggling to get out of bed or out of a chair, and picking something up off the floor can be more difficult than usual. Tasks such as doing up your shoelaces or painting your toenails can seem impossible. You can overcome problems such as these; for example by putting your feet on a stool to tie your shoelaces so you don't have to bend down so far. If you need help, there's no shame in asking. It can be difficult to be reliant on others but remember it's only temporary.

ASK A... MIDWIFE

Can I have a water birth in hospital? This depends on the maternity unit: some have birthing pools; others have facilities for you to hire a pool. Some units may be unable to allow a pool to be used for structural reasons; the amount of water would be too heavy for the floor to hold.

If your maternity unit does have a birthing pool, bear in mind that it may already be in use when you go into labour. Some units may let you labour in a pool, but not allow you to give birth in the water.

FOCUS ON... YOUR HEALTH

A diabetic pregnancy

Whether you develop diabetes in pregnancy (known as gestational diabetes – see p.473), or have pre-existing diabetes, you'll require special care from a diabetic healthcare team and consultant obstetrician. This is because diabetes poses risks in pregnancy.

In the mother, these include high blood pressure, blood clots, pre-eclampsia (see p.474), diabetic kidney disease, and diabetic retinopathy, a condition that affects the retina in the eye. For the baby, there is an increased risk of congenital abnormalities and growth may be too fast or too slow.

The key to a healthy pregnancy and baby when you have diabetes is good blood-sugar control as your insulin requirements will change throughout pregnancy. Controlling blood-sugar levels reduces the risk of birth defects and stillbirth, or of you having a larger than expected baby, which can lead to problems during the birth.

If you have gestational diabetes, you will need to adapt your diet to include more carbohydrates and fibre and reduce your intake of fats and sugar. You may also need insulin injections (see below) to help control your blood-sugar levels.

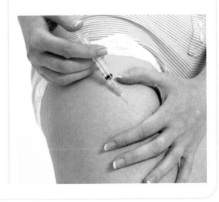

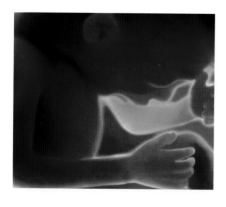

YOU ARE 34 WEEKS AND 2 DAYS

40 days to go...

YOUR BABY TODAY

At the back of your baby's eye, nerve cells that identify either black and white or colour are maturing. The cells that respond to colour signals are the last to develop but will eventually process more than half of the information that the eyes receive.

Your baby is blinking and learning to focus, and his pupils will dilate in response to light filtering through the uterus.

Your baby's eyes first began to develop two weeks after conception and then all of the major eye structures formed over the following four weeks. The eye, however, keeps growing during the pregnancy and the optic nerve continues to develop after birth.

The eyes have been opening since 26 weeks of pregnancy but, until now, eye movements have been poorly co-ordinated. Eye movements are first seen at 18 weeks but they are random and infrequent. Movements become more frequent from 26 weeks and now, in the final few weeks, movements settle into a cycle of rest alternating with rapid eye movements (REM).

Some light does get through into the uterus and your baby is now much more responsive to strong lights.

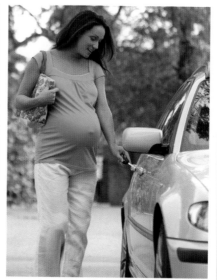

Driving is still an option in late pregnancy, but you may find it uncomfortable to be in the car for long periods.

ASK A... MUM

I'm concerned my maternity leave cover will do a better job than me. Are these fears normal? Yes, completely normal. I remember being worried that the man hired for my position would outshine me. The amazing thing was that once my baby was born, anything to do with work was eclipsed by my new role. Far from losing skills, I think I became an efficient multi-tasker and when I returned to work, found the job easier than caring for a baby.

Try not to worry. Not only do you have legal rights regarding the safety of your job (see pp.348–9), but you will have your chance to shine once again when your baby has settled into childcare. In the meantime, enjoy your leave. It goes quickly, but also presents you with an opportunity to hone some important life skills.

GETTING OUT AND ABOUT

In most cases, it's perfectly safe to drive in the months leading up to the end of your pregnancy. However, if you feel that you're not able to concentrate at the wheel, or driving makes you uncomfortable, then give it a miss. When driving, it's very important that you position your lap belt directly under your bump (see p.253), to ensure that there is no danger to your baby if you are involved in an accident.

Travelling by public transport is fine, too, but make sure you take full advantage of your condition to pointedly request a seat. Being jolted around on a train or bus is not ideal – not because it will damage your baby, but because your centre of gravity has changed and you are more likely to fall or experience embarrassment and discomfort. Long periods of standing can also cause your ankles and feet to swell.

If you're feeling uncomfortable or dizzy, get off the train or bus and sit down in a cooler environment, preferably with your feet up, for about 20 minutes. Always carry water with you on journeys.

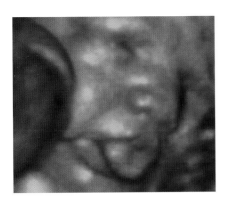

39 days to go...

YOUR BABY TODAY

Your baby will often stick his tongue out, as part of the development of the reflexes needed to suckle. The rooting reflex enables your baby to find the nipple, then the strong suckling reflexes take over to co-ordinate breathing, suckling, and swallowing.

As maternity leave approaches, you might be looking for ways to save money, so here are ways to find baby clothes on a budget.

Dressing your newborn baby doesn't have to be expensive.
Don't be shy about asking friends and family members for hand-me-downs. Those who aren't planning any more children will probably be glad to get rid of them. Get together with your antenatal group, and arrange a swap session – many mums may have older children of a different sex to the new baby, and have no need for pink T-shirts, or rugby shirts! While the idea of your baby wearing "used" clothing may take some getting used to, rest assured that most babywear is hardly worn.

Look on the internet for end-of-season sales, and even on some of the auction sites, where you can often pick up designer goodies for a fraction of the original price. Visit your local NCT sales or, even better, sales at the local "twins club", where there will be double the number of goods on offer! Shop around; you don't have to pay a lot for items such as babygros and will find cheap prices in the supermarket. Make a purchase with your weekly shop and you won't notice the cost as much.

Remember, too, that you will probably receive numerous gifts of clothing when your baby is born. If you know exactly what you'd like, you may like to organize a gift list from a favourite shop or ask people for vouchers for that store. When

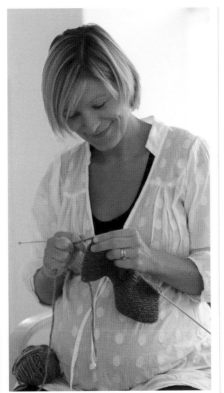

Knitting your own baby clothes is a great way to save money, and it can be rewarding to see your newborn in your own creations.

looking for more expensive items of clothing, head for the three- to six-month-old rail, so that your baby will get plenty of use out of them. It can be disappointing if your newborn only gets a couple of weeks' wear out of an outfit you like.

38 days to go...

YOUR BABY TODAY

This 2D ultrasound has captured the moment that the baby is sucking his thumb. Your baby is gradually learning to co-ordinate this complex activity with breathing movements even though surrounded not by air but by the amniotic fluid.

Inside the uterus your baby is already practising the suckling reflex, which will enable him to feed when he's born.

ASK A... MIDWIFE

My mum has offered to stay with us after the birth. Is this a good idea? Some couples prefer to get to know their baby on their own, taking the first few days to settle in and get used to the idea of being new parents. It's also good to try to do things your own way when it comes to caring for your newborn. Having said that, you'll find an extra pair of hands invaluable.

It really depends on your relationship with your mum: if it's good and you feel she'll be supportive, then it's more likely to help than hinder. However, gently establish some guidelines – namely that while you welcome her help, you'd like to do things your way and have space to bond with your baby. Encourage your mum towards helping around the house, rather than just with the baby, not least so that your partner doesn't feel excluded at this important time.

By this stage of pregnancy you may not feel up to spending hours shopping for equipment and clothes for the baby. You can save a lot of time by getting catalogues from the major stores and making some preliminary decisions from the comfort of your armchair.

The suckling reflex is present earlier in pregnancy but it is known from assessing premature babies that it's usually not until around this time that the baby is strong and co-ordinated enough to suckle with ease. Your baby regularly practises suckling and this, in combination with the rooting reflex, will enable him to feed.

After birth you will see the rooting reflex as your baby turns towards anything that strokes his cheek. The head will turn, and your baby will move his mouth in a series of gradually diminishing circles until the object is found. Once feeding is well established,

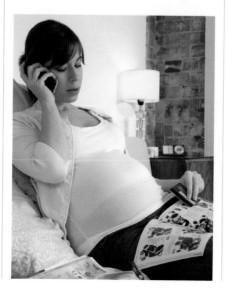

at about four months, the rooting reflex disappears. From this point on, your baby has much more control over the process, and is able to turn and directly latch on (see pp.448–9) to the nipple.

While in the uterus, there is no chance of your baby accidentally swallowing amniotic fluid into the lungs. The lungs are already filled with fluid and the high pressure of this, together with your baby's larynx, keeps out amniotic fluid. After birth, babies have a series of reflexes designed to keep breathing and drinking separate. To help with feeding, babies always breathe through their nose.

ARE YOU READY FOR THE BABY?

You may find that you soon become too tired to shop. Try to buy items gradually, but there are certain things that it's worthwhile purchasing by around 37 weeks, just in case you go into labour. First, buy those small babycare items you'll need straight after the birth (see p.269) plus a car seat and a Moses basket or cot. You won't need a pram immediately after the birth.

If going out shopping becomes difficult in late pregnancy, consider buying some items online.

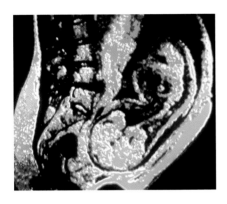

37 days to go...

YOUR BABY TODAY

This is an MRI image showing a cross section of the entire pregnancy. The mother's spine is on the left of the image, and the baby is lying head down within the pelvis. An MRI is rarely needed during pregnancy, but if recommended, it is entirely safe.

You'll probably find yourself analyzing every ache and pain in these final weeks of your pregnancy.

By this stage of pregnancy every time you get a twinge you may worry that it's the onset of labour. This is a normal concern, but try to remember that, even though you're heavily pregnant, most aches and pains are still likely to be due to constipation, or stretching ligaments, rather than labour.

You may begin to have Braxton Hicks' contractions; these practice contractions occur as the uterus tightens as a warm up for labour. They also help to direct more blood to the placenta in the final weeks of pregnancy. Some women are unaware of them, while for others they can be quite uncomfortable. Relaxing the uterine muscles by changing your position, walking around, or having a warm bath can help.

If you're unsure whether the pains you're having are Braxton Hicks', do always consult your midwife.

ASK A... MUM

What will I need if I'm planning to breastfeed? I found all the following items really useful when I was breastfeeding my baby:

■ **Nursing bras** that can be unclipped at the front (see right) or have zip-open cups. Get properly fitted (bearing in mind that your breasts will be bigger once your milk comes in). You'll need at least two nursing bras and, thankfully, it's possible to get some attractive styles.

■ **Nipple cream**: this is soothing if you have cracked nipples.

■ **Breast pads** (disposable or washable). Slip them inside your bra to absorb any leaks between feeds. Alternatively, breast shells slot inside your bra to catch any excess milk.

■ **Breastfeeding pillow:** a V-shaped pillow isn't essential, but it will help you and your baby to get comfortable.

■ **Muslins** to catch dribbles.

■ **Breast pump** and bottles or bags for storing expressed milk.

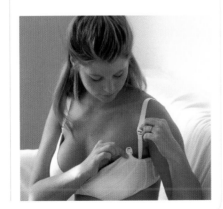

TIME TO THINK ABOUT

Breastfeeding

If you've decided to breastfeed, it's the best choice for you and your baby (see pp.448–9). However, it doesn't always come naturally so make it easier by being prepared:

■ **Read all about it.** If you're expecting some of the discomforts, they won't come as such a shock and you may be able to take measures to prevent them. It can help, for example, to know how to latch on your baby correctly (see p.448).

■ **Address any concerns** before your baby is born: ask your midwife, or friends who've breastfed.

■ **See how it's done** by visiting a breastfeeding café (ask your midwife to recommend one). You may have been concerned about breastfeeding in public, so it can help to see how discreetly it can be done. You could also ask a friend to let you watch her position and breastfeed her baby.

■ **Look for a breastfeeding counsellor** – maybe a friend can recommend one, or contact the National Childbirth Trust or La Leche League (see p.480) for a list of counsellors.

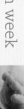

Your rights and benefits

Having a baby is a huge life change and many new parents find time and money are in short supply. Maternity and paternity leave and pay can help to ease the transition, so it's worth finding out what you're entitled to.

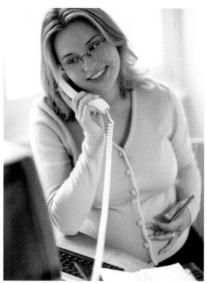

Finding out about your maternity benefits can give you peace of mind that you will have some security during your maternity leave.

MATERNITY LEAVE EXTRAS

Keeping in touch

While you're on leave, you can be paid for up to 10 days' work for your employer, known as "keeping in touch" or KIT days, without losing your statutory maternity pay (see right). How much you'll earn is at your employer's discretion, but at the least they should top up your maternity pay so you receive the equivalent of a day's salary.

KIT days are arranged by mutual consent between you and your employer. They allow you to keep in touch and maintain relationships, keep on top of new developments, and ease yourself back into work.

Your rights

When you have a baby, you can take up to a year off work and retain your right to return, irrespective of how long you've been employed, how many days you work, or how much you earn. The first 26-week block is known as ordinary maternity leave (OML). If you take more time off (up to a further 26 weeks, totalling 52 weeks), it's called additional maternity leave (AML). You are legally obliged to take a minimum of two weeks' leave after the birth. You'll retain your normal employment rights and benefits (apart from pay), such as a company car, gym membership, and accrued annual leave, throughout both your OML and AML. You need to give your employer at least four weeks' notice of when you intend to start your leave and a minimum of four weeks' notice of when you intend to return. The earliest you can start maternity leave and pay is 11 weeks before your baby is due (unless he is born before).

Mothers returning from OML are entitled to go back to the same job. If your employer can't keep your job open, you must be offered a similar, suitable job with equal terms and conditions.

You have a legal right to take time off in pregnancy for antenatal appointments; this includes attending hospital antenatal classes or antenatal relaxation classes.

Maternity pay

According to a survey of just under 2,000 mothers in 2007 by the National Centre for Social Research, around 88 per cent of working mothers received some type of maternity pay. The amount you'll receive depends on what you earn

STAYING UP TO DATE

Sources of information

Maternity and paternity rights, and especially the precise amounts of benefits, can change from one year to the next, as the Government reassesses its budgets and priorities, and responds to the changing needs of the population. The rights and benefits given on these pages are current for the year 2013–14. For the most up-to-date information and further details, see the guides on the Government's website, www.gov.uk.

and how long you've been working for, but most employed mothers will receive around nine months' maternity pay.

There are two types of maternity pay – statutory maternity pay (SMP) and maternity allowance (MA). If you don't qualify for either, you may be able to claim incapacity benefit, jobseeker's allowance, or income support instead.

Statutory maternity pay (SMP) You'll qualify for SMP if you've worked for your employer for at least 26 continuous weeks (full- or part-time) by the 15th week before your baby is due. Statutory maternity pay lasts for up to 39 weeks, and the amount you receive will depend on how much you earn during the eight-week period before the end of the 15th week before your due date.

If you earn an average of at least £109 (before tax) per week, you'll get 90 per

Will I have to pay back my SMP if I change my mind after the birth and decide to stay at home?

No; if you decide not to return to work after maternity leave, you don't have to pay back SMP. This also applies even if you decide to leave your job or you're made redundant or sacked after the 15th week before your baby is due.

What happens about my holiday entitlement when I'm on leave?

You'll accrue your usual number of days' holiday. However, your employer's normal rules about how much holiday you can carry over to the next leave year still apply, which means you'll need to plan carefully so you don't lose out. Ask the human resources department how many days you're entitled to take.

I've just been offered my dream job, but I'm eight weeks' pregnant. Should I keep mum?

You don't have to tell your prospective employer about your pregnancy at this stage. But if you do, they are not allowed to discriminate against you because you're pregnant. You have to tell your employer once you're 25 weeks' pregnant. You may choose to inform them earlier if you want paid time off for appointments, or if there are health and safety issues.

---

cent of your salary for six weeks, and up to £136.78 (before tax) or 90 per cent of your average weekly earnings, whichever is lower, for a further 33 weeks; the last 13 weeks' leave of AML are usually unpaid. Tax and National Insurance are deducted. Some employers have their own schemes and pay contractual maternity pay instead of SMP; this must amount to at least as much as SMP.

Maternity allowance (MA) You can claim this benefit, which is paid weekly by the Government agency Jobcentre Plus, if you're not entitled to SMP (see above) during maternity leave. (If you live in Northern Ireland, contact the Jobs & Benefits Office.)

To qualify for MA, you must have been registered self-employed and/or have been employed (not necessarily continuously or for one employer) for at least 26 weeks out of the 66-week period ending the week before your baby is due.

Maternity allowance is paid for up to 39 weeks. The standard rate is £136.78 or 90 per cent of your average (before tax) weekly earnings, whichever is less. You have to earn at least £30 a week to qualify, so the least you would receive is £27 (90 per cent of £30). You don't pay tax or National Insurance on MA.

Dads at home

Dads who've been employed for at least 26 weeks by the 15th week before the due date can take up to two weeks' paternity leave, which is taken in a one- or two-week block, within eight weeks of the birth. Men who earn at least £109 a week qualify for statutory paternity pay (SPP), paid at 90 per cent of earnings up to £136.78 per week. Dads who don't qualify may be able to claim income support while on leave.

Additional paternity leave (APL) enables fathers to take up to an extra 26 weeks' leave during the first year of the baby's life if their partner returns to work before the end of her maternity leave. Fathers on APL may also qualify for additional paternity pay.

Parental leave (PL)

If you've worked for your employer for a year, both parents can take a total of 18 weeks off work per child up to their fifth birthday. If your child is disabled, you can take up to 18 weeks' leave before his or her 18th birthday. Providing you don't take longer than four weeks in a year, you can go back to the same job. The downside is that PL is usually unpaid.

Going back to work

Before returning, consider the following:
■ Will life as a working mum be easier if you switch to a flexible working arrangement, such as a job share or part-time work? Give your employer ample time to consider any request.
■ If you're breastfeeding, your employer must provide a private, clean, and safe room for you to express and store milk.
■ You're entitled to time off (which may be unpaid) for family emergencies.
■ You may be eligible for working and child tax credits, which can help with childcare costs.

Other benefits

During pregnancy and for up to a year after the birth, you're entitled to free NHS dental treatment and prescriptions. Your midwife can give you a form to apply for an exemption certificate.

Baby and child benefits

■ **The Sure Start Maternity Grant** is a one-off payment of £500 to help low-income families cope with the cost of providing for a new baby.

■ **Child benefit** is a weekly payment of £20.30 for the eldest or only child, plus £13.40 for every other child. It's important to apply sooner rather than later, as claims are only backdated up to three months. You may be liable to a tax charge on this benefit if you, or your partner, has an individual income of over £50,000.

■ **Junior ISAs** are tax-free savings accounts for those under 18. They work like cash ISAs, shielding any growth in cash from income and capital gains tax.

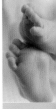

Your rights and benefits

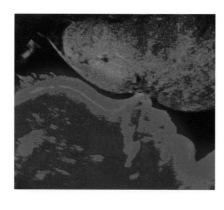

36 days to go...

YOUR BABY TODAY

The placenta, shown in red above the baby's green profile, is now receiving 0.5 litre (18fl oz) of blood each minute from your circulation. In order to accommodate this increase your blood volume expanded dramatically in the first few months of pregnancy.

It's never too late to improve your fitness and whatever you do now will stand you in good stead for labour.

ASK A... DOCTOR

Why are some babies born prematurely? There are certain factors that may increase a woman's likelihood of having a premature baby. These include a previous obstetric history of prematurity of either themselves or a mother or sister; illness during pregnancy; the state of a woman's health prior to pregnancy; having a multiple pregnancy; fetal problems, such as reduced growth, which may be due to lifestyle factors such as smoking, and other fetal disorders.

You might be in the final few weeks but you still need to stay active. Exercising regularly and consistently will enable you to reap the rewards of your efforts: increased fitness, higher self esteem, and much more energy.

Find activities that you enjoy: swimming and walking are often favoured by pregnant women in this late stage. As well as helping to improve fitness, both of these activities will help you to relax and unwind.

It is difficult to put an exact figure on how long you should be exercising for, but bear in mind that this will be determined by how hard you exercise – the two are interlinked. Consider the

difference between a sprint and a marathon – each will have its own energy needs: one is short and has a very intense need for energy, while the other needs slow and sustained energy.

Always listen to your body and stop if you're in danger of over-exerting yourself. It's important to eat plenty if you're exercising: choose snacks that will fuel your body (see p.339), especially given that the third trimester is the most demanding in terms of your baby's nutritional needs.

KANGAROO CARE

If your premature baby goes into a Special Care Baby Unit (SCBU) (see pp.452–3) you may be able to look after him using a method called Kangaroo care. You will be asked to hold your baby on your chest between your breasts with his head turned so that his ear is next to your heart.

Developed in Bogota, Columbia, in response to a lack of incubators, kangaroo care is shown to have many benefits for SCBU babies – mainly that their heart and breathing rates

regularize quite quickly, allowing them to sleep for longer periods. The baby's temperature is regulated by the temperature fluctuations in your breasts, meaning he doesn't have to expend energy keeping himself warm.

This, in addition to the extra sleep, preserves his energy for other vital functions, such as brain development and weight gain. Breastfeeding is also more successful and some kangarooed babies lose none of their birth weight.

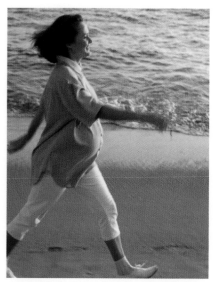

If you go for a daily walk you will feel energized and it will be good preparation for all those strolls you'll be doing with your baby.

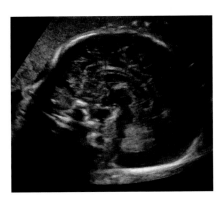

YOU ARE 35 WEEKS EXACTLY

35 days to go...

YOUR BABY TODAY

Your baby's brain continues to mature. This ultrasound image shows that the folding pattern overlying the cerebral hemispheres has now developed, giving rise to the familiar folds and grooves on the brain's surface. The bright reflections are from the bony skull.

The reality of being a mother will begin to hit you in these final weeks, and you have everything to look forward to.

Before the birth, it can be difficult to imagine having a relationship with your baby, even though you may feel a close bond during pregnancy

Fortunately, bonding is a chemical process in your brain when you give birth. Other people's babies may leave you feeling cold, but it's highly likely that your own baby will spark all sorts of feelings that you never even knew you could experience. It's normal to worry about being a mother – coping

with the responsibility, caring for a helpless baby, being "good enough", and making lifestyle changes. However, when your baby is born, your priorities will become abundantly clear, as will your affections – although bonding may not always be instant.

In some cases, postnatal depression (see p.475), or even the short-term baby blues (see p.450), can interrupt the natural progression of feelings a mother has for her newborn baby.

ASK A... MIDWIFE

Will I be able to breastfeed my twins? Yes, but if possible, arrange for a breastfeeding counsellor with experience in feeding twins to be available after the birth. If you get the positions correct and know how to latch on your babies (see p.448) at the outset, you'll feel much more confident continuing on your own.

Many mums of twins find that feeding them simultaneously, using a specially designed breastfeeding pillow, is the easiest way to manage. This is something you may wish to buy now. There is a variety of effective breastfeeding positions for twins that the counsellor or a midwife can show you.

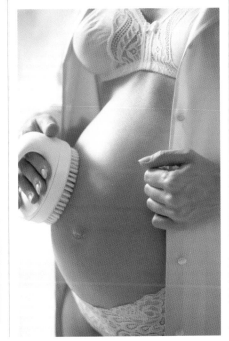

FOCUS ON... YOUR BODY

Pamper yourself

You may not feel particularly lovely, but that's all the more reason to pamper yourself. There's unlikely to be time for beauty rituals once the baby is born.

■ **Treat yourself to a manicure,** but don't have nail extensions for when your baby is born – sharp implements and babies don't mix.

■ **Indulge in a facial:** it will make you feel good and help you to relax.

■ **Have your hair cut** as it may be some time before you get to the hairdresser again. It's worth opting for a style that will be easy to manage once your baby arrives.

■ **If you have aches and pains,** book a massage with someone who specializes in pregnancy.

■ **Have a pedicure** a week or two before the birth. You'll be thrilled once your bump has gone and you're able to see your feet again.

If you're keeping a photographic record of your bump, you'll want it to look as good as possible. Gently exfoliating and moisturizing will ensure the skin is as smooth as possible. It won't, unfortunately, prevent stretch marks but it will improve the appearance of the skin.

Your 35th week

351

Your 36th week

GET TOGETHER WITH YOUR PARTNER AND TALK THROUGH YOUR BIRTH PLANS

Don't leave crucial arrangements until the last minute. Have an action plan ready for when you go into labour – it might be sooner than you think. Babies can arrive ahead of schedule, so make sure you and your partner feel confident about coping. Work out practicalities, such as organizing care for other children, or even the cat. Rope in your parents or friends to help if need be, pack your hospital bag, and relax.

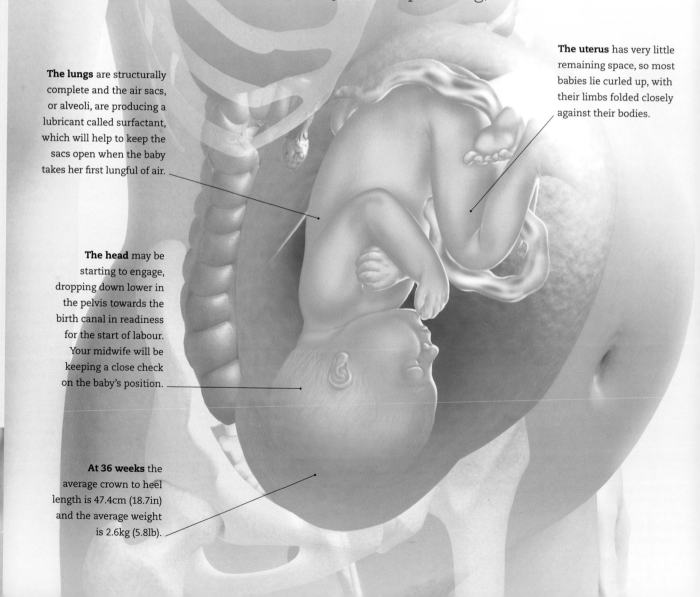

The uterus has very little remaining space, so most babies lie curled up, with their limbs folded closely against their bodies.

The lungs are structurally complete and the air sacs, or alveoli, are producing a lubricant called surfactant, which will help to keep the sacs open when the baby takes her first lungful of air.

The head may be starting to engage, dropping down lower in the pelvis towards the birth canal in readiness for the start of labour. Your midwife will be keeping a close check on the baby's position.

At 36 weeks the average crown to heel length is 47.4cm (18.7in) and the average weight is 2.6kg (5.8lb).

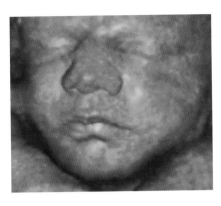

34 days to go...

YOUR BABY TODAY

Your baby's hair and eye colour are both determined genetically and set before birth. Unfortunately, however detailed an ultrasound image is, it can only show the shape of structures and will never be able to show true colour information.

You may be surprised to find that your social life is already changing, and the baby hasn't even arrived yet!

If you've become a home bird recently, be reassured it's quite normal. Wanting to stay at home is common in the final stages of pregnancy. You may be reluctant to plan social engagements for the next few weeks, just in case. For example, you don't want to spend money on a theatre ticket that might not get used. Do, however, pencil in dates with friends because they will understand if you cancel nearer the time. You'll also find that once you're on leave, you're glad to get out of the house in the evenings.

Do take the opportunity to go out with your partner in these last few weeks as dinner dates may not be on the agenda once the baby arrives.

ASK A... MIDWIFE

My feet are swollen and tight; can I do anything about it? Swollen feet and ankles, known as oedema, is due to excessive fluid seeping into the tissues because of the increased volume of blood (see pp.466–7). By late pregnancy, as blood volume continues to rise, this is a common problem. The swelling is usually worse later in the day and when the weather is warmer.

Steps you can take to help reduce swelling include elevating your legs when sitting, rotating your feet, and lying on the floor with your feet up the wall. Wearing support stockings or tights (see p.225) also improves circulation. Make sure you drink plenty, particularly water, as this improves kidney function and reduces water retention. Don't take diuretics – studies have found that these can adversely affect an unborn baby.

FOCUS ON... YOUR BODY

A soothing swim

Although you may feel too big to be exercising, swimming is a great activity for late pregnancy. The water supports the weight of your bump, so you may feel much lighter than you do normally. Try to do some gentle swimming as well as just relaxing in the water. Also consider going to antenatal aquanatal classes, which have exercises tailored for pregnant women.

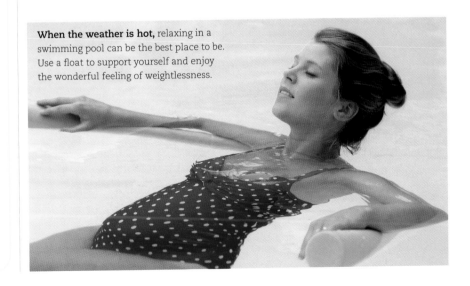

When the weather is hot, relaxing in a swimming pool can be the best place to be. Use a float to support yourself and enjoy the wonderful feeling of weightlessness.

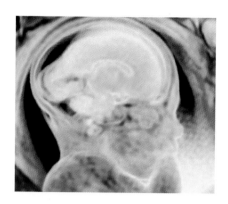

33 days to go...

YOUR BABY TODAY

This MRI scan shows detail of the baby's brain. MRI is particularly good at showing structures within the central nervous system. Taking and interpreting these images remains difficult and time-consuming, however, so they do not form part of routine testing.

Although the colour is developing in your baby's eyes, the final colour will not be known for some time.

What colour will your baby's eyes be? The iris controls the amount of light that enters the eye and gives the eyes their colour. Eye colour is determined by the amount of melanin within the iris; this is the substance in the skin that gives different skin tones.

It certainly doesn't follow that your baby will have an identical eye colour to that of you or your partner. Most fair-skinned babies will be born with only a small amount of melanin in the eye and the iris will appear grey or blue. If dark-skinned then there is a great deal of melanin and the colour is usually dark grey or brown. The colour continues to change after birth as melanin is produced in response to light. Your baby will be a year old before the final colour of her eyes is fully developed.

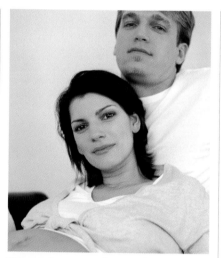

You may have started to wonder whether your baby will have the same eye colour as you or your partner. Her eye colour may resemble either of yours, or it may be different from both of you.

PRACTISING VISUALIZATION

Visualization is an effective and positive way to help prepare for labour. Try practising it in these final weeks, beginning with a basic relaxation exercise. So start at the top of your head and gently contract and relax every muscle down to your toes, concentrating on each muscle, and your breathing, as you do so. Now imagine the birth, with every step given a positive connotation. For example, your baby is floating in water, and is gently rocked as the contractions begin; the tightening you feel is the strong walls of your uterus, guiding your baby into the world; the contractions are waves on which you and your baby are riding, as your baby is washed out – you are both swimming together with the tide.

FOCUS ON... YOUR BODY

Caesarean birth

If you know you're going to have your baby by Caesarean, it's worth being aware of what to expect following the birth. Although you should remain mobile after a Caesarean operation, it's also important to get plenty of rest. Keep in mind that a Caesarean section is major surgery so you will need to avoid lifting and carrying heavy loads for the first few weeks. As this may be difficult if you have other small children or you are at home alone, you should try to recruit as much help as possible after the operation. You should avoid doing any shopping as this usually involves carrying heavy bags. Order online if you can.

The advice is not to drive for six weeks. If you feel up to it before this time, check with your insurance company that it is okay and make sure you're comfortable wearing a seatbelt and doing manoeuvres, including emergency stops.

It is generally thought to take up to six weeks to fully recover from a Caesarean delivery.

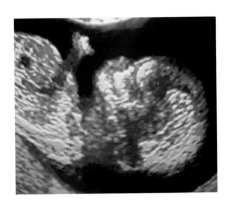

32 days to go...

YOUR BABY TODAY

In this week, the lungs become almost fully functional and able to support the baby if delivered early. However, the baby at this time is still preterm, and will not be mature enough until 37 weeks to be considered full term.

Don't forget this is a life-changing time for your partner, too, so find positive ways to involve him in the run-up to the birth.

There is, understandably, a lot of focus on women in the lead up to childbirth, but it's important not to neglect the dads-to-be. Your partner may be getting anxious about the birth itself, fearing that he might not cope with being in the delivery room or just concerned about how it will affect him to see you in pain. Some men feel guilty that they cannot take their share of the pain and help more during labour.

Aside from thinking about the birth, your partner may be anxious about the fact he'll be responsible for a newborn baby in just a few weeks!

Talk to your partner if he appears anxious and involve him as much as possible – from helping you cope with pregnancy discomforts to preparing for the birth. If you've written a birth plan (see pp.181 and 303), go back over it now and discuss what might happen and how your partner could help on the day.

You could practise positions and breathing techniques for labour so that he feels more confident about helping you cope. If possible, he could attend your final antenatal appointments with you, where he can discuss any concerns he has with the midwife.

(see pp.181 and 303)

ASK A... MIDWIFE

I'm having my twins next week, but will I be able to love them both equally? Although this can be a concern, it is more likely to be the case that rather than favour one child over the other, a parent gives more love and attention to the baby who needs it most at that time.

It is also possible that the strain of having two babies in the house may increase the likelihood of delayed bonding, although this can also happen if the birth has been traumatic; if the mother or indeed the father is exhausted; or if one baby has

taken time to establish feeding, or is more fractious than the other. This does not mean that bonding will not take place over time.

In every family, there are bound to be ebbs and flows of love between parents and children. When a parent has two children born at different times, that parent may love one child differently to the other, but this does not mean that the love a parent has for one child is to the detriment of the other. If once your babies are born you still have concerns, speak to your midwife or health visitor.

FOCUS ON... DADS

Getting ready

Have you done all your dad-to-be jobs? These include:
- **Buying a car seat** and making sure you know how to fit it safely in the car. You can't leave the hospital with your newborn without one.
- **Assembling the cot** if you're going to use one in the early weeks.
- **Ensuring there is storage space** for the baby's clothes, bedding, nappies, and other bits and pieces.

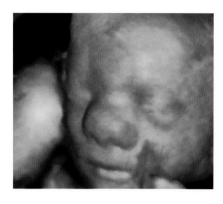

YOU ARE 35 WEEKS AND 4 DAYS

31 days to go...

YOUR BABY TODAY

Your baby's heart will beat quite fast, at between 110 and 160 beats every minute. Even after birth, your baby's heart will continue to beat at this speed. It will be several years before the heart rate is 70 or so beats per minute, the same as an adult.

The lungs don't become fully functional until these final weeks, but important development is taking place now.

If you imagine the lung as a tree, then the windpipe or "trachea" is the trunk of the tree. This then forms several branches or "bronchi", which divide several times, like twigs, to then produce the most delicate structures: the alveoli or leaves of the tree. It is within the alveoli that gas exchange will take place.

The alveoli began to develop at 24 weeks but they continue to increase in number throughout the pregnancy. The alveoli contain surfactant-producing cells to keep them open and these now become fully functional.

PRESCRIBED BEDREST

Towards the end of pregnancy, there are some circumstances when you may need to be admitted into hospital for bedrest.
- **If you have contractions,** but your waters haven't broken.
- **If you develop pre-eclampsia** (see p.474). Measures will be taken to reduce your blood pressure.
- **If you have placental abruption,** where the placenta separates from the uterus (see p.473).

FOCUS ON... YOUR BODY

Getting strong

Maintaining muscular strength, stretching, and doing gentle exercise right up until you give birth will help your posture – minimizing backache, reducing stress on your skeleton, and making you feel more energized and relaxed.

As long as you feel good and adhere to the guidelines set out on page 18, you can continue with your activities.

Most importantly, at this time you should use common sense and listen to your body. If you're in pain, feel fatigued, or have dizzy spells, see your doctor immediately and stop exercising. You'll be feeling tired carrying around all that extra weight so adjust your activities accordingly. This could mean that you lower the intensity of your exercise and exercise for a shorter time, but if you feel good don't stop exercising altogether.

Look at the routines on pages 90 and 250, but don't do any exercises at this stage that require you to lie on your back.

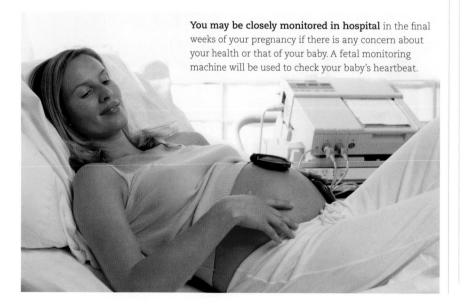

You may be closely monitored in hospital in the final weeks of your pregnancy if there is any concern about your health or that of your baby. A fetal monitoring machine will be used to check your baby's heartbeat.

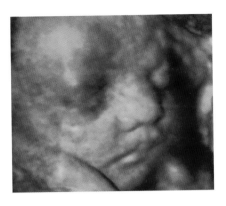

30 days to go...

YOUR BABY TODAY

Many babies will still have a good volume of amniotic fluid around them, but shadows from the placenta or side of the uterus, coupled with the curled up fetal position, will make imaging the baby harder and harder.

It's worth making practical arrangements now for what might happen if you go into labour.

With only around four weeks to go, now is the time to make sure you have all your partner's contact details and know exactly how to get hold of him in case you go into labour when he's at work. He might want to take extra care to ensure he has his mobile phone switched on and to hand in these final few weeks, and that he's not travelling too far away.

If you have other children or other dependants, or a pet, then you should arrange what will happen to them when you go into the hospital. You may want to explain to any older children what is going to happen so that they are prepared for when they go to stay with Grandma, or whoever will be looking after them.

If you're having a Caesarean, you might also want your older children looked after once you're home from hospital.

Reassure your children that you will be coming back and that you're not sick, but that you have to go into hospital when the baby comes. Depending on the age of your children, you could go with them to buy a present for the baby or you could give them a special job such as opening all the new gifts. Presents from the newborn to her elder siblings is also a good gesture.

In the run-up to the birth, ensure your toddler spends time with any family members who will be looking after him while you're in hospital. This will help him to settle and cope without you without getting upset.

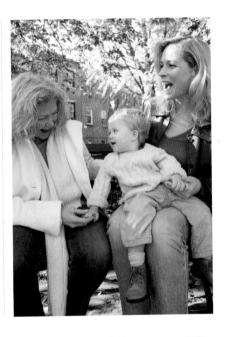

AS A MATTER OF FACT

In one study of women who anticipated that they would not need pain relief, 52 per cent actually used it.

According to recent research from NICE (National Institute for Clinical Excellence), women underestimate how much giving birth will hurt, and don't find out about the pain-relief options available (see pp.402–7).

ASK A... MIDWIFE

If my baby is premature and is in the special care baby unit, should I still express milk? Yes, definitely. Breast milk helps to ensure that the mother's natural immunity is passed on to her baby via her milk. As premature babies are more prone to infection, expressing your breast milk is a great way to help your baby if she is in the special care unit. Breast milk is much easier for a baby to digest: this is important for premature babies since their digestive tract may be less developed than a full-term baby's.

This is also a great way for you to bond and develop a relationship with your baby. This situation could be a time of considerable stress for you and you may feel helpless, so knowing that you're doing such a great thing to help your baby could help.

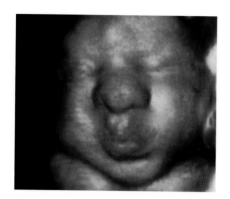

YOU ARE 35 WEEKS AND 6 DAYS

29 days to go...

YOUR BABY TODAY

Most babies will now be positioned longitudinally (lying straight up and down, with their head well in the pelvis). Even now, when space is limited in these final weeks, there is still time for the position to change to head down if your baby is bottom first (breech).

Complex developments are taking place in your baby's lungs that will enable her to breathe unaided once she is born.

The blood flow to your baby's lungs mirrors the development of the airways. Blood leaves the right side of the heart through a one-way valve into the main pulmonary vein. This then divides to give a pulmonary branch to each lung, and also a duct that allows blood to bypass the lungs and travel to the body directly. This will close soon after birth as the lungs expand and their resistance to blood flow falls.

Because your baby doesn't use his lungs for gas exchange in the uterus, the blood supply to them is quite small – only 10 per cent of the post-birth supply. At this stage of pregnancy, the lungs' blood supply has completed its development, branching into finer and finer vessels as they come to lie closer to the alveoli.

When your baby is born, her chest is compressed in the birth canal and this helps to push the fluid out of the lungs in preparation for that incredible first breath. If your baby is born by Caesarean, she will need first to bring the fluid up by herself. This is not a problem but for this reason the first breaths of a Caesarean baby can be full of mucus.

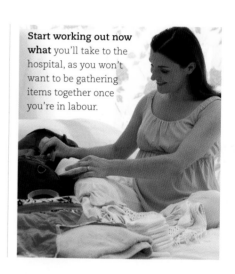

Start working out now what you'll take to the hospital, as you won't want to be gathering items together once you're in labour.

ITEMS FOR YOUR HOSPITAL BAG

Make sure you have all the items you need for your hospital bag. Remember to include items for yourself as well as the baby and, if you know you're having a Caesarean, pack enough items for a few days.

For yourself:
- Nightwear
- Underwear
- Nursing bras
- Slippers
- Dressing gown
- Hairbrush
- Toothbrush
- Toiletries

- Maternity sanitary pads
- Breast pads and nipple cream
- Comfortable daywear in case you stay in and want to get dressed.

For your baby:
- Vests
- Babygros
- Cellular blanket
- Nappies
- Nappy bags
- Cotton wool
- Nappy cream
- Baby wipes if you intend to use them
- Hat and cardigan for going home – you can also use the cardigan if your

baby needs layers to keep warm while she's in hospital.

Other useful items:
- Camera – stills camera and/or video camera
- Music for the delivery room
- Books and magazines
- Massage oil
- TENS machine (see p.399)
- Face flannels.

Your partner should also get a bag ready for himself (see p.338) and ensure the car seat is fitted. Pack snacks and drinks nearer the time, but think about what you might need.

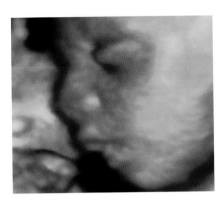

28 days to go...

YOUR BABY TODAY

You may notice a change in the character of your baby's movements, reflecting the reduced amount of amniotic fluid and, consequently, space to move around in. Each movement is more likely to be felt, however, as he touches the side of your uterus.

All pregnant women need support in the final weeks, but if you're single this can be even more important.

Whether you're single by choice, or have unexpectedly found yourself in this position, you may be experiencing mixed feelings about the weeks to come. There is no doubt that going solo involves extra responsibilities and worries, but with a little help from your close friends and family, you can make these final few weeks of your pregnancy positive.

If you're concerned about going into labour alone, line up a close friend or family member who is on call at all times. He or she might want to get permission from their place of work to take leave to be with you should you go into labour. Keep yourself busy before your baby arrives, planning plenty of activities during your maternity leave.

Don't be afraid to ask people for help with shopping for last-minute baby buys or getting your home ready for your new arrival. Most people will be delighted with the honour of being asked to keep you company, and helping you to get things ready.

Most importantly, look after yourself: get organized by preparing meals you can freeze so you have plenty of healthy food in store for the weeks after the birth.

THE LOWDOWN

Baby showers

Throwing a baby shower to celebrate the imminent arrival is a great opportunity to get together with the girls. Organize it yourself, or ask your best friend to do the honours. Note to best friend: surprise parties are great, but consider whether the mum-to-be will want to be the centre of attention.

Think about:
- **A pampering theme:** the guests could give each other manicures and pedicures, or you could even hire a beautician for the afternoon.
- **Clubbing together to buy the mum-to-be something useful,** such as a car seat, or indulgent, such as a relaxing day out at a spa.
- **Games you could play,** such as inviting guests to guess the baby's sex, weight, and date she'll be born.
- **Refreshments:** Champagne, non-alcoholic drinks, nibbles, and a "birth" day cake.

At your baby shower you'll probably receive lots of gifts. It's common for there to be presents for both mum and the newborn.

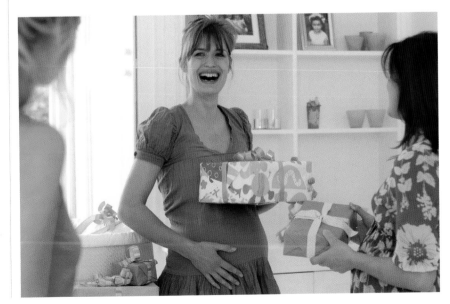

Your 37th week

YOUR BUMP MAY LOOK AS THOUGH IT'S STARTED TO SLIDE DOWNHILL

You're now about as big as you're going to get. Soon – maybe this week – the baby will drop down lower into your pelvis, ready for birth. Your bump may shift downwards, too, giving you a different shape. This doesn't necessarily mean that labour is imminent, so don't worry about the baby "falling out". You're likely to still have some time to enjoy maternity leave and get organized.

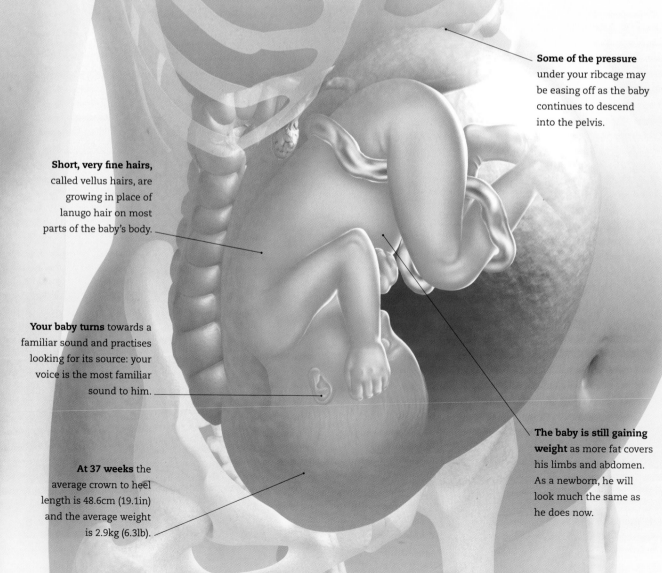

Some of the pressure under your ribcage may be easing off as the baby continues to descend into the pelvis.

Short, very fine hairs, called vellus hairs, are growing in place of lanugo hair on most parts of the baby's body.

Your baby turns towards a familiar sound and practises looking for its source: your voice is the most familiar sound to him.

The baby is still gaining weight as more fat covers his limbs and abdomen. As a newborn, he will look much the same as he does now.

At 37 weeks the average crown to heel length is 48.6cm (19.1in) and the average weight is 2.9kg (6.3lb).

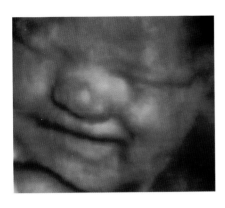

YOU ARE 36 WEEKS AND 1 DAY

27 days to go...

YOUR BABY TODAY

When scanned, this baby was lying with his back to his mother's. This "back to back" position is common at this stage but becomes less so as the pregnancy continues. Your midwife will be able to feel for the position of your baby's back from this point on.

You're likely to begin your maternity leave around this time. This can be a relief, but also a time of mixed emotions.

Going on maternity leave is a significant pregnancy milestone. As you leave your working role, the reality of beginning your role as a mother may hit you – but you hopefully have a few more weeks to get used to the idea!

It can be a welcome respite to take it easy and not have to rush around in the mornings, and you'll feel less tired by not having to travel. Although you need to take it easy, it's worth planning some outings, as not having a routine can take some getting used to.

Although it's good to stay in touch with colleagues, try not to fall into the trap of logging on to work emails or staying up to date with what's happening at work. You might be worrying about losing some of your identity while you're on maternity leave; this is a common feeling but you'll find that before you know it your leave is over and you're settled back into work again.

Try to enjoy this run-up to the birth and make the most of the time (see p.366) to get organized and prepare for your new arrival.

ASK A... MIDWIFE

Will I feel different when my baby engages? You will feel lighter, in that your breathing will be easier, with more room for your lungs to expand. Your abdomen may seem smaller, with your bump shifting down and forward, as your baby's head enters the birth canal. With pressure on your bladder, you may need to urinate more. You may also experience some pelvic pain.

WHEN YOUR BABY ENGAGES

Engagement is the process by which your baby's head moves through the pelvic brim and into the birth canal in preparation for birth, and this can occur any time in these final weeks, until the start of labour. In the last weeks of pregnancy, your midwife will palpate your abdomen to see if the head has started to engage.

The degree to which a baby's head is engaged is measured in fifths. If three- or four-fifths of the head can be felt above the pubic bone, then the baby is not engaged. If only two-fifths of the head can be felt, then the baby is said to be fully engaged, and if just one-fifth is felt, the baby is recorded as being deeply engaged.

When your baby engages you will look and feel slightly different (see above). If you're experiencing discomfort in your pelvis and perineum, try to avoid standing for long periods of time.

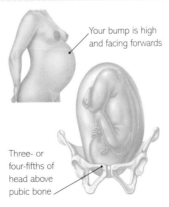

Your bump is high and facing forwards

Three- or four-fifths of head above pubic bone

Not engaged: The baby's head has started to move into the pelvis, but more than three- or four-fifths can be felt above the pubic bone.

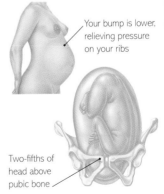

Your bump is lower, relieving pressure on your ribs

Two-fifths of head above pubic bone

Engaged: The baby has dropped into the pelvis in preparation for birth. This causes your bump to change position and shape.

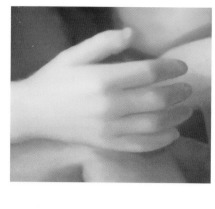

26 days to go...

YOUR BABY TODAY

Although almost invisible in the image, a very thin layer of vernix covers your baby. At first this helped to reduce the amount of water leaving your baby's skin, but now it helps to prevent direct contact between the skin and amniotic fluid.

Have you started nesting? The need to provide a safe, comfortable space for your new baby is a primitive desire.

THE LOWDOWN

On plaster casts!

Preserve your bump for posterity by making a plaster belly cast. You can either buy a kit or (far cheaper) purchase the plaster separately; it's all available online.

You will need:
- Plaster of Paris bandages, cut into several strips
- Large tub of petroleum jelly
- Bucket of warm water
- An assistant or two (not essential, but can be useful for speeding up the process and bringing refreshments).

Here's how to do it:
1. Strip off bar a pair of old knickers (the smaller, the better)
2. Apply petroleum jelly liberally to your bump and breasts
3. Assume a comfortable pose
4. One by one, dip the plaster of Paris strips into the water, then apply, overlapping the layers until you have a thick coating
5. Sit and wait for it to dry – it's a good excuse to have a rest
6. Slip it off when it's rock hard and paint it if you wish.

The nesting instinct usually begins in the final weeks of pregnancy, accompanied by a surge of energy and an uncontrollable urge to get your home shipshape.

Give in to your inner domestic goddess: cook, clean, organize, and de-clutter, but take it easy. If you spend hours on your hands and knees scrubbing, you may find yourself in labour sooner than you'd expected.

Some men develop a nesting instinct, but unfortunately this tends to be associated with cars and garden sheds. If this happens to your partner, at least you can look forward to a sparkling-clean motor, spruced-up patio, and manicured lawn.

Nesting not happening for you? Pay the professionals to do a spring clean. Or forget it: your baby won't care whether the cupboards are clean.

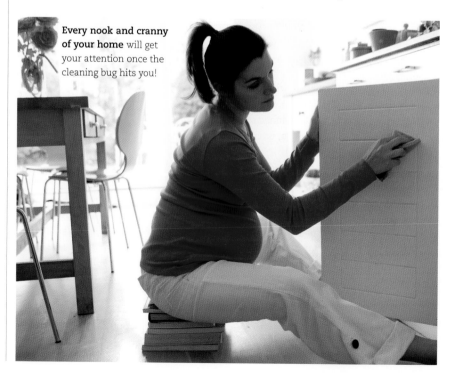

Every nook and cranny of your home will get your attention once the cleaning bug hits you!

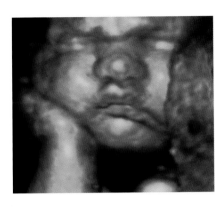

25 days to go...

YOUR BABY TODAY

A short portion of the umbilical cord is lying close to the mouth, which makes this baby appear to have a rather grumpy looking expression. The placenta is seen to the right of the image partially obscuring the view of the face.

You'll find that your beautiful bump is intruding on your life more and more, affecting your movements and eating patterns.

You might be getting a little frustrated by your size around now, which can make everyday activities more difficult. Simple manoeuvres, such as fitting through doors or getting off the sofa, can be more difficult and you may find that everything takes that bit longer to achieve. All you can do is be patient and focus on getting through the next few weeks. You'll soon have your body back to normal.

THE LOWDOWN

Lotus birth

Instead of cutting the cord within minutes of their baby's birth, some parents choose to leave it attached to the newborn and the placenta, until the cord withers and drops off naturally (usually within a few days). It's highly unlikely to be permitted at a hospital birth.

Proponents of "umbilical non-severance" – also known as lotus birth – claim that the baby continues to receive sustenance from the placenta via the cord until it naturally detaches. They also believe the babies experience a gentler birth as they are spared the stress of being suddenly separated from the placenta.

During pregnancy, it's common to eat more often than previously but to eat less at each meal. This is because your uterus has grown so much that all your other organs have moved about and are squashed into much less space. Your stomach simply has less room in it to fit the food so you can't eat as much before feeling full. When your stomach empties you may find yourself hungry again. It's fine to snack, but make sure you're reaching for healthy foods and not the biscuit tin!

Getting comfortable behind the steering wheel will become increasingly challenging in the late stages of pregnancy. Keep journeys as short as possible or take regular breaks if you need to travel for any length of time. Always wear your seat belt (see p.252).

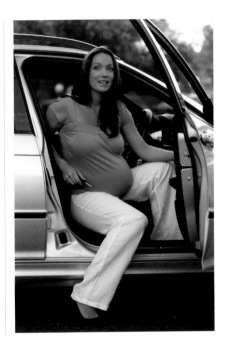

FOCUS ON... YOUR BABY

Working out with Mum

Your baby will usually move several times in the 20 to 30 minutes after you exercise. By keeping the intensity of your exercise at a moderate level you will not affect the oxygen supply to your baby. When you exercise too hard and for too long, you may compromise the oxygen supply and the result is the baby's movements will fall below their usual levels.

If you're concerned and unsure, keep a log of how much your baby is moving and compare this to the activity levels after exercise. If the level falls below what you consider to be "normal", speak to your midwife.

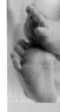

24 days to go...

YOUR BABY TODAY

Your baby is now more suitably equipped for the time after birth. His ears are fully formed on the outside and inside and he is used to hearing the sound of your blood circulating and your heart beating, and he recognizes your voice.

Your baby is losing the downy hair that he's had for several weeks, but if he's born now there may still be some visible.

Lanugo is extremely fine hair that covers your baby's body and, unlike adult hairs on the body, it is not associated with sweat glands. Lanugo hairs begin to be shed now as they are lost into the amniotic fluid in the last few weeks before birth. Your baby then swallows these lanugo hairs in the amniotic fluid but this is not a cause for concern: these hairs provide your baby with an important source of protein, essential to his development. It's been estimated that two-thirds of the protein in the fluid is swallowed and absorbed by the baby's gut each day, providing 15 per cent of his protein needs.

The fine lanugo hairs are gradually replaced by vellus hairs, which are short, soft, non-pigmented hairs (often seen more on women and children). Terminal hair is the thicker, coarser, and longer hair that first grows on your baby's eyebrows, then his eyelashes, then his scalp. In adults, facial hair (beards), armpit, and pubic hair is terminal hair.

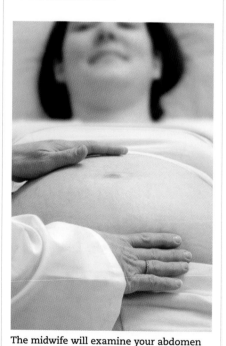

The midwife will examine your abdomen in late pregnancy to check the position of the baby. If the baby is breech, an ECV (see right) may be recommended to turn him into a head-down position. If he doesn't turn, a Caesarean delivery may be necessary.

FOCUS ON... YOUR BODY

Desperate for the loo

In the third trimester you'll be frequenting the loo regularly, as you did in the first trimester. At this stage it's due to the increasingly heavy baby pushing down on your bladder from above. If you find that it hurts when you expel urine, you may have a urinary infection and should contact your midwife or doctor for a test.

ASK A... DOCTOR

I've heard about doctors "turning" breech babies. How does this work? Some obstetricians may try to turn a baby in late pregnancy using external cephalic version (ECV), which has a success rate of around 50 per cent. The obstetrician tries gently to guide the baby into a head-down position by pressing his hands on the mother's abdomen, using an ultrasound as a guide. You may be given a drug to relax the uterine muscles. You will be scanned first and if the baby is in an awkward position the procedure may not continue. If your baby is large this can affect the procedure, as can the amount of amniotic fluid: a low amount of fluid offers less protection to the baby.

If you're rhesus negative, you will have an anti-D injection (see p.123) after the ECV because of a small risk of a bleed around the placenta. An ECV is not recommended if you have a multiple pregnancy, have had bleeding, your placenta is low-lying (see p.212), your membranes have ruptured, or there is a known problem with the baby.

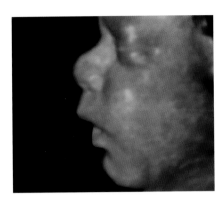

23 days to go...

YOUR BABY TODAY

3D views at this stage of the pregnancy will be extremely clear. Every part of the face is fully developed and your baby will be very expressive. Your baby is only a few days away now from being full term.

Don't be concerned about embarrassing yourself in labour – your carers will have seen it all before.

Many women worry about losing control during labour – for example that they will urinate or defecate when they are pushing. You might well pass a bit of stool when you're pushing but you probably won't notice; your midwife will put on a pair of gloves and use gauze to remove it.

The reality is that when you're in the throes of labour, you really won't care – you'll just want that baby out!

Keep an open mind about pain relief as you won't know how you'll handle the pain or what your pain threshold is until you're actually in labour.

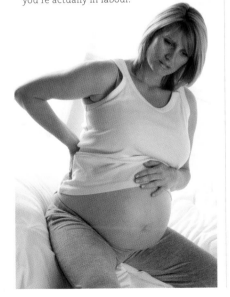

ASK A... PANEL ABOUT PAIN RELIEF

What if I can't cope with the pain of labour?

Doctor: If you're concerned, take time to investigate the pain-relief options in advance of labour, so that you're aware of what's on offer, even if you don't plan to use it.

There's no shame in deviating from what you requested in your birth plan; the ultimate goal is to deliver a healthy baby, and to keep your energy levels and your spirits high. It's also important to ask for pain relief as soon as you feel that things are getting on top of you.

Mum: When I was in labour, the pain literally took my breath away, and I really did feel that I would be unable to carry on. Changing position, walking around, and using a birthing ball proved to be a good distraction, even if they passed the time rather than provided relief, and I chanted to myself, over and over, "You can do it!"

I dimly remembered that when the pain is at its worst you've hit "transition", which signals the beginning of the delivery itself, and it did help to know I was near the end, even if it did seem a long time in

coming. Focus on how much you want your baby in your arms, and view every contraction as one step nearer to that moment.

Midwife: Mums who are prepared for the pain seem to find that it isn't as bad as they thought it might be, and are able to cope using breathing exercises and massage. The best advice is to know your limits. If you find the pain unbearable, then ask for some pain relief. Even a little gas and air can take the edge off the discomfort, and make the process more bearable.

No woman can anticipate how her labour and delivery will proceed, and sometimes babies make things difficult by presenting themselves in awkward positions, or simply enjoying life inside a little too much to arrive promptly. Take things one step at a time, and when you know you've had enough, conserve your energy by getting the help you need. Any woman who delivers a healthy baby has had a successful delivery, and that's what's most important.

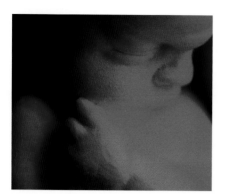

22 days to go...

YOUR BABY TODAY

Your baby will be able to recall and recognize the frequency and pattern of the most familiar sounds he hears within the womb – your voice. Also, you might have noticed that loud noises may startle your baby during these final weeks.

If you're lacking in energy, try carb loading. This is also an effective measure in the days leading up to labour.

The idea behind carb loading comes from endurance athletes, who get 70 per cent of their calorie intake from carbohydrates for three days prior to a big event. This enhances muscle uptake of fuel so that muscles are fully loaded with glycogen, the form in which carbs are stored in the body. If you're feeling tired, and especially prior to being active, ensure you take on plenty of carbohydrates.

In the days before your due date, base meals on carbohydrates, so that this food group provides up to 70 per cent of your total calories. Include cereal or bread for breakfast, sandwiches for lunch, and include pasta, rice, or potatoes at dinner.

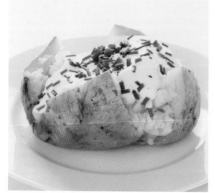

A jacket potato is a great mini-meal, providing you with carbohydrates. Try different carbohydrate foods in the run-up to labour to see which suit you best.

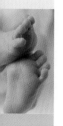

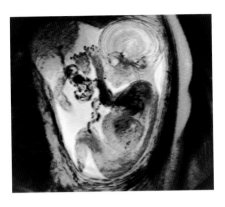

21 days to go...

YOUR BABY TODAY

This baby is lying in the breech position, with the umbilical cord seen as it travels towards the placenta in the top left-hand side of the image. Approximately 3 in every 100 babies will be in a breech position after 37 weeks.

Your baby is now able to hear many sounds that will all be familiar to him once he's born.

In this late stage of pregnancy, sounds penetrate the uterus easily and there is no doubt that the baby can hear and respond to these before birth. Your baby will startle at loud sounds but now also turn towards familiar sounds, and practise looking for the source of the sound. Your baby is not only recognizing a wider range of sound frequencies, but also discriminating between different sounds as well as learning and remembering familiar sounds, such as your voice and that of your partner.

Your baby breathes more quickly when he's concentrating on sounds and his heart rate increases. Although the baby can hear at birth, the ear drum continues to thin out, at the same time becoming more mobile and responsive to sounds. Your voice will be the most familiar sound to your baby at birth.

ASK A... MIDWIFE

What if I can't breastfeed? It's normal to have doubts but be reassured that most women have enough milk, and with some help with positioning the baby can breastfeed without any problems. By this stage, you may even be leaking colostrum (see p.295).

Try to keep an open mind and remember that the breast milk does not come in straight after the birth (see p.448). Even if you have problems, try to persevere and don't feel pressured to give up just because it's convenient for the hospital staff or your partner, or because a friend or family member tells you it's not necessary.

Even if you don't end up breastfeeding, you can still get close to your baby by bottle-feeding.

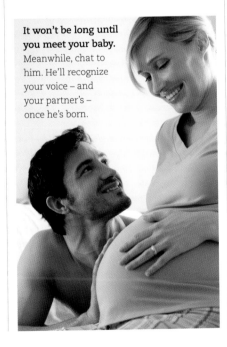

It won't be long until you meet your baby. Meanwhile, chat to him. He'll recognize your voice – and your partner's – once he's born.

FOCUS ON... DADS

The final weeks

You aren't alone if you're a dad-to-be who's feeling a bit bewildered and shell-shocked by the imminent arrival of your baby. To begin with, you can expect a lot of changes at home. Once your partner starts maternity leave, she may start a whirlwind of activity in preparation for the new arrival, and will need your help to get everything ready.

While supporting your partner both practically and emotionally will be important in the coming weeks, do look after yourself, too. Take every opportunity to get some rest. Even if you've agreed that your partner will do the majority of the night-time babycare, your sleep will still be disrupted in the weeks after the birth. Catch up with friends now, but not to the point where you tire yourself out, and keep up your exercise routine, if you have one.

It's normal to feel anxious about what's ahead – both being a birth partner and a dad – but be reassured that somehow everything will fall into place. Focus on the thought of holding your newborn baby.

Your 38th week

EVEN IF YOU HAVE ENJOYED YOUR PREGNANCY, YOU MAY BE LONGING FOR IT TO BE OVER

The baby is nearly ready, you are more than ready, so when is the birth going to happen? Probably not yet – especially if this is your first pregnancy. For another week or so, the uterus is still the best place for your baby while the finishing touches to her development take place. If you have other children, you can tell them that their new brother or sister won't keep everyone waiting much longer.

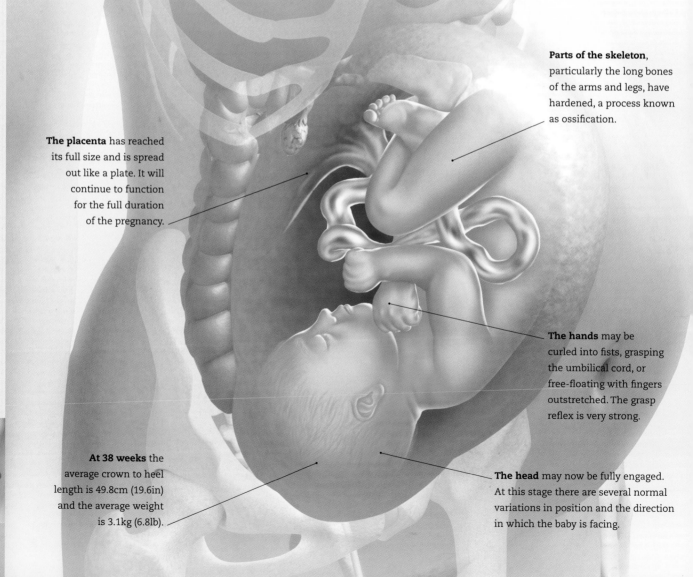

Parts of the skeleton, particularly the long bones of the arms and legs, have hardened, a process known as ossification.

The placenta has reached its full size and is spread out like a plate. It will continue to function for the full duration of the pregnancy.

The hands may be curled into fists, grasping the umbilical cord, or free-floating with fingers outstretched. The grasp reflex is very strong.

At 38 weeks the average crown to heel length is 49.8cm (19.6in) and the average weight is 3.1kg (6.8lb).

The head may now be fully engaged. At this stage there are several normal variations in position and the direction in which the baby is facing.

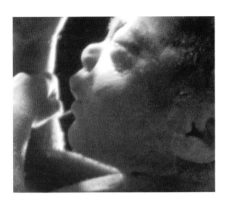

20 days to go...

YOUR BABY TODAY

Full term has been reached and your baby's features are now very clearly formed. To a certain extent from now on your baby is simply growing and putting on weight – factors necessary to provide energy after birth and help with temperature control.

Start preparing for the birth now: by being practical and positive, you can make it memorable for all the right reasons.

AS A MATTER OF FACT

Being hypnotized during pregnancy can make you more confident in the run-up to labour.

A study found that first-time pregnant women also experienced a shorter labour. The average amount of time they pushed in the second stage was one hour, compared with the usual two hours for a first baby.

Probably the most effective way to remember as much as you can about your labour and the birth of your baby is to try to remain as healthy and rested as possible prior to the start of your labour; this will give you the best chance of staying strong and clear-headed throughout.

Feeling strong and having plenty of energy may also help you to remain upright and active during the course of your labour, reducing the need for pain relief such as pethidine (see p.403), which can create a mild state of amnesia that makes it more difficult to remember the finer details of the birth. It's also helpful to have your birth partner with you throughout your labour so that he or she can help to fill in any blanks later. Photographs and videos are also good prompts.

After the birth, if you find that there are parts you can't remember, you can ask your midwife to let you see your birth notes. You might want to write up your experience in a journal.

FOCUS ON... DADS

Health professionals and you

When you get closer to the birth, and especially during labour, you will find that there is inevitably more contact with health professionals. These individuals are a source of reassurance and a font of knowledge, but as a male you may sometimes feel that you're being side-lined or that your opinion doesn't count. This can be very frustrating if you want to be highly involved in the pregnancy and birth.

Bear in mind that the health professionals are trying to provide care for the person who needs it the most – namely your partner. If you want to be heard, it's a good idea to write down any questions that you may have before you meet with health professionals. Midwives will make every effort to help you to feel involved, and support you in supporting your partner.

Try to keep in mind that the most important relationship your partner has is with you, and that a positive attitude on your part can make a substantial difference to your partner's pregnancy and birth. So be patient and persistent but not pushy.

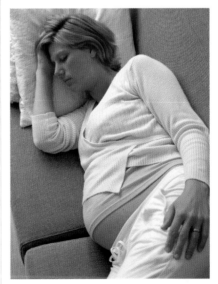

Ensure you get plenty of rest in the next few weeks to get you in the best frame of mind for labour and birth.

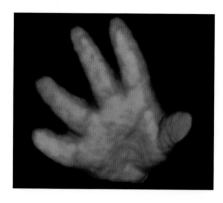

19 days to go...

YOUR BABY TODAY

A 3D close-up of the hand shows the skin folds. Just as fingerprints are unique, so are the deeper skin folds seen on the hands and feet. The grasp reflex is strong and your baby will start to grasp anything that touches the palm of her hand.

Your baby will benefit from extra time in the uterus, but her development is almost complete and she's now "full term".

THE LOWDOWN

Hair down there

One dilemma that's rarely discussed – but much pondered – among mums-to-be is whether they should shave or trim their pubic hair before giving birth.

It's really a personal choice and depends how much it bothers you: just because your best friend had her pubic hair waxed, you shouldn't feel pressured to do the same – aside from anything else, itchy regrowth will not be welcome in the days following the birth of your baby.

You might want to trim your pubic hair or use tweezers or shave any stragglers, though, in the interests of postnatal hygiene. Postnatal blood loss will cling to the hair.

If you're booked in to have a Caesarean, the top inch (at least) of your pubic hair will be shaved in hospital, so you may prefer to do this at home yourself.

Your baby will be very cramped in the uterus. It won't be long, however, until she's positioned head down and begins to engage in the pelvis as she prepares to make her entry into the world.

There is now less space for your baby to move and she will soon, if she hasn't already, settle down into a comfortable head-down position. The shape of the uterus encourages this head-down position and, once in it, turning would be a major effort for your baby. Plenty of amniotic fluid remains to cushion and protect your baby, who will still be attempting to be very active in this more confined space.

Your baby's behaviour is now exactly the same as a newborn: she'll turn towards light and yawn just as much as a newborn, and she'll continue to practise breathing the amniotic fluid in and out with regular rhythmical movements.

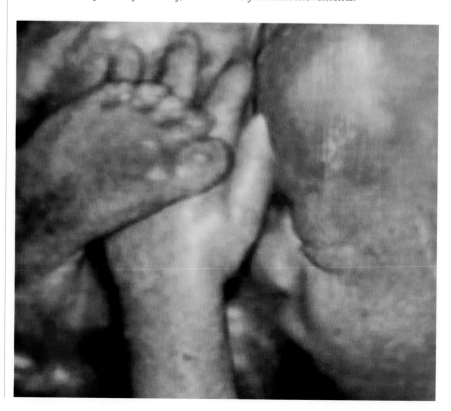

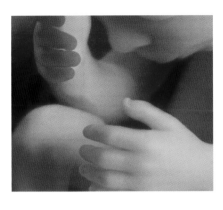

18 days to go...

YOUR BABY TODAY

With each day that goes by delivery is becoming ever more likely. You may experience Braxton-Hicks' contractions, which help to soften the cervix and prepare for labour. The amniotic fluid that surrounds your baby ensures she'll hardly notice these mild tightenings.

It's worth giving some thought to life after the birth, and ensuring you have adequate help and support lined up.

Even at this late stage of pregnancy, it may still be hard to imagine your baby being born and living in your home. You and your partner may settle into life with your newborn with ease, and manage without any help, but it's still worth having back-up support just in case.

What you may not be prepared for is the fact that you're likely to be exhausted after weeks of poor sleep during pregnancy, and the rigours of labour itself. Add to this broken nights' sleep and the whole adjustment to being a new parent, and you may well find you'll need to call on people to help practically and emotionally.

It can help enormously to have a good support network set up in advance. Ideally, this will be close family and friends who you know you can rely on to drop round to help, but who will also know when you need to be left alone. Even an hour's help to prepare you a nutritious meal, or hold your baby while you get a much-needed rest or a shower, can give you some welcome respite.

Have the number to hand for your breastfeeding counsellor and midwife, so that you can ask for advice. Also get on the phone to mums-to-be whom you've met at antenatal classes; they more than anyone will be able to relate to how you're feeling.

Don't be too proud to accept help with housework and shopping. Knowing these tasks are taken care of will help you relax and focus on your baby.

Try to limit the number of guests you have in the early days, and make sure that they are pre-warned that visits will be short. Although you will be desperate to show off your new baby, visits can be draining so it's better to wait until some routines are more established.

FOCUS ON... NUTRITION

Healthy snacking

Large meals are likely to leave you feeling uncomfortably full, especially late in the third trimester. If you go long periods of time between meals, you may become light-headed and feel weak from hypoglycaemia – low blood sugar. This is because the baby is constantly drawing glucose from your bloodstream.

Healthy snacking is the key to eating well and comfortably:

■ **Keep lots of fresh fruit** on display in a bowl so you'll remember to eat it.
■ **Stock your cupboards** with a variety of dried fruits and nuts.
■ **Hard boil eggs** and keep them in the fridge. Try eating them with a sprinkle of salt to quell that salt craving.
■ **Buy or make some frozen juice pops** and keep them in the freezer. Some women also find it refreshing to suck on these during labour.

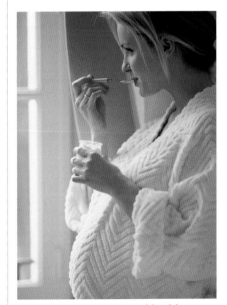

Yogurts are a nutritious and healthy snack for any time of day. For variety and additional nutrients, sprinkle granola or dried fruits on the top.

371

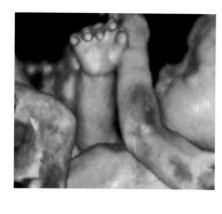

17 days to go...

YOUR BABY TODAY

What exactly triggers the start of labour is still a mystery. Does the signal come from your own body or does the baby play a part in the decision? Every labour is different, and the timing of your first labour can be quite different from your second.

Gradually, each of your baby's bones is becoming strengthened thanks to adequate amounts of calcium.

Your baby's bones are strengthened by the process of ossification in which hard bone is formed from calcium. To meet this increase in demand, you absorb calcium much more readily from your diet.

By this stage of pregnancy, the baby's humerus in the upper arm, femur in the upper leg, and tibia in the lower leg have undergone this process. As ossification occurs at specific weeks in your pregnancy, ultrasound can use these as markers to estimate the date of the pregnancy, if necessary.

The time at which this ossification occurs may be seen a few days earlier in girls than boys and, interestingly, the patella (knee bone), does not ossify until after birth.

ASK A... DOCTOR

I've had a small amount of bleeding. Should I be concerned?
Bleeding in late pregnancy may be serious as it can be due to the placenta partially, or totally, detaching from the wall of the uterus, known as placental abruption (see p.473), or to a low-lying placenta, known as placenta praevia (see p.212). If you have a mucus discharge tinged with blood in late pregnancy, this may be a "show" (see pp.391 and 411).

Always seek medical advice for bleeding at any stage of pregnancy to rule out any problems.

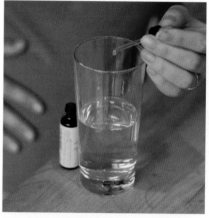

One way to take Bach Flower Remedies (see below) is to put four drops into a glass of water and sip it at intervals. Alternatively, you can put the drops directly on to your tongue using the pipette. Always read the label before using any remedy.

AS A MATTER OF FACT

Just because your partner weighed above average at birth, it doesn't mean your baby will too.

The birth weight depends on the mix of genes your baby inherits. So, if your partner is tall and big-built and you're petite and were a tiny baby, keep your fingers crossed that you have the more dominant genes!

BACH FLOWER REMEDIES

Flower essence blends are designed to calm and centre your energy, which some think can help you relax and encourage you to focus. Rescue Remedy and Emergency Essence, types of Bach Flower Remedy, are thought to be effective when used in labour, and in the weeks prior to and after the birth. Whether you're anxious, shocked, worried, suffering from the effects of stress, distressed, or simply need a boost during a long or painful labour, you may find these remedies have a positive effect.

Take a few drops on your tongue as required or mix them in water, as shown above. Both of these blends also come in cream form, to apply topically, or as a spray, to spritz yourself, and your environment.

Try out different forms now in this late stage of your pregnancy.

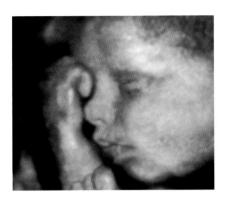

16 days to go...

YOUR BABY TODAY

The size of your uterus may have reduced slightly as your baby's head becomes more deeply engaged within your pelvis, allowing her body to move down. This can take some of the pressure away from your ribs, which is a welcome relief at this stage.

When there's going to be a new arrival on the scene, it's important to prepare the little members of your household.

How you handle introducing the new baby to your children will depend on their age. A toddler might be totally indifferent and unfazed, being more interested in your new baby's toys than the fact that she has a new brother or sister. An older child might be shocked and jealous by the arrival of a new baby, who appears to steal her limelight, and usurp Mummy's and Daddy's attention.

It's a good idea to prepare your little one several weeks in advance, explaining that the new baby will need a lot of time and attention, will need to be fed and changed regularly, and probably not be much fun for a few months. Focus on how your child can be a great helper, and show her what the new baby will need when she is born. Take some books out of the library that explain how families change when a new baby is born, and ask your child to talk about how she's feeling, and how she thinks things will be different when the baby arrives.

Encourage your child to choose a gift to give to the baby, and find something your child really wants as a gift from her new sibling. Ask grandparents or close friends to arrange a few treats or outings for your child both now and after the birth, so that she's occupied, and getting extra attention.

ASK A... MIDWIFE

My mum had a difficult delivery with me. Am I likely to have the same experience as her? Like many women, you're obviously aware of the details of your own birth.

Some say you'll have the same sort of delivery your mum had with you – for example, your baby will be early or late or you'll have a very quick labour or a slow, assisted one. This isn't necessarily true.

Remember, depending on how old your mum is, there have probably been significant developments in obstetrics since your mum's days and, even if you face the same hurdles during your labour, they might be managed differently.

Also, you might be healthier and stronger than your mum was, so don't assume you're in for a difficult labour just because she had one.

Try to encourage a bond between your older child and your baby. Ask your child to imagine what the baby might be getting up to inside Mummy. Encourage her to suggest names, although don't promise to use them!

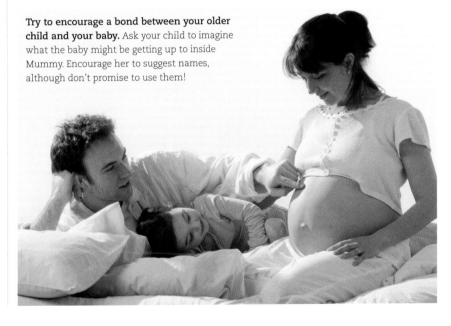

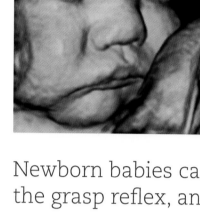

YOU ARE 37 WEEKS AND 6 DAYS

15 days to go...

YOUR BABY TODAY

Estimating your baby's size by measuring from the top of the uterus to the front of your pelvic bone can give you an idea of size, but this is less accurate now. Your baby may not yet have moved down into the pelvis and the amount of fluid around your baby is variable.

Newborn babies can tightly hold someone's finger because of the grasp reflex, and this is already functioning in the uterus.

Inside the uterus your baby has developed a strong grasp reflex. The grip is so strong after birth that it could support your baby's weight. This grasp reflex persists until your baby is about six months old; she will then have more choice over whether to grasp an object or not.

Interestingly, your baby also has a similar reflex in the foot. This is the "plantar reflex" and it causes the toes to attempt to curl around your finger if the sole of the foot is stroked. The plantar reflex takes slightly longer to disappear after birth, typically persisting until 12 months of age. Another reflex action causes the toes to spread out if the side of the foot is stroked. These reflexes and others seem to be quite primitive in nature and although they are thought to protect the baby, the precise function of each reflex is not fully understood.

AS A MATTER OF FACT

Second labours are usually shorter in duration than first labours.

This usually means an easier labour, but a second baby could be bigger than a first, or positioned differently. There are many factors to consider.

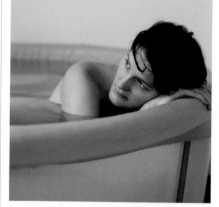

As well as being an effective way to relax, using a birthing pool can speed up labour. It is thought that water sets off a surge of the hormone oxytocin, which triggers contractions.

ASK A... MIDWIFE

Is it true that natural or water births are best for the baby? Most childbirth experts would agree that a straightforward vaginal birth is the safest form of birth for both mother and baby. It is also generally considered safe to use water as a method of relieving the pain in uncomplicated labours.

However, it is sometimes not possible to achieve a straightforward vaginal delivery due to certain situations that can arise during labour and birth. If a problem with either the mother or baby occurs, the medical team will advise on the safest way of delivering the baby.

It's important to think about the type of birth you would prefer and are comfortable with, but be prepared to be flexible and to see how labour unfolds. Do speak to your midwife to find out if there's a birthing pool you can use at your hospital.

THE LOWDOWN

Owls!

Could owls give us an insight into pregnancy and birth? It's doubtful, but these myths are entertaining!

■ **If a pregnant woman** hears the shriek of an owl, her child will definitely be a girl.

■ **An owl living in the attic** of a house will cause a problem with the baby.

■ **When the time comes to give birth** there should be no owls in the delivery room – if they hoot at the moment of birth the child will have a miserable life.

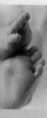

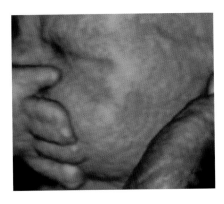

14 days to go...

YOUR BABY TODAY

The back of the hand is held up against the mouth in this image. Your baby will be practising suckling at every opportunity, but this will be with parts of the hands, thumbs or fingers, as it's no longer easy to reach the toes.

If you haven't found out the sex of your baby, the excitement will be building; if you have, you can get very organized!

Knowing the sex of your baby enables you to decide on the name, buy specific outfits, and even decorate the nursery, if you have one, in a certain way. Do, however, remember there's a chance that the scan (see pp.214–15) gave you misleading information. The only way to be absolutely certain of the baby's gender is if you found out following a diagnostic test, such as amniocentesis or chorionic villus sampling (see pp.152–3).

see pp.214–15

THE LOWDOWN

Boys and girls

Still wondering what you're having? Well, to help you guess, you might want to bear in mind a few more old wives' tales...

■ **If you have soft hands** you're having a girl, rough hands you're having a boy.
■ **If the father-to-be is nervous,** it's a girl, if he's relaxed it's a boy.
■ **If the mother picks up her coffee cup** with two hands it's a girl, if she picks it up by the handle it's a boy.
■ **If you have a sensitive belly button** it's a girl, if you have cold feet it's almost certainly a boy!

If you know the sex, you won't have the same incentive of a surprise at the end of your labour, but you may feel you can bond more closely with your baby during pregnancy and picture what he or she will be like as a newborn.

If you don't know the sex yet, then you will have a well-earned surprise after your hard work in labour. Some women who don't know the sex of their babies say that they have a strong instinct that the baby is a particular sex, but may get quite surprised when they have a baby of the opposite sex.

Try to keep an open mind and not raise your hopes about having a baby of a certain gender – the odds are slightly in favour of you having a boy.

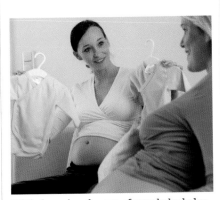

While knowing the sex of your baby helps you make decisions, such as should you buy pink or blue, not knowing gives you a greater sense of anticipation.

ASK A... DOCTOR

My baby is in a posterior position. How will this affect my labour?
In the posterior position the baby faces your tummy instead of your spine (see p.336). This position may prolong your labour, which can be tiring, and cause more backache. If this is the case, you can try the same methods as for turning a breech baby (see p.329) to encourage your baby to move in to an anterior position.

Most of the time the baby turns with the help of contractions when you are in fully established labour. If she doesn't, intervention such as the use of forceps or ventouse (see pp.436–7) may be needed.

AS A MATTER OF FACT

Your body is designed to handle the pain of labour!

Nobody likes pain, but your body's endorphin levels will increase during labour to help you cope with it. So it's reassuring to know that as the intensity of the contractions build, so does your ability to handle them.

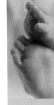

Your 39th week

TIME MAY FEEL AS THOUGH IT'S STANDING STILL AND EVERY SMALL TWINGE HAS YOU ON THE ALERT

Clue up on the signs that mean labour is really about to start. You may have some false alarms, so don't hesitate to call your midwife for advice and reassurance. Excitement will be competing with nerves – and that goes for your partner as well. No one can predict how labour is going to turn out, but before the big day it's helpful to agree on what your partner's role should ideally be.

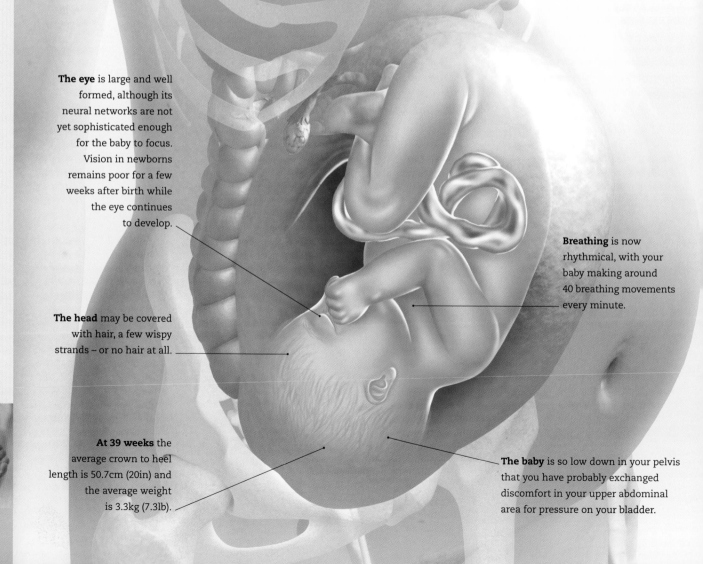

The eye is large and well formed, although its neural networks are not yet sophisticated enough for the baby to focus. Vision in newborns remains poor for a few weeks after birth while the eye continues to develop.

Breathing is now rhythmical, with your baby making around 40 breathing movements every minute.

The head may be covered with hair, a few wispy strands – or no hair at all.

At 39 weeks the average crown to heel length is 50.7cm (20in) and the average weight is 3.3kg (7.3lb).

The baby is so low down in your pelvis that you have probably exchanged discomfort in your upper abdominal area for pressure on your bladder.

13 days to go...

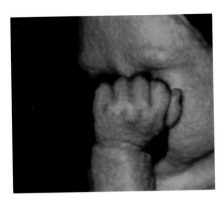

YOUR BABY TODAY

This baby's hand is in the same position as in the image opposite, with the fist held tightly in front of the face. All of your baby's movements help to build muscle strength and aid co-ordination, whether it's a kick or simply curling and uncurling the fingers.

With labour imminent, you'll be playing the waiting game. Staying active will help the time pass much more quickly.

You'll be resting a lot in the next two weeks. As your figure expands and you become more tired, it's natural to want to sit out the remainder of your pregnancy at home with your feet up, and put the answering machine on to field all the "Has it arrived?" enquiries!

It's fine to do this but it's worth remembering that the very best way to stimulate labour is to keep active. What's more, the hormones produced by even gentle walking will lift your mood and help you to feel more positive when your labour begins.

Try giving yourself one or two small tasks each day – perhaps meeting a friend for lunch, taking a very gentle swim, or purchasing some last-minute items for baby – taking care to stop and put your feet up when you feel tired. Be sensible about the type of activities you undertake, and avoid anything that could be overly exhausting or potentially dangerous; for example, bear in mind that your centre of gravity is way off balance at the moment, and that wallpapering the nursery or carrying heavy shopping should definitely not be on your to-do list.

It may feel as though your life is on hold at the moment so that's why it's good to fill your time as best you can. Don't forget, however, that in just a couple of weeks you'll have your newborn occupying all your time.

The power of music

Research has shown that women who listen to music during labour tend to feel less stressed and are less likely to need pain relief. There's also some evidence to suggest that babies born to the accompaniment of music are calmer.

One study compared different beats and found that classical, instrumental sounds were the most relaxing. Familiar tunes and rhythms could distract you from the pain and – if you choose the right track – help you focus on your breathing. Line up a selection of tunes on your iPod well in advance of labour.

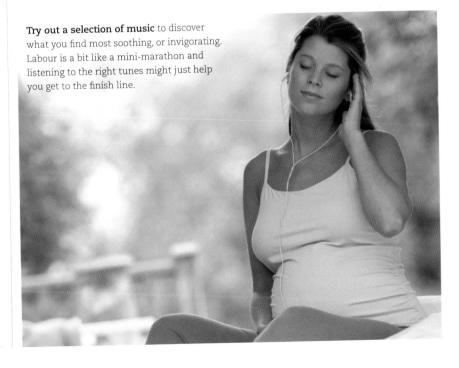

Try out a selection of music to discover what you find most soothing, or invigorating. Labour is a bit like a mini-marathon and listening to the right tunes might just help you get to the finish line.

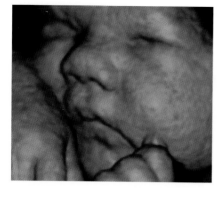

12 days to go...

YOUR BABY TODAY

Although your baby's head is deep within your pelvis, it will remain rounded in shape. It is not until labour starts that the bones of the skull move closer to each other, elongating the shape of the head, and allowing your baby to pass more easily along the birth canal.

Although your baby will be born with beautifully big eyes, it will be some time before he will see clearly at a distance.

Your baby's eyes are almost their adult size at birth. Although the eyes continue to grow very slightly until adolescence, and the lens within the eyes grows throughout life, the eyes are three-quarters of their adult size at birth. Both colour (cones) and black and white visual cells (rods) are present in the retina but vision is still rather poor

Your baby will have gained weight steadily during these final weeks, with fat being laid down under the skin. If born now, he would have a plump, rounded appearance.

– equivalent to being able to just see the top letter of the optician's chart. This is referred to as 20/400 vision. This means than if the baby could read, then he could read a letter at 6m (20ft) that a person with perfect vision could read when 122m (400ft) away. Because of this, your newborn may not seem to pay much attention at first; he'll have some difficulty focusing and his eye muscles will be quite weak. He will, however, be able to see objects 30cm (12in) away; as this is roughly the distance between your breast and face, it means your baby can see your face as he feeds.

He'll be six to eight weeks old before fixing on to and following an object, four months before he can judge distances, and two years of age before his vision has perfected to 20/20.

AS A MATTER OF FACT

95 per cent of babies don't arrive on their due date – of these 25 per cent come early and 70 per cent late.

There's a five-week window between 37 and 42 weeks of pregnancy that's regarded as normal and safe for a baby to be born.

Five weeks is a long time to wait, so put a message on your voicemail along the lines of "We'll be in touch as soon as the baby's arrived." Keep yourself busy: have your hair done (much easier without a newborn in tow), catch up with friends, and, most importantly, get some sleep!

ASK A... MIDWIFE

I don't often swear but is it true that I'm likely to subject my partner to verbal abuse during labour?
Possibly, but no one will blame you if you do! Giving birth can be incredibly painful, and you may feel emotional, irritable, shaky, and even nauseous. Don't worry too much about what you say and do: try to stay focused on the birth and ask for pain relief if you need it. Most birth partners will be forgiving and are unlikely to take the abuse personally. They will realize that you might not quite be yourself during childbirth – and if they've been by your side throughout labour will be fully understanding of what you're going through. You may also be irritable with your carers, but they will be used to this!

11 days to go...

YOUR BABY TODAY

This image demonstrates how your baby will have laid down fat stores, nicely rounding out the cheeks. The exact weight of your baby will depend now on which day you deliver as your baby will continue to grow in the uterus, although at a slower rate than previously.

If you're having a home birth, you can make the midwife's task as easy as possible by being well organized.

If you're having your baby at home, spend this week ensuring that everything is in order and that the room in which you plan to give birth is clean, comfortable, and adequately heated.

Your midwife may bring round a pack about now, which contains all the items she will need. To make her task easier, make sure the bed on which you're going to deliver (if you plan to use a bed) is easily accessible from all sides. You might also want to ensure you have plenty of extra pillows to hand as well as several changes of bed sheets.

Even if you plan to labour in dim lighting, there needs to be a good source of light for the midwife, especially after the birth when you may need stitches.

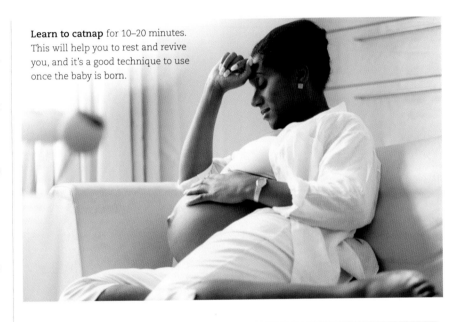

Learn to catnap for 10–20 minutes. This will help you to rest and revive you, and it's a good technique to use once the baby is born.

THE LOWDOWN

On pushing

Is pushing the baby out natural and instinctive? All women will feel an urge to push during labour, but because it's painful they might resist doing so. Medications, such as an epidural (see pp.404–5), will interfere with the sensation of needing to push. Your midwife will help you throughout and guide you as to when it's safe and most effective to push.

ASK A... MIDWIFE

I'm so tired already. How will I ever get through labour? First of all, take every opportunity you can to rest – even if this means napping several times during the day. Every bit of sleep you get will make a difference to your energy levels, especially if you're having broken sleep at night.

When you are feeling active, try to do some gentle exercise as this can encourage healthy, restful sleep. Swimming can be a great way to expend energy and take your mind off things, and it puts little or no pressure on your bump or your aching muscles and joints.

Try eating food containing tryptophan (see p.177) before you go to bed, which can encourage sleep, and make sure that you get plenty of high-energy carbohydrates (see p.92) during the day, to keep your blood-sugar levels stable and prevent energy slumps.

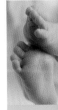

10 days to go...

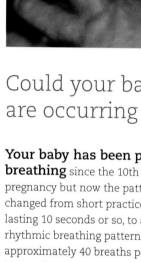

YOUR BABY TODAY

Your baby's neck muscles have strengthened, so the head can be held well away from the chest wall. Once delivered though, the buoyancy provided by the amniotic fluid will be lost and you will need to support your baby's head at all times while holding him.

Could your baby be dreaming already? A lot of his movements are occurring when he's fast asleep.

Your baby has been practising breathing since the 10th week of pregnancy but now the pattern has changed from short practice bursts lasting 10 seconds or so, to a regular rhythmic breathing pattern of approximately 40 breaths per minute, just as the baby will breathe after birth.

Eye movements have also matured with periods of rapid eye movement (REM) lasting for just over 25 minutes at a time and rest periods lasting just under 25 minutes. REM sleep is closely coupled with periods of increased activity and a faster heart rate. So, just because your baby is moving it doesn't always mean that he's awake.

Although your baby cannot stretch out as freely as before, movements at least 10 times a day should continue in the same familiar pattern and are a reassuring sign of a healthy baby.

FOCUS ON... NUTRITION

Fuel for labour

The recommendations by the National Institute for Health and Clinical Excellence (NICE) are that all women should be allowed to drink water in labour, and that isotonic, or sports, water may be slightly more beneficial because of its higher calorie value and quick absorption into the body.

Eating light snacks, even in established labour, is recommended as long as you haven't had opioid painkillers (see p.403), which include pethidine and diamorphine, and there are no other risk factors that might mean you will need to have a general anaesthetic.

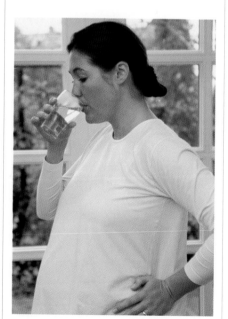

During labour it's essential to stay hydrated. Your body will be working hard and you're likely to be hot.

ASK A... MIDWIFE

What is a membrane sweep and could I have this instead of being induced if I end up being overdue? Prior to an induction of labour, at 41-plus weeks of pregnancy, it is recommended that all women are offered a membrane stretch and sweep to assess the readiness of the cervix for labour.

A membrane sweep involves your midwife or doctor placing a finger just inside your cervix and making a circular, sweeping movement to separate the membranes from the cervix. The aim of this is to stimulate the release of hormones that may start labour contractions. Although this is likely to be an uncomfortable procedure, it should not cause you actual pain; you will also experience a mucus/bloodstained "show" (see p.411) following a membrane sweep, which is quite normal.

Membrane sweeps have been shown to increase the chance of labour starting naturally within 48 hours and therefore reduce the need for other methods of induction (see p.432). Your midwife will advise you nearer the time.

9 days to go...

YOUR BABY TODAY

In many ways you will be the best judge of the likely size of your baby, especially if you can compare it with a previous pregnancy. An ultrasound scan can estimate the weight, but as with all other measurements at this time it has a fairly wide margin of error.

Don't just wait for contractions – it's worth familiarizing yourself now with the signs that may mean labour is imminent.

FETAL MONITORING

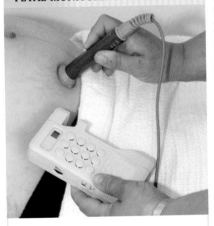

If there are no complications or reasons for concern, your baby's heartbeat will usually be monitored using a hand-held Doppler ultrasound device. Once your labour is well under way, your midwife will listen to your baby's heartbeat for 60 seconds after a contraction every 15 minutes in the first stage of labour and for 60 seconds after a contraction every 5 minutes in the second stage of labour.

If you've had complications in pregnancy, or problems develop during labour, the midwife may monitor the heartbeat using a CTG (see p.418).

When does labour actually start? If it's your first pregnancy, it can be difficult to recognize the signs that the baby is on his way. Some women get lower back pain that is niggling before becoming painful. You might notice a show (see p.411), which can happen well before true labour actually starts. Your waters may break as the sac containing the amniotic fluid bursts open. Even if your waters breaking is not accompanied by contractions you should still inform your labour ward.

Finally, the most obvious sign is contractions: these painful tightenings of your uterus will increase in intensity and become more regular as labour progresses. Contractions are associated with the dilation and shortening of your cervix, so your midwife will examine you to see how far you've progressed (see pp.414–15).

If you do think that you have gone into labour, stay calm and telephone the labour ward at your hospital. Inform them of your symptoms and, especially, describe your contractions. If you're having contractions every 5 minutes that last for one minute (time them), and they're so uncomfortable that you're forced to stop what you're doing, you should think about going to hospital. If you're having your baby at home, you should call your midwife.

ASK A... DOCTOR

How long am I likely to stay in hospital after the birth? In most maternity units, there's a degree of flexibility as to how long you remain in hospital. If you wish to stay for as brief a period as possible, talk to your midwife. The minimum length of time in hospital is six hours after delivery.

Many mothers stay overnight to rest and gain some confidence in caring and feeding their newborn, under the midwives' guidance, especially if it's their first baby.

How long you stay in hospital will largely depend on your type of delivery. If you have a vaginal birth, you should be able to go home after six hours, but a Caesarean may mean you need to stay in for about three days. If your baby is born early, is unwell, or is struggling to feed or maintain his temperature, you'll be advised to stay in hospital. If your baby has to remain in hospital for a long period, you would have to go home and visit him in the special care baby unit (see pp.452–3).

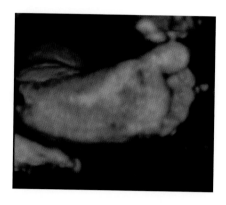

YOU ARE 38 WEEKS AND 6 DAYS

8 days to go...

YOUR BABY TODAY

The movements that you feel will usually be concentrated in a few areas as your baby cannot readily change position. Although the character of these movements will have changed, you should still experience many movements each day.

As you're heading into the final week, you're bound to feel a little anxious, but hopefully excited, too.

It's normal to feel a little jittery about your impending labour, especially if it's your first baby. Try not to keep your feelings bottled up: share anxieties with your partner, as you might find he's in need of reassurance, too. If you have specific concerns, call your midwife. She'll be used to handling these worries and will be able to put your mind at rest. Find ways to occupy your mind, even if it's just doing crosswords, as this will stop you fretting.

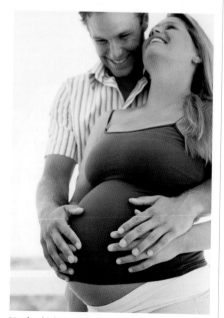

You're in it together and will need each other more than ever in these final two weeks.

FOCUS ON... DADS

The stages of labour and you

There is so much variation in the time taken to complete the first stage of labour (see pp.408–21) that for one pregnancy a woman might be in labour for days, whereas for a subsequent labour it might be a matter of hours.

As your partner's primary support, you have the difficult job of trying to take charge, exude calm, and give emotional and practical support. Don't hesitate to call the midwife for advice – a short discussion with her may help you to gauge how far through the first stage your partner has progressed. You must allow plenty of time to get to the hospital and you should be familiar with the route well beforehand (see box, below).

There may be periods when your partner is not lucid, but you will know what she wants better than anyone else. It's therefore your role to advocate for her and to engage with medical staff when she can't do so herself. You'll also know how to reassure and encourage your partner in the right way.

You'll need to support her in whatever position she chooses to use during the second stage (see pp.422–7) – when she's delivering the baby – and provide lots of encouragement. In the third stage (see pp.428–9), once the baby is born, you may cut the cord and might be holding your new baby while the placenta is delivered.

ASK A... DOCTOR

What are the signs that it's too late to go to the hospital? Generally speaking, if you're having an uncontrollable urge to push, then that's the point where it may be too late to reach the hospital before your delivery. If you do find yourself in this situation, contact your local maternity unit who will arrange for paramedics to attend you for the delivery of the baby. They will also ask an on-call midwife to attend the birth (although the paramedics might get there first). Or you can contact the emergency ambulance services yourself.

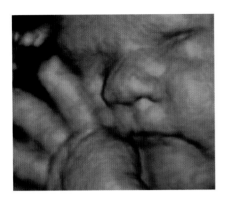

7 days to go...

YOUR BABY TODAY

This baby can easily be seen at this late stage in the pregnancy because there is ample amniotic fluid present. The amount of amniotic fluid at this point is still extremely variable, but it is usually in the region of 0.5 litre (18fl oz).

Use this time in the run-up to labour to get your partner fully up to speed on how he can help you on the big day.

It's a good idea to prepare your partner in advance, and work out what may help the proceedings once labour does begin. For example, if you're planning on using natural remedies, put together a natural medicine kit and explain to your partner when you think you'll need different remedies.

Ask your partner to practise some massage strokes, using a soothing blend of oils (see p.163). Some women can't bear to be touched during labour, but others find it helpful to have their back, or even just their hands and feet, massaged. You won't really know what works for you until you're in labour but trying massage now won't do any harm.

If your partner has been attending antenatal classes with you, he'll be familiar with the breathing and relaxation techniques so practise these together and, if necessary, get advice from your midwife about techniques.

It may be helpful for your partner to speak to male friends or relatives who have recently become fathers. Hearing the experiences of others and learning some dos and don'ts of being a birth partner might be useful.

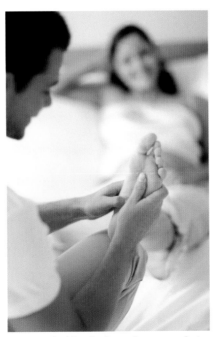

You may find it relaxing to have your feet massaged in the early stages of labour, even if you don't want your back or shoulders touched. A massage helps to relieve tension.

AS A MATTER OF FACT

Whatever their weight, most babies at 40 weeks are approximately the same length.

Ninety-five per cent are between 45cm (17.7in) and 55cm (21.6in) long. The length of newborn babies is remarkably consistent and relates to skeletal growth, whereas birth weight may vary considerably.

FINAL PREPARATIONS

It's amazing that even after 40 weeks of pregnancy, when labour begins there is still a scramble to get everything organized as you head off to the hospital. So to avoid any last-minute panic:

■ **Make sure your bag is packed** (see p.358). You may also want to pin up a list of any extras you need to include at the last minute.

■ **It's advisable to keep a small bag of change** in your hospital bag to pay for parking and drinks from vending machines.

■ **Decide who will do what:** for example, perhaps your partner could prepare snacks.

■ **Do a trial run** of the trip to the hospital – anticipating areas where there is likely to be traffic, seeking out shortcuts, and working out where you are most likely to find a parking space. It can also help to time the run at various points in the day, so that you can avoid school-run hotspots or commuter traffic. Also find out how to get into the maternity unit at night.

■ **Above all, don't panic.** The majority of parents-to-be do get to the hospital in plenty of time.

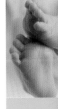

383

Your 40th week

ALL THE MILESTONES ARE SAFELY PASSED AND YOU WILL MEET YOUR BABY ANY DAY NOW

Like many mums-to-be, you may have to linger in suspense beyond the "last" day of pregnancy. Without a doubt, the big event is about to happen very soon and it will be worth the waiting, wondering, and fretting. Once you see and hold your baby, you won't spend much time looking back over the past 40 weeks, but you'll certainly marvel at the miracle of it all.

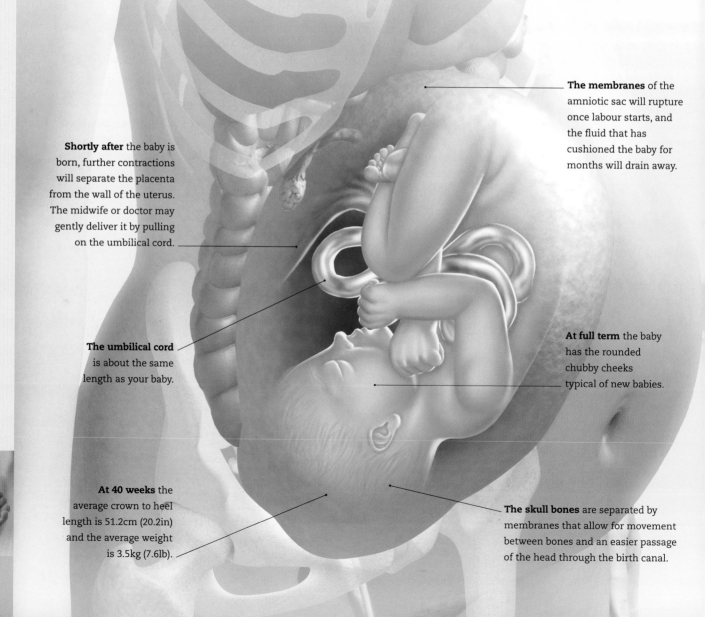

The membranes of the amniotic sac will rupture once labour starts, and the fluid that has cushioned the baby for months will drain away.

Shortly after the baby is born, further contractions will separate the placenta from the wall of the uterus. The midwife or doctor may gently deliver it by pulling on the umbilical cord.

The umbilical cord is about the same length as your baby.

At full term the baby has the rounded chubby cheeks typical of new babies.

At 40 weeks the average crown to heel length is 51.2cm (20.2in) and the average weight is 3.5kg (7.6lb).

The skull bones are separated by membranes that allow for movement between bones and an easier passage of the head through the birth canal.

6 days to go...

YOUR BABY TODAY

If you are to have a planned Caesarean delivery, this is usually offered now – in order to balance the chance of labour starting unexpectedly with that of delivering your baby too soon. It is best for babies to be delivered as close to the due date as possible.

It's worth revisiting your birth plan at this late stage as you may feel differently now about some of the requests you made.

A birth plan is usually filled in earlier in pregnancy, and you may not have given it much more thought since (see pp.181 and 303). Now that the birth is imminent, look over it with your partner to work out whether you've changed your mind about anything. For example you may be veering towards a more natural birth or, conversely, you may now be certain you want an epidural. Adapt it as you wish and discuss it with your midwife, if necessary.

As your partner will be your advocate in labour, putting your requests forward to your midwives and doctors if you're unable to express them, it's important that he understands your wishes and that they're fresh in his mind.

Remember, though, that you won't really know how you'll feel or what you want until you're in labour, so keep an open mind and be prepared to adapt your plans on the day if it's in the best interests of your baby's wellbeing.

Get your partner's view. Remember that this is a big event for him, too: the moment when he'll meet his baby for the first time. He may have anxieties and concerns and want reassurance about what his role will be on the day: tell him how you think he can best help you, whether it be a massage or just holding your hand throughout. Discuss how you both are feeling in the preparation for the birth – your concerns, hopes, and expectations.

ASK A... MIDWIFE

Can I refuse an induction of labour? You have a right to say no to any intervention and when induction (see p.432) is considered, your carers should discuss all your options before a decision is reached.

If you wish to delay induction beyond 42 weeks, then it may be suggested you attend the maternity unit for monitoring, which may include a Doppler ultrasound (see p.285) to check the blood flow in the placenta. You will also be offered an ultrasound scan to check on the amount of fluid surrounding your baby, as this can be a good indicator of how efficiently the placenta is working and your baby's wellbeing.

STAYING CLOSE

It can be difficult to think of anything but the birth and meeting your baby when you are this close to the end of pregnancy. Try to focus on other things, too:

■ **Spend time with your partner:** Enjoy quality time together while it is still just the two of you, before the baby makes demands on your time, and exhaustion sets in. Share your hopes and fears about how your lives are going to change.

■ **Make love:** you might feel you are too big, or too tired, but it is good to remind yourselves of your sexual relationship. And, you never know, making love could just get your labour started (see p.393).

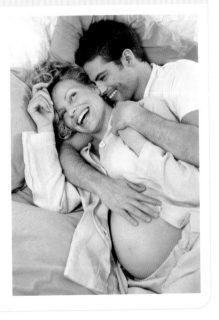

385

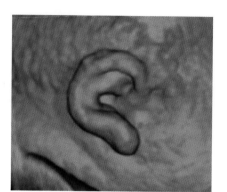

5 days to go...

YOUR BABY TODAY

This close-up 3D ultrasound view shows that this baby's earlobe is particularly prominent. The dark flecks around the ear look like hair, but are in fact shadows (although many babies have hair at this stage).

Your baby's bones have hardened to a certain degree, but this process will continue right up to the teenage years!

Your baby's skeleton has gradually transformed, from soft cartilage to bone, a process called ossification (see p.372). This process starts in the centre of each bone spreading outwards. By the end of pregnancy, ossification is complete along the length of each bone but the ends of the long bones and the tips of the bones in the fingers and toes remain as cartilage. This is necessary to allow later bone growth as the child develops.

The bones in the upper part of the skull are slightly different, developing from membranous structures rather than cartilage. These do not fully fuse until several years after birth and remain separated from each other by connective tissue. This connective tissue forms areas called sutures and where more than two bones meet, wider spaces called fontanelles. Their function is to allow space for movement or "moulding" between the skull bones, making it easier for the head to descend into the pelvis during labour. It is also these suture lines and fontanelles that help your midwife determine the position of the baby's head during labour.

After delivery you will notice that your baby's head shape is often elongated, but this soon changes as the bones realign back into their usual positions.

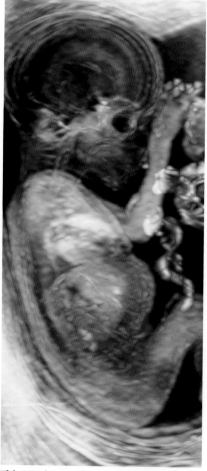

This MRI (magnetic resonance imaging) scan shows a fetus approaching full-term. The baby's brain, spinal column, heart, liver, and lungs are visible, and the umbilical cord can be seen to the right of the image.

THE LOWDOWN

Placenta on toast?

The thought of eating the placenta may turn your stomach, but some women choose to do exactly that. The organ is revered for its spiritual properties, and devotees of placentophagia believe the nutrients it contains, including vitamin B6, will help to prevent them developing postnatal depression. However, the evidence in favour of the health benefits of consuming a placenta is purely anecdotal.

An alternative and less controversial custom involves dressing the placenta with herbs, then burying it at a party to celebrate the baby's birth: this is thought to be an important bonding ritual for the extended family.

Art is another option: press the placenta against a piece of paper and you'll get a tree-shaped print.

Some cultures use the dried organ to make medicinal herbs.

Not sure how to cook placenta? Well just look online and you'll find plenty of placenta recipes, from pâté to lasagne, but, understandably, these might not be to everyone's taste.

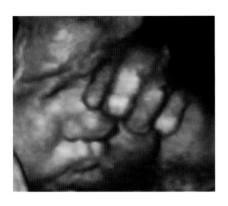

4 days to go...

YOUR BABY TODAY

Once labour starts your baby will no longer have room to place her hands on top of her head or by her face although, interestingly, she is still moving around – you probably won't notice these movements as you will have other things on your mind.

The enquiries may begin flooding in this week and it will feel as though the whole world is awaiting news of your baby's arrival.

In this final week of your pregnancy, the weight of expectation can be immense. It can feel as though everyone is waiting for you to pop, especially if it's your first baby.

You'll no doubt cope with it this week – and you may even enjoy getting all the attention – but if you happen to go overdue you might get frustrated by the constant calls and by having to repeat yourself. Try to be patient and remember people are simply excited for you and are just as frustrated with waiting as you are.

Matters aren't helped by the due date. Everyone will have this estimated date in mind, but unfortunately not many babies stick to a schedule and they enter the world exactly when they are ready (see p.378). Up to 42 weeks isn't really considered that late in medical circles.

If it all becomes too much, rely on others close to you to field all the calls and make it clear that you promise to be in touch with an announcement just as soon as there is any news.

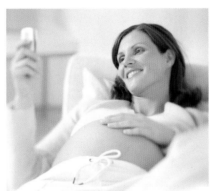

Text messaging can be a useful way of staying in touch with people in the final days. Sending out a circular "baby hasn't arrived yet" message is a good idea.

ASK A... MIDWIFE

I've heard about hospitals being understaffed and women who are in labour not getting a bed. Is this true? There are concerns about shortages of midwives and beds. Many hospitals now employ ancillary staff and maternity support workers to provide back-up for midwives. Unfortunately, there have been times when maternity units are full, although this rarely happens. If no beds are available, a bed will be found at another hospital; many hospitals have "sister" units, to which they will transfer you. Most maternity units are not full for long and will organize for you to be transferred back as soon as possible.

FOCUS ON... YOUR BODY

False labour

You may experience deep and painful twinges, and practice contractions, known as Braxton-Hicks', particularly towards the end of pregnancy. It's easy to mistake these for the real thing, and you may find yourself rushing to the hospital when your body is really still practising. You may also experience regular contractions for a period, which then stop. All of this is normal.

One sign that labour may be imminent is that you lose your mucus plug (see p.411); another is your waters breaking. In some cases, however, neither of these events takes place until labour is established, so don't panic if they don't happen to you.

You'll definitely know you're in labour when your contractions are occurring regularly, approximately every 15 minutes – time the gap between them. True contractions will get longer, stronger, and closer together as time goes on, and won't go away when you walk around or change position.

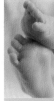

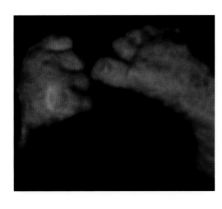

3 days to go...

YOUR BABY TODAY

This image shows that even at this time your baby will be able to reach down and touch her toes (see the foot on the right and the hand on the left). Because there is less space your baby will no longer be able to place her feet on top of her head.

Don't be too concerned if your baby hasn't engaged yet as this won't have any bearing on the final delivery date.

There are many reasons why your baby may not have engaged yet: the shape of your pelvis may mean that you need the pressure of the contractions to get the baby's head to engage. Very athletic women tend to have babies who engage late because their taut muscles hold the baby in a different position. Second and subsequent babies tend to engage later because the tummy muscles are very loose, so the baby may move freely without feeling any need to get her head down. A big baby may not descend into the pelvis until the contractions start.

HOW YOUR BABY IS POSITIONED

Once the baby is head down and moves into the pelvis there are several positions she may adopt: six of the most common are shown below. The position is determined by where her back and occiput (the back of her head) are lying. The most usual position is LOL. If the baby is breech (see p.433), the position is determined by how the bottom is lying.

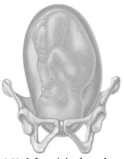
LOL: left occipito-lateral

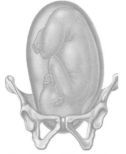
LOA: left occipito-anterior

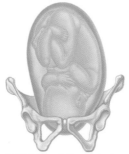
LOP: left occipito-posterior

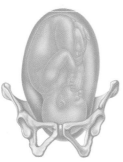
ROL: right occipito-lateral

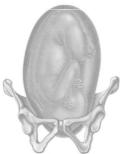
ROA: right occipito-anterior

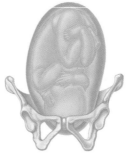
ROP: right occipito-posterior

LOL (left occipito-lateral): the back and occiput are positioned on the left-hand side of the uterus at right angles to the spine.

LOA (left occipito-anterior): the back and occiput are positioned nearer to the front of the uterus on the left-hand side.

LOP (left occipito-posterior): the back and occiput are towards the spine on the left-hand side of the uterus.

ROL (right occipito-lateral): the back and occiput are at right angles to the spine on the right-hand side of the uterus.

ROA (right occipito-anterior): the back and occiput are towards the front of the uterus on the right-hand side.

ROP (right occipito-posterior): the back and occiput are towards the spine on the right-hand side of the uterus.

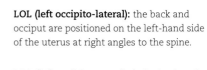
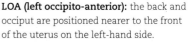

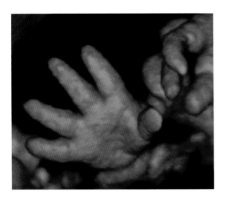

2 days to go...

YOUR BABY TODAY

This great image of the hands even shows the fine folds that have formed in the palms. Every baby has a unique pattern of folds on the palms and on the soles of the feet that you'll see when your baby finally arrives.

You'll be in labour very soon and it's normal to be anxious about what you need to go through to meet your baby.

You're bound to have mixed emotions about going into labour. While you'll want your baby to be born, you may be apprehensive about going through childbirth. Most women are understandably concerned about the pain, and may worry about their health and that of the baby. Remember that the majority of deliveries are normal and without complications and the majority of babies are fit and healthy.

Even though you've spent the past nine months preparing for the birth, you may still feel that you're not ready for the baby and that you won't be able to manage. Some of this will be the fear of the unknown – you have not yet met your baby and it's impossible to predict what the labour – and the weeks that follow it – will be like.

Although you may not feel fully prepared, be confident that you'll know how to care for your newborn. In fact, you'll have probably already started the process of becoming a mother, wanting to nurture and protect your baby even before she's born, and this natural instinct will continue.

ASK A... MIDWIFE

What's the difference between an emergency and elective Caesarean?
An elective Caesarean is when a pre-planned decision is made during pregnancy to deliver the baby by Caesarean section before the onset of labour. This is usually decided upon for medical reasons, although some women may decide to have an elective Caesarean for practical reasons or to avoid having to go through labour.

An emergency Caesarean is when a situation arises, usually in labour, that means the safest route for delivery is by Caesarean section.

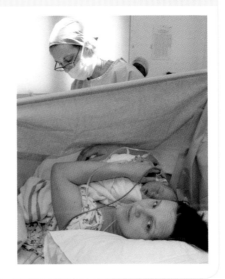

MRSA: IS IT A RISK?

There's a great deal of media coverage of "superbugs", such as MRSA. This is a bacterium that can live harmlessly on the skin of healthy people, but can lead to infection in vulnerable individuals. Good hygiene, particularly in the form of precautions such as hand-washing, is an effective method in the prevention of MRSA and your chances of acquiring the infection in hospital are low. Healthcare workers use antiseptic solutions and more recently many hospitals have alcohol gels for hand cleaning on all wards.

As well as general hygiene measures, hospitals prevent the spread of MRSA by treating those infected with antibiotics, and by detecting cases early so that they can isolate affected patients. Infected patients are moved to a single room or to a room with others who have MRSA.

Many hospitals now screen women before admission for MRSA, particularly if they are having a Caesarean, with the aim of treating those who carry MRSA before they are admitted for surgery.

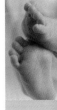

389

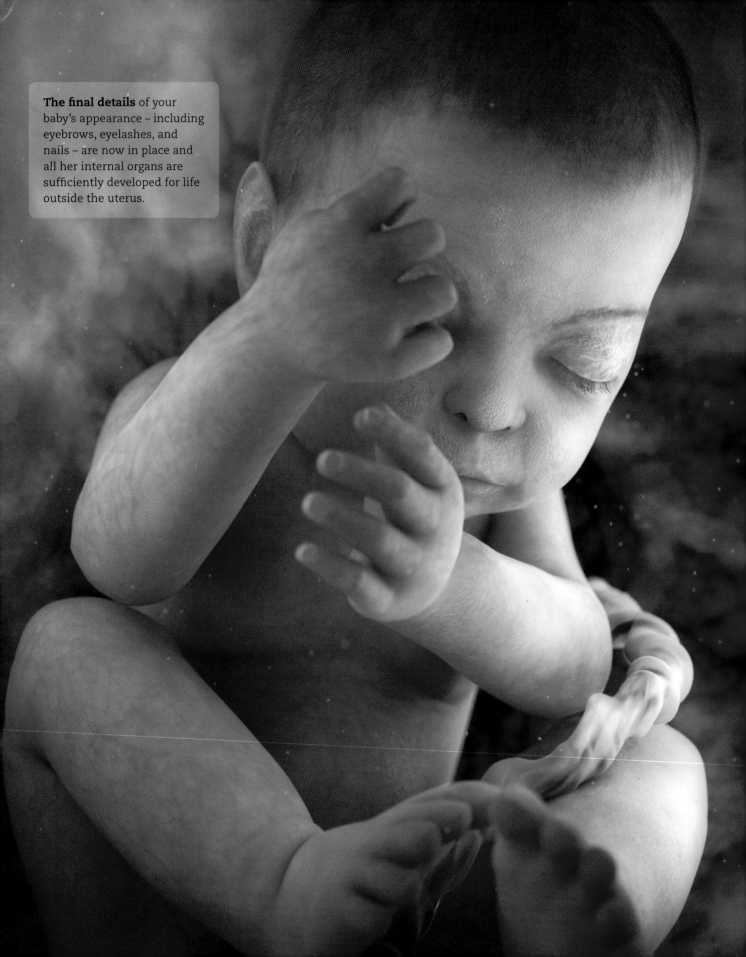

The final details of your baby's appearance – including eyebrows, eyelashes, and nails – are now in place and all her internal organs are sufficiently developed for life outside the uterus.

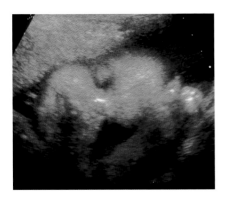

1 day to go...

YOUR BABY TODAY

It's been wonderful to see your baby's progress and facial features as each day of the pregnancy has passed by. 2D and 3D ultrasound images, as well as MRI, have all played a part in giving us a glimpse into the fascinating and complex world of life before birth.

Your newborn's stomach will be fully developed, but low acid levels mean she can only be fed milk for the first few months.

RASPBERRY LEAF TEA

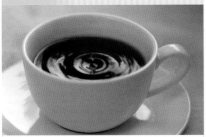

Raspberry leaf tea has been proven to facilitate labour by helping the muscles to contract more efficiently. Studies have found that drinking this in the months prior to delivery (not before week 30) helps to shorten the second stage of labour by making the contractions more effective. It also appears to reduce the risk of having an assisted delivery, such as emergency Caesarean or ventouse (see p.437).

Best of all, raspberry leaf tea is enormously nutritious, containing vitamins A, C, E, and B, and the minerals calcium, magnesium, and iron, all of which are required for a healthy pregnancy.

Drunk after the birth, this tea can help the uterus to contract back to its normal size, and encourage the flow of breast milk.

Unlike an adult, your baby produces little gastric acid and keeps amniotic fluid in the stomach longer; it is this fluid that helps to keep the acid content of her stomach low. While your baby is in the uterus hiccupping, turning upside down, and trying to co-ordinate breathing with swallowing, not having much hydrochloric acid in the stomach is a good idea.

After birth the acid content of your baby's stomach will increase quickly in the first 24 hours but not reach adult levels until three months. This is why solids aren't introduced until a baby is at least four months old, although six months is the current advice on when to start weaning. Some studies show that breastfed babies given solid food before six months are more likely to get diarrhoea and chest infections, and may be more prone to developing allergies. There is less research on formula-fed babies, but there is no evidence that they need solid food any earlier.

THE LOWDOWN

Take a babymoon

Getting to know your newborn can be difficult if there's a constant stream of visitors bearing gifts and good wishes. Why not shut out the world and spend a few days home alone? Your newborn baby will sleep a lot, so take the opportunity to do the same. There will be plenty of time for people to meet the new member of your family.

Your hormones will be all over the place, so expect to experience lows as well as highs, especially when your milk comes in (see pp.448–9).

Your partner also needs time to bond with his baby, nurture you both, and get to grips with nappy changing.

So stick a message on the front door, switch on the answer phone, and snuggle up with your new family.

ASK A... MIDWIFE

What exactly is a "show"? During pregnancy, a plug of jelly-like mucus seals the lower end of your cervix and this prevents infection getting into your uterus (see p.411). This "plug" comes away towards the end of pregnancy – known as a "show" – and although this can mean that labour is going to start soon, it can also dislodge up to six weeks before your labour actually starts.

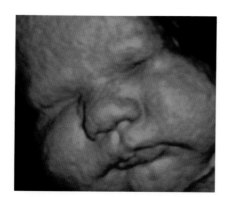

0 days to go...

YOUR BABY TODAY

Your baby is now ready for the outside world. Sudden changes will take place with that first breath after delivery, as she immediately adapts from her time within the fluid-filled environment of the uterus to life in the air outside.

You've reached 40 weeks exactly! It may have seemed like a long wait, but it will be worth it once you're holding your baby.

Congratulations! If you don't yet have your newborn baby in your arms, you soon will, and your life will be changed forever. Even the longest pregnancy seems unaccountably short when your labour begins, and the reality begins to hit that you'll soon be holding your newborn.

You'll get through the labour; and you'll forget about the discomfort after a few good sessions detailing it to family and close friends. In fact, everything that precedes that moment when you hold your newborn baby for the first time becomes inconsequential when you realize that you have created the most wondrous thing of all: a new life. So good luck and well done! This is only just the beginning of the most amazing years of your life.

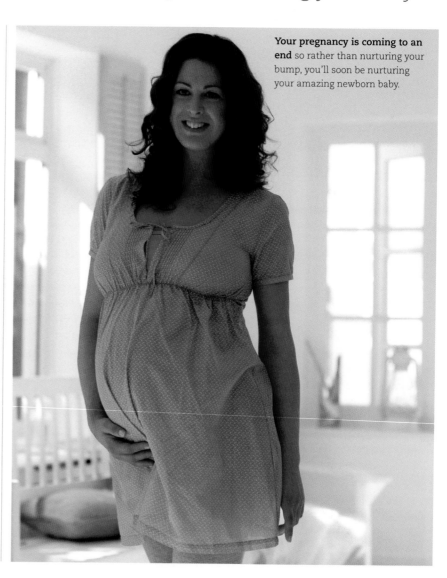

Your pregnancy is coming to an end so rather than nurturing your bump, you'll soon be nurturing your amazing newborn baby.

AS A MATTER OF FACT

58 per cent of parents questioned in a recent survey believed that the name they gave their baby would contribute to his or her success in life.

More found it easier to name a boy than a girl, and just 3 per cent said they would change the name they'd given their baby if they could.

Overdue baby

Your baby is described as being overdue if you have not gone into labour by the time you are 40 weeks pregnant. This is not unusual as most women do not go into labour at exactly 40 weeks, and anything between 37 and 42 weeks is considered to be normal.

Why labour is late As the exact trigger that sets off labour is unknown, it's not clear why some women go overdue. You are more likely to go overdue if this is your first baby, if you've had an overdue baby before, or if the condition runs in your family. Some think it's more common in well-nourished women, and there is even evidence that pregnancies are longer in the summer than in the winter. If your due date was worked out from an early ultrasound, this gives a more accurate dating of pregnancy than the date of your last menstrual period, and you'll be less likely to be classed overdue.

What will be done

After 41 weeks, there is a slightly increased risk to your baby's heath that may be due to the reduced efficiency of the placenta. After 42 weeks the risk increases, but is still small. Depending on hospital policy, you will be offered an induction between 41 and 42 weeks (see p.432). The following may also be done.

Sweeping the membranes After 40 weeks, your midwife may do an internal examination to "sweep the membranes". She'll insert a gloved finger into the cervix and pull the membranes in a circular pattern. This can soften the cervix and increase the chance of you going into labour in the next 48 hours by 30 per cent. It's safe for you and your baby, but can cause cramp and slight bleeding.

Assessments after 42 weeks If your pregnancy goes beyond 42 weeks and you don't want to be induced, most hospitals offer monitoring with scans to

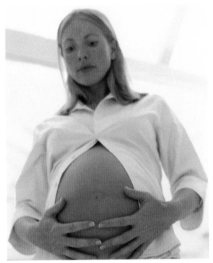

Going over your due date can be stressful, but it may help to remind yourself that it's also extremely common and quite normal.

measure the baby's heart rate and volume of fluid around the baby; or you may have a CTG (see p.418) once or twice a week until labour to pick up any signs that the placenta is failing. If a problem is found, you'll be advised to have a Caesarean or an induction of labour (see p.432).

How you're feeling

You might find the physical and mental stress of being pregnant over your due date considerable, but it can help to know that unless you have a medical condition, going overdue does not significantly increase the risks to your health. You may be worried, too, that your baby will grow too large, causing difficulties in labour. However, your baby is unlikely to put on enough weight in the last week or so to make a big difference and most overdue babies have a normal birthweight.

AT-HOME STRATEGIES

Bringing on labour

Although no "home" or alternative remedy has been proven to bring on labour, there are several harmless techniques that are thought to assist the body's natural processes.

■ Probably the most enjoyable way to try to bring on labour is to make love with your partner. Sperm contains prostaglandins that may act as a natural uterine stimulant, although the evidence that this works is inconclusive. Making love is not dangerous to your baby, unless your doctor has specifically told you to refrain from intercourse for a medical reason, such as fetal growth restriction or placental bleeding.

■ Nipple stimulation during sex or by itself can release oxytocin from your pituitary gland, which is linked to contractions and cervical ripening.

■ Walking and exercise may cause a mild increase in uterine contractions by helping the baby to move down the pelvis, putting pressure on the cervix.

■ Raspberry leaf has been associated with increased uterine activity (see p.391). It is fairly mild and hasn't been linked with pregnancy complications, but neither has it been shown to be effective in any well-designed study.

■ Some homeopathic remedies are recommended.

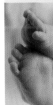

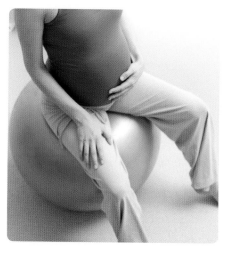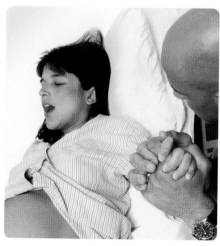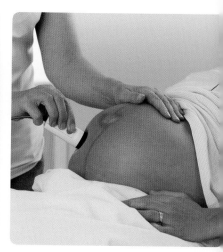

As the moment you've so eagerly anticipated approaches, you may have increasing concerns about what lies in store for you during the labour and delivery, and doubts as to whether you'll be able to cope with the physical and mental demands during this crucial time. Being as informed as possible about both the progress of labour and your options for pain relief are important first steps in enabling you to face labour and birth with a positive mindset.

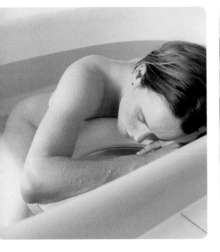
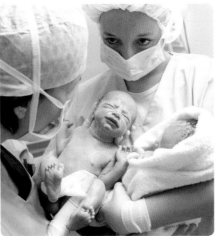
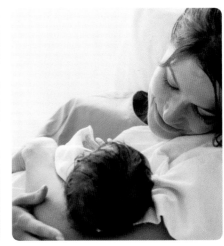

Labour
and birth

Pain relief options

A PRIOR KNOWLEDGE OF PAIN RELIEF WILL HELP YOU TO MAKE INFORMED CHOICES IN LABOUR

Once in labour, as well as needing emotional and physical support, which your midwife and birth partner will provide, you may also need some form of pain relief to help you cope. The midwife will help you to work with your labour pain by employing natural methods such as breathing techniques. If you require stronger pain relief, she will advise you on medical methods, such as analgesics or an epidural (see pp.402–7).

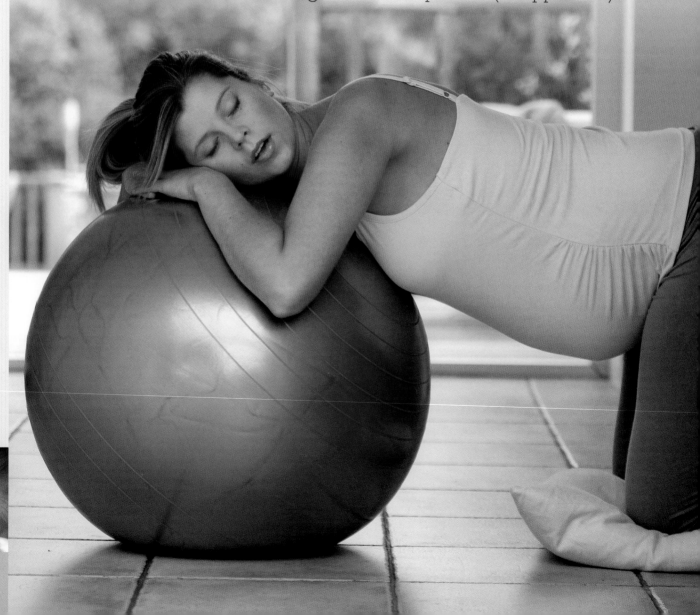

Coping with pain

To help you cope with labour and birth, it's important to have an understanding of the progress of pain during labour.

Labour pain is unique and quite different from everyday chronic and acute pain. Generally, pain is a warning sign that something is wrong, but labour pain acts as an "alert" that the birth process is underway and that you need a safe environment in which to give birth. Some women prefer a home-like environment, which has been shown to have many benefits, including reducing the need for medical forms of pain relief such as pethidine. For this reason, many labour rooms in maternity units and especially birth centres have homely decoration and furnishings to make them feel less medicalized. Other women need the reassurance provided by hospitals that stronger forms of pain relief and medical backup are available.

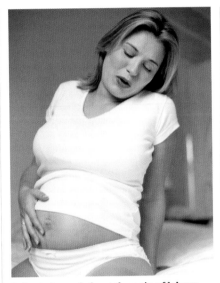

Being informed about the pain of labour can reduce your anxiety and help you to cope.

How women react to pain

No one really knows what starts labour and every woman's labour is unique. Likewise, the pain associated with labour can vary enormously between women. Some women have relatively painless labours, while some describe the pain as moderate, and others experience severe pain. One thing that does seem clear is that anxiety and fear increase the levels of adrenaline, which in turn can increase the intensity of the pain experienced. The strength of labour pain can also be affected by factors such as your emotional state and anticipation of labour; your previous experiences, if any; cultural beliefs; and, in particular for first-time mothers, the fear of the unknown. Thorough preparation before the onset of labour and sensitive and caring support throughout the labour and birth can help to reduce anxiety and fear considerably.

Thinking ahead

The sensation of pain is different during the different stages of labour, and as labour progresses the intensity and duration of the pain increases. The most effective methods of dealing with pain will also change as your labour progresses (see box, left).

The more familiar you are with the methods of coping with pain and with the several natural and drug-induced methods of pain relief available (see following pages), the easier it will be for you to manage during labour and birth. To make decisions about pain relief, you will also need to understand the changes that take place in your body during the three different stages of labour (see pp.408–29).

PAIN RELIEF THROUGHOUT LABOUR

Your pain-relief requirements may change during labour, so it helps to be aware of when different types of pain relief can help.

Early first stage In this phase, the cervix begins to dilate. Contractions are mild, and you may find that natural methods, such as massage and breathing, are helpful. If you need stronger pain relief, you may be given analgesics, such as gas and air or pethidine (see pp.402–3), which dull pain, but allow you to remain active.

Active first stage The cervix now starts to dilate more quickly and contractions are stronger and closer together. Some women are happy to continue with natural or analgesic pain relief; others may need stronger relief and an epidural may be given at this point (see pp.404–5).

Transition Contractions are intense and frequent as the cervix dilates fully. Analgesics such as entonox can be useful, but pethidine isn't usually given this close to the birth as it could affect the baby. If you have an epidural in place, this can be topped up.

Second and third stages The second stage lasts from full cervical dilation until the birth; contractions are strong and longer-lasting, but easier to cope with as you start pushing. Gas and air can be used. In the third stage, delivery of the placenta, contractions are mild and you shouldn't need pain relief.

Natural pain relief

Many women opt for natural pain relief in labour, or choose to complement medical pain relief with natural methods.

During your labour, encephalins and endorphins (feel-good hormones) are released to provide you with some naturally induced pain relief. Many women now are also more aware of natural techniques, such as staying active, and of the availability of complementary therapies that they can use in addition to, or instead of, medical pain relief during pregnancy, childbirth, and following the birth. Some of these therapies are self-administered and some are practitioner-administered. A knowledge of the benefits of different therapies and how to use them is important if you are considering using them to cope with pain in labour.

Staying active

Being active in labour has been shown to help women cope with pain and reduce the length of labour. Historically, women have been active in labour for centuries, but a medicalization of childbirth in the West led to an acceptance that women lay in bed, and the most common image of labouring women in the UK is "on the bed". The National Institute for Health and Clinical Excellence (NICE) recently advised that women should be helped to move around in labour to find comfortable positions.

Although during labour you may want to rest on a bed between contractions, many women find that when they feel supported, they instinctively move around and do not cope well lying down, which can increase pain and hamper the progress of labour as your baby pushes against gravity. There are certain interventions, such as the use of electronic fetal monitoring (see p.418), intravenous drips, and some types of analgesia, that will limit your mobility.

RELAXATION TECHNIQUES

There are various techniques you can use to help you relax during labour; if you're relaxed, it will be easier to stay calm and in tune with your body. These techniques include focusing on your breathing (see below); listening to music (perhaps humming to the beat of a favourite tune during a contraction); and listening to a meditation CD.

Learning how to breathe slowly and steadily in labour helps you to focus and stay calm. Usually, your breathing responds to how you're feeling and may increase slightly during a contraction, or you may hold your breath, which can make you feel light-headed. If this happens, you need to focus and steady your breathing. Your midwife will remind you to breathe slowly and steadily. Breathing in for five and out for seven slows your breathing down, helps you relax, and stops you panicking.

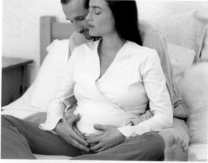
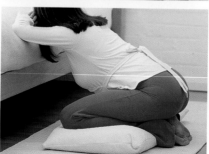

Concentrating on your breathing in labour is calming and helps you to focus (top). **Leaning forwards while breathing steadily** can be comforting during contractions (bottom).

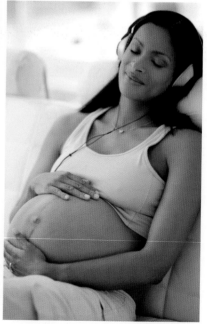

Listening to some of your favourite music in the first stage of labour is a great way to relax between contractions, enabling you to let go and reserve energy for later in labour.

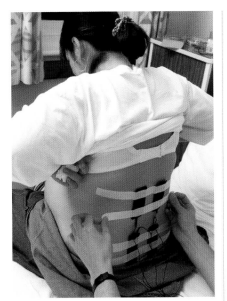

Once the electrodes for TENS are positioned on your back, you will be free to move around and find comfortable positions.

TENS

TENS stands for Transcutaneous Electrical Nerve Stimulation, and is a small electrical device that reduces pain signals sent to the brain. As well as being used in labour, the device can also be used at the end of pregnancy (after 36 weeks) if you have backache or uncomfortable Braxton Hicks' contractions (see p.410).

The battery-operated machine has thin wires that are connected to four electrodes, or sticky pads, which are taped to the lower back. The machine works by sending electrical impulses from the machine along nerve roots to the pain pathways in the brain, thereby blocking pain impulses. It's also thought to stimulate the brain to produce "feel-good" encephalins and endorphins, which can modulate the pain.

TENS is most effective in early labour, particularly for lower-back pain, and it is therefore important to have the device available at the start of labour. It's worth finding out if your hospital loans TENS machines or whether you need to hire one in advance. TENS is popular partly because you can hold the device or have it near you in labour and can increase the strength of the electrical impulse with a button as your contractions get stronger.

There are several advantages to TENS. It has no known side effects and is completely safe for you and your baby; it allows you to remain active; and it can be used in combination with other types of pain relief, such as gas and air or pethidine (see pp.402–3). The disadvantages are that it is generally effective with just mild to moderate pain; the sticky pads mean that a back massage is more difficult; and it isn't possible to labour in water or have an epidural fitted while using the device.

Water

Many women find being in warm water during labour very soothing and an excellent way to cope with labour pains. The warmth of the water soothes muscles, promoting relaxation, and being in water aids buoyancy, which can help to relieve the pressure on your pelvis. Over the last decade or so, this natural method has become more available for women and many birth centres and maternity units in the UK provide birthing pools. Whether or not you can actually deliver your baby in the water will depend on the hospital's policy and whether there are any midwives trained in water births (see p.427). You can also hire a birthing pool to use at home.

Hypnosis

Self-hypnosis, using visualization and breathing techniques to induce a state of deep relaxation and banish fear, is an increasingly popular means of coping with labour, and is referred to as "hypnobirthing". This is based on the "fear-tension-pain" syndrome of

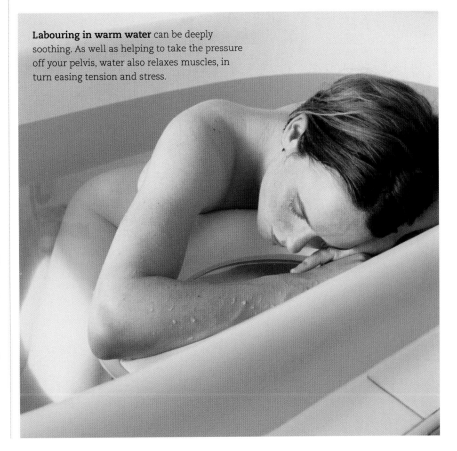

Labouring in warm water can be deeply soothing. As well as helping to take the pressure off your pelvis, water also relaxes muscles, in turn easing tension and stress.

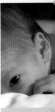

Will I be able to stay active in labour?
Yes, most women are able to remain active through labour and are encouraged to do so, perhaps using props such as a chair, bean bag, or birthing ball. Staying active can help to keep your labour on track, and changing your position can help you cope with labour pain. When you arrive at hospital or the birth centre, discuss your birth plan with the midwife and inform her that you want to be as active as possible.

Will I lose control if I use hypnosis during my labour?
No, you'll feel deeply relaxed, but will still be in control and know what you're doing. Don't worry – self-hypnosis will help you to be less anxious and frightened during your labour, which will help you to cope with labour pain. With preparation, your partner can help you to stay focused and use some hypnotic techniques, too.

I've had a previous Caesarean section. Does this mean that I won't be able to labour in water this time?
Unfortunately, you'll be advised not to labour in water. This is because, after a Caesarean, the midwives will want to monitor you and the baby continuously during labour, which they can't do in a birthing pool. Close monitoring is needed because there is a very small chance that your uterus may rupture. If this happens there can be sudden, acute pain and a rapid pulse, but often it's only detected through a change in the baby's heartbeat.

When can I get into the birthing pool?
This is up to you. Relaxing in warm water is often suggested in the early stages of labour, although some midwives do recommend waiting until you are around 4cm dilated, as it's thought that the water may be so relaxing that your contractions slow down. However, there is little evidence to support this.

childbirth first described by the British obstetrician Grantly Dick-Read (see p.303), who believed that fear prevents the release of the "feel-good hormones", endorphins and encephalins. He maintained that when fear is eliminated, most women can give birth naturally. With hypnobirthing, you are fully aware of what is happening around you, but may feel as though you're day-dreaming or drifting off to sleep. You and your birth partner can attend hypnobirthing classes from around 25–30 weeks of pregnancy to learn the techniques before labour. Ask your midwife for further information about local classes.

Acupuncture
This uses fine needles placed at specific points on the body to reduce pain by stimulating the production of endorphins. Acupuncture is a traditional form of Chinese medicine that believes there are channels within the body through which energy, or "chi", runs. Blockages can occur in these channels, and so by inserting needles at certain points, energy is unblocked, relieving pain and restoring balance to the body. Many women find acupuncture helpful to treat mild pregnancy symptoms, and some women use this therapy during labour. Acupuncture has no harmful side effects for the mother or baby and in labour needles will usually be inserted in points that do not restrict your movement, for example in the ear. If you wish to have acupuncture during labour, you will need to look for an acupuncturist who specializes in this area and arrange to have him or her with you during labour.

Many women find massage helpful in labour to induce relaxation, bring about a sense of wellbeing, and alleviate pain. Your birth partner may find it relaxing and therapeutic too. Ideally, he or she will have had a chance to see a midwife demonstrate massage techniques in antenatal classes and to practise before labour. Massaging the lower back helps to relieve pain in this area; head, neck, and shoulder massage is beneficial for relieving tension and fatigue.

The touch therapies shiatsu and acupressure can also relieve pain and tension. They involve the application of pressure to specific points to increase endorphin levels. You or your partner will need to learn the techniques from a trained practitioner. Ask your midwife if she can put you in touch with a practitioner.

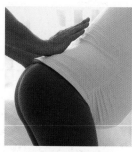
Your partner can use the heel of his hand to apply firm pressure to the base of your spine. The hands can be alternated to stroke around the lower back.

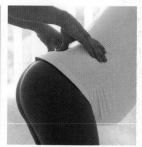
Using the thumbs to massage the lower back in a circular motion, working from the base of the spine down to the buttocks, can release tense muscles.

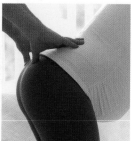
Applying deep pressure to the buttocks and lower back with the thumbs can help you partner to focus and release held-in tension during contractions.

Homeopathy

This is based on the principle of treating like with like. There are several homeopathic remedies that are safe to use during labour and birth and childbirth kits are available that you self-administer. These kits have ampoules with remedies and a guide to which remedy to use when. Some remedies need to be repeated quickly and regularly to stimulate a response. Or a registered homeopath can prescribe remedies based on your individual needs. There is a lack of scientific evidence on the effectiveness of homeopathy, although many women find the remedies helpful.

Aromatherapy

Aromatherapy (essential) oils are derived from plants and used for their therapeutic properties. The use of these oils in childbirth can stimulate, refresh, and soothe you, and to some extent your partner. There is some evidence that oils, such as lavender, reduce anxiety in labour, which in turn helps you cope with pain. Hot and cold compresses with essential oils added to the water used to wet the cloth can be soothing, and massaging diluted essential oils (in a carrier oil) into the skin is also therapeutic. Some midwives have further training in aromatherapy; ask your maternity unit if they are able to offer this service, or if they have information and contact details for qualified aromatherapists in your area.

Reflexology

Reflexology involves massaging reflex zones on your feet that correspond with different parts of your body to improve your blood circulation and relax any tension you may be feeling. Reflexology is gaining some popularity as a coping technique in the early stages of labour. However, as many women naturally want to be active and move around during their labour, this may be more helpful in between early contractions.

BIRTH STORY A NATURAL HOME BIRTH

Gemma is a 31-year-old mum and this is her second labour. She had a straightforward birth with her little girl, now aged three. This pregnancy was uneventful, so she decided to have a home birth this time.

Gemma's birth story: When I was eight days' overdue, my midwife did a "stretch and sweep" (see p.393) of my cervix to encourage labour. I then had a couple of shows (see p.411) and irregular contractions. In the night I woke with contractions 20 minutes apart. I couldn't get back to sleep, so had a warm bath, took a couple of paracetamols, and went back to bed. My little girl woke at 06.45am and we had breakfast. My contractions were every 10 minutes and getting stronger, so my partner stayed at home.

By 8.00am, my contractions were every five minutes, stronger, and lasting 50–60 seconds. My partner called the midwife. She said she was on her way and advised me to stay active. I started to use the TENS machine (see p.399) on a low setting, which helped me to focus. I found standing and rocking my pelvis back and forth and from side to side helpful and I used a birthing ball. My partner was supportive, massaging my shoulders and under my abdomen where it hurt most; I found the heat from his hands soothing. My little girl held my hand.

At 8.40am, the midwife arrived. She checked my blood pressure, pulse, and temperature, felt my tummy, listened to the baby's heart, and took a urine sample, which relieved some pressure in my pubic area. She confirmed I was in established labour as my cervix was 5cm dilated. My cervix was thinning, the head was pressing down, and my waters were intact. I remained active, using TENS, and leaning forwards. My partner put on a relaxing CD.

At 9.50am my contractions were every two minutes, very strong, and lasting 60 seconds. I tried walking and then marching on the spot. My mum arrived and took my little girl to the park. I felt hot and so I had a cold drink and my midwife dabbed my face with a cool, wet cloth. I found kneeling on all fours, rocking and arching my back, helpful.

By 10.30am my contractions were very painful and I had some gas and air (see p.402). I used this for every other contraction and continued to walk around and use TENS. My midwife listened to the heartbeat intermittently.

By 11.00am I felt an urge to push. My waters broke and my contractions were very strong and each minute. I felt panicky, but my midwife encouraged me, saying she thought the baby would be born soon; my partner helped me to focus by breathing slowly. My midwife confirmed that I was fully dilated and ready to push. I somehow found the energy to bear down and felt the head emerge. I took a breath, concentrated, and pushed my baby out. My baby boy was born at 11.14am, 8lb 2oz, and my partner cut the cord once it had stopped pulsating. I delivered my placenta without drugs (see p.429). My midwife advised me to put my baby to my breast to stimulate the hormone oxytocin, which causes contractions and helps the placenta to come away. My placenta was delivered at 11.40am.

The midwife's comments: Gemma and her partner prepared well and worked as a team. Gemma was active for most of her labour, and stayed focused. Her feelings of panic in the transition period were normal, but her partner and I gave her extra support. By working with her instincts she found inner strength and had a normal birth. Her labour was nine hours, about average for a second-time mum.

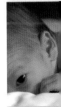

Drugs for pain relief

Various types of medication are available for pain relief during labour; many can be used alongside natural forms.

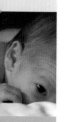

AS A MATTER OF FACT

Up until 150 years ago there were few options for pain relief during childbirth.

The history of modern obstetric pain relief began in the mid-19th century with the discovery of chloroform. Nitrous oxide and opioids followed, and at the start of the 20th century enthusiasm for pain-relief was so great that they were overused, with women in labour in a state of near-unconsciousness. The natural childbirth movement in the '60s and '70s was a reaction to such overuse of drugs. In the '70s another revolution was at hand as epidurals became available.

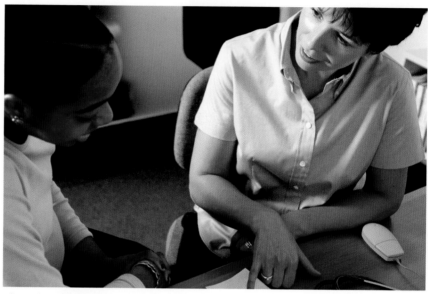

Discussing different pain relief options with your midwife prior to labour can help you assess the merits of each type and to think about what type of pain relief you would prefer.

For some, natural pain relief may not be suffficient to enable them to cope with the increasing intensity of contractions, and they may choose to use medication in combination with natural techniques. In some situations, for example if labour is induced (see p.432) or augmented (see p.415), contractions may start strongly rather than build up gradually and a stronger type of pain relief may be needed.

There are several types of medical pain relief available, which fall into two groups. Analgesic drugs, such as entonox and pethidine, dull the perception of pain, while anaesthesia, which is regional or general, numbs pain totally. In regional anaesthesia, also known as a nerve block, a local anaesthetic is injected around nerves that supply a particular area. There are several types of regional nerve block: epidurals and spinal blocks numb sensation in the abdomen and are used

to reduce the pain of contractions; a pudendal block numbs sensation in the vagina and perineum and may be used in a forceps delivery. Occasionally, a general anaesthetic is given during a Caesarean.

As all labours are different, it's not possible to have a "one size fits all" approach to pain relief. Being flexible and informed will help you to feel in control. Read any literature from your midwife, attend antenatal classes, and ask questions. You can minimize worries by increasing your knowledge, for example by asking to attend the anaesthetic clinic.

Entonox (gas and air)

This comprises 50 per cent nitrous oxide gas and 50 per cent oxygen, with nitrous oxide being the pain-killing component. It's delivered either through a pipe on the wall or from a cylinder by the bed, and is available in all UK maternity

PROS AND CONS

Entonox (gas and air)

Advantages

- Gas and air is an effective method of pain relief for many, particularly in the early stages of labour.
- It can be used throughout labour.
- It wears off quickly so you don't stay affected.
- As it's short-acting, it's completely safe for both you and your baby.

Disadvantages

- Gas and air reduces pain, but doesn't remove it. Some use it with other forms of pain relief, such as TENS; some need stronger medication as labour proceeds.
- It can cause sleepiness and nausea, so some use it for a short time only.

units and at home births. It's used by taking deep breaths through either a face mask or a mouth piece.

You need to inhale the gas at the start of a contraction to ensure that you get its maximum effect when the contraction is at its peak. As the effect is rapid and wears off almost instantly, taking it between contractions won't have any benefit for the following one. Some women report feeling light-headed and/or nauseous.

Opioids

These belong to a group of drugs called narcotics (which literally means sleep-inducing), and are similar to morphine. They attach themselves to receptors in the brain or nerves and block the transmission of pain. The most commonly used is pethidine, although diamorphine is used increasingly in many units.

Pethidine This synthetic form of morphine is given as an injection into a muscle in the buttock or thigh. It takes about 20 minutes to work and lasts for three to four hours. Pethidine sedates, but doesn't give a feeling of wellbeing, and many women dislike the disassociated, out-of-control feeling it creates. Also, many feel it sedates them between contractions without providing effective pain relief at the peak of a contraction. It can also cause nausea and vomiting, so an anti-nausea injection may be given.

Pethidine crosses the placenta rapidly and can affect the baby's breathing, so it shouldn't be given in the two to three hours before birth. If it causes breathing problems, an antidote called naloxone can be given to the baby after the birth.

Many studies show that babies of mothers who've had pethidine are often slow to establish breastfeeding. However, there are no long-lasting adverse effects.

Diamorphine This semi-synthetic morphine derivative is injected into a muscle. It produces better pain relief than pethidine and a sense of euphoria. It can cause nausea too (but less than pethidine), so may also be given with an anti-nausea injection. It crosses the placenta too and can cause breathing problems in the baby, so its administration needs to be carefully timed.

REMIFENTANYL: A PATIENT-CONTROLLED PAIN MEDICATION

Remifentanyl is a relatively new narcotic drug that isn't in mainstream use in maternity units, but which is sometimes given as an alternative to epidural pain relief where this isn't recommended (see p.404). It's a very potent painkiller that is rapidly broken down in the bloodstream, and its effects are short-lasting, which makes it ideal in labour. However, as a result of its potency, it can reduce the rate and depth of the mother's breathing and can therefore only be safely offered if you are continuously accompanied by a midwife. Also, in common with all narcotics, it crosses the placenta to the baby; however, because it's quickly metabolized, its effects are small.

As remifentanyl is such a fast-acting drug with a short-lasting effect, if it is offered in labour it is most likely to be given by means of a patient-controlled analgesic (PCA) device that allows self-administration of a drug. The PCA device is connected to a vein by means of a small tube and allows the woman to control the amount of pain medication she receives. When a button is pressed, a preset amount of medication is delivered directly into the bloodstream. The device can also be programmed to deliver a continuous low dose of medication while allowing the woman to give herself an extra top up dose if needed. It's programmed to avoid giving too much medication so that an overdose is not possible.

Opioids (pethidine and diamorphine)

Advantages

■ Opioids help you to relax during labour, which can help you to conserve your energy between contractions.

■ Opioids can be administered by a doctor or a midwife. A doctor can give an advance prescription at around 36 weeks so that an opioid can be given by a midwife at a home birth.

■ Diamorphine produces a feeling of wellbeing, which many women find beneficial during labour.

Disadvantages

■ Many women report feeling nauseous with opioids. Pethidine in particular has side effects of nausea and vomiting.

■ Opioids can cause dizziness, which can be disorientating during labour.

■ Some women report feeling out of control with pethidine and therefore out of touch with how their labour is progressing.

■ Opioids cross the placenta easily and pass into the baby's bloodstream. This can have the effect of sedating the baby and can affect the baby's breathing after the delivery. The administration of these drugs therefore needs to be carefully timed during labour so that they are not given too near the time of the delivery of the baby.

■ Opioids can depress the mother's breathing during labour. However, this side effect is more common when the mother has a pre-existing respiratory illness, such as asthma or emphysema.

■ Opioids cause a delay in emptying the bowels; if general anaesthesia is needed later, this increases the small risk of stomach contents being inhaled into the lungs under anaesthesia.

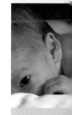

Drugs for pain relief

403

Considering an epidural

Pros

■ An epidural provides absolute pain relief in 90 per cent of cases; 10 per cent of women have some degree of residual pain, but still have a marked improvement in their overall discomfort.

■ Epidurals do not pose any risk to your baby.

■ The presence of an effective epidural means that if intervention is needed at any time, the epidural can be topped up with anaesthetic for either an assisted delivery with forceps or ventouse (see pp.436–7), or a Caesarean delivery (see pp.438–9). This also reduces the likelihood that a general anaesthetic will be needed.

Cons

■ Around 1 in 10 women do not experience absolute pain relief with an epidural.

■ Some women develop a headache that persists after the epidural has worn off (see p.406).

■ A rare complication is patches of heaviness in the legs or feet.

There are a few very rare risks with an epidural

■ In common with all invasive procedures, inserting an epidural can result in infection. Meningitis occurs in around 1 in 100,000 women and an epidural abscess occurs in about 1 in 50,000 women.

■ There is a 1 in 170,000 risk of developing a blood clot in the epidural space (epidural haematoma).

■ There is a 1 in 100,000 risk of the epidural tube moving into the fluid around the spine and resulting in unconsciousness, and there is a 1 in 250,000 chance of the epidural causing some form of paralysis.

Epidurals

An epidural is a regional anaesthetic that can be given at any stage of labour to numb the abdomen and therefore block the pain of contractions.

How epidurals work A hollow needle is inserted between two vertebrae in the lower back. A tiny plastic tube is then passed through the needle and into the epidural space surrounding the spinal cord. A local anaesthetic is injected into the needle and flows through the tube into the epidural space so that the nerve roots carrying the pain stimulus to the brain are coated with anaesthetic and pain is reduced or completely blocked.

Mobile epidural Some units offer a combination of a local anaesthetic used in a low dose and an opioid (painkiller), which allows you to walk about and adopt different positions and use aids such as a birth ball so that labour can be assisted by gravity. If the contractions are too strong, the epidural can be topped up with a higher dose of opioid.

High-dose epidural If your unit does not offer mobile epidurals or it's not suitable for you, a stronger anaesthetic is used. This will affect sensation in your legs so that you need to remain in bed and your baby will be closely monitored. A stronger epidural also affects sensation in your bladder, so you will need to have a catheter. Used late in labour, a stonger epidural may mean that you need help to push the baby out, as the pelvic floor muscles will be heavy and ineffective. In this case, your midwife will put a hand on your abdomen to feel when a contraction starts and will tell you when to push. In some cases, an assisted delivery (see pp.436–7) becomes necessary.

When are epidurals used? Epidurals can be used throughout labour, as early or late as you choose. As everyone has varying pain thresholds, the time when one is requested varies. There are factors to bear in mind should you opt for an epidural late in labour. To minimize the risks, you must remain completely still during the placement of the epidural tube. If your labour has progressed too far to enable you to do this, the anaesthetist may refuse to proceed with an epidural in your own interests. Also, if you choose to have an epidural late in labour, it may be necessary to give a high dose so that it takes effect in time, which has disadvantages (see left).

If you're considering using an epidural, inform your midwife early in labour so that she can consult the anaesthetist. The anaesthetist may then discuss this with you and take a brief medical history to ensure that it's safe for you to have an epidural. She will discuss any risks, and answer any questions that you or your partner has, all of which can save time later on if you decide to go ahead.

There are occasions when an epidural is not advised. These include cases where a woman has had spinal surgery or is taking blood-thinning medication. Rarely, a woman may have an infection that could be exacerbated by an epidural.

Side effects There are a number of minor side effects with epidurals. The medication can cause blood pressure to fall, so this will be monitored (see right). If it does fall, you'll be given fluids and medication, and subsequent doses may be reduced.

It's common to experience itching with epidurals, caused by the release of histamine from the opioid component of a mobile epidural. Histamine is a substance released by the body during an allergic reaction that can cause itching. The itch can be treated, but in most cases it gets better on its own. If you develop an itch, a greater concentration of local anaesthetic alone will be used.

It's not unusual to shiver with an epidural, although this is a more common side effect if a concentrated local anaesthetic is used, as is the case for a Caesarean delivery.

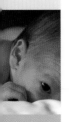

Labour and birth

If you opt for an epidural, the midwife or doctor should explain the procedure to you, and you should have the opportunity to ask the anaesthetist any questions.

Getting ready for an epidural

Before starting the epidural, a plastic tube will be placed in a vein in the back of your hand or in your arm, to which a drip containing fluid will be connected. You are given fluids during an epidural to stop your blood pressure dropping. The midwife will then help you into the correct position to receive the epidural, which will either be sitting up with your legs over the side of the bed leaning forwards, or curled up on your side on the edge of the bed. The position may depend on the preference of the anaesthetist.

Your lower back will be cleaned with antiseptic and a drape placed over the rest of your back to reduce the risk of infection. Before the epidural needle is inserted into the back, a local anaesthetic will be given into the skin and surrounding tissues. This creates a numb patch to ensure that the insertion of the epidural needle is not painful. When the local anaesthetic is injected, you may feel a scratching sensation and experience a very short-lived sting in the area between the vertebrae bones.

The procedure

As it's important for you to remain still during the procedure, the anaesthetist will insert the epidural between your contractions. If this is difficult, you should try to concentrate on your breathing and remain as still as possible until the procedure is completed. You will feel a pushing sensation in your back while the anaesthetist is trying to find the very small epidural space with the hollow needle. When the space is located, a tiny plastic tube will be fed into it through the needle. The epidural needle is then removed and the tube, which is secured onto your back with sticky tape, remains in the epidural space. The tube remains in place until your baby is delivered and, as it is very thin, soft, and pliable, it is perfectly safe to lie on the tube and to move around.

Managing the epidural

Once the epidural tube is successfully in place, the anaesthetist will give the first dose of medication through it by means of a syringe. Once she is satisfied that the epidural is in the correct position and is working effectively, all subsequent doses, or "top ups", will be given by a midwife. Your blood pressure will be taken once the epidural is in place and will be monitored for the next half an hour or so, and then regularly thereafter, including after each top up. Each dose of medication takes around 20 minutes to take its full effect and can last between one and two hours. The epidural will be topped up regularly as required, usually around every three to four hours, to keep you comfortable throughout your labour. An anaesthetist should be available 24 hours a day to manage any concerns or problems that may arise with the epidural.

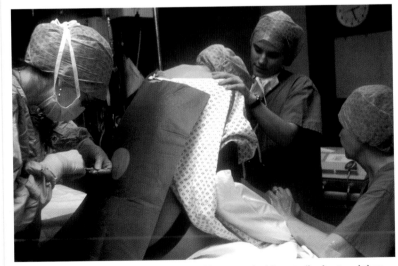

Before the epidural is given, your back will be covered with a sterile sheet and then a local anaesthetic will be given to numb the area so that you don't experience pain when the larger epidural needle is inserted.

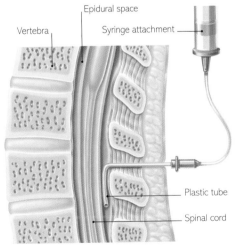

Epidural space

Syringe attachment

Vertebra

Plastic tube

Spinal cord

The anaesthetic is given through a tube that is inserted into the epidural space, avoiding the spinal cord and its covering.

Drugs for pain relief

405

Epidural pain relief can cause a rise in temperature. If this occurs, you'll have a blood test to eliminate an infection as this can also cause your temperature to rise. You will be given preventative antibiotics while waiting for the blood test results, and paracetamol to bring your temperature back to normal.

Problems with epidurals As well as side effects, there can occasionally be problems with the effectiveness of an epidural. The anaesthetic may not spread evenly in the epidural space, which may be caused by the epidural tube sitting on one side of the epidural space. This can mean that pain relief only occurs on one side of the body. If this occurs, the anaesthetist will try to reposition the tube and give another dose of anaesthetic. If this doesn't work, the only other solution is to redo the entire epidural.

Sometimes, one spot can remain painful, usually in the groin area or low down in the front of the tummy, which is referred to as a "missed segment". This results from a single nerve root not being coated with the local anaesthetic.

Again, the anaesthetist may reposition the tube. Sometimes, a stronger local anaesthetic or an opioid is used to numb the area. If a persistent missed segment is too uncomfortable, the anaesthetist may do a combined spinal epidural block, known as a CSE (see below).

It's thought that epidural pain relief may prolong the second stage of labour. It also increases your chances of having an assisted delivery with forceps or ventouse, especially if a high dose of anaesthetic is given towards the end of labour, which will affect your ability to push. Also, despite common misconceptions, epidurals do not cause long-term backache after the birth.

Spinal block

This is similar to an epidural in that a needle is put in your back and pain relief is achieved by blocking nerve fibres that supply the pelvic organs. However, in a spinal block, the needle is passed through the epidural space to pierce the membrane covering the spinal cord (the dura) so that anaesthetic can be injected into the fluid around the spinal

cord; no tubes are left in place. The needle used for a spinal block is smaller than that used for an epidural, which means it's less painful to insert. There is also less risk of a headache than there is with an epidural (see box, below) because insertion of the smaller needle is less likely to result in leakage of spinal fluid.

A smaller dose of anaesthetic is needed and it works very quickly: pain relief is almost immediate, whereas an epidural takes 20–30 minutes. However, the use of a spinal block is limited because only a single dose of medication can be administered. As a result, spinal blocks are usually reserved for use during a Caesarean section, or for an assisted delivery when an epidural isn't in place.

Combined spinal epidural (CSE)

This involves both a spinal injection and putting an epidural in place. It's sometimes done when problems are encountered with an epidural (see left) and is also used for a Caesarean. A CSE gives pain relief for about two hours. However, it's a specialized technique and isn't offered in all units.

Pudendal blocks

This type of regional anaesthesia involves injecting a local anaesthetic into the vagina where the pudendal nerves are located to reduce pain in the vagina and perineum. The pudendal needle is quite long and thick, so before the injection is given, a cold anaesthetic spray is applied to the area. The anaesthetic has no effect on the baby and can be used with pethidine or entonox. It takes effect very quickly and is sometimes used just before birth to aid an assisted forceps delivery.

General anaesthesia

Most Caesareans are conducted using regional anaesthesia. However, in some cases general anaesthesia, where the mother is put to sleep, is necessary. This may be because of a failure of regional

---

AN EPIDURAL "HEADACHE"

Some women report a headache after an epidural, which can develop more than 24 hours after the delivery and tends to be at the front of the head. It is made worse by sitting up and moving about and is much improved by lying down. This occurs in around 1 in 100 women and is caused by the epidural needle moving too far forwards and cutting the dura sheath, the membrane maintaining the fluid around the spinal cord and brain. This small hole results in a loss of fluid from the sheath, which causes a headache. The risk is hugely reduced by remaining still during the placement of the epidural. In around 70 per cent of women, the hole heals on its own.

You will be advised to drink plenty of fluids and to take simple painkillers, such as paracematol and ibuprofen and you will be reviewed at regular intervals by an anaesthetist.

If the headache persists, a procedure called a "blood patch" will be done. This is carried out in the sterile environment of an operating theatre by two anaesthetists. One places an epidural needle in your back, while the other takes around 20ml of blood from a vein in your arm. The blood is then passed down the needle into the epidural space. This forms a clot that seals the hole and prevents further leakage of fluid from around your spine, therefore relieving the headache.

Labour and birth

Alice was having her first baby. Her pregnancy had been uncomplicated and she had written a birth plan with her partner outlining her desire for a natural childbirth by keeping active and using TENS and then warm water to deal with contractions. Alice also stated that she wished to avoid an epidural if possible.

Alice's birth story: My partner and I arrived at the delivery suite in early labour. I started to use a TENS machine for pain relief. However, as my labour progressed, I became very distressed as I hadn't anticipated that the contractions would be so painful. When I was around 3cm dilated, I decided to remove the TENS machine and get into the bath. My partner gave me a back massage and provided emotional support. However, I think he struggled to understand my discomfort and he needed support from the midwife. After 15 minutes, I decided to get out of the bath as it was providing little pain relief. I used a birth ball to stay active and my partner gave me more massage and acupressure. I coped well for the next hour, but then became increasingly exhausted and upset. When I was

examined, I was only 5cm dilated. We both felt despondent as we had hoped I was further along.

My midwife then suggested that I talked to the anaesthetist regarding my options for further pain relief, and as a result of my conversation with the anaesthetist, I decided to have an epidural. I told the anaesthetist that I'd had an epidural a few years ago for a knee operation and how the epidural had provided excellent pain relief, but that I had itched for hours afterwards. The anaesthetist surmised that the itch was caused by one of the painkilling medications (fentanyl) in the epidural top up and agreed that this medicine wouldn't be used.

The anaesthetist agreed to perform a low-dose combined spinal epidural that gave absolute pain relief within five minutes. My legs were a little heavy at first, but they felt fine within an hour. I felt that we were both able to take time out after the epidural and that I was able to refocus on my labour. I felt pleased that I'd managed a large part of my labour without pain relief, and was happy with the decision to have an epidural when I did. I had an unassisted delivery later that evening and gave birth to a beautiful baby girl.

The anaesthetist's comments: Alice kept an open mind regarding pain relief and understood that different methods of pain relief could be used at different times during labour. After the epidural, she no longer felt that her labour was an endurance test and was able to focus again on her labour and on delivering a healthy baby.

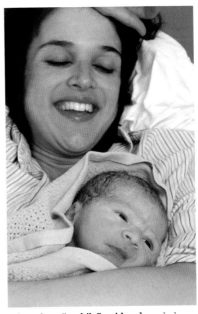

A low-dose "mobile" epidural can help you to manage pain and maintain some control so that you can focus on the birth.

anaesthesia, blood-clotting problems in the mother, an infection in the mother's bloodstream, or severe fetal distress.

The procedure Precautions are taken to minimize the risks to you and your baby. You'll be given a sodium citrate drink to reduce stomach acid. Often a catheter is inserted into the bladder and antiseptic is applied to the abdomen before you're put to sleep to minimize the baby's exposure to the anaesthetic.

As you are put to sleep, an oxygen mask is held tightly over your nose and mouth. Pressure is applied to part of

your neck to reduce the risk of food or acid from the stomach coming up the oesophagus and going into the lungs. This can feel alarming, but you're asleep within 30 seconds. Once asleep, an anaesthetist inserts a tube through your mouth and down your throat so that oxygen can easily reach your lungs. You may therefore have a sore throat when you wake up.

During the operation the anaesthetist looks after the mother, giving painkillers and anti-sickness medicine when needed. The baby is looked after by the midwife. Depending on hospital procedure, the

partner may or may not be present for the birth. However, no hospitals allow the partner to be present while the mother is being put to sleep.

After the operation The procedure takes about an hour. The mother is woken 5–10 minutes after the operation. The baby is kept with the mother at all times unless he needs extra care.

As general anaesthesia doesn't give localized pain relief, it's normal to need pain relief afterwards. Tablets will be given regularly and morphine-based medication may be given for a day or two.

1st stage of labour

WAITING FOR YOUR LABOUR TO START CAN BE BOTH FRUSTRATING AND EXCITING

You may be anxious to get your delivery over with, or feel that you aren't ready for labour. This can be an emotional time, so try to stay calm. This section helps you to identify the symptoms and signs of labour and takes you through the changes that occur as your body gets ready to give birth.

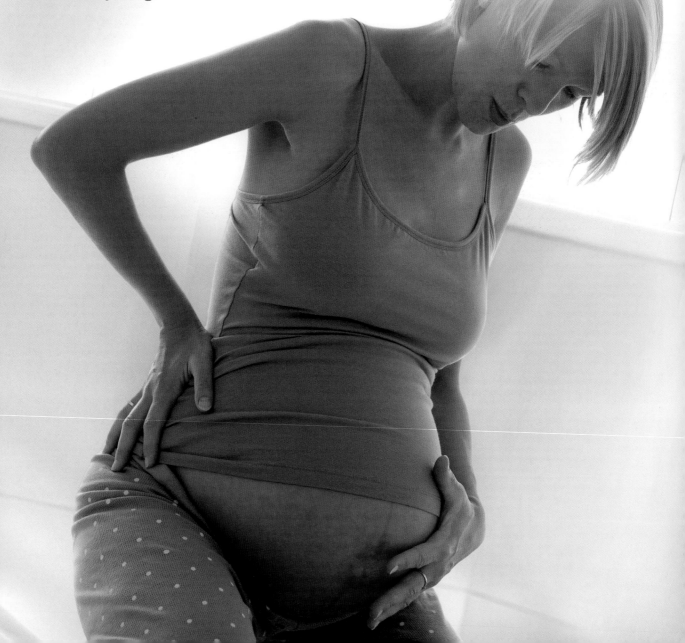

Approaching labour

As your pregnancy comes to an end, your cervix starts to soften and your body prepares for the forthcoming labour and birth.

As labour approaches, your body starts to prepare itself for the task ahead and you may notice various physical symptoms and signs that labour is about to start. Not every woman experiences labour in the same way, and certain signs can occur either before labour starts or during labour.

Common physical symptoms

Towards the end of your pregnancy, you may experience a sensation of building pressure or cramping in your pelvic or rectal area. This pelvic cramping can feel very similar to monthly menstrual cramps. A dull pain in your lower back that comes and goes is common, too. You may also notice an increase in heartburn (acid reflux) and gassiness. Unless you have a high-risk pregnancy, there is no need to go to the hospital or call your midwife if you experience any of these symptoms in the later stages of your pregnancy.

Your emotional state

This is a time of waiting and many women busy themselves with household tasks. These bursts of activity are often thought to be instinctive, as the mother prepares the home for the new arrival, referred to as "nesting". The anticipation of what will happen during labour can give rise to a mixture of emotions, from fear and anxiety to excitement and impatience. Women may feel fearful about how much pain they might feel or how uncomfortable they will be with bodily functions. Nothing can prepare you fully for how you will feel in labour, but the more you understand about pain relief options (see pp.396–407) beforehand, the more confident you will feel about your ability to cope. It's also thought that by being informed and prepared, you are likely to reduce your anxiety during labour, which in itself can enable you to cope better with the pain of contractions.

CHECKLIST

Preparing for labour

The period before labour starts can last for hours or even days, particularly with a first labour. So that you can cope when you do go into labour, you need to look after yourself during this pre-labour stage.

■ **Stay well rested** so that you aren't completely exhausted when you go into labour. If you're having trouble resting due to anxiety, try practising relaxation techniques.

■ **Trouble sleeping is usually due to physical discomfort,** such as being too hot, not being able to get into a comfortable position, or having trouble breathing from congestion. Measures that can help include body pillows, a dehumidifer, and fans or air conditioning in the summer.

■ **Carry on eating to keep your energy levels up** and provide fuel for the days ahead. You may not feel like eating a large meal; instead eat little and often.

■ **If you're suffering with back pain, try showering in warm water or having a warm bath.** However, take care when showering, as pregnancy increases your chances of feeling dizzy, and avoid a prolonged bath in very hot water as this may not be good for your baby.

■ **A lower back masssage is comforting** and a good way to relax and ease discomfort – ask your partner to give you a soothing massage.

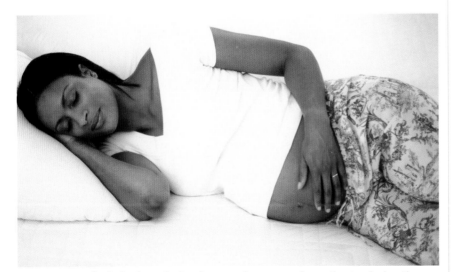

To prepare your body for the task ahead, ensure that you get plenty of rest and relaxation. As well as getting a good night's sleep, have a cat nap during the day if you feel fatigued.

No one is sure exactly what triggers labour, but it seems the process varies with each species.

In sheep, a drop in progesterone signals the start of labour. In mice, babies release proteins to signal their maturity, which in turn triggers labour. In humans, little is known about the signals that start labour although there are many theories. Studies suggest that the production of hormones such as corticotrophin-releasing hormone (CRH) by the uterus and placenta may play a role. It's also thought that an increase in pro-inflammatory substances known as cytokines may be involved. Whatever the trigger, it's likely that the onset of labour involves a biological communication between your baby and your body to indicate that your baby is ready to be born.

Braxton Hicks' contractions

One of the most common symptoms of approaching labour is an increase in the strength and frequency of Braxton Hicks', or practice, contractions, which may occur up to four times an hour. The purpose of these practice contractions is to prepare your uterus to deal with real labour contractions so that labour progresses smoothly. It's also thought that they may help to soften and shorten the cervix. Some women find Braxton Hicks' relatively painless, while others find these contractions fairly uncomfortable, especially if the baby is quite low and contractions increase pelvic pressure.

Apart from the level of pain, one of the main ways to distinguish Braxton Hicks' from real contractions is that Bracton Hicks' are irregular and they fade away, whereas labour pains occur at regular intervals and gradually become stronger, more intense, and closer together. The other main difference between Braxton Hicks' contractions and real ones is that, unlike Braxton Hicks', real contractions cause your cervix to dilate, which indicates that labour is beginning.

Engagement of the head

With a first baby, dropping down of the baby's head into your pelvis, known as engagement, can happen as early as 36 weeks. In second and subsequent pregnancies, engagement may not occur until the start of labour.

You can usually tell that your baby's position has changed in two ways. First, you may notice that you have less discomfort in your upper abdomen or around your ribs because the downwards movement releases some pressure. Second, you may notice increased pressure or pain in your pelvic or vaginal area as the baby's head moves into position. Your walking may become more of a waddle and you may have to pass urine more frequently than before. In some cases, your baby's head may pinch some of the nerves that run through your pelvis and you may

SIGNS OF APPROACHING LABOUR

Although each woman's experience of labour differs and there are no hard and fast rules as to what will happen when, there are signs that indicate that labour is likely to start either imminently or within a matter of days. One of the classic signs that labour isn't far away is a "show" (see opposite), when you lose the plug of mucus that has protected your baby from infection during pregnancy. The other indisputable sign that labour will be shortly underway is that your cervix begins to dilate, although of course this will only be apparent during an internal examination.

One other sign that labour may be about to start is if your waters break (see opposite). However, for the majority of women this happens later on during established labour.

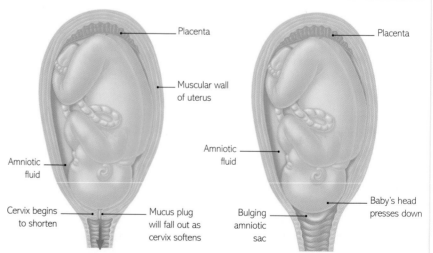

Placenta

Muscular wall of uterus

Amniotic fluid

Cervix begins to shorten

Mucus plug will fall out as cervix softens

Placenta

Amniotic fluid

Bulging amniotic sac

Baby's head presses down

As the cervix starts to soften and shorten, the thick plug of mucus that protected your baby from infection during pregnancy comes away and falls out of the vagina, known as a "show". You may notice a clear, yellowish jelly-like discharge that may be bloodstained.

The amniotic membrane bulges through the cervix as the baby's head presses down. When the membranes break (waters breaking), labour is imminent, or may have already started. The amniotic fluid may pass out as a gush of fluid or a trickle.

When to seek help

Make your way to hospital or seek advice if any of the following occur:

■ **You have vaginal bleeding** that is like a period or heavier.

■ **You're leaking amniotic fluid** or leaking greenish fluid that could indicate the baby is distressed.

■ **The baby isn't moving as expected** (ask your midwife for advice).

experience sciatica, a sharp electric pain that runs down the outside of your leg to your outside toes (see p.470).

The "show"

In pregnancy, a plug of mucus forms within the cervix to prevent infection entering the uterus. At the end of pregnancy, as the cervix softens and widens, this plug is dislodged and comes out through the vagina. When this occurs, you may see a discharge known as the "show", although some women don't notice anything. The discharge may appear as a thick, clear or yellow clump that looks like mucus from your nose. It's common for small amounts of blood to be present due to small tears in the cervix as the plug comes away.

Many women think that losing the plug means that labour is imminent, but this is not necessarily the case. In fact, it may be many days before labour starts. However, if loss of the plug is accompanied by other symptoms, such as painful, frequent contractions, heavy bleeding, or leaking fluid (indicating your waters have broken), you should call your midwife or hospital immediately.

Waters breaking

Rupture of the amniotic membranes, called the waters breaking, usually occurs once labour has started, but it can happen earlier. If this happens, it often means that labour is imminent. For some, a big gush of fluid is a clear sign that their waters have broken, while for others there may be a trickle and it can be hard to determine if the amniotic fluid is leaking. Also, as many women have trouble controlling their bladder in pregnancy, telling the difference between urine and amniotic fluid can be hard. One way to tell is to wear a sanitary pad. If the pad quickly becomes soaked, your waters have probably broken. Amniotic fluid also has an odour that is quite different from urine, even to non-professional noses.

Monitoring after the waters break If you think your waters have broken but contractions haven't started, contact your midwife or the hospital for advice. If you're due, there are no complications, and your baby's head is engaged, you may be advised either to stay at home for a while to see if labour starts, or will be asked to be seen by a midwife at home or at hospital. This is because, once your waters have broken, your baby has lost the protective membrane surrounding him, which means there is an increased risk of an infection reaching your baby. The midwife may take a vaginal swab to check for potentially harmful bacteria. She may also monitor your baby's heartbeat (see p.418) to check that your baby isn't distressed.

If she is happy that all is well, you may be able to return home, or stay at home, for a set amount of time and an appointment will be made to see how you're progressing. If labour doesn't start within 24 hours (the timescale may be longer in some hospitals), the hospital may suggest an induction (see p.432).

Early contractions

As your body prepares to go into labour, you will start to experience mild and irregular contractions. These differ from Braxton Hicks' as they build gradually and will soften and dilate the cervix.

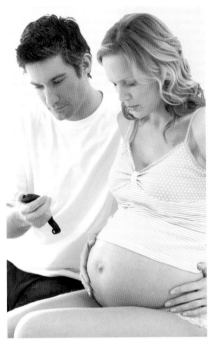

As you approach labour, you will experience irregular contractions; these will increase in strength and regularity as labour progresses.

When am I in labour?

A common concern of many women is how they will know when they are in labour. The following are indications that labour is truly underway.

■ **You are having contractions that are becoming stronger** and more intense, lasting longer, and the interval between the contractions is getting shorter.

■ **Changing your position or** walking around doesn't ease the intensity of the contraction.

■ **The contractions start high in your abdomen and** move down through the uterus and lower back, rather than occurring only in the lower abdomen.

■ **Your waters break** (see left) while you're having contractions.

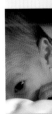

How labour progresses

Stronger and more regular contractions continue to stretch your cervix until, at around 10cm, it is fully dilated.

SUDDEN BIRTH

Although uncommon, labour and birth can occur unexpectedly fast, resulting in an unplanned homebirth or a birth on the way to hospital. Sudden birth is more likely to happen in second and subsequent labours, or if you've had a previous sudden birth.

If you're at home If your contractions start coming very rapidly and you begin to feel some pressure in your bottom try to stay calm and phone the emergency services for an ambulance. Also ask them to contact your midwife. Try to contact a friend, relative, or neighbour who can help. If someone is with you, ask him or her to contact the ambulance and midwife.

Wash your hands and gather flannels and towels or tea towels, or if you have an assistant ask him or her to prepare in this way. If there is time, the floor or bed should be covered with a plastic sheet or newspapers; have a plastic bowl to hand for the placenta.

If you have an urge to push, breathe slowly; panting and blowing can help. Sit or kneel on the floor or your bed on top of a clean towel so that your baby doesn't fall onto a hard surface. Your waters may break and an assistant can watch for a sudden bulging of the perineum and for your baby's head to appear, at which point you can push.

Once the head is delivered, you will feel another contraction and can push the body out. You may be able do this alone, or an assistant can put his or her hands either side of the head and apply gentle pressure. If your baby is born in the amniotic bag, this can be punctured with fingers; the baby's face will need wiping so that the airway is clear. Try to record the time of birth.

Give your baby immediate skin-to-skin contact to keep her warm; then dry her and wrap her in a towel or blanket. Putting her to your breast stimulates contractions to deliver the placenta. An assistant can watch for a gush of blood or lengthening of the cord, a sign that the placenta has come away. Put the placenta in a towel in a bowl to be checked. Clamp the cord with string or a shoe lace; the midwife or paramedic will cut it when he or she arrives.

If you're in a car If you feel an urge to push, your partner should pull over and put the hazard lights on. If your baby is born in the car, your partner can put him on your tummy for warmth. If you have towels, dry your baby, wrap him in a clean towel, and call an ambulance.

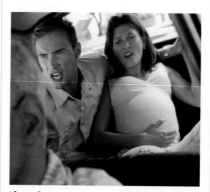

If you have an uncontrollable urge to push on your way to hospital, you may need to pull over and call the emergency services.

As every woman's experience of labour is different, it's hard to say exactly what your experience will be like. However, the stages of labour are common for all women. The first stage, when labour becomes established, starts when contractions start to open, or dilate, the cervix (see box, p.415). For some women, especially those who don't want strong pain relief, this is the hardest part of labour. Waiting for the cervix to dilate can be a long process with your first baby, and there isn't much you can do to hurry the process. The first stage of labour can be broken down into different phases, referred to as the early, or latent, phase, and the active phase (see below). After these phases comes transition, when your cervix becomes fully dilated and before you start to push your baby out (see p.416).

The early (latent) phase During the early phase, which can last for over a day or so in a first labour, your contractions gradually become more uncomfortable, but still relatively mild, and occur more frequently, although they may be irregular. During this phase, your cervix gradually shortens, a process known as effacement (see box, p.414) and begins to dilate. When the cervix is approximately 3–4cm dilated and you're having regular, strong contractions, the active phase has begun (see below). The changes to your cervix during the early phase can be slow or fast and are hard to predict.

The active phase The active phase of the first stage is the individual point for each woman where cervical change happens more quickly and predictably.

Many couples feel unsure about when to go to hospital. If your pregnancy is low risk, you will almost certainly be more comfortable at home at the start of labour and should wait until you're in active labour, when your contractions are regular, occurring every 5 minutes, and painful, before going to hospital. At this stage, the hospital will want to assess how your baby is responding to strong contractions, and you may want some medication for pain. This needs to be administered in a setting where you can be monitored and, in the case of an epidural (see p.404), can only be given in hospital.

If your pregnancy is high risk, you have had a prior Caesarean, have a breech baby, or carry the streptococcus B bacterium, call the maternity ward to discuss when to go to hospital.

Once you're in active labour, a final reason to go to hospital is to make sure your baby is born there. An unplanned home (or car) birth is not best for you or your baby. This is unusual in a first pregnancy, but with subsequent births, women are more likely to arrive at the hospital quite dilated or to have an unintended home birth.

Getting to hospital Arrange for someone to drive you to hospital, either your partner, or a friend or relative; do not consider driving yourself. Map out the route ahead of time, consider a dry run before the big day, and have a bag packed with everything you will need for you and your baby (see p.358).

Admission procedure When you get to hospital, you'll be checked in and will be put into a labour room if you look like you're in active labour, or into an assessment bed if this isn't clear. Usually you will be asked for a urine specimen, and a midwife will check your temperature, pulse, and blood pressure, check your cervix, and review your pregnancy history. If you're in early labour, you may be sent home. This doesn't mean you were unwise to come in; it's good to ensure all is well.

Once you've been admitted to the ward, you and your baby will be assessed and you'll be assigned a midwife. You can make your room comfortable with items from home. Some units limit the number of visitors allowed in your room.

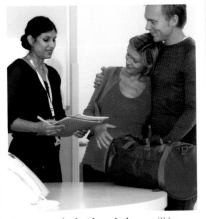

On your arrival at hospital you will be assessed to see if you are in established labour and should remain at the hospital.

However, exactly when you enter active labour can be hard to establish, even for a midwife. For most women, active labour occurs at around 4cm dilation. Your contractions are regular and may be every 5 minutes or so and getting closer together until they're 2 to 4 minutes apart and lasting from 45 seconds to one minute or more. From the start of active labour to the birth can last for around 10 to 12 hours, although this may be considerably shorter in a second labour.

In active labour, the nature of your contractions change, with pain becoming less concentrated in the lower abdomen, instead starting higher in the abdomen and moving down towards the pelvis and lower back as your baby is pushed down. Contractions are caused by a painful tightening of the muscles that may start off feeling like a severe period pain and

FOCUS ON... A HOME BIRTH

As labour begins

If you're having a home birth, your midwife will have talked to you in advance about how to contact her once you're in labour. This may be via her mobile phone or pager, or via the maternity unit. As she will be travelling to you, bear in mind local traffic conditions. If the roads might be busy, it's worth phoning her in early labour. She may ask you to phone again when your contractions are closer together.

While waiting for the midwife, you may want to move around, or relax in a warm bath. If you've hired a birthing pool, ensure that this is ready to use. Ask your partner to lay down old sheets or plastic sheeting over the floor. Eating small, nourishing snacks and drinking water will provide energy for the hours ahead.

It's usual for two midwives to attend a home birth in the UK. Either both will be present throughout, or one will be present in labour and will call the other one closer to the delivery, so that both are present for the birth. Rarely, if a midwife is held up and your labour progresses rapidly, you may have to call the maternity unit who will arrange for paramedics to attend the birth.

How labour progresses

413

CHANGES TO THE CERVIX

The cervix is comprised of firm muscle that forms a strong base at the bottom of the uterus. For your baby to be born, the cervix needs to stretch and soften so that it can open, or dilate, and your baby can pass out of the uterus and into the vagina.

Towards the end of pregnancy, substances in your blood called prostaglandins start to soften the cervix so that it becomes more malleable. While you are pregnant, your cervix is usually around 2 to 3 cm long. In late pregnancy or early labour, Braxton Hicks' practice contractions start to shorten, or thin, the cervix, known as effacement. Most women have a cervix that has shortened to 1cm in the very early stages of labour. This is also referred to as 50 per cent effaced. As the cervix continues to shorten, it is drawn up by the uterus. Eventually the cervix is fully dilated (see box, opposite), and the baby can be pushed out. In second and subsequent pregnancies, the effacement and dilation of the cervix can occur simultaneously.

As labour approaches, the cervix loses its firmness and softens in response to the presence of prostaglandins in the blood and Braxton Hicks' contractions.

Lower segment of uterus

Cervix

Once the cervix has softened, it starts to shorten, a process known as effacement. This occurs either before the cervix begins to dilate or at the same time as dilation.

Cervix being drawn up by uterus

Cervix shortened

THE "STATION"

The "station" refers to the position of your baby's head in relation to your pelvis. This is recorded as a number between -5 and +5. Zero station means the head is "engaged" and has entered into the pelvic cavity. A negative number (-5 to 0) means that the head isn't engaged in the pelvis. A positive number (0 to +4) means that your baby's head is moving down the pelvis and +5 means your baby is crowning (being born). Ideally, you should not push until the head is engaged in the pelvis, even if you're fully dilated.

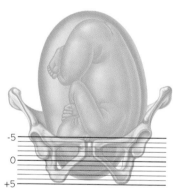

-5

0

+5

The position of the head in relation to the pelvis is marked on a scale of -5 to +5.

---

increase in intensity as they reach their peak. Your midwife will assess if you're in active labour by observing your pain levels, the frequency and strength of contractions, and by using a tool called a labour curve, which plots cervical change and the position of your baby's head in relation to your pelvis over time (see partograms, p.419).

It's important for your midwife to determine when you enter active labour so she can assess how labour is progressing. For first labours, 90 per cent of women have a cervical dilation of about 0.5cm per hour, whereas labour moves faster in subsequent births. If you've had an epidural (see p.404), labour may be slower. Once it's established that you're in active labour, the midwife or doctor can predict when you may deliver. However, as women vary widely in how long it takes them to have a baby, bear in mind that this is only an estimate.

During active labour, you may wish to have medical pain relief if you haven't so far, such as gas and air, pethidine, or an epidural (see pp.402–6).

Abdominal and vaginal examinations

Your abdomen is palpated to assess the baby's position and, in a first labour that progresses normally, you may have two to three vaginal examinations with your permission; in a second labour you may have just one vaginal examination. If the midwife is assessing whether amniotic fluid is leaking, a speculum examination may be done. Usually, the midwife uses her index and middle fingers to assess the baby's presentation and position. She'll try to check you often enough to ensure that labour is progressing, but not so often that it increases the risk of infection or causes extra discomfort. The following are assessed during a vaginal examination.

The station The midwife will check how far the head has descended into the pelvis (see box, above).

Cervical effacement The midwife will assess how your cervix is shortening, known as effacement (see box, opposite).

Cervical dilation The midwife assesses how dilated, or open, your cervix is (see box, below). Active labour is established at 3 to 4cm dilation and full dilation occurs at around 10cm. You can't push your baby out until you're fully dilated.

Fetal position Fetal presentation refers to the part of your baby that is coming out first. Babies can be born head first or bottom first (breech, see p.433). Your midwife will also assess which way your baby is facing in the birth canal. The easiest way for a baby to be born is head down with the back of the baby's head (occiput) and spine towards the front (anterior) of your uterus, known as an occipito-anterior position. Your baby can also be born vaginally from an occipito-posterior position (the back of the baby's head and spine towards the back of your uterus), but this can take longer and be more painful. Vaginal tears are more common when babies are born in the occiput posterior position. A final position is when your baby faces your side, known as occiput transverse. Full-term babies can't be born in the transverse position as the head is too big to deliver this way. It's not uncommon for babies to rotate during labour, although this would need to happen before you give birth. If this doesn't happen, delivery may need to be assisted with forceps or a ventouse cup (see pp.436–7).

Descent with contractions Although most of the time your midwife will try to examine you in between contractions, sometimes it helps to see how much the baby's head comes down in the pelvis during a contraction, referred to as the descent. If there is a good descent during contractions, this means that the baby is fitting well into your pelvis and that your contractions are efficient.

DILATION

Once your cervix is stretched and softened (see box, opposite), it begins to open, or dilate, so that your baby can pass through into the vagina to be born. Regular contractions cause the cervix to dilate, and in first labours the cervix dilates at an average of 1cm per hour; this rate is often faster for subsequent labours. You cannot push your baby out until you are fully dilated, which occurs at 10cm.

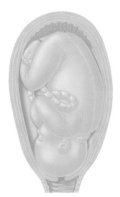

At 2cm dilation, the cervix has shortened and is beginning to open. Contractions may still be irregular.

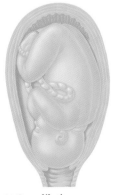

At 6cm dilation, you are in active labour. Your contractions will have become more frequent, regular, and stronger.

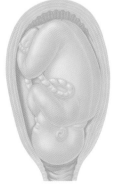

At 10cm dilation, you are fully dilated. Contractions may be almost continuous and you are nearly ready to start pushing your baby out.

QUESTIONS AND ANSWERS

Am I likely to have medical interventions in labour in hospital?
The reality of a hospital birth is that medical interventions may be suggested, some of which may be more helpful than others. Procedures that can be carried out include artificially breaking the waters; inserting a catheter; inserting an intravenous (IV) drip into a vein in your hand or arm through which fluids or medication can be given; and speeding up labour with drugs.

Is manual rupture of the membranes routine in hospital?
Manually breaking the bag of waters, known as amniotomy (see p.432), isn't routine, but may be offered if labour isn't progressing. It's a painless, low-risk procedure that is thought to shorten the time of labour by one to two hours, reduce the chance of a low early APGAR score in the baby (see p.428), and decrease the chance that you'll need drugs to speed up labour (see below). Amniotomy does, however, increase the intensity of contractions. The one time it's necessary is if a fetal scalp electrode is put on the baby's head (see p.419) as this can't be done without breaking the waters. It may also be done as part of the induction process (see p.432).

How is labour speeded up with drugs?
A slow labour may be speeded up with the drug oxytocin, a procedure known as augmentation. Oxytocin is naturally released from the pituitary gland in labour. Synthetic oxytocin is given via an IV drip to strengthen contractions. When this is done, it's usual to have continuous fetal monitoring (see p.418) as, if contractions become too strong, your baby may show signs of distress. Oxytocin is cleared quickly from your system once the drip is turned off, so contractions that are too strong can be weakened quickly. Oxytocin is also given in an induction (see p.432).

Transition

Transition is the time between the end of the first stage of labour and the start of the second stage, when you get ready to start pushing. It can be very quick or can last for up to two hours; on average it lasts for about 30 minutes. This can be one of the most challenging parts of labour as your contractions intensify and can begin to feel continuous as they now occur every 30–90 seconds and last for 60–90 seconds. If you don't have an epidural, transition can be especially difficult as you may feel a lot of pressure in your lower back and rectum and have an overwhelming desire to push, but will be unable to push because your cervix is not fully dilated. Even if you've had an epidural, you may notice increasing pelvic pressure. If you do push before your cervix is ready, you may tear your cervix or cause your cervix to swell and thicken, which will prolong the process of labour.

It's not uncommon to vomit now, a side effect of the stretching of your cervix and the pelvic pressure. You may also tremble or shake and have hot flushes.

How you can cope You may feel very uncomfortable during this period as your contractions become stronger and you try to hold back from pushing. Significant pelvic pressure during the transition phase can make it difficult to relax between contractions, and you will therefore need plenty of support from your birth partner and midwife at this time, as you may be feeling exhausted, out of control, possibly frightened, and may even think that you can't continue.

Work with your midwife to find the best position for you. This is the one stage of labour where it can be helpful not to adopt an upright position, as you can take some of the pressure off the pelvis. Sitting or being on all fours with your bottom raised may help. Keep breathing during your contractions; your midwife may show you how to pant and breathe shallowly to help resist the urge to push. If possible, moving around during contractions can sometimes help as you will be focusing on doing something else until you can actively push. You could try rocking on a birthing ball or in a rocking chair. If there is time between your contractions, ask your partner to massage your lower back if this helps to relieve pressure.

It can be easy to lose sight of the purpose of labour at this point, so try to focus on the fact that your baby will soon be born.

Pain relief Your midwife may not give you intravenous pain relief medications now, as these can cause your baby to be too sleepy if they are given close to the birth. Depending on hospital procedure, you may or may not be able to have an epidural now (see p.404).

Support in the first stage

During the first stage, your partner has a varied and important role. As well as helping you to feel comfortable and assisting you with positions, your partner can also support you mentally. This is especially important at the end of the first stage, when you reach transition (see above), a point when women often feel panicky and out of control. Your partner can offer reassurance that you're doing well and that the delivery of your baby is not far off. He can also improve your comfort, for example by applying a damp, cool flannel to your face and neck, and he can help you to focus on your breathing, reminding you to pant or blow to help you resist the urge to push before the cervix is fully dilated.

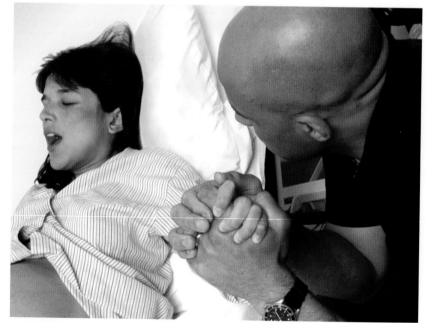

During transition, you may be overwhelmed by the strength and frequency of your contractions. Your partner's support is crucial during this stage and his encouragement can help to keep you focused on your labour.

If your cervix is not dilating, or your baby is not descending, as quickly as expected during the first stage, your midwife will try to assess why this is and whether something can be done. Usually, your midwife will assess the three P's: the passenger (the size of the baby and his position in the womb); the powers (the efficiency of your contractions); and the passage (the size and shape of your pelvis). These three elements work together and each one is important for your labour to progress smoothly.

There are several reasons why a labour may not progress. These include if the baby's head is too large for the mother's pelvis, known as cephalopelvic disproportion (CPD); if contractions are inefficient; and if the baby is in a posterior position with his back facing the mother's back.

Cephalopelvic disproportion

Sometimes CPD may be suspected before labour, in late pregnancy. This may be the case if the midwife thinks that you have a narrow pelvis or a prominent sacral bone, both of which may make birth slower or more difficult. However, an assessment of the pelvis alone is not an accurate way to predict if you'll be able to have a successful vaginal birth and, even if the pelvis is not an optimal shape, the midwife or doctor may be happy for you to continue trying for a vaginal birth. This is because it's not the shape of your pelvis alone that is important, but the interaction between your baby (the passenger) and your pelvis.

If CPD is suspected, but the baby's head has engaged, a vaginal birth can still be attempted. The labour will be monitored with a partogram (see p.419) and if there are signs that the baby is in distress or progress in labour is slow, a Caesarean may be carried out. Also,

if the head hasn't engaged near the end of labour, a Caesarean may be offered.

If your midwife suspects CPD in labour, she will reassess the baby's size to check if she originally underestimated the baby's weight. Even though the combination of a large estimated weight and a slow labour can suggest that there may be delivery problems, often labour proceeds normally.

Inefficient contractions If labour isn't progressing because the cervix is dilating slowly or has stopped dilating, your midwife will offer emotional support and assess the frequency of your contractions, which should be every 2 to 3 minutes. She'll also assess the strength of the contractions by palpating the abdomen: the firmer it is during contractions, the more likely they are to be effective. If contractions are more widely spaced than they should be and their strength indicates they're unlikely to be effective, she may use one or two techniques to speed up labour, known as augmenting labour.

First, she may manually rupture the membranes if they haven't already ruptured, a process called amniotomy (see p.432). This can shorten labour by

around one to two hours, but can mean that stronger pain relief is needed. If amniotomy has no effect, you may be given the drug oxytocin to increase the strength and frequency of contractions (see p.432). Initially, a small dose is given and then increased over time until you're having three or four moderately strong contractions every 10 minutes. If this is done, you'll have continuous electronic fetal monitoring (see p.418) to check that the baby is not distressed by the sudden onset of stronger contractions.

If, several hours after the drugs are started, labour is still not progressing a Caesarean may be recommended.

Posterior presentation The best position for your baby in labour is an occipito-anterior position with the back of the head (occiput) facing your front. If the back of the head faces your back (occipito-posterior) this can make it hard for the baby to turn and move down the birth canal. The midwife may suggest that you change position to help the baby to turn, but the baby usually turns anyway during fully established labour; if not, ventouse or forceps may be needed (see pp.436–7).

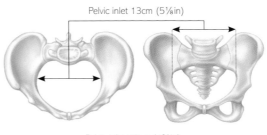

Pelvic inlet 13cm (5⅛in)

A gynecoid pelvis is the name given to a pelvis that has a circular shape. The generous proportions of this more typical "female-shaped" pelvis provides room for the head to pass through during the birth.

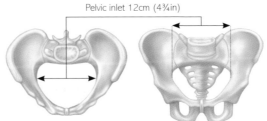

Pelvic inlet 12cm (4¾in)

An android pelvis is the term used to describe a pelvis that has a more triangular shape. This reduces the room available for the baby's head to pass through and is more likely to cause problems during a vaginal delivery.

How labour progresses

417

Monitoring during labour

Throughout established labour, your baby's heartbeat and your contractions will be monitored to make sure that your labour is progressing as it should and that the wellbeing of you and your baby is not threatened.

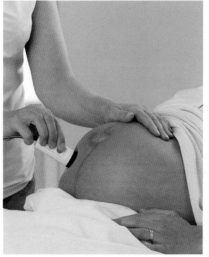

A hand-held device can monitor your baby's heartbeat at intervals, leaving you free to move around during labour.

Your baby's heart rate is an indication of how well your baby is coping with labour and it is monitored at regular intervals, using intermittent auscultation. If there's a problem or your pregnancy is high risk, electronic fetal monitoring will be advised, in which the baby's heart rate and your contractions are monitored continuously by a cardiotocograph (CTG) machine (see box, below). The information about your labour is recorded on a chart, called a partogram (see opposite).

Intermittent auscultation

This is done using a hand-held battery-operated device known as a Doppler sonicaid, which is held against your abdomen to listen to your baby's heartbeat. When you are pushing in the second stage of labour, the fetal heart needs to be monitored more frequently.

Electronic fetal monitoring

In this type of monitoring, two devices monitor your baby's heart rate and the strength and frequency of contractions. Your baby's heart rate is monitored with a circular ultrasound-like device. If you wish, you can hear the heartbeat, or ask that the volume be turned down if it's distracting. Contractions are monitored with a small plunger on a plastic circle. One or two elastic belts are put around your abdomen to secure the monitors. You should be able to stand, sit or squat with the monitors in place; some hospitals have monitors that allow you to walk around and be monitored by radio signal.

HOW MONITORING IS DONE

External electronic fetal monitoring

The baby's heartbeat and the strength and frequency of your contractions are measured by devices strapped to your abdomen. Wires from the devices connect to a machine that produces a printout of the readings called a cardiotocograph (CTG).

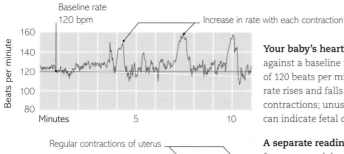

Baseline rate 120 bpm — Increase in rate with each contraction. Beats per minute 160 140 120 100 80. Minutes 5 10. Intensity of contractions — Regular contractions of uterus. Minutes 5 10.

Your baby's heartbeat is recorded against a baseline measurement of 120 beats per minute. The heart rate rises and falls naturally with contractions; unusual variations can indicate fetal distress.

A separate reading records the frequency and duration of each contraction. This can detect infrequent or irregular contractions and can be useful with an epidural when you can't feel contractions.

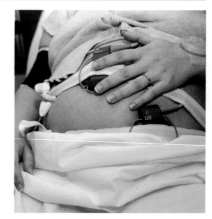

Continuous monitoring of your baby's heart rate and your contractions is carried out by means of two monitors strapped to your tummy.

INTERNAL MONITORING

Scalp electrode

If there are concerns about the baby's heartbeat, a small electrode attached to the scalp can give a more precise reading than external electronic fetal monitoring. The electrode is passed through the cervix and attached to the head.

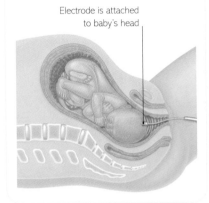

Electrode is attached to baby's head

Internal monitoring If your baby's heart-rate reading indicates that your baby is distressed, or the signal from an electronic monitor is poor, the midwife or doctor may suggest internal fetal monitoring. In this technique, a small electrode is attached to your baby's scalp and detects the electrical impulses of his heart. A wire from the electrode comes out via the cervix and attaches to the CTG machine, which produces a trace of the heartbeat. You still wear a strap around your abdomen, which holds the device for detecting the rate and strength of your contractions.

The electrode is placed during a vaginal examination and is no more uncomfortable than this. Placing a scalp electrode may be mildly uncomfortable for your baby and there is a small risk that your baby could get a scalp infection, which can be treated with antibiotics after the birth. Even though these risks are small, a scalp electrode should not be placed routinely. Your

midwife should discuss how the device works before it is placed, and you should understand why it is being done. Scalp electrodes should not be used if you have a viral disease, such as hepatitis B or C, or HIV, that could be transmitted to your baby during labour and delivery. Once a scalp electrode has been placed, you can't move far from the monitor, although you may be able to change position.

If a CTG reading from the scalp electrode indicates that your baby is distressed, a blood sample may be taken from the scalp to check acidity levels. If these are high, a Caesarean or assisted delivery may be suggested.

Partograms

A partogram is a large chart used when you're in established labour. It contains several graphs that provide information on your labour, allowing the midwife to monitor your progress. One of the most useful tools in this chart is a graph showing your labour curve. This plots cervical change and the position of your baby's head in relation to your pelvis over time. The graph enables the midwife to establish when your labour became active. Also recorded are your blood pressure, pulse, and temperature, your baby's heart rate, and the rate of your contractions, as well as your pain levels and the strength of your contractions.

RISKS AND BENEFITS

Should you have electronic fetal monitoring?

Although monitoring during labour is an important part of the care of you and your baby, there is some debate as to the benefits of continuous monitoring and some believe there may be associated maternal risks. As a result, most hospitals suggest intermittent fetal monitoring. Although you can refuse monitoring entirely, the staff may be unhappy about this and ask you to sign a form or statement releasing them from liability if anything goes wrong during labour and birth.

Risks Studies suggest that women who are monitored continuously are more likely to have a Caesarean section or an assisted delivery with forceps or ventouse (see pp.436–7). This is because your midwife may see changes in the fetal heart rate that concern her. Some changes, such as a faster heart rate (more than 160 beats a minute), known as tachycardia, or decreases in the heart rate that occur after your contractions, can be caused by decreased oxygen to your baby. If

your midwife sees these changes, she may be unable to determine if they were caused by low oxygen or if your baby is actually fine.

If it's thought that your baby may be at risk, an emergency Caesarean section may be recommended. If there are fetal heart rate changes while you are pushing, a forceps or vacuum delivery may be offered.

Benefits The benefits of continuous electronic fetal monitoring are not entirely clear. You are able to hear your baby's heartbeat and some women may find this comforting. Also, experts agree that continuous monitoring reduces the chance that your baby will have a seizure after the birth, a symptom of brain injury from low oxygen. Seizures are rare, occurring in around 2.5 per 1,000 births with monitoring and 5 per 1,000 births without monitoring. Electronic fetal monitoring may possibly prevent rarer complications such as cerebral palsy or fetal death, but this is harder to prove.

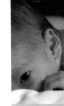

Positions for 1st stage of labour

Being active during the first stage of labour is thought to help labour progress. If you're well prepared and practise different postures and positions for labour during pregnancy, you will instinctively be able to use these during childbirth.

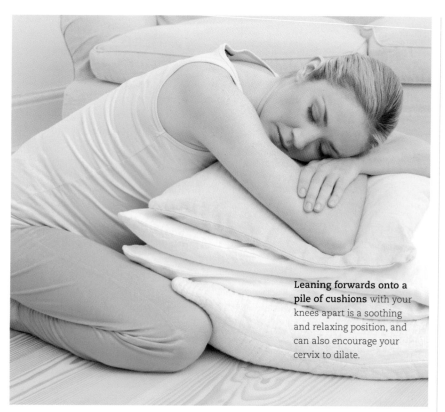

Leaning forwards onto a pile of cushions with your knees apart is a soothing and relaxing position, and can also encourage your cervix to dilate.

Many different postures and positions can help you in the first stage, and there is evidence that changing your position in this stage increases the effectiveness of your contractions and reduces the pain. Assuming upright positions in particular uses gravity to assist the descent of the baby.

Active positions

Positions that allow you to remain active are thought to help labour to progress. Some women find rocking the pelvis backwards and forwards, and then rotating the pelvis in a clockwise and then anti-clockwise direction while standing or sitting on a birthing ball, helps ease the pain. Adopting an all-fours position on your hands and knees can help you to stay focused and also allows you to rotate your pelvis. Moving backwards and forwards in a rocking chair can also be comforting. Many women find marching on the spot and walking around helpful.

Supported positions

Supported positions can be especially helpful if your baby is in an occipito-posterior position (baby's back to your back). Leaning forwards with your hands on a table or chair during a contraction and breathing slowly and steadily helps you to focus. If you find it comforting, your partner can massage your shoulders and back at the same time. A lot of women find either sitting astride a chair facing the back of the chair or sitting on a toilet and facing the cistern with a pillow for their head and arms, a comfortable position. This also allows you to "cat-nap" between contractions.

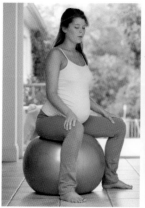 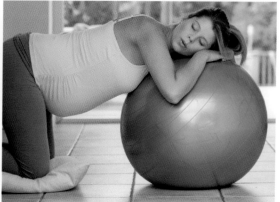

Using a birthing ball during labour enables you to adopt upright positions while feeling supported (left). While sitting on a birthing ball, or adopting a supported kneeling position with one, you will be able to rotate your hips to encourage the progress of labour (right).

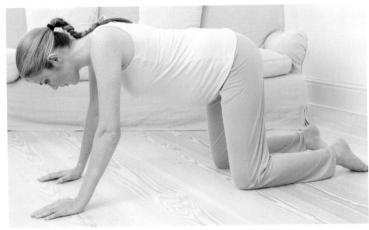

Kneeling in an all-fours position helps to take the weight off your back. This position also allows you to move your hips back and forth or rotate them, which can be comforting during early contractions.

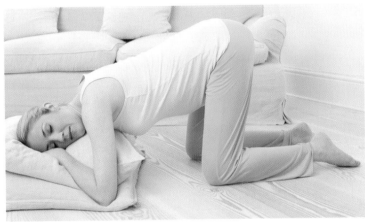

Kneeling and leaning forwards onto cushions with your bottom raised also helps to ease backache and can be a helpful position to adopt during transition (see p.416) when you may need to resist the urge to bear down.

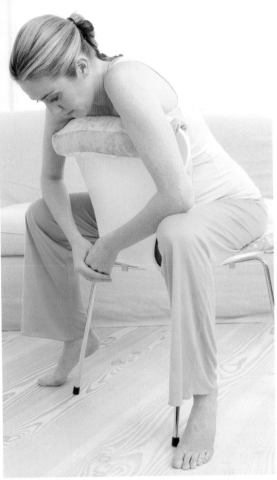

Sitting astride a chair can be a restful position as this enables you to lean forwards with your legs astride while remaining supported.

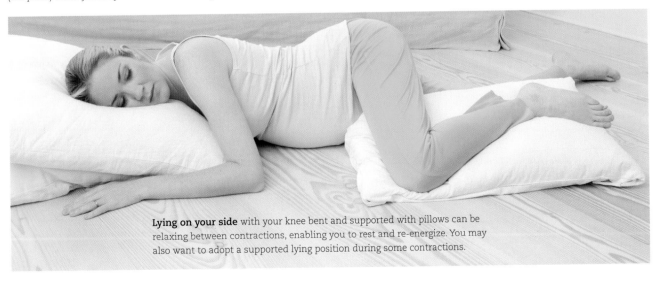

Lying on your side with your knee bent and supported with pillows can be relaxing between contractions, enabling you to rest and re-energize. You may also want to adopt a supported lying position during some contractions.

2nd & 3rd stages

THE MOMENT OF DELIVERY IS WITHIN SIGHT AND YOU WILL SOON MEET YOUR LONG-AWAITED BABY

The second stage begins when your cervix is fully dilated and your baby has moved deep into the pelvis. These signs may be accompanied by an overwhelming urge to bear down and, once your midwife is happy that you are ready to do so, you will be able to push your baby out. The third stage, the delivery of the placenta, marks the end of labour.

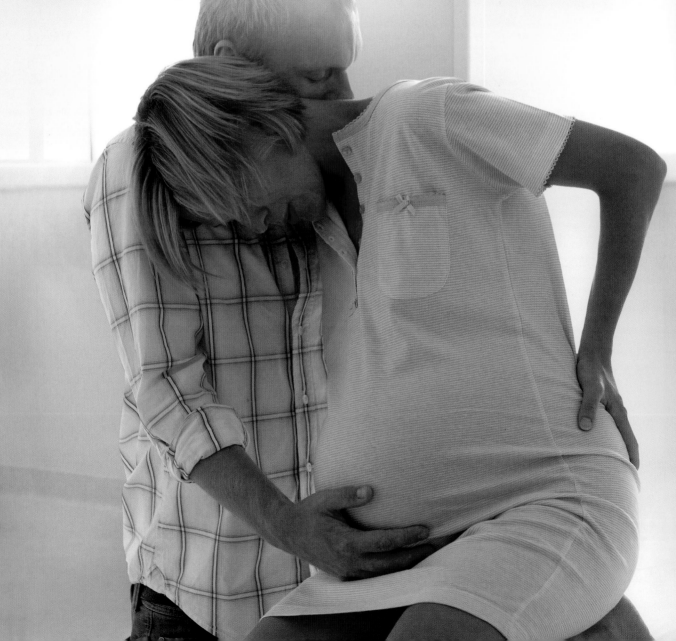

Labour and birth

Delivering your baby

In the second stage, your labour starts to accelerate as you actively push your baby out into the world.

As you enter the second stage of labour, you will probably experience an overwhelming desire to bear down. Once your midwife has established that you are fully dilated and is happy for you to start pushing, you may start to feel more in control of your labour as your pushing helps to move your baby further down into the pelvis.

The second stage

The second stage of labour starts when your cervix is completely open, at 10cm, and ends with the birth of your baby. This stage usually lasts for 45 minutes to two hours for a first labour and 15–45 minutes in subsequent deliveries. It lasts even longer if you have an epidural. The second stage is intense and during this time your contractions will become stronger, but may occur less frequently, around every two to five minutes. At this point you may feel a sensation of fullness in your vagina or bowel and have a strong urge to push. Many women find labour pains more

AS A MATTER OF FACT

The birth passage, far from being straight, involves a series of rotational manoeuvres known as the "mechanisms of labour".

This curve, known as the "curve of Carus", is thought to result from the evolution of humans from being on all fours to being upright. This caused the spine to curve, the pelvis to tilt, and gave a curve to the birth canal. Your pelvic floor muscles help the head to rotate through the birth canal.

Support in the second stage

In the second stage, your partner's support is invaluable. His or her role is to make you feel supported and safe and to offer lots of encouragement.

Your birth partner can provide verbal support to help you cope with the strenuous task of pushing your baby out with each contraction. There may be times when you're not lucid and your partner will need to speak for you and liaise with medical staff.

As well as emotional support, your birth partner can act as your physical support in whatever position you adopt in the second stage, whether this is a squatting position or another position that you find comfortable. Your partner will be able to massage your back if this is helpful, and can hold you and comfort you and help you to focus on your breathing during and between each contraction.

Your partner can also watch as your baby's head crowns and describe what he or she can see, or hold a mirror for you to see the baby's head. This can be deeply reassuring as you realize that the end is in sight.

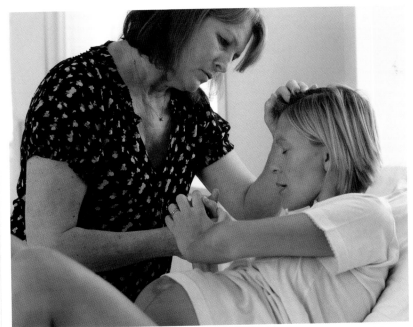

The emotional and physical support provided by your birth partner can be crucial during the second stage of labour, the time when you are having to exert yourself physically to push your baby down in your pelvis and out through the birth canal.

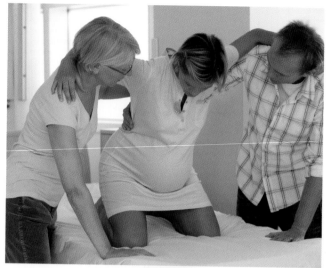

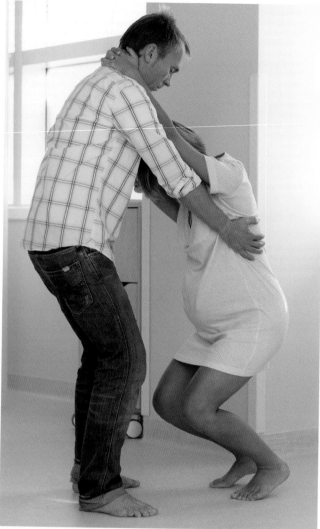

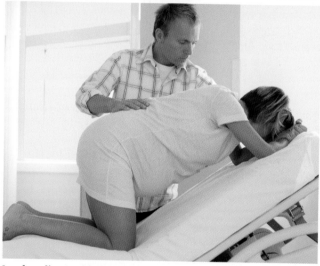

In a kneeling position, both your partner and the midwife can support you as you bear down (top). **Being on all fours** with the hospital bed for support can be a comfortable position (bottom).

An upright squatting position is good for pushing and can be adopted if you have firm support from your partner. He can support you under the arms while you put your hands around the back of his neck.

bearable in the second stage as they can now actively work with the contractions and push their baby out. Other women find this a particularly hard part of labour as they start to feel exhausted from the effort of prolonged pushing.

Second stage positions

Although you may be tired and want to lie down, it's recommended that you resist this urge in the second stage. Your partner and midwife can give you plenty of support to help you to adopt the most comfortable position.

Staying upright Adopting an upright position during the second stage of labour has several advantages. The main one is that you are using gravity to assist your baby's descent, which will also help you to bear down and push. Being upright can also improve the alignment of your baby in the birth canal; can increase the efficiency of your contractions; and widens the passageway through the pelvis.

There is also evidence that adopting upright positions in the second stage of labour can reduce the length of time

you take to bear down and give birth, and make it less likely that you will have an instrumental delivery or episiotomy (see pp.436–7 and p.427).

Which positions to adopt Upright positions during the second stage of labour include upright sitting and squatting positions.

If you prefer a sitting position, try to sit in an upright or semi-recumbent position. If you adopt a sitting position on a bed, sitting at a 45-degree angle can help your breathing and reduce the risk of a condition known as aortocaval compression, which can affect how well your blood is circulated around your body and to your baby. This is caused by the weight of your womb and the baby pressing on major blood vessels (the aorta and vena cava), reducing the amount of oxygen that circulates around your body, which makes you feel light-headed and dizzy. If this happens, you will be advised to lie on your left side to relieve pressure and increase the amount of oxygen circulating.

Because kneeling or squatting increases the pelvic outlet, many women will naturally adopt a squatting or all-fours position to give birth as they find that this is the most comfortable and easy position in which to deliver their baby. Upright squatting and kneeling positions help to increase your pelvic outlet by around 28 per cent compared to when you're in a lying-down position. This means that there is more room for your baby to descend through your pelvis and into the birth canal. Some women find it hard to squat down comfortably as they are not used to being in this position and tire easily. If this is the case, ask your partner to support you as you squat.

Alternatively, you may find that lying on your side is your preferred position; your partner can help you by supporting one of your legs to keep your pelvis as open as possible. There is also some evidence that lying on your side can protect your perineum from tearing.

Using props Some women find using props such as a bean bag, birthing ball, pillows, or a large cushion, while kneeling and leaning forwards helpful.

When to push
Your baby will start to rotate her head and shoulders to enable these to descend through your pelvis to be born, and you will feel the urge to bear down and push as this is happening. Your midwife will help you to focus and

Coping in the second stage

The second stage of labour can be a time when instinct takes over and you may find that you are oblivious to everything around you as you follow the overwhelming urge to push. You may have been concerned before labour about how you would behave during the delivery. Some women are worried that they will defecate while they are pushing. This is actually very common and it's natural to pass a stool during the delivery; you should rest assured that the midwives and doctors will be completely used to this. You may not even notice yourself that this has happened.

Rather than be concerned about how you will act, try to take encouragement from the fact that you now have more control over your labour and are actively pushing your baby out. You may find that you make a lot of noise while pushing, or you may push quietly and intensely. Focusing on the imminent arrival of your baby will help you to persevere.

encourage you to push when you feel the urge, which will come naturally with a contraction. With each contraction, you will need to concentrate on pushing down deep into the pelvic area and bottom. It can help to put your chin on your chest and to bear down for as long as possible during a contraction, during which time you may need to take several steady breaths. You may feel like grunting and making noises when bearing down, or you may prefer to breathe deeply and quietly; you should do whatever you find helpful and works best. You will need to work with your body's instincts and adopt the position you find most comfortable and easy to give birth in (see left). Pushing your baby out into the world takes a huge amount of effort and energy, but you have the ability and are very capable of doing this.

Your midwife and birth partner will encourage and support you throughout this stage and help you to believe in your ability to give birth.

Your baby's descent
The time it takes to push your baby out once she is deep within the pelvis can be around 30 minutes to two hours for a first labour, although this time may be considerably reduced in subsequent labours, sometimes taking just a few minutes. The combined force of the contractions (which are now around every two to five minutes) and your pushing moves your baby further down into the pelvic outlet. As this occurs, the pressure on your back and rectum will intensify and you may experience a stinging sensation as your vagina becomes fully stretched. Your midwife may tell you to stop pushing at this point so that your perineum can thin further and so that the baby's head isn't delivered too suddenly, which could

PUSHING WITH AN EPIDURAL

If you have had an epidural, this can affect your awareness of when to bear down and push. If this is the case, your midwife will first check that your baby isn't showing signs of distress, and may then decide to wait a while for the epidural effect to wear off slightly so you can feel when to bear down and push. Alternatively, the midwife will feel the top of your uterus so that she is aware of when a contraction is starting and will then guide you to bear down and push.

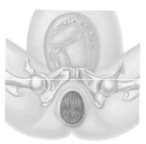

The crowning of the head means that the delivery of your baby is imminent and witin one or two contractions the head will emerge.

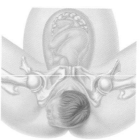

Your baby's neck will extend backwards as the head is delivered and your baby will turn to one side to aid the delivery of the first shoulder.

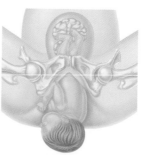

Once both shoulders are safely delivered, the rest of your baby's body will slip out fairly quickly.

SHOULDER DYSTOCIA

This is an emergency situation in a delivery that occurs when the baby's head has been successfully delivered, but the shoulders are stuck. As the head may be delivered fairly easily, the problem is often not discovered until this point in labour. Urgent action is then needed because if the baby is not delivered rapidly, she may be starved of oxygen. The midwife or doctor will move quickly to lie the mother flat and push her legs upwards and outwards to widen the birth canal; if this does not work then various other manoeuvres are used. An episiotomy (see opposite) may need to be performed to assist the rapid delivery of the baby.

Shoulder dystocia is more likely if the baby is particularly large or the mother has a small pelvis and in women with diabetes or who are obese. If the condition has occurred in a previous pregnancy, this will be recorded in the maternity notes and an obstetrician will be present at the birth or a Caesarean section may be offered.

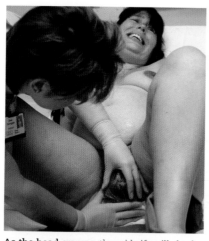

As the head crowns, the midwife will check that the cord isn't around the baby's neck, and may then apply gentle traction to the sides of the head to help deliver the shoulders.

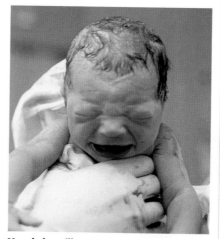

Your baby will emerge covered in blood and the thick, greasy substance known as vernix that provided a protective covering for your baby's skin in the womb.

cause serious tears. She may tell you to pant or blow instead to help you resist the urge to bear down.

Crowning Initially, the head will descend with each contraction and then move slightly back up the birth canal. Eventually, it will descend far enough to be visible through the vagina at the height of a contraction, known as "crowning", before it once again moves back up and disappears. As contractions continue, the head finally stays in the vaginal opening, and from this point it won't be long before your baby is born.

As your baby descends, the chin will be tucked down towards the chest and the head will rotate slightly so that your

baby is facing your back; this enables the largest part of your baby's head to pass through the widest part of the pelvis. As the head passes out of the vagina, it extends backwards so that it almost touches her back. The midwife or doctor will check whether the cord is around the baby's neck. If this is the case, it will be lifted up and away from the neck. The midwife will remove any mucus from your baby's nose and mouth. Once the head has been delivered, it will return to its normal position.

Rest of the body After the delivery of the head, your baby will turn slightly so that the first shoulder can be delivered in the next contraction. Your midwife

may help by applying gentle traction to your baby's head at the side to help the first shoulder emerge. Once the first shoulder has been delivered, your baby will turn again slightly so that the second shoulder can be delivered. After this, the rest of the body will slip out and the delivery of your baby will be complete.

Monitoring you and your baby

In the second stage, the midwife monitors the baby's heartbeat and your contractions. If the second stage is becoming prolonged, with the possibility of you becoming tired from pushing, an assisted delivery may be suggested with forceps or ventouse (see pp.436–7).

Episiotomies

An episiotomy is a cut made in the perineum to aid the delivery of the baby. Around 30 years ago, episiotomies were routine as it was assumed that a cut prevented worse tears occurring. This has been shown since not to be the case, and today an episiotomy is only done by a doctor to aid a forceps delivery; in an emergency, for example if the baby is in distress; if the baby is large; or if the perineum is particularly tight. Before carrying out the procedure, the midwife or doctor should explain why they think it is necessary and should obtain your verbal consent.

Before you're cut, you'll have a local anaesthetic to numb the area. The cut is usually done at an angle between the vagina and the rectum and will be stitched after the birth. The midwife or doctor will stitch all of the layers of the cut in one long absorbable stitch, bringing together the posterior wall of the vagina, your perineal muscle layer, and your skin layer.

You may be given a suppository for pain relief straight after you've been stitched, and paracetamol and anti-inflammatory medication may be recommended. Bathing in warm water can be soothing.

Perineal tears

Some women tear naturally during the delivery of their baby, and this tends to be more common in a first labour. Spontaneous tears are classified by the severity of the tear and the tissue layers involved. A first degree tear involves the skin layer only; a second degree tear involves the skin and muscle-tissue layers; and a third degree tear involves skin, muscle, and the anal sphincter. A first degree tear doesn't need stitches, but second and third degree tears do. Second degree tears are the most common; fortunately, only a small number of women sustain third degree tears, which are usually associated with assisted deliveries.

BIRTH STORY WATER BIRTH

Becky is a 22-year old woman in her first pregnancy. She'd had no problems and at her 36 week appointment she discussed her birth plan and told her midwife that she wanted a waterbirth at the local birth centre.

Becky's birth story: By the time I was two days overdue I was having irregular contractions. I'd had a show and had backache. The next day I woke at 6.30am with regular contractions. I coped using breathing techniques, stayed active, and used a birthing ball. Once my contractions were every 5 minutes and lasting a minute, I rang the birth centre as I felt that I needed to use the pool. The midwife said she would get it ready.

At 11.35am, my partner and I reached the centre and met the midwife. She felt my contractions, listened to the baby's heartbeat and did a vaginal examination. She said that I was in established labour as I was 5cm dilated and the head was descending. Once in the pool, I was able to move around and change my position and the warm water eased my backache and contractions. I felt calmer and started to relax. I found kneeling in the water and rocking my pelvis back and forth and from side to side helpful. My partner supported me and periodically the midwife listened to my baby's heart rate.

At 3.20pm, my contractions were every 1 to 2 minutes and very strong. The midwife and my partner reassured me and I managed to focus. I began to feel the urge to bear down. At 3.50pm, my baby's head was born and a couple of minutes later I pushed my baby out into the water. The midwife gently lifted my baby up to me and we stayed in the water a few moments. I got out to deliver the placenta, which I did without drugs. At 4.20pm my placenta was delivered and I didn't need stitches.

The midwife's comments: Becky found the warm water helped her cope with contractions, and she stayed calm. She tried different positions and the water kept her buoyant. She and her partner were focused. Her labour progressed well and was just under 10 hours. It was wonderful to observe.

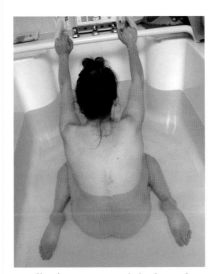

Kneeling in warm water helped ease the pain of Becky's contractions.

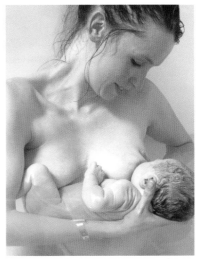

After the birth the midwife lifted the baby to Becky's breast so she could breastfeed.

After your baby is born

Shortly after your baby's birth, the cord will be cut and your uterus will start to contract again to deliver the placenta.

The third stage

This is from the birth of your baby until the delivery of the membranes (the amniotic bag that surrounded your baby) and placenta. The delivery of the placenta can be actively managed with the help of drugs or delivered without drugs, known as a physiological (natural) third stage. Your midwife will discuss these options with you before labour.

Cutting the cord

Cutting the cord After your baby's birth, the cord may be left to pulsate for two to three minutes before it's cut. This means your baby receives more placental blood, which boosts his oxygen supply and blood volume. The cord is clamped in two places, about 1cm and 4cm from the baby's tummy, and is cut with scissors between the clamps. Your partner may be able to cut the cord on request.

Active delivery of the placenta

Active delivery of the placenta After your baby is born, you will be offered an intramuscular (IM) injection of an oxytocic drug (often Syntometrine) in your thigh to make the uterus contract so that you can deliver the placenta and membranes quickly. Helping the uterus to contract in this way reduces the risk of heavy bleeding occurring during the third stage, known as a postpartum haemorrhage (see box, opposite) and speeds up the delivery of the placenta, which can happen within 5 to 15 minutes after the birth of the baby. The risk of a postpartum haemorrhage occurring is the reason many units advise an active third stage. If you have a fibroid, active delivery will be advised as there is an increased risk of bleeding.

Your midwife will place one of her hands just above your pubic bone to prevent the uterus being pulled downwards when she pulls on the

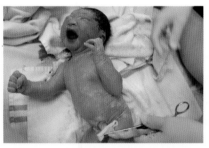

The umbilical cord will be clamped and cut a few minutes after the birth, severing the link between your baby and the placenta.

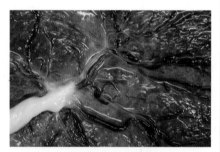

The disc-shaped placenta, weighing around 500g (1lb 2oz), has a network of blood vessels surrounding the umbilical cord in its centre.

FIRST CHECKS

Apgar score

At 1, 5, and 10 minutes, your baby's breathing, pulse, movements, skin colour, and responses are assessed. (In Asian and black babies, the colour of the mouth, palms of the hands, and soles of the feet are checked.) Each is given a score between 0 and 2, called the Apgar score. A total of 7 or more at 1 minute is normal; under 7 means help is needed.

Apgar score	2	1	0
Skin colour	Pink all over	Body pink; extremities blue	Pale/blue all over
Breathing	Regular strong cry	Irregular, weak cry	Absent
Pulse/heart rate	Greater than 100 bpm	Less than 100 bpm	Absent
Movements/muscle tone	Active	Moderate activity	Limp
Reflexes after given certain stimuli	Crying or grimacing strongly	Moderate reaction or grimace	No response

cord. With her other hand, she will then apply gentle traction to the cord to help deliver the membranes and placenta. This is known as "controlled cord traction" (CCT).

Delivering the placenta naturally

If you decide to deliver your placenta without drugs, known as a physiological third stage, this can take up to an hour. Your midwife will encourage you to bear down and you may find squatting helps. After the delivery of the placenta, the midwife will check it to ensure that it looks complete and that none of it stays in the womb, which can cause a postpartum haemorrhage (see below).

How you feel after the birth

After the huge effort of giving birth, it's common to have a physical reaction. Many women shake or shiver uncontrollably, and some feel nauseous and may even vomit. As well as your physical reaction, you are also likely to be feeling overwhelmed and emotional. Once you and your baby have been given the all clear, you should be given some quiet time alone to get to know each other.

POSTPARTUM HAEMORRHAGE

A postpartum haemorrhage describes the loss of up to 500ml (17 oz) of blood after the delivery. This is often associated with a retained placenta, when the placenta remains in the uterus for a prolonged period of time, which is most likely to occur during a natural delivery of the placenta. It can also occur after an assisted forceps delivery; after a prolonged labour; or following a Caesarean. Improvements in the treatment of this condition with antibiotics and blood transfusions has meant that the incidence of complications following a haemorrhage has fallen considerably over the years.

YOUR BABY'S APPEARANCE

Newborn babies are usually surprisingly unattractive. Fortunately, as parents, we think they are beautiful. Newborns are covered in a waxy substance called vernix, together with amniotic fluid and blood from the birth canal. Babies who have passed meconium before the delivery may also have green-stained skin and nails.

In addition, newborn babies often have a moulded, elongated head, with a swollen area on top known as a "caput", which is due to the pressure on the baby's head as it passes through the birth canal. Also, the nose may be squished to one side and the eyes may be swollen. Sometimes the genitals are swollen, too. Rest assured that all of these features are temporary and within 24 hours or so the moulding will sort itself out and your baby will

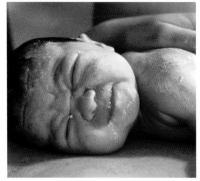

Your newborn baby may have a squashed appearance, but this will smoothe out within a day or two.

begin to look more like the baby you were expecting to meet.

Many babies are born with birthmarks that are referred to as "stork marks". These are red birthmarks on the eyelids and at the nape of the neck, which fade in time.

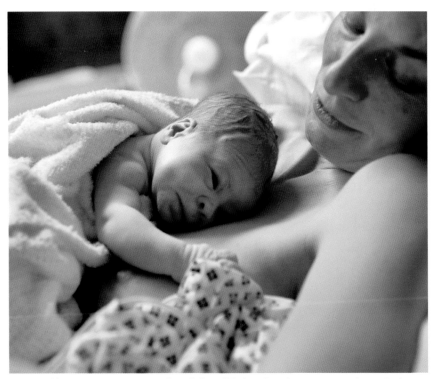

Skin-to-skin contact with your newborn baby will help to keep her warm – newborns don't have very good temperature control – and will also help the two of you to start bonding.

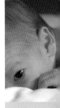

Special cases

EACH LABOUR IS DIFFERENT AND THERE ARE TIMES WHEN SOME TYPE OF INTERVENTION IS NEEDED

You may know in advance that a condition or factor in your pregnancy means that intervention, such as an induction or a Caesarean section, will be needed. At other times, events can occur in labour that mean assistance is needed, or a premature labour can mean that your baby needs special care. In all cases, rest assured that procedures are in place to ensure your own and your baby's safety.

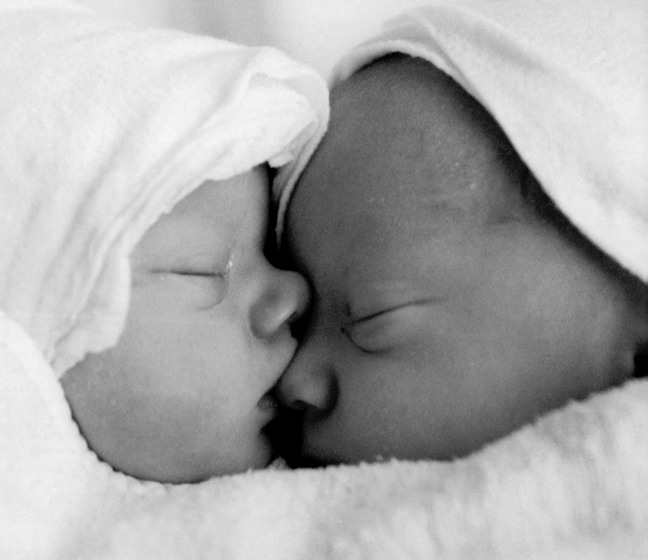

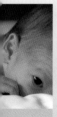

Premature birth

The term "premature" describes both the time of birth, before 37 weeks, and how prepared your baby is for life outside of the womb. Premature births account for seven per cent of UK births.

Your baby may be born prematurely either because an early delivery is advised on medical grounds (see below), or because you go into spontaneous preterm labour. The earlier the birth, the higher the chance of complications in the baby, such as breathing problems or infections. Nowadays, however, huge advances in the care of premature babies means that babies born as early as 22 weeks may survive. If your baby is premature, she may need to spend time in a special care baby unit (see p.452).

Advising an early delivery

A decision may be made to deliver a baby early as the mother's or baby's health is in danger. For example, an early delivery may be recommended if the mother has a medical problem, such as a heart condition that could increase her physical stress, or pre-eclampsia (see p.474), which could endanger her own and her baby's health. An early delivery may also be advised if a scan shows that the placenta is not functioning well and the baby is not receiving enough oxygen. Most babies delivered before 32 weeks on medical grounds are born by Caesarean; after 32 weeks, an induction of labour (see p.432) may be possible.

Spontaneous preterm labour

The cause of spontaneous labour before 37 weeks is often unknown. However, it is more likely if a woman has a major abnormality of the uterine wall, such as large fibroids (see p.218), or a weakness in the cervix. Infection or inflammation within the amniotic membranes around your baby can also set off contractions.

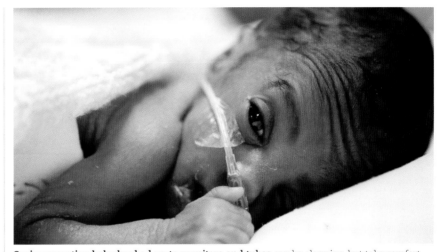

Seeing your tiny baby hooked up to monitors and tubes can be alarming, but take comfort from the fact that these are helping your baby to breathe and feed, and in turn to develop.

What might be done? If you are at high risk of preterm birth you may be given the hormone progesterone as a pessary or gel to reduce the risk. Once preterm labour has started, it can't be stopped, but medication can slow the process and reduce some risks.

Steroids can promote the production of surfactant, a natural chemical in the baby's lungs that reduces the effort of breathing. They must be given 24 to 48 hours before birth for maximum benefit.

You may also be given tablets or an injection to reduce the frequency of contractions. This can prolong pregnancy for a few days, during which time the steroids can take effect. Also, if necessary, you can be transferred to a hospital with special care baby facilities.

Finally, you may be advised to have injected antibiotics as premature babies are susceptible to bacterial infections caught via the cervix during birth.

PREDICTING PREMATURE LABOUR

It's hard to predict who will go into labour prematurely. However, if you've had a previous premature birth, tests may be done to find out if it is likely to happen in your current pregnancy. A cervical scan may be done around 23 weeks as a shorter cervix increases the risk of early labour. Vaginal swabs detect bacteria that are linked to premature labour, and a test called a "fibronectic swab" shows if the membranes and cervix are under stress, which can trigger early labour. Sometimes, a short cervix is strengthened with a stitch. Antibiotic creams can be given if abnormal bacteria are found, and progesterone pessaries may be given to stop contractions, although this treatment is in its infancy.

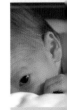

Induction of labour

For one in five women in the UK, a decision is reached to start labour by artificial means, a procedure known as induction.

An induction may be offered if it's felt that continuing the pregnancy poses a risk to your health or to the health of your baby. The most common reason for an induction is the continuation of a pregnancy beyond 41 or 42 weeks, in which case the placenta may begin to fail. Induction may be offered earlier if you have twins, or a medical condition such as diabetes. Before setting a date for induction, your midwife may offer to sweep your membranes (see p.393) to help you go into spontaneous labour.

Induction is not the same as an augmentation of labour, which is when drugs are used to increase the efficiency of your contractions when you've already gone into labour spontaneously (see p.415).

Assessing the cervix

Before an induction, you'll have an internal examination to assess the cervix. Induction is easier if your cervix is short and soft, described as "favourable" or "ripe", rather than long and firm. The findings may be logged in a table called the Bishop's Score, which also assesses how far the cervix is dilated (see p.415), the position of the cervix, and the station of the fetal head in the pelvis (see p.414). A total score over six indicates good conditions for an induction of labour.

Softening the cervix

If your cervix isn't ripe, it can be softened with prostaglandins. These are naturally occurring chemicals that help to stimulate contractions. Artificial prostaglandins can be given in the form of vaginal tablets of gel, which are placed at the top of the vagina near the cervix. This is usually effective, but sometimes prostaglandins fail to soften the cervix, even after several doses, in which case this may be tried again after a few days. On the other hand, some women experience dramatic effects after a small dose.

Breaking the waters

Manual rupture of the membranes, or amniotomy, is one of the most important steps in the induction process. This is often referred to as "breaking the waters" and it's done once the cervix is soft and slightly dilated, and the head has started to enter the pelvis. A thin plastic probe is passed through your cervix and used to make a small hole in the amniotic membranes, which allows some of the fluid around your baby to leak out. This softens the cervix even more and can provoke contractions in the wall of the uterus. If contractions don't become established after the procedure, then you'll require treatment with the drug syntocinon (see below).

Oxytocin and syntocinon

Oxytocin is a natural hormone that stimulates the uterus, increasing the frequency and strength of contractions. A synthetic form called syntocinon is used with the same effect. It's diluted in clear fluid then dripped into a vein in your arm. This is safe and effective when used correctly; however, it needs to be used with care as excessive contractions can reduce your baby's oxygen supply in labour. As a precaution, the contractions and your baby's heartbeat will be continuously monitored (see p.418).

QUESTIONS AND ANSWERS

Are medical interventions more likely with an induction?

If your labour is induced, the chance that you will need an assisted delivery with forceps or ventouse (see pp.436–7) or a Caesarean is increased. This is even more likely if you are having your first baby, if the cervix is unfavourable (see right), or if you're being induced relatively early in your pregnancy. The reason for these medical interventions is usually that the labour is proceeding too slowly, or that it cannot be started off at all, despite all of the steps taken. Also, concerns about the baby's wellbeing during the induction process can sometimes lead to intervention.

Is induction of labour more painful than a spontaneous labour?

Some women find that they experience strong contractions very quickly after an induction. As they haven't been able to build up gradually to more painful contractions, they may be less able to tolerate the pain, which can result in an increased need for stronger types of pain relief, such as an epidural.

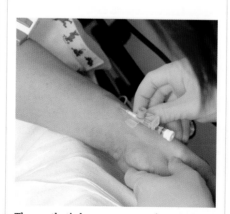

The synthetic hormone syntocinon is given via an intravenous drip to stimulate the strength and frequency of your contractions.

Breech baby

At 32 weeks, 15 per cent of babies are breech (bottom first). With time most turn, and just 3 to 4 per cent remain breech at term.

Breech labours and births are usually more difficult, so if your baby is still in a breech position in late pregnancy, you may be offered a procedure to turn your baby (see below).

Turning your baby

The procedure to turn your baby is called external cephalic version (ECV) and is usually offered at around 37 weeks if a baby is still in a breech position. The doctor or midwife presses on the lower part of your tummy to elevate your baby's bottom out of the pelvis. Pressure is used to rotate your baby until she is head-down. The procedure may feel uncomfortable, and you may be given medication to relax the uterus. A scan is done during the procedure for guidance.

The success rate for ECVs is often over 40 per cent. There can be complications, such as bleeding behind the placenta and uterine rupture, but these are rare. If an ECV is unsuccessful and you want to try for a vaginal birth, you will be advised to deliver in hospital so that help can be provided quickly if needed. In some cases, the position of a breech baby is likely to make vaginal delivery difficult and a Caesarean will be advised.

Breech diagnosed in labour

Occasionally it isn't discovered that your baby is breech until you're in labour. This happens because it can be hard to distinguish between a baby's head and bottom by feeling your tummy alone.

If a breech presentation is diagnosed in labour, you can still have an ECV, but when it's done this late it has a lower success rate. It may not be possible to offer an ECV in labour if the waters have broken, if you're in advanced labour, or if there's no one to do the procedure.

Delivery of your baby

If you try for a vaginal birth, you should have one-to-one care from a midwife. An obstetrician is likely to be present at the birth, and another nurse or doctor may be there to look after your newborn baby in case resuscitation is needed.

You'll be advised to have your baby's heartbeat monitored throughout labour, and you may have a drip in your arm or hand, in case you need a Caesarean. To prepare for the delivery, you may be asked to sit with your feet in stirrups so that the doctor can access the baby. Alternatively, you could stand or be on all fours. Your bladder may be emptied with a catheter and an episiotomy may be done (see p.427) to ensure there's sufficient access to the vagina if forceps are needed. The midwife or doctor may apply gentle pressure to the baby's arms or legs during birth, but you're unlikely to notice this. Apart from these differences, the birth should feel the same as the birth of a head-first baby. The head will be eased out of the birth canal, either by hand or with forceps, to control the speed of the birth, which should be neither too fast nor too slow.

A Caesarean is likely if complications arise. For example if the baby shows signs of distress; the cord slips below the baby's bottom; the cervix dilates too slowly; or the baby isn't descending.

POSITIONS OF A BREECH BABY

A breech baby can lie in one of three positions, known as extended (frank); flexed (complete); or footling. With an extended breech, the hips are flexed, knees extended, and the feet are by the head. A vaginal delivery is most likely with this type of breech. With a flexed breech, the hips and knees are flexed, with the feet above the buttocks, and a vaginal birth may be possible. In a footling breech, the hips are extended with the feet below the buttocks, so a vaginal delivery is unlikely.

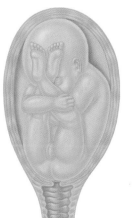
Extended (frank) breech

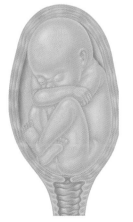
Flexed (complete) breech

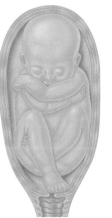
Footling breech

Multiple births

Carrying twins or more increases the risk of complications during birth and you and your babies will be closely monitored.

Multiple pregnancies occur naturally in around 1 in 90 women, but some factors increase the chance of you conceiving twins or more, including the use of some fertility treatments, becoming pregnant when you're older, already having children, and having a family history of twins.

Monitoring during pregnancy

As multiple pregnancies are high risk, you'll receive extra monitoring; the type of delivery will depend on the position of your twins and any other complications. A concern is whether twins will be born prematurely with a small birth weight, which can mean they will need to spend time in a special care baby unit (see p.452).

Towards the end of pregnancy, you may have extra scans to monitor the babies' growth, as the ability of the placenta to provide oxygen can be reduced in a twin pregnancy. The volume of fluid around each baby may be measured and the heart rates recorded to check their wellbeing.

Possible complications

Certain complications with the babies or the mother can influence the delivery and mean that a Caesarean is planned.

Fetal complications Twin-to-twin transfusion syndrome (TTTS) is a condition unique to identical twins who share a placenta (see p.51). It occurs if

there is a direct link in the blood supply between the babies and can put the lives of both at risk. Babies with TTTS need specialized treatment that may involve reducing the fluid around one baby or using a laser to separate the circulations.

Rarely, twins can develop in the same sac, known as monoamniotic twins. The main risk of this condition is that the cords become tangled, affecting the oxygen supply. The twins may have heart traces at the end of pregnancy and are usually delivered early by Caesarean.

Maternal complications When you're carrying twins, you're at a higher risk of complications, such as pre-eclampsia

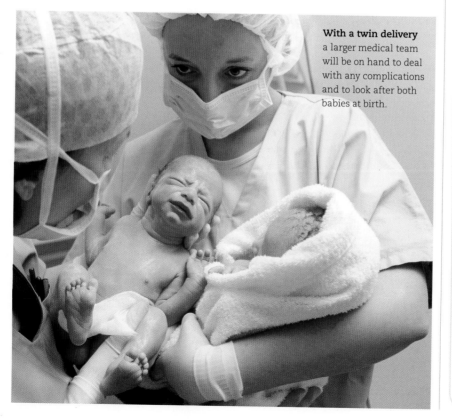

With a twin delivery a larger medical team will be on hand to deal with any complications and to look after both babies at birth.

Gillian found out she was having twins at an early scan. At first she was worried that the pregnancy and birth would be hard, but her confidence grew as she saw her babies growing well. She went into labour at 35 weeks.

Gillian's birth story: I was shocked when they told me I was carrying twins, as none of my family have had twins. The pregnancy was quite tough as I was very tired and I had such a big bump. I enjoyed the scans though as they were really reassuring.

I went into labour at just over 35 weeks. After initial contractions, my waters broke at 2am. My partner got me to hospital in 15 minutes; I think he was in a bit of a panic. Jonathan, our first twin, was born just after 4pm, so the first part of my labour was quite long. I managed with gas and air, plus an injection of diamorphine.

Celia came 20 minutes later. They broke my second bag of waters as her heartbeat was low, but she was fine at birth. I remember the birthing room being crowded, and even though people introduced themselves to me, I couldn't have told you who they were. However, they all disappeared soon after the birth and left us to spend some time alone with our babies. That was the best time. All the worries disappeared and we could just get on with being a mum and a dad.

The midwife's comments: Like many women with a twin pregnancy, Gillian was worried about what might happen to her and her babies during labour. She had talked at length to me and the doctor during her pregnancy, but still felt anxious. When she arrived on the labour ward however, she could see that the people caring for her were highly

professional and experienced. This gave her the confidence to deal with events as they unfolded. Both babies were doing very well when they left hospital and Gillian was making an excellent recovery, too.

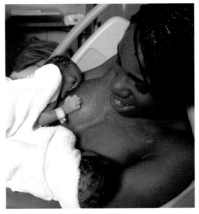

Despite being higher risk, a twin birth is most likely to conclude with the safe delivery of both babies.

(see p.474), possibly because of the additional strain on the kidneys; the liver condition obstetric cholestasis (see p.473), for reasons that are unclear; and thrombosis, as there is an additional strain on your circulation. These conditions may also mean that an early delivery is recommended.

Going into labour

You're more likely to go into labour early and your babies may be lighter than average. With twins, you're likely to go into labour around 37 weeks; with triplets around 34 weeks; and with quadruplets around 32 weeks. The average birthweight for twins is 2.5kg (5.5lb); triplets 1.8kg (4lb); and quadruplets 1.4kg (3lb).

Labour and birth with twins

Current recommendations are that an obstetrician should attend a twin birth. If you're planning to have a vaginal

birth, the labour should be almost as quick as it is with one baby.

Continuous monitoring of both heartbeats with a CTG machine (see p.418) is recommended during a multiple labour. This is usually done by putting one strap around your tummy for each baby, but sometimes the second baby is monitored in this way and the first baby may have a clip put on his head (see p.419), which gives a clearer picture of the first baby's heartbeat if it has been difficult to find.

Delivering the first twin For your first baby, the chance of using forceps or ventouse is the same as for a singleton birth, although the birth of the first twin may need to be assisted so that the doctor can gain quick access to the second twin. After the first twin's delivery, his cord is clamped and cut, but the placenta usually remains in the uterus until the second baby has been born.

Delivering the second twin The medical team will confirm whether your second baby is head- or bottom-first, either by feeling your abdomen, doing an internal examination, or by scanning you. As the second baby's head or bottom enters the pelvis, the second bag of waters may be broken to encourage strong contractions. A normal birth should follow in about 30 minutes, and forceps or ventouse are only used if problems arise. If the second twin is bottom-first, a doctor should be at hand to help. It's unusual for the first twin to be born vaginally and the second to be born by a Caesarean, but this may happen if the second baby needs an urgent delivery and a vaginal birth seems unsafe.

Delivering the placenta There is a greater risk of postpartum haemorrhage with twins, which means that an active management of the third stage is usually advised (see p.428).

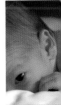

435

Assisted birth

In the UK, around 1 in 10 babies have an assisted birth. These are considered safe and can prevent further complications.

CHECKLIST

Reasons for an assisted birth

There are several factors that can make an assisted birth more likely.

■ **Your baby has an abnormal heart rate,** which suggests that she might be in distress.

■ **You have been pushing a long time,** but your labour is progressing slowly.

■ **You're exhausted** and can't manage any more pushing.

■ **You've a medical condition** and have been told not to push for long.

An assisted birth is one in which either forceps or a ventouse suction cup (also called a vacuum extractor) are used to aid a vaginal delivery. There may be some mild side effects such as bruising after an assisted birth, but major complications are rare.

As with all medical interventions, the use of forceps or a ventouse suction cup will be offered only when it is thought to be necessary for the health of the baby and/or mother.

The procedure

First, the doctor looking after you will explain the need for the procedure and may also explain the potential complications. You may be asked to sign a consent form, although not all hospitals insist on this. Before the birth takes place, your legs will be put into a pair of stirrups called lithotomy poles. The end of the bed will then be removed so that the doctor has access to your baby and you will be cleaned with a little water. Fresh covers are often placed over your legs and tummy and a catheter will be inserted to empty your bladder. The doctor will place the forceps around the baby's head or attach the ventouse cup and will encourage you to start pushing again when you have a contraction. Your baby should be born within around another 20 minutes from this time. On some occasions, a specially trained midwife will carry out a ventouse birth, which has the advantage that, during your labour, you will probably have had time to get to know the midwife.

Forceps

Modern surgical forceps were invented by the British doctor Chamberlen in the 17th century and so have been in use for hundreds of years, although they have been modified over time. They are an effective and reliable way to assist a delivery, but they have to be used with care by a trained doctor.

The forceps are placed so that they hold the sides of the baby's head near the ears and cheeks. The operator then gently pulls the baby's head downwards while you push during a contraction, and then guides the baby out of the birth canal.

Forceps can also be used to adjust the the baby's head before the birth if the baby is lying in an occipito-posterior position, with his back facing the mother's back (see p.417), towards the end of labour. After turning the baby's head, delivery is then completed as described above.

METHODS OF ASSISTING BIRTH

Assisting your baby's birth with ventouse or forceps is a safe, well-practised procedure, which can prevent the need for an emergency Caesarean. Whether you have forceps or ventouse may depend on the particular expertise and experience of the doctor carrying out the procedure.

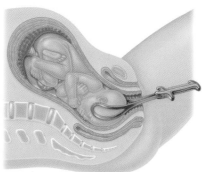

With forceps, your baby's head is cradled on either side with metal tongs that guide him down in time with your contractions.

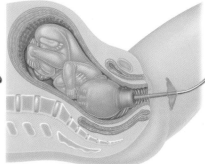

With ventouse, a soft suction cup is attached to your baby's head and then your baby is gently guided out.

436

Pros and cons of forceps There are several advantages of forceps over ventouse. They work well even if your contractions are weak or if you are finding it hard to push due to exhaustion. Also, forceps have a low failure rate: if the doctor can get the forceps around your baby's head easily, he will usually be able to complete the vaginal birth of your baby without having to resort to an emergency Caesarean. The disadvantage of forceps is that you may be more likely to have vaginal or perineal damage than you would with ventouse.

Ventouse

The ventouse, or vacuum extractor, was invented in the 1950s. It consists of a cup attached to a tube that connects to a suction pump. The cup, which can be hard or soft plastic or metal, is placed on top of the baby's head and held in place while the suction creates a vacuum that makes the cup adhere to the baby's scalp. The doctor or midwife pulls downwards while you push during a contraction.

Ventouse births are known to be very safe as long as you are at least 34 weeks' pregnant. Before this time your baby's head may be too fragile to cope with the suction and few doctors use a ventouse before 32 weeks.

Pros and cons of ventouse This has some advantages over forceps; it's often a little easier to apply and may be less uncomfortable; it's less likely to cause vaginal and perineal damage and you'll be less likely to need an episiotomy; and it can be used before you're fully dilated if there are signs of fetal distress. There is a small risk of bruising of the scalp, but serious complications are rare; if your baby needs to be delivered these small risks must be balanced against the risk of not delivering your baby.

Ventouse fails in up to 20 per cent of cases, and it's especially likely to fail if the baby isn't in an ideal position for birth. If a ventouse comes off during the

POSSIBLE COMPLICATIONS

In the majority of cases, both the mother and baby are perfectly well after an assisted birth, but occasionally complications are encountered.

Problems during the delivery A condition known as shoulder dystocia, in which the baby's shoulders become stuck during the birth (see p.426), is more common with a forceps or ventouse delivery. If the shoulders get stuck, simple manoeuvres usually release them without great difficulty, but very rarely a shoulder dystocia can turn into an emergency, and a doctor with specialized expertise has to be called to complete the baby's birth.

How your baby may be affected Forceps can leave a temporary bruise on the side of your baby's face and can even put pressure on a nerve near the eyes, stopping the baby from being able to blink properly for a day or two. In contrast, the ventouse tends to leave a bruise on the top of the head rather than on the face (and the head may apppear elongated at first where the suction pressure was applied). This can look a little alarming, but it will disappear after a couple of weeks. More severe complications for your baby, which can include a fractured skull bone after a forceps delivery, or bleeding inside the skull after a ventouse, are very rare.

How you may be affected You're more likely to be given an episiotomy cut, particularly during a forceps delivery, to protect your back passage from more severe damage during the birth. This is usually successful, but in some cases an extra tear may occur in the back passage and careful stitching, often done in an operating theatre, is required to repair the area. Stitches may also be used if you get other tears in or around the vagina.

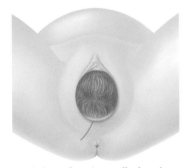

A medio-lateral cut is usually done into the muscle, angled away from the vagina and the perineum.

birth, it can be reapplied, or a pair of forceps can be used instead. Sometimes, however, a Caesarean has to be carried out if the ventouse fails.

Pain relief

It can be painful having an assisted vaginal birth, so it is important that you have sufficient pain relief to help you cope with the delivery. In some situations, an injection of a local anaesthetic in and around the vagina is sufficient to help you cope with the pain, particularly if the doctor and midwife are anticipating the birth to be fairly quick, and if your baby has already travelled most of the way through your pelvis. For more difficult assisted births, for example if the baby is not in an occipito-anterior position (see p.417), an epidural may be given (see p.404). This is especially useful if you're going to give birth in the operating theatre instead of the delivery room because the doctor feels that forceps or ventouse has a high chance of failing, leading to the need for an emergency Caesarean. Finally, if you already have an epidural in place, this can be topped up with additional medication if needed.

Caesarean section

A Caesarean section may be suggested if there is a potential benefit to your own or your baby's health, or sometimes both.

A Caesarean section is the delivery of your baby by means of a cut in the abdomen. A Caesarean rate of around 10–15 per cent is thought to be reasonable, although in most Western countries the rate has risen well beyond 20 per cent and around a quarter of all babies in the UK are now delivered by Caesarean.

It's not clear why Caesarean rates have increased, but some hospitals may feel that their practice is less likely to be criticized if they advise a Caesarean when a problem arises. Some women may think that Caesareans are safer for the baby than a vaginal birth. In fact, if you've had an uncomplicated pregnancy, a Caesarean is hard to justify on medical grounds.

Types of Caesarean
Caesareans are either emergency or planned procedures. The doctor assesses urgency with a grading scheme. A Grade 1 Caesarean is one that is carried out if there is an immediate threat to the baby's or mother's life. A Grade 2 Caesarean is one where there is concern for the baby's or mother's wellbeing, but no immediate threat to life. A Grade 3 Caesarean is done when there is no immediate concern for the mother or the baby, but an early delivery is advised, perhaps because of a condition in the mother or baby. A Grade 4 Caesarean is an elective delivery planned to suit the woman and the hospital.

Emergency Caesareans A Grade 1 Caesarean is most commonly carried out when the baby is thought to be at risk, for example if the baby's oxygen supply has been reduced and there are signs of fetal distress. In this case, the staff will try to carry out the Caesarean rapidly – within 30 minutes when possible, although it's important that shortcuts aren't taken that could put your own health at unnecessary risk.

Grade 2 and Grade 3 Caesareans take place when there's no immediate threat to life, and these are more common than Grade 1 procedures. A Grade 2 Caesarean may be done if your baby's heart rate is causing concern very early in labour and the prospect of a vaginal delivery taking place within a reasonably short time is low. An example of a Grade 3 Caesarean is one that is carried out because of a failed induction of labour.

Elective Caesareans Around one third of Caesareans are elective, or Grade 4, procedures, and the number of these has increased greatly in recent years. Reasons for an elective Caesarean

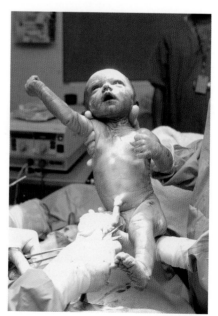

Your baby is gently lifted out of the uterus and the cord is clamped and cut.

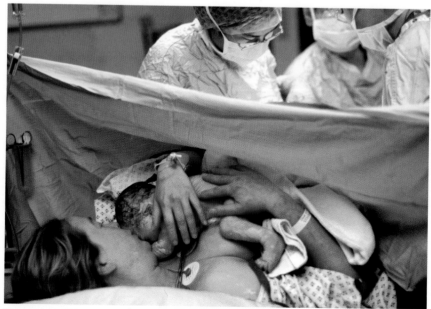

You or your partner can enjoy the first hold of your baby while the surgical team complete the operation by delivering the placenta and stitching the wound.

include a breech baby; a tear involving the back passage, or another traumatic event, during a previous vaginal delivery; a previous Caesarean; a larger than average baby; and maternal choice. In these situations, although a Caesarean is reasonable, an attempt at a vaginal birth is also reasonable with the right precautions. It's uncommon for maternal choice to be the sole reason for a Caesarean, and there's likely to be another factor, such as one of those cited above.

In some situations, it would be hazardous for either you or your baby if you were to try for a vaginal birth; for example you've had multiple previous Caesareans or other major operations on the uterus; the baby can't be moved from lying horizontally; the placenta is lying very low (see p.212); or there are severe pelvic abnormalities in the birth canal. Some maternal medical conditions also mean that vaginal birth is not advisable.

Giving your consent

The doctor will need your consent prior to carrying out a Caesarean. He should tell you why the procedure is being proposed, and what its benefits and risks are. Ideally, you should have plenty of time to decide whether you want the operation or not, although with an emergency Caesarean, the time to think things over may be limited. Even so, you are always within your rights to say no to a Caesarean, even if this means that your life or that of your baby is at risk.

Your anaesthetic

Before the operation, you will meet an anaesthetist, who will make sure that you have no pain during your operation, and will help you with pain control afterwards. Most women are awake during a Caesarean. An injection of medication into the spinal fluid in your back, called a spinal block, numbs any sensation of pain (see p.406). Or, if you've been using an epidural for pain relief in labour (see p.404), this can be used for the operation. After your anaesthetic

has been given, the anaesthetist will check that it is working properly.

Being awake usually means that your birthing partner can stay with you and it's also a little safer for you and for your baby than a general anaesthetic. Very occasionally a general anaesthetic is needed (see pp.406–7).

The operation

Before the operation, a drip will be put in your hand or your arm so that fluids or medications can be given intraveneously if necessary. Also, the pubic hair on your tummy will be clipped downwards by about 3cm (1in) to clear the way for the cut. Both of these may be done before you go to the theatre or after you arrive there.

Once the anaesthetist is happy that you're pain free, a catheter will be inserted into your bladder and will stay in until the next day while your sensation recovers. Your tummy will be cleaned with an antiseptic solution and sterile drapes will be placed over you, which also stop you and your partner seeing the operation.

During the operation, a 10 cm- (4in) long cut will be made, usually horizontally, on the tummy wall, across the bikini line, although occasionally an up-and-down cut below the belly button is done. Your bladder will be pushed down and the front of the uterus opened so that the doctor can access the baby. If your waters haven't already broken, this will be done now before the baby and placenta are delivered. The surgeon will release the head from the pelvic brim and lift the baby out. Sometimes another member of the team needs to put pressure on the uterus to assist this. You'll be able to see your baby when the cord has been cut, and once initial checks have been done on your baby, you or your partner should be able to hold him and have skin-to-skin contact while the operation is completed. You'll have an injection of syntometrine to help deliver the placenta (see p.428).

To finish the Caesarean, the uterus will be closed up with one or two layers

POSSIBLE COMPLICATIONS

There are several common, but minor, problems associated with Caesareans. These include bleeding during the operation, or a day or so later; needing a blood transfusion; or getting a minor infection in the bladder or in the wound. A major infection is far less common and having to have a second operation because of a life-threatening wound infection is rare. The chance of a blood clot in the pelvic veins is higher if you don't have medication to thin the blood afterwards. If you're generally well and you're given this medication, the chance of a life-threatening blood clot on the lungs is small. There's a small risk that the bladder, or even the baby, could be cut. The bowels are less likely to be damaged and other internal organs are highly unlikely to be injured.

Long term, there's evidence that you have a higher risk of postnatal depression (see p.475) after a Caesarean, and an increased risk of fertility problems in the future.

of stitches, then the tummy wall will be stitched in separate layers. This takes about half an hour, although it can take longer, especially if you've had previous operations. You may have dissolvable stitches, or stitches that have to be taken out after five or six days; less commonly, small staples may be used. The choice is usually made by the doctor, but if you have a preference, make this known to the team looking after you before the operation starts.

Your recovery

Your midwives will encourage you to get out of bed the following day, and by the day after this you may be well enough to do most things for yourself, with help. Women usually go home on the third day after the Caesarean with pain relief.

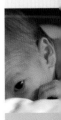

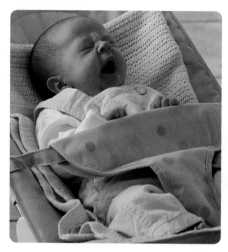 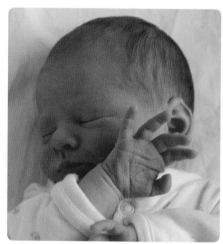 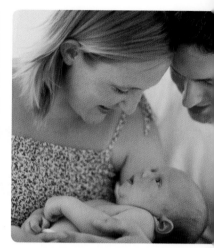

You've spent the last nine months anticipating this moment, but nothing can quite prepare you both for how you'll feel when you meet your baby. In the coming weeks, you'll recover from the birth, but your world will change dramatically as you grapple with your baby's everyday care. You may feel an array of emotions, from pure joy to frustration at your level of exhaustion. Most importantly, you'll be getting to know your tiny baby and marvelling at this new addition to your family.

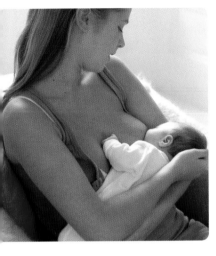
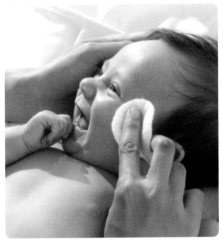
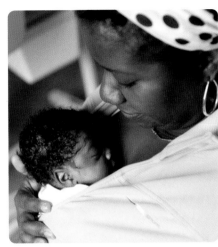

Life with your new baby

The first 12 hours

A few minutes ago you were a couple – and now you are parents! The moment you have been dreaming of for nine months has finally arrived... so what happens next?

Of course, your experiences will depend on your labour and birth and local procedures, but here is what usually occurs in your first 12 hours after birth.

🕐 **1–2 hours** As long as she is well, your baby can be placed in your arms immediately, and you can cuddle her and make the most of these first magical moments. The midwife or your partner will cut the umbilical cord after a few minutes, or once it stops pulsating. You may feel elated, relieved, or just exhausted. Don't be alarmed if you start to vomit, shake vigorously, or feel too shattered even to hold your baby at first. These are all very normal post-birth sensations.

If your baby is fine and you want to breastfeed, put her to the breast, but she may just nuzzle at first. Snuggle her close, skin to skin: the warmth of your body is all she needs right now. At 1, 5, and 10 minutes, your baby will be observed and given an Apgar score (see p.428). She will be wiped with a soft towel and her fingers and toes checked. She will then be weighed and her head circumference measured.

But you also have work to do. Shortly after your baby is born, the placenta will need to be delivered. You will have a choice to deliver the placenta naturally, without drugs, or to have an injection of either syntocinon or syntometrine, to speed up this third stage (see p.428).

If your perineum tore, or you had an episiotomy (a cut to ease your baby out), you may need stitches. You'll be given a local anaesthetic first so you don't feel a thing. Your partner can hold your baby and sit close by while you are stitched.

In the first hours following delivery, your baby will have a hearing test. It is also recommended that he be given an injection of vitamin K. Stores of this vitamin, needed for blood clotting, are often low in newborns. You can also opt for the vitamin to be given orally.

🕐 **2–3 hours** Time to refuel: many women say their first cup of tea and slice of toast after giving birth are the best they've ever tasted... enjoy.

🕐 **3–4 hours** After the exertion of giving birth, you'll be sweaty, sticky and in need of a shower, which you can have now if you didn't have an epidural. Ask a midwife or your partner to walk with you if you're wobbly. Afterwards you'll feel like a new woman and can put on a breastfeeding bra for comfort.

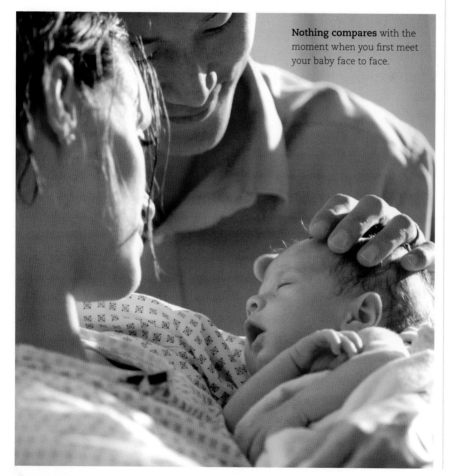

Nothing compares with the moment when you first meet your baby face to face.

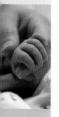

5 hours Off to the loo? The first time you pass urine it can sting, especially if you had stitches, so pour a jug of warm water over the area as you pee. The midwives need to know everything is in good working order before you leave their care. You'll need maternity towels to soak up the vaginal blood loss (lochia). Alert your midwife if this is very heavy.

6 hours If you feel fine, you've had a postnatal check (see p.444), and you've been signed off by the doctor and your baby by the paediatrician, you may return home. You'll be given contact numbers to call if you have any worries. Otherwise, you'll be relaxing in the postnatal ward. You'll be taken there in a wheelchair while holding your baby.

7 hours This might be the first chance you've had to look at your baby's tiny toes, scrunched-up legs, or fine head of hair. There may be traces of greasy vernix on her skin. Perhaps she has long, flaky fingernails that need trimming (nibble them off with your teeth), or a downy fuzz of hair called lanugo on her back. She's unique and gorgeous.

8 hours Keep your breast exposed as much as possible and lie your baby next to you under your arm so that she can feed easily. You're producing nutrient-rich colostrum that contains antibodies. Your baby should open her mouth wide and take the whole of the areola, known as "latching on" (see p.448). Breastfeeding stimulates the release of the hormone oxytocin, which contracts the uterus. This causes afterpains, often more noticeable in second and subsequent births, which feel like contractions. The consolation is that with each contraction, your uterus, and hence your abdomen, shrinks back down.

9 hours If you're up to it, you might be ready for visitors, either at home or on the ward. But don't let them tire you out.

THE FIRST MEDICAL CHECK

In the first 12 hours a midwife or paediatrician will give your baby a checkup. As well as a head-to-toe examination, there will be checks on skin colour, temperature, and muscle tone, and on reflexes, such as sucking and grasping.

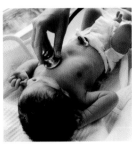
Heart and lungs are checked to ensure they sound normal.

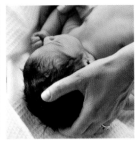
Head shape and fontanelles (soft areas between the skull bones) are examined.

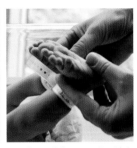
Hands and feet are checked for reflexes, and fingers and toes are counted.

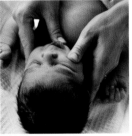
Mouth and palate – the separate sections should have fused together.

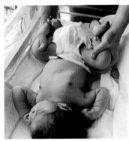
Hips are rotated and the legs are bent upwards to check for signs of dislocation.

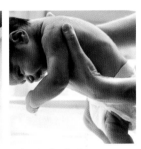
Spine is checked to ensure it is straight and free from abnormalities.

10 hours Your baby's newborn checks will take place when she is between 4 and 48 hours old (see above).

11 hours If you went to the postnatal ward and you and your baby are doing well, you could be sent home today. You may feel a bit vulnerable if you have any worries about stitches or piles or if feeding is difficult. However, help is close at hand: you can call a contact number if you have a problem and a midwife will visit you at home.

12 hours After a whirlwind of agony, ecstasy, and sheer hard labour, you need to rest when you can. If your baby is sleeping, fend off visitors, draw the curtains round your bed, turn off your phone, and sleep.

AFTER A CAESAREAN

Your recovery

Although you've had major surgery, the midwives will encourage you to rotate your ankles to get your circulation going. After an epidural, this will be as soon as you've regained feeling in your legs; after a general anaesthetic, when you're no longer sleepy. You'll be encouraged to get up the following day. You won't be able to shower yet, but your midwife can give you a bed bath to help you freshen up.

You'll probably feel very tired and sore, so ask for help with positioning your baby at the breast, and take painkillers when you need them.

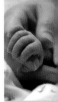

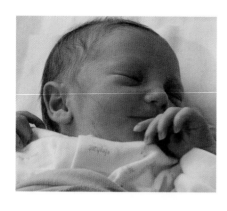

Going home

YOUR BABY TODAY

In the first 24 hours, your baby should pass urine and meconium, the first greenish-black, sticky faeces. Meconium is made of mucus, amniotic fluid, bile, and cells shed from the baby's skin and intestinal lining while he was in the womb.

Finally, your baby is in your arms! If all is well today, you and your baby will be able to return home together.

CHECKLIST

Safe sleeping

Cot death is a concern for all new parents. Following the guidelines from the The Lullaby Trust can minimize the risks.

■ **Place your baby on his back** with his feet to the foot of the cot, to stop him wriggling down under the covers.

■ **Don't let him get too hot,** and keep his head uncovered. To check if your baby is too hot, check if he is sweating or feel his tummy. Don't worry if his hands and feet feel cool: this is normal.

■ **Don't let anyone smoke in** the same room as your baby.

■ **Never sleep with your baby on a sofa or armchair.** The safest place for your baby to sleep is in a crib or cot in your room for the first six months. Avoid taking him into your bed, especially if you or your partner smoke; if you've drunk alcohol; if you've taken medication or drugs that make you drowsy; or if you feel very tired. It is also important not to take your baby into your bed if he was born before 37 weeks or weighed less than 2.5kg (5½lb) at birth.

At last, you're a mum! You may feel love at first sight, when you first hold your baby after the birth, but for many women bonding takes place over the next few days or weeks. For both parents, skin-to-skin contact with your baby helps the bonding process and is particularly beneficial for premature babies (see p.452). Try not to be anxious when you pick up your baby. In the first few weeks, your baby has little head control, so support him with a hand under his head and shoulders, or both hands under his arms and with your fingers supporting his head.

The midwife or doctor will carry out a postnatal check before you go home. He or she will check that the womb has contracted and is reducing in size; check that your blood loss (lochia) isn't too heavy; and will check any stitches. You'll be asked if you've passed urine and opened your bowels, and will be given help with breastfeeding if needed. You'll be asked about support at home and travel plans and will be given postnatal leaflets and a summary of your care for your doctor. Before leaving, warmly wrap up your baby. If you're travelling by car, you'll need a baby car seat.

YOUR BABY'S REFLEXES

Newborn babies have reflexes that form part of their survival skills. As well as the rooting and grasping reflexes shown here, babies also have a startle reflex, whereby they will fling out their arms if unsupported, and a stepping reflex, which means they will step their feet up and down if held upright on a surface.

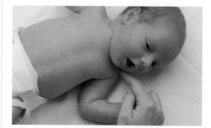

Rooting reflex: If you touch or stroke your baby's cheek, he will turn towards that side with his mouth open in search for food.

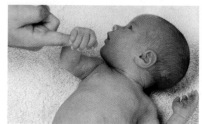

Grasping reflex: If you place your finger in the palm of your baby's hand, he will instinctively tightly grip your finger.

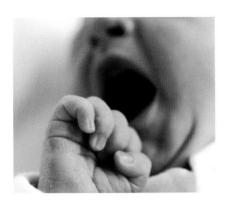

1st WEEK: DAY 2

Settling in

YOUR BABY TODAY

Newborn babies sleep for around 16 hours a day, although some sleep for most of the first few days while others seem awake and fretful. If your baby is very sleepy, you may need to wake her for feeds, which should be at least every six hours.

You may be feeling anxious about your new responsibilities, but be reassured by the support network around you.

Your community midwife will usually visit today. She'll ask how you're coping, check that you have emergency contact numbers, and that you are aware of the risks of cot death (see opposite). She will also examine both you and your baby and you will be able to talk to her about any concerns you may have.

It's important that you eat a healthy diet and rest during the day whenever possible. Pelvic floor exercises (see p.69) are vital to strengthen your muscles. If you were given painkillers or anti-inflammatory tablets take these as necessary, and accept any offers of help that enable you to get some rest.

Your first full day at home with your tiny new baby can be daunting. Apart from the responsibility of your new role, you are probably feeling tired and disorganized after getting up to feed and change your baby in the night.

Keeping your baby's cot close to your bed can help to make life easier for you when you get up at night to feed or change her. A cot with a side that can be lowered placed next to your bed enables you to pick your baby up to feed her when she wakes and place her back in her cot without actually getting out of bed. Try to deal with night wakings with the minimum of fuss. Keep the lighting low and don't talk much or stimulate

WINDING YOUR BABY

Winding simply means helping your baby to burp after a feed. Once your baby has fed, air bubbles in her stomach need to rise to the top and you can help this happen by sitting her on your lap or holding her upright against your shoulder. You don't need to rub or pat her, but this often feels right and babies seem to like it! It's worth winding half way through a feed and again at the end, especially for bottlefed babies, as air fills up the stomach, slows down the feed, and makes a baby more likely to vomit.

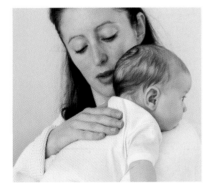

Holding your baby upright over your shoulder after a feed can help your baby to burp and therefore ease discomfort.

your baby. Only change your baby's nappy if this is really necessary and, once the feed is finished, lay her straight back down in her cot.

You'll rapidly discover that babies don't like being dressed, and they especially don't like having clothes pulled over their heads. Keep life simple by buying machine-washable, front-fastening babygrows and only changing outfits if a nappy leaks or your baby vomits down it. In the first few weeks, there is no need to change your baby into a daytime outfit. If she is cold, simply add layers, wrapping her in a shawl or adding a cardigan.

TIPS FOR EASING DISCOMFORT

Stitches and haemorrhoids

The following can increase comfort:

■ Sit on an inflatable ring.

■ Have a warm bath or spray water on your stitches with the shower head.

■ When you go to the toilet, pour a jug of warm water over the area to ease stinging, or urinate in the bath.

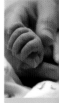

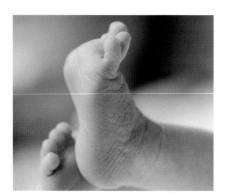

Everyday care

YOUR BABY TODAY

A new baby's skin is often quite dry in the first few weeks. This is normal and the skin will eventually correct itself. Although you don't need to put moisturizer on a baby's skin, if you wish you could gently massage in some baby or olive oil.

Once your breast milk arrives, your baby may start to appear more relaxed and contented and go for longer between feeds.

Today, you may notice that any swelling in your hands and feet begins to subside (although you may still have problems wearing rings) as you start to pass good amounts of urine. However, you still need to drink plenty of fluids – around two to three litres a day – to prevent bladder infections, avoid constipation, and help the production of breast milk. Today or tomorrow may be the first time you open your bowels since giving birth, which is normal. Eating plenty of fresh fruit and vegetables and an adequate amount of fibre will also help your bowel movements return to normal.

Up until now, your breasts have been producing colostrum, the watery premilk that is rich in nutrients and antibodies. By the end of the third day your milk will come in and your baby will start to feel more satisfied.

Once your milk is in, your breasts may feel engorged and uncomfortable. As feeding becomes established over the next few days this discomfort should start to recede.

A midwife or maternity support worker may visit you today or in the next couple of days depending on your physical, emotional, and social needs.

Fathers are now entitled to up to two weeks' paternity leave, which provides a great opportunity for dads to bond with their baby in the early days. Apart from breastfeeding, dads can be involved in all other aspects of babycare, including settling their baby, changing nappies, and bathing and dressing.

Your baby's cord stump, which is the end of the umbilical cord, shrivels up and falls off naturally around 7–10 days after the birth. Many parents feel uneasy about touching the stump and are unsure whether or not to clean it. If it appears clean, there is no need to touch the stump. However, as the moist area around the stump can harbour potentially harmful bacteria, if it gets dirty it should be cleaned with damp cotton wool. If the cord stump or the surrounding area becomes sticky, inflamed, or smelly, contact your midwife or doctor for advice.

TOPPING AND TAILING

Babies don't need frequent baths; as long as you keep their bottoms and faces clean, known as topping and tailing, you can get away with a bath every few days. To top and tail your baby, you need a bowl of warm water, a clean flannel, and cotton wool. Start by cleaning your baby's face and clean the bottom last, using damp cotton wool for the eyes and bottom and a flannel elsewhere. If you wish, use a gentle baby bath product.

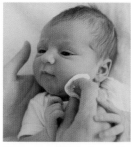

Clean your baby's face with damp cotton wool, using a fresh piece for each eye.

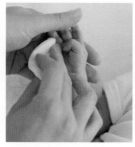

To clean her hands, wipe the backs and palms and between the fingers.

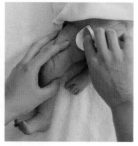

Wash the nappy area last, taking care to clean between the creases in the skin.

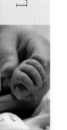

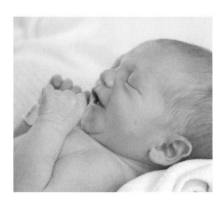

First outing

YOUR BABY TODAY

Almost all babies lose weight initially, and by day 4 they are usually at their lowest weight. When your midwife visits you on day 5, she will weigh your baby, and if your baby has lost over 10 per cent of her weight, will give you advice on feeding.

Your body is gradually recovering from the birth, and you may be starting to feel like facing the world once again.

Today, you might feel emotional and weepy, known as the "baby blues". This is caused by hormonal changes and exacerbated by tiredness and a feeling of anti-climax after the build up to the birth. The baby blues last a day or so and with rest and emotional support you will start to feel better. If the feelings fail to subside after a few days, talk to your midwife as you may be suffering from postnatal depression (see p.475).

Your breasts will still feel tender and full today. Feeding your baby on demand (see p.448) helps relieve this. Feeling tired interferes with the "let down" reflex (see p.449), so it's vital to rest or sleep during the day when your baby sleeps to make up for broken nights. You should also continue to breastfeed on both sides at night to prevent milk stagnation, which can lead to problems such as abscesses and mastitis (see p.475). Your blood loss should have started to ease off, although it may be heavier first thing in the morning and while you're breastfeeding.

You may think it's the last thing you can deal with, but getting out of the house may be just what you need to help you feel better emotionally and physically. Don't overdo it though: you still need plenty of rest.

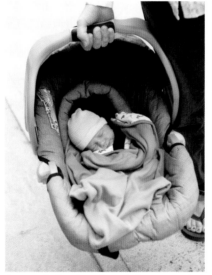

A properly fitted newborn baby car seat is a legal requirement when you're transporting your baby by car.

AS A MATTER OF FACT

By the fourth day about a third of all babies are visibly jaundiced.

Jaundice in newborn babies is usually harmless and is due to an elevated level of the waste product bilirubin in the blood, caused by the baby's immature liver. Very high levels of bilirubin can cause problems and are treated with light therapy (see p.477).

CHECKLIST

Taking your baby out

If you haven't been out yet, cabin fever may be setting in. Make sure you have everything you may need before venturing out on a trip.

■ **Pack a nappy bag with** two nappies, wipes or cotton wool, a few nappy sacks, a spare babygrow, a muslin, and a bottle of formula if you're bottle-feeding.

■ **Take layers of clothing** on outings, including a vest, babygrow, and cardigan. In winter, add an all-in-one babysuit and a blanket in a pram.

■ **A third of a baby's heat is lost through his head,** so on cool days, add a hat or hooded top. Socks and booties are easy to lose; babygrows are more practical; gloves are only needed in cold weather.

■ **In hot weather, make sure your baby is covered** and protected from direct sunlight at all times.

■ **Take time in advance to work out how to** put on a baby sling or, if travelling by car or public transport, how to fold or unfold a pushchair.

■ **Do not carry your baby too far in a car seat** as it's bad for your back.

Feeding your baby

Breastfeeding provides your baby with the best nutritional start in life and has a range of other benefits, outlined here. If you decide to bottle-feed, you can also be confident that your baby will thrive. The key to both methods is preparation.

QUESTIONS AND ANSWERS

How often should I feed my baby?
If you have a healthy, term baby you should feed him on demand, which means feeding him when he cries and seems hungry. This can mean that sometimes he will feed every couple of hours and sometimes he'll go for four to six hours without a feed. Although you may not feel as though you're producing much milk initially, your baby only needs small quantities of colostrum, the first watery milk. His demands will grow after the first few days, which will coincide with your milk coming in (see right).

Will I be able to breastfeed my twins?
Milk is produced on a supply and demand basis, so it's perfectly possible to breastfeed twins and more. If your babies are born early, breast milk is beneficial as it protects against infections, which premature babies are more susceptible to, so it's worth breastfeeding, even for a few weeks, but you'll need rest and ample nutrition. Start by feeding your twins separately. If you then want to feed them together, take time to position them well. An under-arm hold works well and supportive cushions and a willing helper are useful. Expressing (see opposite) means the babies can be fed together, alternating on the breast. If you think that they aren't getting enough milk, consult your midwife. The local twins club, a breastfeeding advisor, and the twins' organisation TAMBA (see p.480), all offer support, too.

The benefits of breastfeeding

Breast milk is the perfect first food for your baby; it contains all the nutrients your baby needs and works on a supply and demand basis, so that as your baby feeds, your body responds by producing more milk. Breast milk is thought to reduce a baby's risk of developing allergic conditions, such as asthma and eczema; to make childhood obesity and diabetes less likely; and to reduce the long-term risk of heart disease.

Breastfeeding also provides benefits for you. It helps you get back into shape quicker after the birth as your body uses additional energy to produce breast milk, and it reduces your risk of getting breast and ovarian cancer.

It can also help prevent your bones becoming weaker later in life.

Lastly, and importantly, breastfeeding helps you and your baby to be close both physically and emotionally.

When your milk comes in

In the first few days your breasts produce colostrum, a watery yellow substance that contains essential nutrients and antibodies that help your baby to fight off infections such as those of the ear, chest, and gastrointestinal tract.

At around day three, or sometimes a bit later, you will start to produce milk, which contains all the nutrients your baby needs. Your breasts may feel uncomfortably full and tender at this

THE RIGHT TECHNIQUE

Latching on

Taking the time to ensure that your baby is latched on properly before a feed is important because you could otherwise develop sore nipples. A baby that is properly latched on has his mouth wide open, with the whole areola (the area surrounding the nipple) in his mouth; his bottom lip will be curled back and he will be noticeably sucking. You'll feel a sucking effect over the entire area.

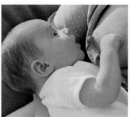 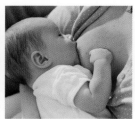 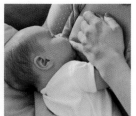

Once you've positioned your baby so that he is level with your breast, hold him with his nose and mouth facing your nipple.

When your baby opens his mouth wide, bring him to the breast, ensuring that he takes all of the nipple and the areola into his mouth.

To remove your baby from the breast insert your finger into the corner of his mouth to break the seal so that he doesn't pull the nipple.

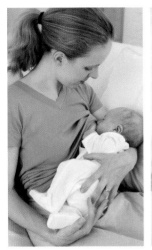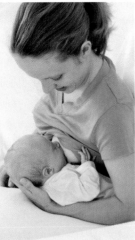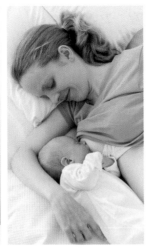

Holding your baby tummy-to-tummy is a comfortable position for you both, enabling your baby to latch on well (top, left). **An under-arm "rugby" hold** can help to keep a restless baby still (middle). **Lying side-by-side** is often recommended after a Caesarean section (right).

time, and you'll need to make sure they're properly emptied at each feed to prevent them becoming engorged.

Successful breastfeeding

Despite the fact that breastfeeding is a natural process, it can prove difficult. Getting comfortable before a feed, positioning your baby well, and ensuring that she latches on properly (see box, left), are all prerequisites for successful feeding.

For your baby to latch on properly, it's important that you're both positioned well. Ensure that you're comfortable with your back well supported; supportive cushions can be helpful. Cradling your baby at chest level can be comfortable with her tummy facing your tummy. A rugby hold with your baby under your arm is a good position if your breasts are sore, as it stops your baby dragging on the breast. Some find it helpful to lie on their side to latch their baby on. You'll soon discover which positions suit you best and will gradually gain confidence in your ability to feed.

Once your baby is latched on, the "let down" reflex is triggered. You will feel a tingling sensation as milk is released, which in turn stimulates the production of more milk. Your baby will pause during feeds and stop when he is full.

It's advisable to always have a drink during or just after a feed to replace the fluids lost from breast milk.

Bottle-feeding

This involves more preparation, but your partner can help and become involved with feeding. You'll need in advance four to six bottles: larger 250ml (8fl oz) bottles, and smaller 125ml (4fl oz) ones; newborn teats; a bottle brush; and newborn formula milk. You'll also need a sterilizing system: either an electric

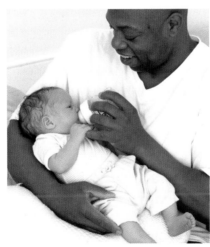

Bottle-feeding helps dads to strengthen the bond with their baby and allows you to have some welcome time off from feeding.

An extra supply

Expressing your milk boosts your milk production and enables you to go out or have an unbroken night's sleep while your partner feeds the baby. You can express milk as soon as you like after the birth, although women often wait until feeding is established, at about four weeks. Your milk can be stored in the fridge in a sterile bag or bottle for up to 24 hours and can be frozen for three months and then defrosted in a bowl of warm water.

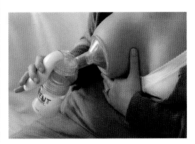

Most women use a breast pump, either electric or manual, to express milk. You can also express manually.

or microwave sterilizer, or sterilizing tablets. Wash the bottles in warm, soapy water with a bottle brush, then rinse and sterilize them. Put cooled boiled water in the sterilized bottle, then add the formula according to the manufacturer's instructions. Test the temperature of the milk by squeezing a drop on your inner wrist: it should feel warm, but not hot. Cool the milk if necessary by placing the bottle in a jug of cold water, or running it under cold water while shaking the bottle all the time. When ready, hold your baby half sitting with his head in the crook of your elbow and his back along your forearm. Gently put the teat into his mouth and tip the bottle so that the milk covers the teat to stop him swallowing air. Make up feeds individually and discard any milk left in the bottle.

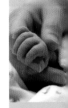

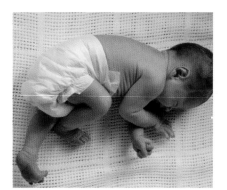

Getting checked

YOUR BABY TODAY

The midwife will examine your baby today. She will ask if he is alert and check for any signs of jaundice. She will also weigh him and will ask how he is getting on with feeding and whether there are any problems.

Try to spend some time focusing on the needs of older children, too, and helping them to adapt to the new arrival.

A midwife may visit you today to carry out a postnatal check to see if you're well, that there are no signs of infection, and that you're coping well with breastfeeding. Your breasts should be starting to feel more comfortable now as feeding becomes established, and your womb will be steadily reducing in size, but can still be felt by pressing on your tummy. The midwife will also ask whether you have any particular concerns,

such as painful stitches, which she can offer help and advice on (see p.445).

The midwife will check your baby, too, and will look for signs of jaundice (see p.477), although this isn't a problem if your baby is otherwise fit and healthy. She will also look for signs of dehydration, such as your baby not having plenty of wet nappies, and any feeding problems. Your baby's unique NHS number will be recorded in your maternity notes.

Your baby's arrival is a major adjustment for an older child, but there are ways to help him welcome the baby. Give your child a gift from the baby and encourage him to help with the baby's care as is appropriate for his age. For example a two-year-old may want to stroke the baby, hold her hand, and fetch things for you, while a five-year-old can hold the baby with some support and sing to her.

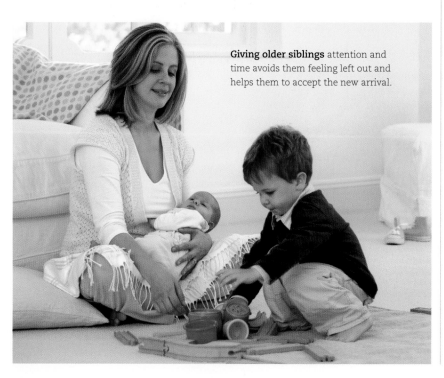

Giving older siblings attention and time avoids them feeling left out and helps them to accept the new arrival.

TIPS FOR COPING

Twins or more

Setting yourself some guidelines can help you cope with the added demands of twins or more.

■ Make time to be with your babies.

■ Prioritize activities ruthlessly, enlist practical help whenever possible, and do grocery shopping online.

■ Don't bathe your babies daily unless you and they enjoy it.

■ Let visitors make their own tea.

■ Consider using dummies if your twins cry a lot. This helps you attend to the twin most in need.

■ Make time for yourself every day.

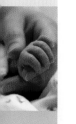

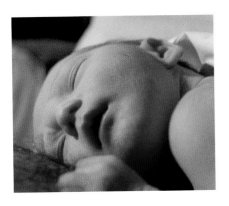

Finding your way

YOUR BABY TODAY

It's likely that both you and your baby are becoming more confident with feeding. It's common for new babies to bring up some milk after each feed, known as posseting, and this is unlikely to cause any harm. Talk to the midwife if you're at all concerned.

By now, you and your partner will be starting to feel more confident about holding, handling, and feeding your baby.

Many parents feel uneasy about giving their baby a bath as they worry about dropping a slippery baby. Many also find that their baby objects strongly to being undressed and immersed in water. Bathing should be fun, so if your baby hates baths at first, top and tail her most of the time (see p.446). Make bathtime as stress-free as possible by gathering everything you need before you start and make sure the room you undress your baby in is warm and draught-free. After the bath, dry and dress your baby immediately.

Nappies will be a part of your life for the next couple of years. There is no need to routinely change a nappy before or after feeds – just when there is a stool or it is heavy with urine. After opening a nappy, wipe away all visible faeces with the nappy. Clean your baby's bottom thoroughly with wet cotton wool, wiping from front to back to avoid spreading germs. If using a terry nappy, use a barrier cream to avoid nappy rash; avoid using too much cream with disposables as this interferes with urine absorption into the nappy. Put a new nappy on, ensuring that it's secured.

CHECKLIST

Exercise basics

You can start gentle exercise as soon as you feel able, but wait until the six-week check (see pp.462–3) before starting a strenuous programme.

- Maintain good posture.

- Continue pelvic floor exercises (see p.69) after giving birth.

- If you had a Caesarean, wait until at least six weeks before starting a general exercise programme.

- Start with low-impact exercises, such as walking and Pilates. Gradually increase the duration and intensity. You can also begin to strengthen your abdominal muscles (see p.456).

- If you have any bleeding or feel faint, stop and consult your doctor.

- Set realistic goals.

BATHING YOUR BABY

Warm the room and have a towel ready and a clean nappy and change of clothes to hand so that your baby doesn't get cold after the bath. Half fill a washing-up bowl or baby bath with water that feels tepid to your elbow (37°C/98°F on a thermometer). After bathing, dry her quickly. Don't use talcum powder, which she could inhale.

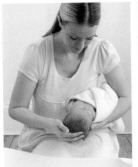

Wrap your baby in a towel, and support her head and shoulders while you wet her head with the other hand.

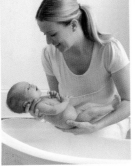

Remove the towel and lower your baby into the bath, supporting her head, shoulders, and bottom.

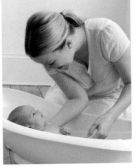

Still supporting her head, wash her with a flannel or sponge; start with the face and end with the bottom.

Special care babies

Around 10 per cent of all babies born in the UK need to spend time in a special care baby unit (SCBU) or in neonatal intensive care. Babies most often need extra care to assist them with breathing until their lungs have matured.

There are many reasons why your baby may need special care, the commonest one being prematurity (being born before 37 weeks). Babies may need to spend days, weeks, or sometimes months in a special care unit until they are big enough and well enough to go home.

The special care unit

If your baby is in a special care unit, this is a particularly stressful time. It helps to understand a bit about who will be looking after your baby, what they will be doing, and how to make sure you're fully informed at all times.

In the UK, most hospitals have a unit to provide special nursing and medical care for babies; these are divided into three levels depending on the degree of care offered. Level one is the most basic level. These units don't provide long-term ventilatory support, but they are expert at looking after babies who are slightly premature, need frequent nursing, or have previously been ventilated and are ready to be transferred to less intensive care. Level two units ventilate and give intensive care to babies from 26 weeks' gestation. Level three units offer intensive care for babies born as early as 23 weeks, and can often carry out neonatal surgery.

All these units are staffed by specialist nurses and doctors who will be happy to show you around the unit before the baby is born if there is time.

Ward rounds Most units have a ward round each morning, and the more intensive units will have another round later in the day. Some allow parents to be present and to ask questions during rounds, while others prefer parents to wait outside and will then make time to talk to them afterwards.

Communication and visiting You should be able to spend some time with your baby before he is sent to a SCBU. However, if your baby needs to be on a ventilator, he will be sent straight to neonatal intensive care, and you may not have much time together after the birth. You'll be encouraged to see your baby as soon as she has been transferred, and if you're unable to go immediately, you may be given a photo of your baby.

You will be able to see your baby any time of the day or night and the nurses will be happy to update you regularly. The consultant will also be happy to give you an update on an ad hoc basis or arrange to meet you for a more formal chat. Other family members may be able to visit the unit with your permission.

THE ROLE OF PARENTS

How you can help your baby

For most, the experience of having their baby in a special care unit is extremely stressful. Parents may feel that they have no role in the care of their baby, even though this is not the case. The most important thing you can do for your baby is to start expressing breast milk. Breast milk will nearly always be the best milk for a premature baby and can be stored in a freezer until needed.

You can both touch and stroke your baby and can be helped to cuddle her while she is on a ventilator. Babies thrive on skin-to-skin contact, called kangaroo care. You'll be encouraged to tuck your baby down your front so that she can enjoy a close bond. Talking, reading, and singing to your baby helps her become familiar with you. You can also change her nappy and help with feeds, even if these are through a nasogastric tube.

Spend plenty of time with your baby, especially when you're still breastfeeding as this may help the let-down reflex (see p.449), but save some time for yourself, too, so that you conserve energy for when you return home with your baby.

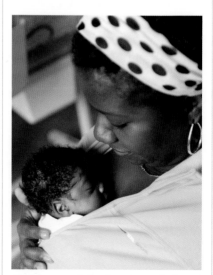

Carrying your baby close to your body and enjoying skin-to-skin contact together will help your tiny baby to thrive.

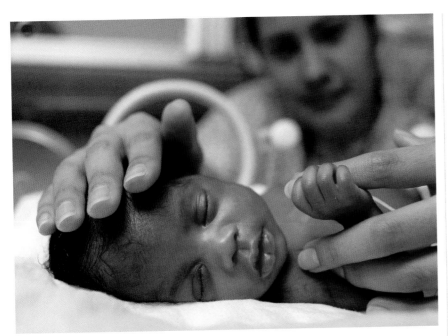

You will both be encouraged to touch, stroke, and caress your small baby, and to spend as much time as possible talking and singing to her.

Your baby's care

While your baby is in the SCBU, she may be treated with medication and have various tests and checks. In some cases, she will need to be on a ventilator.

Tests and X-rays Your baby may have blood tests to check for infection and anaemia, to check kidney function, oxygen and carbon dioxide levels, sugar levels, and to identify her blood group. The frequency of these depends on how ill or premature a baby is. Neonatal intensive care babies need blood tests at least once a day. Most need an X-ray while in special care; very premature babies may have many chest X-rays and sometimes abdominal ones.

Assisting your baby Some babies need a little extra oxygen; others need constant oxygen through a nasal tube. For very premature babies, a tube may be placed in the trachea (windpipe) and connected to a ventilator that blows oxygen into the lungs. Babies are monitored to see when they can be weaned off the ventilator.

Most babies in intensive care need one or more drips to give fluids, blood, and antibiotics. Very small babies may be fed through a long, fine tube connected to a vein. They may also need at least one blood transfusion, as frequent blood tests remove a significant amount of blood, and the bone marrow is too immature to replace red blood cells fast enough.

Antibiotics are often given to prevent infection. Some babies need drugs to keep their blood pressure up; many who are ventilated need drugs to sedate them and to prevent or treat pain. Babies may be given a sugary liquid before a procedure as this is thought to reduce pain.

Who's who on the neonatal unit

Neonatal nurses Most of the care is carried out by highly trained nurses. Some units also have advanced nurse practitioners who carry out many procedures usually preformed by doctors.

Doctors Apart from consultants (see below), two tiers of doctors work on neonatal units. Senior house officers, or SHOs, have at least five years' medical school training, followed by at least two years as a doctor. Registrars, the next tier up, have at least five years' medical school training followed by at least five years' experience as a qualified doctor; some have up to eight years' experience in paediatrics. Registrars supervise the SHOs and work in shifts, staying in the hospital day and night to provide immediate care for babies.

Consultants These are the most senior paediatricians in the unit. There may be several who take it in turn to be the "attending consultant". This may be for a week at a time, or in some level three units for up to a month. This means that the parents of babies who spend many weeks on the unit get to know several consultants. At nights and weekends, the consultant will usually be on call from home and come in rapidly if called in by the registrar or nurses.

Other members of staff A neonatal unit depends on a number of other staff members. These include a dietician, physiotherapist, health care assistants (who do much of the day-to-day baby care), pharmacists, and, in some units, a psychotherapist to offer much needed emotional support to parents and staff.

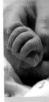

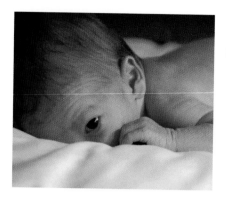

1st WEEK: DAY 7

Tuning in

YOUR BABY TODAY

Vitamin K is given to babies as it's essential to help blood clot. If your baby had an oral dose at birth rather than an injection (which is usually recommended), he will receive another dose today. If your baby is breastfed, a further dose is given at 28 days.

As the bond between you and your baby continues to grow, you will start to feel more intuitive about his needs.

CHECKLIST

Your baby's cries

Follow the checklist below to help you identify the cause of your baby's cries. If your baby cries for three hours or more a day, consult your health visitor or doctor. Helplines offer advice and support (see p.480).

■ **Hunger is the main reason** for crying; he will stop once he is offered the breast, a bottle, a finger, or a dummy.

■ **A cry of pain** is easy to interpret as your baby may be inconsolable, draw up his legs in pain, or arch his back. If you're unsure how to remedy the pain, consult your midwife.

■ **A wet or dirty nappy** can be uncomfortable and cause crying.

■ **Your baby may want a cuddle** if you can see no other reason for his crying. Babies can't be spoilt by too many cuddles. Carrying him in a sling while you go about tasks may comfort him.

■ **Your baby may be overstimulated.** If nothing else works, put him down in a quiet room; in our anxiety as new parents, it can be easy to forget that babies need quiet time.

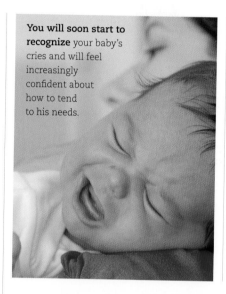

You will soon start to recognize your baby's cries and will feel increasingly confident about how to tend to his needs.

Crying is the only way your baby can gain your attention. Parents-to-be often worry about how they'll know what their baby wants. Although his cries may seem indistinguishable at first, you'll soon start to interpret them (see box, left).

Ideally, you'll have continued doing pelvic floor exercises (see p.69) in this first week. It's important to carry on doing these as they strengthen the muscles that support your bladder, helping to prevent stress incontinence (see p.475). They also help to promote healing and ease discomfort if you've had stitches as they increase the blood flow to your perineum.

THE GUTHRIE (HEEL PRICK) TEST

Some babies are born with conditions that if detected early and treated can result in a better quality of life for the baby than if they were left undetected until symptoms developed. The Guthrie (heel prick) test, done on days 5–8, involves pricking the baby's heel and placing a few drops of blood onto a card that is sent to a laboratory. The blood is analyzed and the results are available in a few days. If there are abnormal findings, further tests will be arranged to confirm the diagnosis. If it is confirmed, a specialist will explain the findings and what will happen next.

Many conditions can be diagnosed in this way, although those routinely tested for varies. In the UK, the following are tested for: phenylketonuria (PKU), a metabolic condition; congenital hypothyroidism; sickle cell disease; cystic fibrosis; and MCADD (medium chain acyl-co-dehydrogenase deficiency), a rare enzyme deficiency.

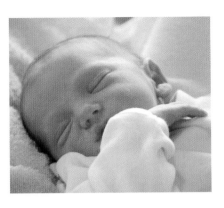

Healthy living

YOUR BABY TODAY

Whether you're breastfeeding or bottle-feeding has an effect on your baby's stools. The stools of breastfed babies tend to be runnier, yellowy in colour, and can have a fairly sweet aroma, while bottle-fed babies may have firmer, stronger-smelling, brown stools.

A healthy lifestyle benefits your physical and mental wellbeing and helps you to cope with the demands of parenthood.

It's important to eat a well-balanced diet (see pp.14–17) to help you cope with the demands of motherhood. If you're breastfeeding, you'll need an extra 500 calories a day. Drink plenty of water and take care to limit your caffeine intake. If you were anaemic during pregnancy, or had a heavy blood loss after the birth, eat lots of iron-rich foods, such as broccoli or spinach. Foods and drinks rich in vitamin C will help you to absorb iron.

If you smoke and didn't manage to stop during pregnancy, this is an ideal time to try again. Ask your midwife or doctor to refer you to a local smoking cessation group. Limiting your alcohol intake is also wise, and drinking while breastfeeding isn't recommended.

It can be easy to take over your baby's care, but it's important that your partner is involved, too, and doesn't feel left out. Your partner is adjusting to fatherhood and may have his own anxieties and concerns. Sharing the practical care will help him to forge his own bond with the baby. As his confidence grows, you'll be able to take some time out while he cares for the baby. Keeping the lines of communication open is vital as this is a time of huge change for you both. It takes time to adjust to being a family, but if you work together you'll manage the transition more smoothly.

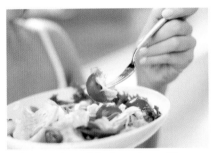

Eating a variety of fresh produce will ensure a good intake of vitamins and minerals.

AS A MATTER OF FACT

If you live in England, Wales, or Northern Ireland you have six weeks to register the birth; in Scotland you have just 21 days.

Your baby's birth is registered in the county or borough where she was born, which may not be where you live.

YOUR BABY'S NAPPY: WHAT'S NORMAL AND WHEN TO WORRY

The colour and consistency of a baby's stools are highly variable, but most are normal and not a cause for concern. However, some types of stool can indicate a problem and it's important that you know what to look for. A change in the colour of urine or the presence of blood might also alert you to a problem.

What's normal
- Once your baby has passed the first dark meconium (see p.444), stools may become dark green, green-yellow, bright yellow, orange or brown; all are normal and may vary in the same day.
- If your baby is breastfed, stools may be loose, seedy, and bright yellow.
- If your baby is bottle-fed, stools tend to be smooth, firmer, and brown.

- Frequency of stools varies from after every feed to every 2–3 days.
- Urine may be yellow or clear.
- A pink or red-orange stain on the nappy due to urate crystals (which form from concentrated urine); these are common in the first few weeks, especially in breastfed babies and are nothing to worry about.

What's not normal
- White or putty-coloured stools, which could indicate a liver problem.
- Blood mixed in the stools, which could suggest a milk allergy.
- Dark urine could be a sign of dehydration or jaundice.
If you notice any of these signs, ask your midwife or doctor for advice.

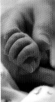

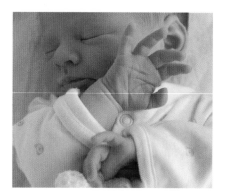

Focus on you

YOUR BABY TODAY

If your baby vomits large amounts and isn't thriving, this may suggest a problem such as gastro-oesophageal reflux (see p.477). This is caused by the immaturity of the stomach muscles and does disappear over time and with treatment.

Now you've begun to adapt to the topsy-turvy world of motherhood, try to carve out some time for yourself each day.

To help you deal with broken nights and constant demands, you need to develop coping skills, such as having an afternoon nap. You may also be dealing with feelings of isolation and may even find it hard to keep track of what day it is as days and nights merge into one. To revive your spirits, arrange for a friend or relative to look after your baby while you have a break. You and your partner also need to make an effort to make time for each other.

TIPS FOR MUM

Tummy-flattening

Strengthening your abdomen enables your body to work more efficiently during any activity and helps you regain your pre-pregnancy tone.

- Sit up straight; pull in your tummy for 60 seconds at least once each hour.

- Stand tall and straight to keep your abdominal muscles firm.

- Massage your abdomen with oil or body lotion in circular movements.

- When you feel able, you can start doing gentle curl-ups to strengthen your abdomen, but wait for at least six weeks after a Caesarean section.

BREASTFEEDING PROBLEMS

For some women, breastfeeding is a straightforward process that both mother and baby take to without a hiccup. However, for many women breastfeeding can be surprisingly hard and extra support is needed to overcome problems. Engorged (swollen) breasts and sore nipples are a common complaint; knowing how to avoid or treat these problems can be the difference between continuing with breastfeeding or giving up.

The secret to avoiding sore nipples is to make sure that your baby latches on to your breast properly (see p.448).

Engorged breasts can make it hard for your baby to latch on; expressing a bit of milk (see p.449) before a feed can relieve some pressure. Whenever possible, let the air get to your nipples, and use breast pads at other times to keep the nipples dry. Placing a chilled cabbage leaf on your breast helps to soothe sore nipples and engorged breasts.

You can relieve engorged breasts by continuing with breastfeeding and expressing milk frequently in between feeds to relieve the pressure. Placing a warm, clean flannel on your breast can also be soothing.

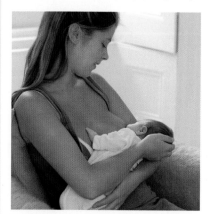

Positioning your baby well at the breast and ensuring that he latches on properly will help to avoid sore, painful nipples.

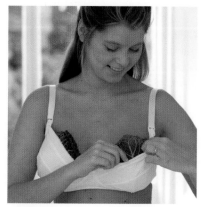

Putting a chilled cabbage leaf inside your bra can be surprisingly soothing, especially if your breasts are feeling inflamed.

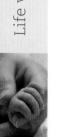

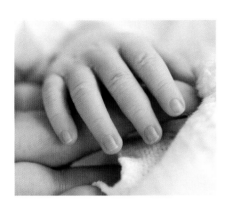

Baby time

YOUR BABY TODAY

Your baby is checked and usually weighed today to see if she is back to her birth weight. Sometimes babies develop skin rashes or irritations and sore bottoms around this time and, if this is the case, you will be given advice on how to relieve these minor problems.

By the second week, you should find that your body is starting to return to its pre-pregnancy state.

You will usually have a postnatal visit today – either a midwife will visit you at home or you can visit a midwife at a postnatal drop-in centre. These centres have been introduced recently and mean that you don't need to wait in for the midwife. The midwife will feel your abdomen to check that your womb has reduced considerably. She will ask about your blood loss, which by now is usually minimal. As long as it is not sudden or heavy with clots or an offensive smell, it isn't anything to worry about. As many women suffer from stress incontinence (see p.475), especially when they sneeze, cough, or laugh, you will be reminded to continue pelvic floor exercises. Your midwife will also check that you are drinking plenty of fluids and have adequate fibre in your diet to avoid constipation. She will check that any stitches are healing well and that there is no swelling or bruising.

Your baby loves to be stimulated. She can focus about a foot away and will watch a simple object such as a mobile. Babies soon recognize familiar faces and she will love to watch you talk. Being part of your daily life provides plenty of stimulation. Tell her what you are doing and your plans for the day, read her stories, and listen to music together. When she is awake, give her time on her tummy to develop strength in the arms and prevent a "flat" head, a common problem in babies who spend a lot of time on their back. Always supervise your baby while she is on her tummy.

SLEEPING BABES

Newborn babies have a least two naps each day and many simply rotate sleeping and eating throughout the day. In the early days, you'll find that there is little routine to your baby's sleep pattern as she can't go for a long period without a feed.

You'll probably find that your baby isn't fusssy about where she naps and that this can be wherever it's convenient for you, whether it's in the car, the buggy, or in a baby sling. If you're at home, you may prefer to put your baby somewhere quiet for a nap, such as in her cot, or you might want to keep her close by in a play pen or on a towel on the floor, if this is safe.

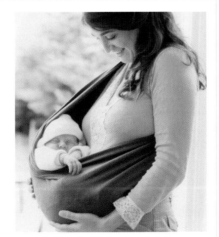

Many babies find being carried close in a baby sling deeply comforting and may sleep happily while being transported.

TIPS FOR BABYCARE

Nails and scratching

Babies' nails grow very quickly and are very tricky to cut! However, to stop your baby scratching her face, you will need to keep them trimmed. Take care not to rip the edge of the nails as this can cause infection.

■ You can buy special baby scissors, although these may not cut the nails short enough to stop her scratching.

■ Biting off the nails keeps them short.

■ You may wish to put mittens on your baby until she is past the scratching stage.

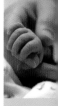

457

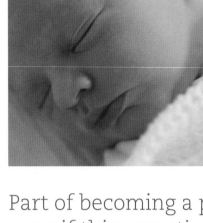

2nd WEEK: DAY 11

Taking stock

YOUR BABY TODAY

Many babies have spots known as milia, or "milk spots". These tiny, whitish-yellow spots appear on the face in the first two days and disappear by four weeks. Occasionally, babies have spots resulting from the mother's hormones that take longer to disappear.

Part of becoming a parent is learning to trust your own instincts, even if this sometimes means ignoring the advice of others.

There are many approaches to baby care, and once you have a baby you may find that everyone has a tip to offer. Although many of these suggestions are helpful, the advice can become a bit overwhelming and is often conflicting. One area where there is a great deal of advice is breastfeeding (see p.448). If you are struggling with breastfeeding and wondering why it all seems so much harder than it looks, you may find that advice from professionals, friends, family, and books is increasingly unhelpful. It can help to take a step back, decide which of your friends or relatives has a similar approach to yours in other areas of life and pay most heed to their advice. Above all, have confidence in your own ability and trust your instincts, reminding yourself that there are many right ways to do things.

(see p.448)

CHECKLIST

Your first trip to the supermarket

Some forward planning and management can help to take the stress out of a supermarket shop.

■ Giving your baby a good feed before setting out may mean that he sleeps peacefully in the supermarket.

■ Supermarkets can be very cold, so dress your baby appropriately.

■ Check if your car seat clips onto a trolley as this can make life easier. Otherwise, use the supermarket's own trolley with a baby seat or put your baby into a sling while you walk around the supermarket.

■ Write a shopping list before you go so that you don't forget essentials if you're distracted by your baby crying.

BABY MASSAGE

Babies love to be touched and massaging your baby can be a great way to bond with your baby. All you need is some olive oil (avoid nut or aromatherapy oils) and a towel on the floor or bed. Ensure the room is warm and that your baby isn't hungry or too full. Undress your baby, rub some oil into your palms, and gently rub his tummy, limbs, fingers, and toes, watching his face to check that he is enjoying the massage. A baby massage class is a good way to make friends with other mums in your area.

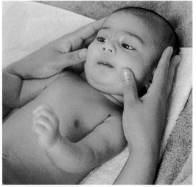

Lie your baby on a soft towel and then use the tips of your fingers to gently stroke your baby's head, avoiding the soft areas, or fontanelles, at the top of the head.

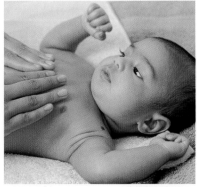

With gentle downwards strokes, massage your baby's chest and then use your fingertips to rub his tummy with clockwise circular strokes outwards from the navel.

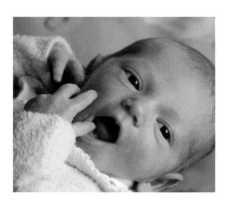

Looking back

YOUR BABY TODAY

By now, you may feel that your baby is begining to interact a bit more as you notice that she loves to gaze at faces and enjoys watching you talk and smile. However, she won't be able to smile back for a few weeks yet.

For some, reliving a traumatic birth is painful and you and your partner may need support to work through difficult memories.

ASK A... MIDWIFE

My baby's eye is constantly sticky. What should I do? Many newborn babies wake up with sticky eyes. This is due to a temporary blockage of the tear ducts, which are tiny in newborn babies. Clear her eye by wiping it with cotton wool soaked in cooled boiled water, using a fresh piece for each wipe. The problem usually clears with time, but if the secretions become yellow and look infected, tell your doctor or health visitor as your baby may need antibiotic eye drops.

FOCUS ON... YOUR BABY'S SENSES

Your baby's world

Your baby will focus on your face when she is feeding. She has been able to hear since she was in the womb, and loves the sound of voices and music. She is startled by sudden noises, but can't locate them yet. She can taste; she loves the sweetness of breast milk, and can tell if you've eaten something different! She can recognize your smell, and loves being cuddled, stroked, and carried close to you in a sling.

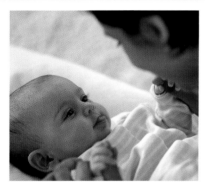

Your baby is fascinated by your face and loves making eye contact with you.

Once the acceptance and realization that you have had had a baby sinks in and you are beginning to adapt to your new role as a mother, you may start to reflect on your birth experience and may want to share this with your relatives and friends. You will remember your birth story for the rest of your life and later share it with your baby.

Sometimes the labour and birth may not have gone as you wanted or anticipated. For example, you may have gone over your dates and had to be induced, and this may have led to interventions and possibly an instrumental delivery or an emergency Caesarean section. You may feel some disappointment and be unsure about why certain things happened and whether you could have done anything to avoid them happening.

Occasionally, some women, and their partners, who had a particularly difficult birth experience can suffer from post-birth trauma. If the birth was traumatic and you feel upset and unsettled, make an appointment with your midwife to discuss your birth experience. She will be able to explain events that you are unsure about and, if necessary, will be able to arrange for you to see the midwife or consultant obstetrician who cared for you during labour. The maternity staff at the hospital will be able to go through your notes and help you to understand why certain decisions were made. If your partner feels traumatized by your birth experience and felt helpless during the process, he can also talk to the midwife or, if he prefers, to the doctor.

Talking to your partner about the labour and birth can help you to relive good memories and to come to terms with the more unsettling ones. Your partner is one of the best placed people to reassure you about how you coped during labour, and talking together can help you to open up and express your feelings about the birth.

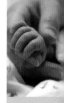

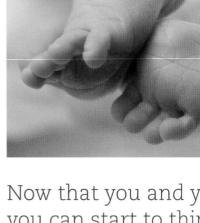

Feeling close

YOUR BABY TODAY

It's inevitable that your baby will be exposed to viruses and some believe this reduces the risk of allergies later on. However, small babies can be quite unwell with a cold so try to avoid people with colds. Breastfeeding provides some protection against viruses.

Now that you and your partner are adapting to your new roles, you can start to think about how to make time for each other.

Finding time alone together can be hard and resuming your love life can take time. Some women resume their love life without any problems, but for many it takes a little longer, especially if they had stitches and are sore. Also, a difficult birth can affect you emotionally, as can tiredness from lack of sleep. It's recommended that you wait two to three weeks after giving birth before having sexual intercourse, to let your womb reduce in size and for the bleeding to stop. Many women prefer to wait until after their six-week check (see pp.462–3). Initially, cuddles and non-penetrative sex can help you and your partner experience closeness. When you both feel right you can resume sex, but the first time needs to be gentle and you may need a lubricant as your hormones can cause vaginal dryness, especially when breastfeeding. If intercourse is painful, talk to your doctor, who can check that you are healing.

You will need to consider contraception now (see p.463). If you're undecided as to what to use and wish to resume intercourse, it's a good idea to use condoms until your six-week check when you can discuss the issue further.

Adapting to family life can mean learning to juggle your time to meet each other's needs.

GETTING YOUR FIGURE BACK

Most women lose around 4–7kg (10–15lb) in the first two weeks after the birth as, in addition to the loss of the weight of the baby, placenta, and amniotic fluid, you will lose the water that you retained in pregnancy. This water will be mobilized from your tissues and reabsorbed back into your bloodstream, and you'll eliminate it through your urine. Women can often feel more swollen after the delivery than they were before, but this extra fluid will be eliminated naturally in the next two weeks as they will probably pass large amounts of urine.

After two weeks, your weight loss will slow down. It's important not to try to lose weight too quickly after the birth, especially if you're breastfeeding, when you need around 500 extra calories each day. If you don't meet these extra nutritional needs, you will probably find that your energy will be low from a lack of calories. Eat a balanced diet that consists of whole grains, fruits, vegetables, and protein, and drink plenty of fluids to avoid constipation.

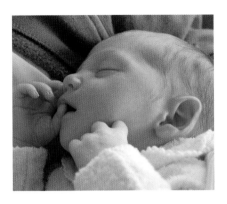

2nd WEEK: DAY 14

New beginnings

YOUR BABY TODAY

At your final check, your midwife will ensure that you and your baby are fit and well. Your baby needs to be back to her birth weight, feeding well, and thriving. Your midwife will check she's had the Guthrie (heel prick) test and that there are no signs of jaundice.

Life will never be the same again and by now you will understand the unconditional love of a parent for their child.

Around this time your midwife will visit you at home or see you in a postnatal drop-in-centre for a final check. As well as checking that you and your baby are physically well, she will also check that you have registered your baby with your GP practice and make sure you have your baby's unique NHS number. She will ensure you have all the information you need and that you have contact numbers if you need to reach her over the next week or so.

If all is well, the midwife may transfer your care over to the health visitor, which happens 10 to 28 days after the birth of your baby. Your health visitor may have already contacted you to arrange a home visit in the next couple of days. If, for any reason, you or the midwife feel you need further checkups, she will arrange this with you over the next week or so.

You may now be getting out more by yourself as your partner may be back at work. Ask your health visitor about times and venues for support groups in you local area and any pram-walking clubs or baby massage classes as these are excellent ways to meet other mums.

At two weeks, you'll be getting the hang of being parents. Life will never be the same again, and although this means that you will always have to put your baby first and will not have as much time for yourself, in return you have the most beautiful, fascinating child with her own personality whom you'll always love unconditionally. There is nothing that compares with the love of parent and child, and by now you will understand exactly what that means.

ASK A... MIDWIFE

Should I try to get my baby into a routine? In the first few weeks, it's too early to establish routines. To establish breastfeeding, newborn babies need to be fed on demand and most, in time, will sort out their own routine. If you want to try to establish set feeding times, you will have to consider how you will cope with a screaming baby. However, it's worth starting a night-time routine early on. Bathing your baby, singing to her, giving her a feed, and putting her down in her cot to sleep will help her develop good sleep patterns later on.

RECORDING YOUR BABY

It's tempting to take photos and videos almost constantly when your first baby is born. Subsequent children often remark on how relatively few photos there are of them! Digital photography means that you can email family and friends immediately with new baby photos, however, try not to go overboard as, although you will never tire of looking at your own baby, other people's baby photos are of more limited interest.

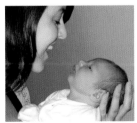

The first pictures together provide precious memories.

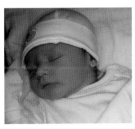

You'll be fascinated by your new baby's every moment.

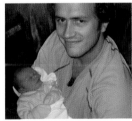

Don't forget to include pictures of the proud dad.

Your six-week check

At about six to eight weeks following the birth, you will be offered a postnatal checkup with either a doctor or a nurse practitioner at your doctor's surgery. This checkup is to see if you are physically and emotionally well. Your baby will also have a physical and developmental check around this time.

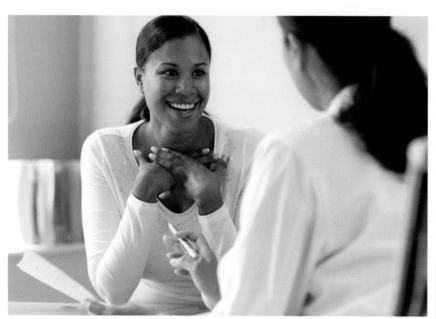

Your six-week postnatal check is the ideal time to talk to your doctor about any problems or concerns you have, and to receive reassurance that you have recovered well after the birth.

Your assessment

In the first couple of months following the birth of their baby, the majority of women don't experience any major health concerns and will revert back to their pre-pregnant health status. However, it's good practice to have a general assessment to reassure you that you are well and coping with the early transition to motherhood.

Your postnatal checkup is an ideal opportunity for you to consult your doctor or nurse practitioner about any concerns you have following the birth. Any worries about yourself or your baby can be discussed, and your doctor can then liaise with your health visitor if necessary. If you do have a particular problem, your doctor will offer you advice and possibly treatment, and will be able to refer you to a specialist for further treatment if necessary.

Your physical checkup

Your doctor will carry out routine checks, such as taking your blood pressure. He or she will also ask if you have any concerns, how you're feeding your baby, and, if you are breastfeeding, whether you've had any problems with your breasts and lactation.

Your womb will have returned nearly to its pre-pregnancy size (about the size of the palm of your hand) and will not be able to be felt. However, your doctor may check your abdomen to see if the muscles are returning to normal, as occasionally the abdominal muscles separate after birth, known as "*diastasis recti*" (see p.250). If the muscles are more than four fingers apart, you may be referred to a physiotherapist. Pilates and core conditioning exercises (see p.250) can help and your doctor may talk to you about these exercises.

Backache can be a problem after the birth, exacerbated by the pregnancy hormone relaxin, which softens muscles and ligaments and remains in the body for a few months after pregnancy. If you're suffering with backache, your doctor may talk to you about your posture, particularly when you're carrying or feeding your baby, and about the benefits of exercise.

If you had a Caesarean, your wound will be looked at to check that it has healed well. You may still feel numbness around the site of the wound, but sensation will gradually return as the nerve endings renew themselves.

If you haven't had a cervical smear in the last three years, you will be asked to have one done in three months' time.

Checking your bladder You will be asked if you have problems urinating, and may be asked for a urine sample if you have symptoms such as frequent urination or stinging when passing urine. Stress incontinence, or leaking urine when you cough, sneeze, or exercise (see p.475), is common after childbirth, so don't feel embarrassed to mention this to your doctor. He or she may encourage you to do pelvic floor exercises (see p.69), and if the problem persists you may be referred to a physiotherapist for bladder-training exercises.

Your stitches If you're still sore from stitches, your doctor will check that these are healing properly. Although most stitches are absorbable, they can take up to three months to completely absorb. Bathing can sometimes help the stitches absorb, but if you continue to have problems your doctor may refer you to a gynaecologist, or to a special clinic known as a perineal trauma clinic (see also Perineal problems, p.475).

Your emotional wellbeing

As well as checking you physically, the doctor will also assess your emotional and mental health. Many women feel extremely tired in these early weeks, as night feeds and constant demands begin to take their toll. However, if you are feeling low, over-tired, or depressed a lot of the time, you may be suffering from postnatal depression (see p.475), so it's important not to ignore these symptoms. Talk to your doctor or nurse about how you are feeling; they will be able to offer support and liaise with your health visitor.

Looking at your lifestyle

Your doctor will advise you on healthy eating and lifestyle measures. If you smoke, you'll be given information about support groups in your local area to help you stop smoking.

Is it true that I don't need to worry about getting pregnant again while I'm breastfeeding?
If you are breastfeeding, you may not have a period for a while after giving birth. Although this means you are less likely to conceive, you can still ovulate, so you shouldn't assume that you don't need to use contraception. The doctor or nurse will discuss contraception and sexual health with you and may recommend the progesterone-only pill, which can be prescribed from 21 days if you're breastfeeding.

I'm bottle-feeding my baby and am worried about getting pregnant again. How soon could this happen?
If you decided to bottle-feed, you will probably have had your first period prior to this check and so certainly could become pregnant again. Although your midwife or health visitor will have already discussed contraception with you, this will be addressed again at your six-week check. The doctor or nurse will want to check that you have contraceptive measures in place; if not, he or she will offer you guidance and advice.

I had stitches and have felt too anxious to have sex since the birth. Is this normal?
Yes, plenty of women feel this way and many wait to resume sex until after their postnatal checkup. During this check, the doctor or nurse will be able to confirm that your wound has healed, and offer reassurance about resuming sex. On the other hand, there is nothing wrong with having sex before this checkup as long as you have stopped bleeding. When you do have sex, you may need to use a lubricant such as KY jelly, particularly if you're breastfeeding, as your hormones can cause some vaginal dryness.

Your baby's check

The doctor will also want to meet your baby at around six to eight weeks to carry out a physical check and look at how your baby is growing and developing.

The doctor will carry out a similar examination to the newborn check (see p.443). He or she will examine your baby's hips, spine, eyes, heart, and the pulses at the top of the legs. In boys, it's important to check that the testes are located in the scrotum. This is also a chance to look for subtle problems such as a heart murmur, which can develop after birth. Your baby will be weighed and his head circumference measured. The doctor will ask how your baby is feeding and check for signs of jaundice. Your baby's development will be checked too: whether he has head control, is starting to smile, and can focus on an object or face a foot away, and follow a moving object. All of these findings will be recorded in the red book, a record of your baby's growth and development, which you will have received from your health visitor.

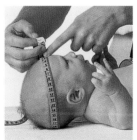

The head circumference is taken and the fontanelles, the soft areas on your baby's head, are checked.

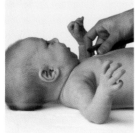

Your baby's heart rate will be listened to and the doctor will monitor and check his breathing.

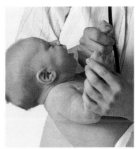

To check head control, your doctor will gently lift your baby up by his arms to see how he holds his head.

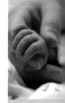

Your six-week check

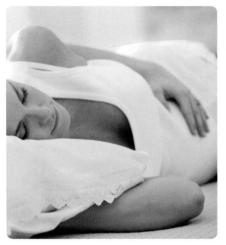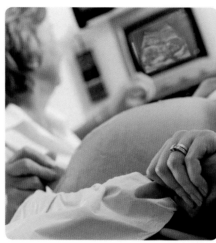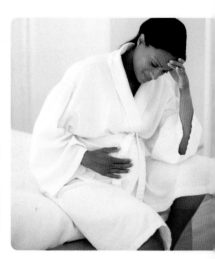

Rarely does pregnancy pass without some complaint. The majority of problems are minor and due to normal pregnancy changes. Some, however, are more serious and require medical attention. Today, high-quality antenatal care means that potentially serious conditions are usually successfully managed, both during pregnancy and in labour. Problems after the birth, either in the baby or the mother, may need medical attention with careful follow-up and sometimes referral to a specialist.

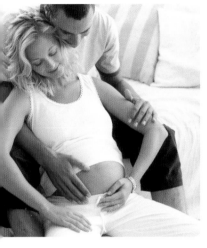
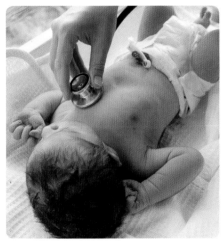
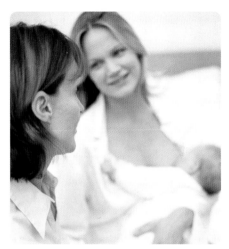

Concerns and complications

Common concerns in pregnancy

Pregnancy hormones affect every system in your body. In this section, you will find a list of common concerns with an explanation of the adaptation process that may cause these symptoms, information on whether medical help is likely to be required, and advice on measures you can take yourself to alleviate symptoms.

General symptoms

Tiredness

An overwhelming feeling of tiredness is often one of the earliest signs of pregnancy. Such feelings usually subside during the second trimester, but are likely to return in the third trimester.

CAUSES The main causes of extreme tiredness in early pregnancy are massive hormonal changes and the extra demands on the body made by an increase in blood volume of up to 50 per cent. It's this increase in blood volume that helps the lining of the uterus to thicken and the placenta to develop. In the second trimester, energy levels usually return to normal as hormone changes settle down. Late in pregnancy, tiredness may recur because your extra size and weight and the demands of the growing baby mean that your body systems need to work harder. In both early and late pregnancy, difficulty sleeping (see below) can contribute to feelings of tiredness. Tiredness in pregnancy can also be caused by anaemia (see p.472).

WHAT TO DO If you are working, take regular breaks and get some fresh air at least once a day. Ensure that your fluid intake is adequate; caffeine is not helpful as it dehydrates your body and will leave you feeling worse. Take more time for sleep if you need to; housework can wait and you may need to cut back on social commitments.

Difficulty sleeping

It's very common to have sleeping difficulties in pregnancy, especially in the first and third trimesters.

CAUSES A common cause of disturbed sleep is the need to urinate frequently. Early in pregnancy this is due to the amount of blood in your body, leading to the kidneys filtering out more fluid, which ends up in your bladder. As pregnancy progresses, another factor is expansion of the uterus within the pelvic cavity, so that it competes for space with the bladder. This leads the bladder to require more frequent emptying, which will interrupt your sleep. Many women also feel hungry during the night and need to snack, while others find that nausea and vomiting interrupt their night or lead to early waking. From about 20 weeks of pregnancy, the uterus moves up out of the pelvis, taking pressure off the bladder, and nausea often subsides, which means that sleep improves. Towards the end of pregnancy, sleep patterns can once again be disturbed. Unborn babies are often active just when you want to rest; your body is bulky and finding comfortable sleeping positions becomes difficult; and as the baby becomes bigger and heavier pressure on the bladder may return.

WHAT TO DO If frequent urination is keeping you awake, don't drink large quantities of fluid close to bedtime, and to avoid waking up hungry include foods high in unrefined carbohydrates, such as wholemeal bread, in your evening meal. If you do wake up, don't lie there for long periods, as this is frustrating and may lead to habitual sleeplessness. Get out of bed and engage in a simple activity that won't overstimulate your brain, have a warm, caffeine-free drink, and return to bed when you're sleepy. Later in pregnancy when you find it difficult to get comfortable, experiment with different sleeping positions: use plenty of pillows, under your head and bump and between your knees. A rest in the day is essential during late pregnancy, but limit this to a 20-minute power nap or an hour reading or watching television with your feet up. If you sleep for long periods in the day, you will further lessen your ability to sleep at night.

Headaches

Headaches are common in pregnancy, especially in the first trimester.

CAUSES Most headaches are unlikely to be a cause for concern and are probably due to hormonal changes and the need for additional fluids. Headaches occurring in the third trimester that are accompanied by other symptoms, such as abdominal pain or nausea, may be a sign of pre-eclampsia and should be assessed by a doctor (see p.474).

WHAT TO DO Making sure you drink enough clear fluids (around 2 litres/4 pints a day) and avoiding caffeine should help reduce the number and severity of headaches. If you're working or concentrating on a task, have a break every two to three hours, and take some gentle exercise in the fresh air. From 12 weeks, it's safe to take one gram (two 500mg tablets) of paracetamol every four to six hours; no more than four doses in any 24-hour period. If your headache is caused by a cold or flu, powdered drink remedies and all other cold remedy preparations are not advised, and ibuprofen or aspirin should not be taken except where specifically prescribed by a medical practitioner. Always discuss your symptoms with your doctor or midwife before taking medication.

If you have a headache in late pregnancy that is accompanied by swelling of the legs and ankles, generalized body swelling, abdominal pain, or nausea and vomiting, contact your midwife or doctor immediately.

Swollen feet and ankles

Some women experience a small amount of swelling in their feet, ankles, hands, and wrists, which can be particularly pronounced in hot weather.

CAUSES Swelling is the result of fluid retention, which in turn results from the extra blood produced during pregnancy to provide for the growing baby.

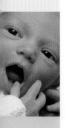

Swollen feet and ankles can be a sign of other problems such as pre-eclampsia (see p.474), so always tell your midwife or doctor who can check for other symptoms.

WHAT TO DO Swelling of the feet and ankles is best managed by alternating light activity with periods of rest during which your feet are elevated. However, you should avoid staying in bed or sitting in a chair for very long periods as this may increase the risk of deep vein thrombosis (DVT) (see p.186). Wearing maternity stockings (see p.225) may also help to reduce swelling.

Skin changes

Itching and dry skin

Many pregnant women suffer from itchy, dry patches of skin that worsen in late pregnancy. Such skin irritation is a reaction to hormonal changes and can be eased by a perfume-free moisturizer. Rarely, itching in late pregnancy may be due to a serious condition called obstetric cholestasis (see p.473). Itching caused by this condition is much more severe, usually constant, and often concentrated on the hands and feet.

Spider veins

Clusters of broken capillaries (tiny red blood vessels) called spider veins may appear during pregnancy, mainly on the cheeks. These occur as a result of increased blood circulation and the softening effect of pregnancy hormones on blood vessels. Spider veins are painless, but if you are worried about their appearance you can cover them with make-up. They usually disappear soon after the birth.

Increased pigmentation

An increase in skin pigmentation is common in pregnancy, due to the increased production of hormones. Most women notice a darkening of the area around the nipple (the areola), and a dark line, called the linea nigra, forming vertically through the middle of the bump from the umbilicus to the pelvis. Also common are dark patches on the cheeks, nose, and chin, known as chloasma or the "mask of pregnancy". On women with dark skin, the patches may

apppear lighter than surrounding skin. Exposure to sunlight can make the patches more obvious, so use a high-protection sunscreen cream on your face.

Stretch marks

Rapid stretching of the skin during pregnancy often leads to the development of pink or purple lines, known as stretch marks. These marks, which can look quite alarming with a scar-like appearance, usually appear in late pregnancy, commonly on the abdomen, hips, thighs, and upper breast. There is no clear evidence that any cream will prevent or remove stretch marks, although a light unscented moisturizer can help to keep the skin supple, as will staying well hydrated and avoiding excessive weight gain. As time passes after the birth, stretch marks become silvery and almost invisible.

Breast problems

Breast tenderness

For many women, breast tenderness and an increase in the size of their breasts are the first signs of pregnancy. Sometimes breasts are so painful that you can't bear them to be touched, and they may also throb and feel hot. Breast tenderness usually subsides by the end of the first trimester.
CAUSES Tenderness is a sign that the breasts are preparing for their role of feeding your baby after the birth: the milk ducts are starting to enlarge and blood flow increases.
WHAT TO DO Wearing a properly fitted bra will help to support your breasts and reduce discomfort. An ill-fitting or tight bra will be uncomfortable and may put pressure on the milk ducts. You may also find it helpful to wear a soft sleep bra at night. If your breasts feel hot, applying a cool facecloth to them may bring relief.

If you have a painful or red patch on a breast you should report this to your midwife or doctor as it could be a sign of mastitis (see p.475).

Nipple problems

There is a huge variation in the size and shape of women's breasts and nipples. Women who have flat nipples that do not protrude or whose nipples are inverted

(concave) may worry that they may not be able to breastfeed. However, all healthy women can breastfeed because babies feed by taking in a mouthful of breast, not just the nipple.
CAUSES Inverted or flat nipples are thought to be due to shorter ligaments in the underlying breast tissue that pull the nipples inwards.
WHAT TO DO If you have any concerns about the suitability of your nipples for breastfeeding, talk to your midwife or doctor who can refer you to a breastfeeding specialist (sometimes known as a lactation consultant). There are also products available that will help to draw out your nipples in preparation for breastfeeding. However, these are not essential because when babies latch on to the breast they are able to draw out even a flat or inverted nipple (although you may need help to show you the best way to help your baby do this).

Digestive problems

Nausea and vomiting

Approximately 80 per cent of women are troubled by the unpleasant symptoms of nausea and vomiting in early pregnancy. During this period it can be difficult to eat large meals, and strong smells and tastes can become unbearable. Many women also find some vegetable and acidic foods more difficult to digest and worry that their usually healthy eating pattern has deteriorated. Early pregnancy nausea and vomiting usually subside between 12 and 20 weeks; however, it's not uncommon to experience some return of these problems late in the pregnancy.
CAUSES Early in pregnancy, the pregnancy hormones interact with hormones that control other body systems, particularly those involved with blood-sugar regulation, and this results in feelings of nausea and vomiting. Late in pregnancy, problems with digestion may occur because the uterus takes up most of the space in your abdomen, displacing your intestines and stomach and leaving little room for the digestion of large amounts of food.
WHAT TO DO The best way to manage the nausea and vomiting of pregnancy is to

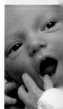

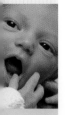

drink plenty of water throughout the day and eat small amounts of food on a regular basis, avoiding long gaps between meals and snacking on complex carbohydrates such as wholewheat and wholemeal products, wholegrain cereals, and brown rice dishes. Avoid snacks with a high sugar content because, although these will give you a quick boost, they will soon leave you feeling worse than before as your blood sugar plummets. Reducing your overall intake of the refined sugar found in sweets, cakes, biscuits, and sugary drinks will help to reduce the symptoms of nausea and vomiting, and will also lessen your risk of developing gestational diabetes.

The "little and often" principle coupled with healthy snacks is equally good advice for the late phase of pregnancy.

Gastroenteritis

This is inflammation of the lining of the stomach and intestines, most commonly due to infection. It causes vomiting and diarrhoea that usually come on suddenly. In most cases, the condition clears up on its own and is not a cause for concern. However, if it's severe, you could become dehydrated, and this can affect blood flow to your baby through the placenta. Infection with listeria bacteria can, rarely, cause late miscarriage.

CAUSES Gastroenteritis is caused by infection contracted either through contact with an infected person, or by consuming contaminated food or drink (food poisoning). Food poisoning is often the result of poor food hygiene.

WHAT TO DO Drink plenty of water, and try to avoid cross infection with other members of the household (see right). If you're unable to retain even small sips of water, or your vomiting and diarrhoea have lasted for 24 hours, you should seek medical advice from your doctor or the local maternity unit. If you cannot access help easily through those channels, go to your nearest accident and emergency department. If you have a pre-existing medical condition such as diabetes, you should seek help immediately. You may be treated with intravenous fluids if you are dehydrated, and fetal monitoring may be carried out to check the health of your baby. Infection with listeria is treated with antibiotics.

AVOIDING GASTROENTERITIS It is important that you try to avoid gastroenteritis by practising good food hygiene (see p.17).

If someone else in your household has gastroenteritis, avoid infection by using separate soap, towels, cutlery, and crockery. If you have more than one toilet, get the infected person to use a separate one to the rest of the household. Wipe toilets, basins, and taps with a mild bleach solution after each use. Infected individuals should also avoid preparing food for others.

Indigestion and heartburn

Many women start to experience episodes of indigestion and heartburn during the second trimester.

CAUSES Indigestion results from slower movements of the digestive tract under the influence of pregnancy hormones combined with reduced space in the stomach from the growing baby. The musclar valve at the top of the stomach is also softened by hormones and this can allow acid from the stomach to flow upwards into the oesophagus, causing the pain of heartburn.

WHAT TO DO Avoiding large meals, especially late at night, helps to prevent indigestion and heartburn. If you suffer from heartburn at night, try sleeping in a propped up position with your head higher than your feet. For relief from heartburn, a liquid antacid preparation can be helpful; ask your doctor or midwife for advice on which medications are safe. Some women find that slowly drinking a glass of milk eases the discomfort.

Constipation

During the second trimester, constipation often becomes a problem.

CAUSES Under the influence of the softening effect of pregnancy hormones, the digestive tract becomes less active. As a result, faecal matter spends longer in the large intestine, allowing reabsorption of fluids and leaving stools hard and difficult to pass. Not drinking enough fluids increases the likelihood of constipation.

WHAT TO DO Dietary fibre in the form of vegetables and whole foods along with an increase in fluid intake usually corrects the problem. Mild laxatives taken on the advice of a medical practitioner or pharmacist are useful as a last resort.

Haemorrhoids

Haemorrhoids, or piles, are dilated blood vessels around the inside of, or protruding from, the anus. Their constriction by the anal muscles and sensitivity to the acidic environment leads to a feeling of discomfort in mild episodes and pain in more severe cases. They are more likely to occur during the third trimester.

CAUSES The hormonal softening of the tissues around the anus increases the risk of developing haemorrhoids. Pressure from the baby's head on the blood vessels is also a factor, as is constipation.

WHAT TO DO Treatment of constipation and avoiding pushing or straining to pass a stool are important in the prevention of haemorrhoids. Cold packs and over-the-counter creams for relieving discomfort are available. If haemorrhoids are protruding and causing great discomfort, a health professional may be able to "reduce" them by pushing them gently back into place.

Heart & circulation problems

Dizziness and faintness

Throughout pregnancy, occasional dizziness or feelings of faintness can be a problem.

CAUSES In early pregnancy, feeling faint may occur even when you are sitting down and is likely to be due to low blood sugar. This can happen as a result of not eating enough, a common problem at this stage of pregnancy when many women suffer from morning sickness. In the second trimester, dizziness or faintness that comes on when getting up from a sitting position or as a result of standing for long periods is likely to be caused by low blood pressure. Blood pressure is lowered in pregnancy because the pregnancy hormone progesterone softens blood vessels to enable blood to flow more freely to your baby. When you stand, the low blood pressure may mean that not enough blood reaches your brain, leading to dizziness and faintness.

As pregnancy advances, you may find that you feel dizzy lying on your back. This happens because in this position the heavy uterus puts pressure on the main blood vessels running through the trunk and reduces the blood flow to the brain.

WHAT TO DO To help prevent low blood sugar, have small snacks of foods high in complex carbohydrates (see p.92). Staying well hydrated, taking regular breaks from work, not standing in one position for too long, and getting fresh air are also helpful in preventing faintness. If you start to feel dizzy, sit down and put your head between your legs, which will relieve the unpleasant feeling. Stay seated until you feel completely recovered and then get up slowly. If you feel well after the episode, there is no need to go to hospital, but you might like to seek the advice of a doctor or midwife if these episodes are frequent. If you have fainted and bumped your head or injured any part of your body then you should go to hospital for a checkup.

If you experience dizziness when lying on your back, turning onto your side will quickly help you to feel better. Lying on your left side is preferable because this helps to pump blood around the body.

Palpitations

A feeling that your heart is racing or beating irregularly is common in pregnancy, particularly between 28 and 32 weeks, but can occur at any time.

CAUSES The reasons for palpitations remain unclear and hypotheses range from the effect of progesterone on the heart muscle to the heart coping with the extra blood flow needed to maintain both mother and fetus.

WHAT TO DO Palpitations are usually fleeting and nothing to worry about. However, if you have frequent palpitations or they are accompanied by chest pain or breathlessness, you should consult your midwife or doctor. If you have a history of heart disease or a heart abnormality, seek advice urgently.

Nosebleeds

Nosebleeds occur frequently in pregnancy, and although they are a nuisance they are rarely a serious problem.

CAUSES As with all other blood vessels in the body, those in the nose are softened and expanded during pregnancy. In addition, your body has an increased blood volume in pregnancy, which puts pressure on these delicate structures. You are more likely to have a nosebleed if you have a cold or sinus infection or if your nasal membrane is dry, which can happen in cold weather or air conditioned rooms.

WHAT TO DO To manage a nosebleed, sit down, keep your head in a normal position and apply pressure to the bottom of the nose with your thumb and forefinger. You will need to maintain this pressure constantly for about 10 minutes before checking to see if the bleeding has stopped. Do not be tempted to tip your head back or lie down, as this will cause you to swallow the blood, leading to nausea and possible vomiting. Ice or a cold compress applied to the nose and facial area in conjunction with the nasal pressure can help to constrict the blood flow and halt the bleeding. Seek medical advice if the nosebleed results from a head injury or if heavy bleeding continues for more than 20 minutes. Mention frequent small nosebleeds at your antenatal appointment to enable the elimination of more serious conditions.

Bleeding, tender gums

Bleeding from the gums and gum tenderness are both common complaints during pregnancy.

CAUSES These problems occur as a result of increased blood volume coupled with the softening effect of pregnancy hormones on blood vessels. Allowing plaque to accumulate may exacerbate these symptoms and also makes the start of gum disease more likely.

WHAT TO DO Good dental hygiene is vital; don't be tempted to avoid brushing your teeth if they feel tender, but switch to a softer brush. Also, make sure that you visit your dentist regularly during pregnancy and the postnatal period. In the UK, dental care is available free on the NHS during this time.

Varicose veins and vulval varicosities

Varicose veins are enlarged, distorted veins that may develop in the legs or around the vulval area. Varicose veins in or around the anus are known as haemorrhoids (see opposite). Varicose veins may become troublesome during the later stages of pregnancy, causing discomfort and sometimes itching; they may also be unsightly. Varicosities in the vagina or vulval areas does not inhibit a normal birth and are not at risk of rupture during the birth.

CAUSES The increased blood flow and softened vessels mean that many women experience varicose veins and vulval varicosities during pregnancy. The growing uterus puts pressure on veins in the pelvis which, in turn, leads to increased pressure in the legs and vulval area.

WHAT TO DO Support tights designed for pregnancy can be helpful, and physiotherapists can prescribe specially designed support underwear. As with all conditions, varicose veins should be reported to your doctor or midwife for assessment and advice. Varicose veins usually disappear after the birth of the baby.

Aches and pains

Backache

Lower generalized backache is extremely common during pregnancy, particularly in the third trimester; around two thirds of all pregnant women suffer from backache.

CAUSES As pregnancy progresses, the increased weight of your abdomen tends to pull on the lower spine so that it curves inwards and your centre of gravity shifts forwards. As you try to correct this, you may strain the lower back muscles. In addition, pregnancy hormones soften your ligaments, causing them to stretch and providing less support for your back.

WHAT TO DO Maintaining good posture (see p.249) and avoiding tilting your pelvis forwards will help relieve pressure on your back, and help both to prevent and alleviate backache. Regular, moderate exercise to keep your muscles toned and supple is also beneficial. See pages 90 and 250 for suggested exercise routines. Yoga, pilates, and aqua aerobics are also recommended.

Try to avoid standing in one position for too long and vary your daily tasks, if possible breaking them down into shorter stints. If your work involves standing or sitting for long periods, take regular short breaks, and while sitting make sure your lower back is supported. Take care when lifting heavy objects.

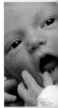

Massage and warm water can help to relieve backache. If back pain is very troublesome, talk to your doctor or midwife about wearing a supportive maternity belt (see p.278).

Pelvic girdle pain (PGP)

Also known as symphysis pubis dysfunction, pelvic girdle pain (PGP) refers to discomfort and pain felt in the pelvic area and groin. The pain may be concentrated in the buttocks or travel down one leg, and for this reason is sometimes mistaken for sciatica (see right). PGP is often worse when carrying out activities such as walking or going up stairs; it may also be troublesome at night, but this is usually related to activities carried out in the day. PGP is most common towards the end of pregnancy and may range in severity from mild to serious enough to need a walking aid.

CAUSES Various factors may contribute to PGP. The pelvis is made up of three bones: the sacrum and the two iliac (hip) bones. The bones are connected at the front by the symphysis pubis joint, and at the back by the sacroiliac joints. The joints are stabilized by ligaments and usually move very little. During pregnancy, however, ligaments soften and stretch more easily so that there is more movement at these joints. This results in instability of the pelvis. In addition, postural changes due to the enlarging abdomen may mean that one joint is more mobile than the other, putting extra strain on the joints. The result is inflammation of the joints and discomfort or pain.

WHAT TO DO If there is increased movement in one side of your pelvis, a pelvic support belt may be recommended, which often gives instant relief. You may be referred to a physiotherapist who will show you how to modify everyday activities, such as walking and getting up, in order to avoid pain, and may also recommend abdominal and pelvic floor exercises (see p.69). Acupuncture can help relieve pain, and aquanatal classes are helpful. Preventative measures include avoiding activities that cause pain, and avoiding heavy lifting, lying on your back, and sustained periods of activity. It's also important to get plenty of rest.

Round ligament pain

The two round ligaments run from the top of the uterus on either side and attach to the side walls of the abdomen. As the uterus enlarges, the round ligaments gradually become stretched, which can cause an ache or brief, sharp pain on one or both sides of the lower abdomen or in the groin. Round ligament pain usually starts during the second trimester.

WHAT TO DO See your midwife or doctor, who will rule out other causes for the abdominal pain. Once you have been reassured, you should find it easier to deal with the pain. When you have an attack, try to rest and relax. Lying on your side and bringing your knees up towards your chest may be helpful, as is taking a warm bath.

Sciatica

This is pain in one or both buttocks that may radiate down one leg. There may also be tingling or numbness in the legs, although this occurs only in a small percentage of women. Sciatica is most likely to occur after the second trimester.

CAUSES Sciatica is caused by trapping or compression of the sciatic nerve as it runs through the spinal column. The pain is termed referred pain, that is, pain felt in an area away from the problem site. Sciatica is not caused by compression of the nerve by the fetus's head. The causes of sciatica in pregnancy are the same as in women who are not pregnant and include poor posture, wear and tear on vertebral joints, and poor lifting techniques.

WHAT TO DO Specific exercises can help to stretch muscles gently and release pressure on the sciatic nerve. Your midwife may be able to advise you on exercises or may refer you to a physiotherapist for help.

Coccygeal pain

The coccyx, or tailbone, is the small bone found at the base of the spine. This bone is usually fairly immobile; however, in pregnancy it becomes more mobile, which facilitates the passage of the baby through the birth canal during labour. Pain in this area can make sitting for long periods extremely uncomfortable, particularly at work or during travel. Coccygeal pain can occur throughout pregnancy.

CAUSES Coccygeal pain may predate pregnancy due to a previous injury to the area; the discomfort may then be exacerbated by the hormonal and mechanical changes of pregnancy. Alternatively, coccygeal pain may arise in pregnancy, as increased movement in the coccyx during this time makes injury more likely. Sometimes the coccyx is injured during labour by the baby's head, and coccygeal pain therefore develops after the birth.

WHAT TO DO Moving around frequently and gently massaging the area can help to relieve discomfort, as can taking simple analgesics, such as paracetamol. The condition usually gets better within 6 weeks of delivery.

Leg cramps

Cramps in the legs, particularly in the calf muscles, are a common problem during pregnancy. These occur most commonly at night, but may sometimes come on when walking, and their frequency can increase as your pregnancy advances.

CAUSES There is debate as to the cause of leg cramps in pregnancy. They are likely to be caused by a combination of factors including maternal posture, increasing body weight, restriction in the blood flow to the legs, and the pressure of the uterus on the pelvic nerves. Some suggest that leg cramps in pregnancy may be due to a lack of salt in the diet. However, research demonstrates that low levels of salt are healthy in pregnancy, and that it is very unlikely that anyone who is eating a balanced diet will suffer from salt depletion.

WHAT TO DO Leg cramps may be relieved by changing position, flexing the toes of the affected leg upwards, and massaging the cramped muscle. If cramps are particularly troublesome, a physiotherapist or massage therapist will be able to suggest suitable exercises and offer advice. Stay well hydrated and alternate regular periods of moderate exercise with periods of rest.

If you have persistent pain, redness, or swelling in your calf, this may be a sign of deep vein thrombosis (DVT) (see p.186), which requires prompt medical attention.

Restless legs syndrome

Restless legs syndrome is an uncomfortable feeling or unpleasant tingling that creates an overwhelming desire to move your legs, or causes legs to jerk uncontrollably,

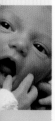

especially during sleep. Sufferers describe the sensation as being like an electric current passing through the legs or like having itchy bones. During pregnancy, the problem is most likely to occur during the third trimester.

CAUSES Restless legs syndrome is frequently triggered or aggravated by pregnancy. The cause is unknown, but some studies indicate that it might be related to low iron levels. Many sufferers have a family history of the condition.

WHAT TO DO If you're suffering from restless legs syndrome, talk to your doctor about having a full blood count to check your iron levels. If levels are low, a simple iron supplement will be prescribed. Some women find it helpful to exercise or stretch their legs, to use hot or cold compresses, or to have a leg massage. If the condition occurs for the first time in pregnancy, there is a very good chance that it will disappear after the baby is born.

Carpal tunnel syndrome

The carpal tunnel is a small tunnel in the wrist through which nerves run from your forearm into your hands and fingers. Carpal tunnel sydrome occurs when the nerves are compressed, resulting in tingling and pain in the fingers, which is often worse at night. In severe cases, there may be considerable discomfort and a reduced grip. In pregnancy, this is most likely to occur in the second and third trimesters.

CAUSES Carpal tunnel syndrome is caused by pressure on nerves running through the tunnel due to swelling of surrounding tissues. During pregnancy, swelling in the hands and feet is common as a reuslt of the extra fluid and blood volume.

WHAT TO DO If you think you may have carpal tunnel syndrome, talk to your midwife or doctor. You may be referred to a physiotherapist, who will recommend specific exercises to help relieve the discomfort. You may also be advised to wear a lightweight splint to support the wrists, which can be especially beneficial if the pain is disturbing your sleep. Carpal tunnel syndrome usually disappears after the birth of your baby. However, if it persists, a simple operation can be carried out to relieve pressure on the nerves.

Urinary and vaginal problems

Thrush (candidiasis)

During pregnancy, an increased vaginal discharge is normal. However, if the discharge is creamy and thick, and you have some soreness and itching in your vaginal area, you may have thrush, a fungal infection. If you have a vaginal discharge with an odour, you could have trichomoniasis or bacterial vaginosis, which are sexually transmitted infections that can lead to premature delivery if not treated with antibiotics. You are more prone to thrush during pregnancy, particularly during the third trimester.

CAUSES Thrush is caused by the yeast-like fungus *Candida albicans*. The organism exists normally in small numbers in the intestines and vagina, and doesn't cause problems. During pregnancy, the vaginal environment changes, causing overgrowth of the fungus. If you are under stress, feeling generally unwell, taking antibiotics, or have diabetes, you are more likely to develop thrush.

WHAT TO DO If you think you have thrush, contact your midwife or doctor, who can take a vaginal swab to confirm the diagnosis. Antifungal pessaries or a cream may be recommended. Other ways to relieve symptoms include bathing the vulval area in water with a few drops of vinegar added, or smearing the area with live yogurt. Wear cotton underwear and always wipe from front to back after a bowel movement.

Stress incontinence

If you have stress incontinence, you pass small amounts of urine unintentionally, particularly when coughing, sneezing, or laughing, and when exercising or lifting heavy objects. Stress incontinence can happen at any time during pregnancy, but is most common in the last trimester.

CAUSES The pelvic floor muscles are under an additional strain during pregnancy and are also affected by hormonal changes. Therefore any increase in abdominal pressure caused by coughing, sneezing, laughing, or other activities that puts these muscles under pressure may result in leakage of a small amount of urine.

WHAT TO DO Stress incontinence can be embarrassing and distressing; however, you should mention the problem to your midwife who will be able to advise you on pelvic floor exercises (see p.69), which should help reduce the problem if you practise them regularly. It's important, too, to empty your bladder whenever you need to. You may wish to wear a sanitary pad for additional reassurance.

Urinary tract infections

During pregnancy, you're more susceptible to urinary tract infections. Most commonly, such infections are confined to the badder, when they are known as cystitis. Symptoms of cystitis include a frequent, urgent need to urinate, and a painful burning sensation when passing urine; there may be some blood in your urine. Occasionally, an infection can travel up from the bladder to the kidneys. In this case you may also have pain in your lower back on one side (over the kidney area), a high temperature, and you may feel nauseous or vomit. Sometimes a urinary tract infection is present but causes no symptoms. Prompt treatment of urinary tract infections is especially important in pregnancy because if an infection reaches the kidneys, it can trigger early labour.

CAUSES Urinary tract infections are caused by bacteria entering the body through the urethra (the outlet from the bladder) and multiplying. Such infections are probably more common during pregnancy because the effect of hormones on the urinary tract slows the passage of urine.

WHAT TO DO If you have any symptoms of a urinary tract infection, see your doctor or midwife right away. You will be asked to provide a mid-stream urine sample, which will be sent off to the laboratory to identify the type of bacteria that is causing the infection. You will be started on antibiotics immediately and then switched to a different type of antibiotic, if necessary, once the results are in. Symptoms usually improve a few days after the start of treatment. Because some urinary tract infections are asymptomatic, all pregnant women have urine tests at every antenatal visit, and if bacteria are found, appropriate antibiotics are prescribed.

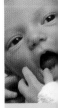

Complications of pregnancy & labour

Certain conditions that are specific to pregnancy and some that occur in pregnancy will classify the pregnancy as high risk. A high-risk pregnancy is closely monitored with more antenatal appointments and possibly additional scans. In labour, certain complications require immediate intervention.

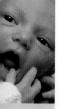

Pregnancy complications

Miscarriage

The loss of a baby before it can survive outside of the uterus is the most common complication during early pregnancy, affecting up to a quarter of all pregnancies (see p.94).

Ectopic pregnancy

This occurs when a fertilized egg implants outside of the uterine cavity. The vast majority of ectopic pregnancies are in the Fallopian tube, but they can occur on an ovary, in the cervix, or in the abdominal cavity at the site of a previous Caesarean section scar.

CAUSES Any woman can have an ectopic pregnancy. However, the risk is increased if you have had a pelvic infection; became pregnant with an IUD in place, while taking the mini-pill, or as a result of fertility treatment; have endometriosis; have had abdominal surgery such as a Caesarean section; or a previous ectopic pregnancy.

SYMPTOMS Most women who have an ectopic pregnancy notice pain and light bleeding at 6–8 weeks (2–4 weeks after a missed period). The pain is usually felt on one side of the lower abdomen and may be severe and persistent. If an ectopic pregnancy is not recognized early and an embryo growing in the Fallopian tube ruptures the tube, there may be sudden severe pain that spreads across the abdomen. Internal bleeding from a ruptured tube can also irritate the diaphragm, causing shoulder-tip pain. If you have severe lower abdominal pain, go immediately to either an accident and emergency department, or an early pregnancy unit.

WHAT MIGHT BE DONE If the tube has ruptured, then you will be taken straight to surgery. Usually, an ectopic pregnancy is suspected before this stage. In this case you will have an ultrasound scan, usually performed through the vagina, which often diagnoses the problem; there will be no baby in the uterus; blood may be seen in the abdomen; and sometimes the ectopic pregnancy itself can be seen. You may also have blood tests taken over a period of 48 hours to monitor the levels of hCG (the pregnancy hormone); if levels of hCG plateau or rise slightly, this indicates an ectopic pregnancy. If an ectopic pregnancy has not been confirmed by these investigations, you will probably be taken to theatre for a laparoscopy, a procedure where a telescope is inserted through a small incision in the tummy button, allowing the surgeon to see exactly what is happening.

If there is an ectopic, the surgeon may remove the tube either using keyhole surgery, or occasionally through a small cut at the bikini line. Occasionally, ectopics may be treated medically with a drug called methotrexate, which stops the pregnancy developing. This is only suitable if the hCG levels are low and the tube hasn't ruptured. The advantage is that surgery is avoided; however, the treatment doesn't always work, can be associated with significant pain, and close follow-up is vital.

Hyperemesis gravidarum

Most women experience some nausea during pregnancy. Occasionally, vomiting may be very severe, known as hyperemesis gravidarum. If you are unable to hold down any food or drink for more than 24 hours, you should see your doctor or midwife.

WHAT MIGHT BE DONE Your urine may be checked to ensure there is no infection, and you may have a scan to check that all is well with the pregnancy. You should be weighed, as if you lose more than 10 per cent of your body weight, you're at risk of complications. If you're very dehydrated, your doctor may advise a short hospitalization so that you can receive intravenous fluids, and you may be given anti-sickness drugs and a vitamin supplement. Hyperemesis usually disappears by 13 weeks.

Anaemia

Anaemia is a low level of haemoglobin, the oxygen-carrying component of red blood cells. Mild anaemia is common in pregnancy because the extra fluid content of blood dilutes the number of red blood cells. Also, the baby uses some of your iron stores. If you have anaemia you may feel tired and breathless and look pale.

CAUSES Usually, anaemia is due to iron deficiency. Occasionally, it's due to a lack of folic acid, vitamin B12, or rarer other problems. An analysis of your blood test result will help to identify the cause.

WHAT MIGHT BE DONE Anaemia is usually remedied with an iron supplement. These can have side effects, including constipation and black stools, so some women prefer to top up their iron intake through diet (see p.154).

Weak cervix

Rarely, a woman may have a weak cervix, previously known as cervical incompetence, which can lead to a miscarriage after 13 weeks. Usually, these miscarriages are relatively painless: you may feel well and perhaps notice some extra vaginal discharge, and then quite quickly miscarry the baby.

CAUSES Risk factors for a weak cervix include a previous late miscarriage; cervical surgery (such as a cone biopsy for an abnormal smear); or a previous late termination of pregnancy.

WHAT MIGHT BE DONE If you are thought to be at risk, the doctor may suggest you have a scan to check the length of your cervix as a shortened cervix makes miscarriage more likely. However, the interval between shortening and miscarriage can be very short, so relying on scanning alone for deciding on treatment is not always helpful. The doctor may recommend that you have a cervical suture (stitch) put in at around 12–14 weeks to strengthen the cervix. The suture is inserted under general anaesthetic and is usually successful in preventing miscarriage. It is left in until you're about 37 weeks; removal is straightforward and does not require anaesthesia.

Obstetric cholestasis

This is a rare condition affecting liver function that causes a build-up of bile acids in the bloodstream. The main symptom is severe itching without a rash that is usually most intense on the palms of the hands and soles of the feet. It usually occurs after 28 weeks.

CAUSES The exact cause of obstetric cholestasis is not clear, but genetic factors are probably involved as the condition tends to run in families and a woman who has the condition in one pregnancy will usually develop it in future pregnancies. Increased sensitivity to pregnancy hormones, which affect the way bile is processed, is also thought to play a role.

WHAT MIGHT BE DONE If a woman has itching without a rash, the doctor or midwife will do a blood test to check her liver function and bile acids. If they're abnormal, then obstetric cholestasis will be suspected. The doctor may recommend a drug called ursodeoxycholic acid to reduce the itching and improve liver function. You may also be treated with vitamin K because levels of this vitamin, which is essential for blood to clot, are often reduced in people with liver and bile problems. Women with severe obstetric cholestasis are usually induced at around 37 weeks because there is an increased risk of late stillbirth. There is also an increased risk of postpartum haemorrhage (see p.474).

Gestational diabetes

Diabetes that develops for the first time in pregnancy is called gestational diabetes and affects one to three per cent of pregnant women. In this condition, the pancreas produces insufficient insulin to move glucose (sugar) from the blood to be stored, resulting in high levels of glucose in the blood. It usually begins at 20–24 weeks. The risk is greater if you have a family history of late-onset diabetes, are overweight, have had several babies, or have previously had a large baby, a stillbirth, or gestational diabetes.

CAUSES Insulin levels become inadequate due to the extra demands of the fetus and because hormones produced by the placenta block the effects of insulin.

WHAT MIGHT BE DONE Between 24 and 28 weeks, you will be offered a glucose tolerance test. If you have risk factors, you may be offered this test earlier. The test involves having a blood test in the morning after fasting, then drinking a special sugary drink and having a repeat blood-sugar check two hours later. If gestational diabetes is diagnosed, you will be referred to a specialist antenatal clinic where you will see a dietician, diabetic specialist, and obstetrician. You will be taught how to test your blood glucose at home. In most cases, the diabetes can be controlled through diet and exercise. However, if these measures prove inadequate you may need insulin injections until the end of pregnancy. Extra scans will be done to check the baby's growth, and early induction (see p.432) may be advised.

If you've had gestational diabetes previously, it's important to ensure that your weight is normal before you become pregnant again.

Amniotic fluid problems

POLYHYDRAMNIOS This describes an excess of amniotic fluid. Symptoms include a stretched feeling in the abdomen; breathlessness; heartburn; swelling in the legs; and constipation. This condition is more likely with diabetes; twins; with an infection; or where there is a congenital abnormality in the baby. Polyhydramnios increases the risk of premature labour and cord prolapse. You will therefore be carefully monitored and advised to rest. In severe cases, the fluid may be drained.

OLIGOHYDRAMNIOS Too little amniotic fluid may be due to a tear in the membranes; placental problems; fetal abnormalities; or problems with the baby's growth (see pp.284–5). A reduction of amnioic fluid is most likely towards the end of pregnancy. If a scan confirms that levels are low and there are concerns about the baby's development, an early delivery may be advised.

Placental insufficiency

Placental insufficiency is the term used when the placenta is not functioning well enough to meet the baby's needs. The signs of this condition are a reduction in the amount of fluid around the baby, a fall off in the growth of the baby's abdomen and hence his weight, and abnormalities seen in a Doppler scan (see p.285).

CAUSES Placental insufficiency is more common in women with pre-eclampsia, those who have an underlying medical problem, and in women who smoke. It also occurs more often in babies with a chromosomal abnormality such as Down's syndrome, or a structural congenital abnormality such as a heart defect.

WHAT MIGHT BE DONE Placental insufficiency is usually picked up by the doctor or midwife noticing that the baby appears small and referring you for a scan. If the baby isn't growing well, the doctor will monitor you closely, and may recommend early delivery. If the placenta is working very poorly, your baby may not be able to cope with labour, so a Caesarean may be recommended.

Bleeding in late pregnancy

If you experience bleeding, it's important that you and the baby are assessed in hospital immediately. If the bleeding is caused by a problem with the placenta, this can be a serious threat to your baby.

CAUSES The most serious causes of late bleeding are placenta praevia (see p.212) and placental abruption. Placenta praevia, in which the placenta lies low in the uterus, is responsible for one in five cases of antepartum haemorrhage. The bleeding usually starts from 28 weeks; it is painless, usually recurrent, and is sometimes severe.

In placental abruption, which accounts for another one in five cases of late bleeding, the placenta starts to separate from the uterine lining, leading to severe abdominal pain and bleeding. The bleeding may not be obvious if the blood is trapped between the

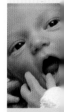

placenta and uterine wall. Placental abruption is potentially very harmful for your baby as the placenta may not be functioning well.

Bleeding can sometimes be due to cervical erosion, especially after intercourse, or to a cervical polyp. In many cases, no cause is found.

WHAT MIGHT BE DONE If you have minor to moderate bleeding without pain, you'll be admitted to hospital for observation and given steroids to help the baby's lungs mature in case an early delivery is necessary. If bleeding is heavy or painful, or the baby is distressed, an emergency Caesarean and a blood transfusion may be needed.

Pre-eclampsia

Pre-eclampsia (also known as toxaemia, or pre-eclamptic toxaemia) is a pregnancy-induced condition characterized by high blood pressure, protein in the urine, and oedema (swelling). Occasionally, women have symptoms such as headache, flashing lights, abdominal pain, or nausea. If left untreated, it can lead to eclampsia, an extremely serious condition that causes convulsions and coma. If you are diagnosed with pre-eclampsia, your pregnancy will be watched very closely and a decision will be made as to the best time for delivery. Around five per cent of women develop pre-eclampsia in their first pregancy.

CAUSES Pre-eclampsia is more common in multiple pregnancies; in very young and older mothers; in women with pre-existing high blood pressure or kidney disease; in women who've had severe pre-eclampsia before, necessitating delivery by 32 weeks; and in women who've had an egg donation.

WHAT MIGHT BE DONE Although the only cure for pre-eclampsia is delivery of the baby, the baby may need longer to mature in the uterus. The mother and baby will be closely monitored with the aim of prolonging the pregnancy as long as possible. The mother may be prescribed drugs to lower blood pressure and will probably be advised to rest as much as possible. As pre-eclampsia can affect blood flow to the placenta, regular ultrasound and Doppler scans (see pp.214–5 and 285) will be done to check the baby's growth and to look for signs of placental insufficiency (see

p.473). If your doctor is worried that your blood pressure is dangerously high despite medication, you're losing a lot of protein in your urine, or there are anxieties about the baby, urgent delivery will be recommended. This would mean either an induction (see p.432) or a Caesarean (see pp.438–9)

Group B Streptococcus

Around 20 per cent of women carry group B Streptococcus (GBS) in their vagina, which is completely normal, and does not cause any symptoms. However, 1 in 1,000 women will pass GBS to their baby once the waters are broken, and the baby may develop a severe GBS-related illness.

WHAT MIGHT BE DONE If a woman is known to carry GBS, and there are risk factors such as prolonged rupture of the membranes, or the baby is premature, intravenous antibiotics may be recommended once she is in labour, which usually prevents further problems. At the moment, routine screening of women for GBS is not done.

Labour complications

Premature labour

The normal length of pregnancy is 37 to 42 weeks. A baby born before 37 weeks is called premature or preterm (see p.431).

Fetal distress

In labour, the baby is monitored for signs of distress that indicate a reduced oxygen supply. One sign of fetal distress is meconium-stained waters (meconium is the baby's first dark green bowel movement). This alone doesn't always indicate fetal distress, but if combined with a slowing of the baby's heart rate, fetal distress is more likely, and steps will be taken for a prompt delivery. If thick meconium is present, there is a danger that the baby could inhale meconium at birth, which can lead to breathing problems and lung infection. The baby will be monitored continuously and delivered promptly if the heart rate slows.

Slow progress of labour

Sometimes the cervix fails to dilate as expected during the first stage of labour.

There are several factors that can hamper the progress of labour: the baby's head may be too large for the pelvis; there may be inefficient contractions; or the baby may be in a posterior position (see p.336).

Cord prolapse

Rarely, the umbilical cord lies below the baby. This is more likely in a breech birth, or where the baby lies in a transverse position. In these cases, when the waters break, the cord can slip through the cervix. This is an obstetric emergency because the cord may be compressed and restrict or cut off the baby's oxygen supply.

WHAT MIGHT BE DONE Unless an immediate assisted vaginal delivery is possible, an emergency Caesarean will be carried out.

Shoulder dystocia

This is when the baby's head is born, but the shoulders become stuck so that the body cannot be born. It's more common if the baby is big, or if the mother has diabetes.

WHAT MIGHT BE DONE If the head is delivered, and there are signs that the rest of the baby isn't coming, the midwife will summon help urgently. The mother's legs will be lifted to help release the baby's shoulders and an episiotomy may be done (see p.427). If the baby still doesn't come easily, there are manoeuvres the doctor or midwife will do to help release the shoulders and aid delivery (see also p.426); adopting an all-fours position can sometimes be helpful.

Primary postpartum haemorrhage

This is said to occur if a woman loses more than 500ml (17 oz) of blood within 24 hours of birth. It can be due to the uterus not contracting quickly enough, to incomplete delivery of the placenta, or to vaginal tears. Active management in the placenta's delivery (see p.428) makes it less likely. Factors that increase the risk include a large baby or twins; prolonged labour; or bleeding before delivery.

WHAT MIGHT BE DONE It's often possible to control bleeding with drugs to help the uterus contract, or by correcting problems such as retained bits of placenta, or by suturing tears. If the bleeding continues, a "balloon" may be put in the uterus. Rarely, an operation is done to check inside the abdomen.

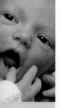

Concerns after the birth

Following the birth, you may have everyday concerns about you and your baby (see pp.441–63). However, few of these are serious and are usually easily remedied or are part of the normal development of your baby or your recovery process. The concerns in this section may require more attention from yourself or a health professional.

Maternal problems

Mastitis

This painful inflammation of breast tissue most commonly affects breastfeeding women. There may be localized redness, hardness, and soreness in the breast; the breast may feel swollen and hot; and there may be flu-like symptoms. Research shows that 10 per cent of women experience mastitis within the first three months of giving birth, although it can occur up to two years after the birth.

CAUSES Mastitis is either non-infectious or due to a bacterial infection. Non-infectious mastitis is caused by a blocked milk duct that allows milk to stagnate in the breast tissue. If bacteria get into the blocked duct, infectious mastitis can occur. If not treated, an infection can develop into a painful abscess.

WHAT TO DO It's important to carry on breastfeeding to help remove the blocked milk. Massaging the breast from under the arm (axilla) towards the nipple while feeding can also help, as can expressing milk after a feed. Rest is advised and it's important to drink lots of fluids. A warm flannel on the breast and mild analgesia such as paracetamol can relieve pain. If an infection is present, treatment with antibiotics is required. An abscess will need to be surgically drained.

Bladder problems

After a vaginal birth, you may have problems controlling your bladder. You may leak urine when you cough, sneeze, laugh, or move around, known as stress incontinence, or you may have a sudden, intense need to pass urine, referred to as urge incontinence.

CAUSES Both conditions are caused by the stretching and weakening of pelvic floor muscles and are exacerbated by excess fluid from pregnancy. Bladder problems should improve in the days and weeks after the birth as your pelvic muscles start to tone up.

WHAT TO DO Pelvic floor exercises (see p.69) to strengthen and tone muscles are recommended. If problems persist, your midwife or doctor may check that you're doing the exercises properly and that there are no other symptoms, such as cloudy urine, pain on passing urine, or an odour, that could indicate an infection and require treatment with antibiotics. Sometimes, referral to a urodynamic clinic is required.

Postnatal depression

This affects about 1 in 10 new mothers. It usually develops four to six weeks after the birth, but can come on any time in the first year. If left untreated, it can persist and have a serious effect on a woman's life.

Emotional symptoms include anxiety; irritability; tearfulness; panic; a prolonged low mood; an inability to cope; a lack of interest in appearance; difficulty in concentrating or getting motivated; and not bonding with the baby. There may also be feelings of inadequacy, guilt, rejection, and isolation. Physical symptoms include not sleeping; tiredness; headaches; lack of appetite; loss of libido; stomach pains; and feeling unwell.

CAUSES The causes are unclear, but there are several factors than may increase the risk of postnatal depression. These are having a previous history of depression or mental health problems; experiencing a traumatic birth; or having relationship problems.

WHAT TO DO In mild cases, emotional and practical support may be sufficient. More serious cases are often treated with antidepressants, and counselling or psychotherapy may be recommended.

Puerperal psychosis

This is a severe psychotic illness that affects 1 in 500 women and occurs in the first two weeks after the birth. The mother may be confused, unable to cope, may neglect her appearance, and forget to care for her baby. In severe cases, she may have suicidal thoughts and could possibly harm her baby.

WHAT TO DO The condition needs treatment from a psychiatrist, and the mother may be admitted to a specialized mother and baby unit and will need follow-up care.

Perineal problems

In a vaginal delivery, the perineum, the area between the vagina and anus, may stretch and subsequently feel sore. If you had a tear that needed stitches or an episiotomy (see p.427), this can be especially painful. If, after stitches, the area becomes red and swollen or you have throbbing pain, you may have an infection.

WHAT TO DO Anti-inflammatory suppositories after stitching reduce discomfort. Warm baths are soothing; some advise putting arnica oil in the water to reduce inflammation. Pouring warm water over stitches when urinating eases stinging. Paracetamol is advised for mild to moderate pain and anti-inflammatory drugs such as ibuprofen may help. Cooling gel pads can reduce swelling and bruising, and a pillow or inflatable swimming ring can make sitting easier. If you have signs of infection, antibiotics will be prescribed. If you experience perineal pain for a prolonged period, you may be referred to an obstetric physiotherapist for specialist treatment.

Secondary postpartum haemorrhage

Excessive bleeding more than 24 hours and up to six weeks after the delivery occurs in around one per cent of pregnancies. The most common cause is retained bits of placenta, which may in turn become infected. The bleeding may be accompanied by symptoms such as fever, abdominal pain, and feeling generally unwell. Infection is treated with antibiotics and retained tissues are removed under anaesthetic.

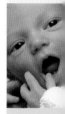

Congenital problems in babies

Down's syndrome

This is the most common chromosomal abnormality, affecting 1 in 1,000 newborn babies. Babies with Down's have some developmental delay and learning difficulties, and an increased risk of other congenital abnormalities such as heart problems. Down's causes a number of typical features, such as floppy muscle tone at birth; distinctive facial features such as upward slanting eyes; a single skin crease running across the palms; and a rather flat back to the head.

CAUSES Down's is due to an extra chromosome 21. Increasing maternal age makes Down's more likely, although most are born to younger mothers, because overall more babies are born to younger women.

WHAT MIGHT BE DONE Some parents who are told they are expecting a Down's baby choose to have a termination. Parents who continue with pregnancy usually find that their child has a good quality of life with advances in education meaning that many enjoy a degree of independence when older; life expectancy with Down's is around 60 years.

Talipes

Talipes describes the condition when a baby is born with one or both feet turning down and inwards. It's also known as club foot.

CAUSES The problem is usually due to the position of the baby in the uterus.

WHAT MIGHT BE DONE If the feet can be held in a normal position, known as positional talipes, this will correct itself in time. Physiotherapy may be needed and the physiotherapist will advise and monitor progress. A few babies have a more severe form of talipes when the foot is stuck in a position that cannot be rectified simply by holding it in the right position. This requires surgery by an orthopaedic surgeon to lengthen the tendons and the baby will wear plasters and/or splints for some time after the surgery. The results are usually excellent, resulting in a normally functioning foot and ankle.

Hip dysplasia

About 1 in 1,000 babies is born with a hip socket that is too shallow, meaning that the hip is easily dislocatable. It's more common in girls than boys. After birth, the midwife or paediatrician will check the hips by moving them around and making sure they're well situated within the sockets. If the condition is suspected or there is an increased risk of the condition, an ultrasound may be done.

CAUSES The risk is increased if there is a family history of congenital dislocation of the hip, if a baby is breech, or if a baby has tallipes (see left).

WHAT MIGHT BE DONE Treatment involves keeping the hips in a splint to hold them in position and allow the sockets to develop properly. If the problem goes undetected until the baby is walking, she will walk with a limp and will probably require surgery.

Cleft lip and palate

In this condition, which occurs in 1 in 700 babies, the two halves of the face don't join up properly, causing a gap in the upper lip and/or palate. A cleft lip can be symmetrical or, more commonly, asymmetrical, with the cleft on one side of the lip distorting a nostril. This may be detected antenatally but isn't always, so can be a shock initially. There's evidence that extra folic acid in pregnancy can reduce the risk of having a baby with cleft lip and palate.

WHAT MIGHT BE DONE Parents usually meet a member of their local cleft lip team after the birth and special teats may be used to aid feeding. Usually, at around three months, surgery is done to close the gap in the lips, and surgery to close the gap in the palate at about nine months. Further cosmetic surgery may be done once the child is older.

Congenital heart disease

Any abnormality involving the structure of the heart chambers or connections between the chambers can affect the function of the heart. Some heart problems are detected antenatally and you will be given advice about where your baby should be delivered and what will happen after the birth

SEPTAL DEFECTS These holes in the heart consist of a small hole between two heart chambers; some types may cause a murmur that is picked up at birth. In many babies, a hole closes on its own.

BLUE BABY Some babies are blue at birth because they have a major problem involving abnormal heart connections. This is an emergency and the baby will be transferred as soon as possible to a specialist centre for heart surgery.

PATENT DUCTUS ARTERIOSUS If the duct between the lungs and the heart fails to close after birth, oxygenated and deoxygenated blood mix. Treatment may be needed in the form of medication and sometimes surgery.

Undescended testicles

This occurs in around 1 in 125 boys. In most cases, just one testicle is undescended. Testicles often descend naturally within a year. Otherwise, surgery is advised as undescended testicles can affect sperm production and fertility and increase the risk of testicular cancer later in life.

Syndactyly

Sometimes babies are born with two digits, either the toes or fingers, joined together. This condition, called syndactyly, is usually caused by the soft tissues fusing together and may be linked to other congenital abnormalities, such as Down's syndrome. Treatment is surgical and skin grafts are used.

Birthmarks

Marks present at birth may be long-lasting, although they often fade over time.

STORK MARKS These pink skin patches on Caucasians often fade by two to five years.

MONGOLIAN BLUE SPOTS Some babies, particularly of Asian or Afro-Caribbean origin, have extensive grey markings on the lower back, buttocks, and other areas, that resemble bruises. Known as Mongolian blue spots, they fade over a few years. They do get mistaken for bruises, so it's worth asking your health visitor to record them in your baby book.

PORT WINE STAINS These permanent marks are caused by abnormal blood vessels in the skin and may occur anywhere on the baby. If one occurs on the face, your baby may be referred to a specialist for laser treatment.

STRAWBERRY NAEVUS This is an overgrowth of blood vessels, but is not permanent and usually needs no treatment. The naevus looks like a strawberry, and although it can be upsetting, it vanishes in a few years. It appears days after the birth and grows over a few months. If it's in a critical area, such as obstructing an eye or nose, your baby may be referred to a specialist.

Problems in babies after birth

Spots and rashes

Spots and rashes are common in newborns, and usually disapppear fairly quickly. Birth marks (see opposite) are longer-lasting and may be of more concern.

CAUSES Small white spots called milia are caused by blocked sebaceous glands, while neonatal acne is caused by the mother's hormones remaining in the baby after the birth. Both disappear in time without treatment. *Erythaema toxicum* is a rash of unknown cause that appears in the first day or two and disappears within a few days. It consists of red splodges with raised yellowish centres. The spots shift positions and eventually vanish with no treatment. Some babies get angry-looking red spots, sometimes in the armpits or groin, with pus-filled centres. These may be septic spots and may need treatment with antibiotics.

Slow weight gain

All babies lose weight in the first days after the birth, but most are back to their birth weight by the 10th day. After that, most babies gain about 30g (1oz) each day. Breastfed babies may take a little longer to regain their birth weight and generally gain weight more slowly. If a baby loses more than 10 per cent of his initial birth weight or is not putting on weight as expected, you will need to see a doctor to check why this has happened and what you should do.

CAUSES Slow weight gain is occasionally due to problems with breastfeeding; for example there may be problems with positioning the baby and latching on, which mean that both mother and baby find it hard to establish breastfeeding. Another possible cause of poor weight gain is excessive vomiting (see right).

WHAT TO DO If you're breastfeeding, check that you have an adequate intake of fluids and calories (you need an additional 500 calories a day), as too little of either of these can affect milk supply. Getting enough rest is also important for a healthy milk supply. You may be asked to give your baby top-up feeds until breastfeeding is well established, and you will need advice on how to do this and maintain a good supply of breast milk.

Jaundice

This is a common condition in newborns that gives the skin a yellowish hue. Neonatal jaundice is usually caused by an excess of bilirubin, which is a substance normally produced during the breakdown of red blood cells. There are several types of neonatal jaundice: physiological jaundice, pathological jaundice, and breast-milk jaundice (see below).

PHYSIOLOGICAL JAUNDICE This is the most common type of jaundice in newborns and is rarely of concern. Newborn babies have an excess of red blood cells. As the baby's liver is immature, it is unable to metabolize red blood cells quickly enough, which leads to a build-up of bilirubin. This type of jaundice often resolves on its own without treatment. However, if bilirubin levels are very high, this can damage part of the brain, so to avoid this, treatment is given with phototherapy lamps. The younger and more premature the baby, the lower the level of bilirubin at which treatment is given. Treatment continues until bilirubin levels fall sufficiently, and the baby is usually kept in hospital until at least 12 hours after treatment stops to check that the level hasn't risen again. The most common time for jaundice to need treatment is three to four days after birth.

PATHOLOGICAL JAUNDICE This is a more serious type of jaundice that is due to a rapid breakdown of the red blood cells and is usually due to an incompatibility between the mother's and the baby's blood. This may need urgent treatment in a neonatal unit.

BREAST-MILK JAUNDICE The most usual cause of prolonged jaundice is breast milk. This is thought to be caused by hormones in the milk affecting the ability of the baby's liver to metabolize bilirubin. It requires no treatment and causes the baby no harm.

If jaundice continues beyond two weeks of age and is not thought to be due to breast milk, this should be investigated to exclude rare causes such as a liver condition that, if found, would require specialist treatment before the age of six weeks.

Vomiting

All babies vomit to some extent in the first weeks after the birth, but you should contact your doctor if your baby has prolonged or excessive vomiting, isn't gaining enough weight, or you're concerned. Serious vomiting can have several causes, including conditions such as gastro-oesophageal reflux and pyloric stenosis (see below).

Other symptoms that may accompany vomiting can suggest particular conditions and will need investigating. If a baby seems lethargic or floppy, this could indicate an infection; if his abdomen is swollen, this could suggest an intestinal obstruction; if vomit is bright yellow or green, there could be a twisted bowel; and if there is also diarrhoea, there may be gastroenteritis.

Gastro-oesophageal reflux

If your baby is miserable, in pain, arching his back, refusing feeds, or vomiting large amounts after each feed, he could be suffering from gastro-oesophageal reflux. This occurs when the valve between the bottom of the oesophagus (gullet) and top of the stomach is immature, allowing the stomach contents to come back into the oesophagus. Acid from the stomach can burn the lower end of the oesophagus, and if the reflux is severe, a baby can go off feeds.

WHAT MIGHT BE DONE Mild gastro-oesophageal reflux that involves vomiting but no problems with weight gain or pain, usually needs no treatment. More severe reflux will need treatment, usually with medicines to thicken the milk, stop the acid production, and prevent the vomiting. For bottle-fed babies with mild reflux, it's worth asking your chemist for an anti-reflux milk.

Pyloric stenosis

In this condition, which occurs most commonly in first-born male babies, the exit at the bottom of the stomach is thickened, meaning that milk cannot leave. It causes so-called projectile vomiting in which a feed is vomited with so much force that it can land a foot or so away from the baby. The baby is constantly hungry and will demand another feed straight after vomiting. Vomiting becomes progressively more severe.

WHAT MIGHT BE DONE Pyloric stenosis is diagnosed with a blood test and ultrasound, and treatment is surgical. The operation is straightforward and the improvement remarkable. Babies usually leave hospital within two or three days.

Glossary

Active birth An approach to childbirth that involves upright positions and movements during labour.

Alphafetoprotein (AFP) A substance produced by the embryonic yolk sac, and later by the fetal liver, which enters the mother's bloodstream during pregnancy.

Amniocentesis The surgical extraction of a small amount of amniotic fluid through the pregnant woman's abdomen. This procedure is usually carried out as a test for fetal abnormalities.

Amnion The thin membrane surrounding the fetus and the amniotic fluid. It's also known as the amniotic sac.

Amniotic fluid The fluid that surrounds the fetus in the uterus. Ultrasound scans may be done in late pregnancy to ensure that enough is present.

Amniotomy The surgical rupture of the amniotic sac, often done to speed up labour. This is referred to as ARM (artificial rupture of the membranes).

Anterior position See *Occipital anterior*.

Anti-D An injection of antibodies given to women who have a rhesus negative blood group if they may have been exposed to rhesus positive fetal blood cells.

Apgar score A general test of the baby's wellbeing carried out at 1, 5, and 10 minutes after the birth to assess the baby's heart rate and tone, respiration, blood circulation, and nerve responses.

Areola The pigmented circle of skin surrounding the nipple.

ARM See *Amniotomy*.

Bilirubin Broken-down haemoglobin, normally converted to nontoxic substances by the liver. Some newborn babies have levels of bilirubin too high for their livers to cope with (neonatal jaundice).

Blastocyst An early stage of the developing egg after fertilization when it has divided and subdivided into a group of around 100 cells.

Braxton Hicks contractions Practise contractions of the uterus that occur throughout pregnancy, but which may not be noticed until towards the end of pregnancy.

Breech presentation When the position of the baby in the uterus is bottom down rather than head down.

Cardiotocograph (CTG) An electronic monitor that is used to measure the progress of the mother's contractions and the baby's heartbeat during labour.

Catheter A thin plastic tube that is inserted into the body through a natural channel to withdraw fluid from, or introduce fluid into, a particular part of the body. This can be used to drain urine from the bladder after an operation, or to maintain a constant input of fluids into a vein, or to introduce anaesthetic into the epidural space.

Cephalic presentation (Vertex presentation) The position of a baby who is head down in the uterus. The most common presentation.

Cephalopelvic disproportion A state in which the head of the fetus is larger than the cavity of the mother's pelvis. Delivery of the baby must therefore be by Caesarean section.

Cervical dilation See *Dilation*.

Chorion The outer membranous tissue that envelops the fetus and placenta.

Chloasma Pigmentation of the skin that causes darker patches, often on the face.

Chorionic gonadotrophin See *Human chorionic gonadotrophin (HCG)*.

Chorionic villus sampling A method of screening for genetic disease by analysis of tissue from the small protrusions on the outer membrane enveloping the embryo that later form the placenta.

Chromosomes Rod-like structures containing genes occurring in pairs within the nucleus of every cell. Human cells each contain 23 pairs.

Colostrum A kind of milk, rich in proteins, formed and secreted by the breasts in late pregnancy and gradually changing to mature milk some days after delivery.

Corpus luteum A glandular mass that forms in the ovary after fertilization. It produces progesterone, which helps to form the placenta, and is active for the first 14 weeks of pregnancy.

Crowning The moment when the baby's head appears at the entrance of the vagina and does not slip back again.

CVS See *Chorionic villus sampling*.

Dilation The progressive opening of the cervix caused by uterine contractions during labour.

Dizygotic See *Twins*.

Domino scheme A scheme operated by some hospitals in which community midwives provide antenatal care and are present at hospital for the delivery.

Doppler A method of using ultrasound vibrations to listen to the fetal heart.

Doula A supportive woman helper who provides physical and emotional support during childbirth.

Drip See *Intravenous drip*.

EDD The estimated date of delivery.

Electroencephalogram (EEG) A test where electrodes are placed on the scalp to record the electrical activity of the brain.

Embryo The developing organism in pregnancy, from about the 10th day after fertilization until around 10 weeks of pregnancy, after which it is termed a fetus.

Engorgement The over-congestion of the breasts with milk. If long periods are left between feeds, or the baby is not well latched on, painful engorgement can occur. This can be relieved by putting the baby to the breast or expressing the excess milk.

Episiotomy A surgical cut in the perineum to enlarge the entrance to the vagina.

External cephalic version (ECV). The manipulation by gentle pressure of the fetus into the cephalic (head down) position. This may be done by an obstetrician at the end of pregnancy if the baby is breech or transverse.

False labour Braxton Hicks (rehearsal) contractions, which are so strong and regular that they are mistaken for the contractions of the first stage of labour.

Fetal distress A shortage in the flow of oxygen to the fetus, which can arise from numerous causes.

Fetus The developing baby in the uterus, from the end of the embryonic stage at around 10 weeks of pregnancy, until birth.

Hormone A chemical messenger in the blood that stimulates various organs to carry out specific actions.

Human chorionic gonadotrophin (hCG) A hormone released into the woman's bloodstream by the developing placenta from about six days after the last period was due. Its presence in the urine means that she is pregnant.

Hypnobirthing A type of self-hypnosis using visualization and breathing techniques to achieve a deep state of relaxation during labour.

Hypotension Low blood pressure.

Identical twins See *Twins*.

Implantation The embedding of the fertilized ovum or egg within the wall of the uterus.

Induction The process of artificially starting off labour and keeping it going.

Intravenous drip The infusion of fluids directly into the bloodstream by means of a fine catheter introduced into a vein.

Intravenous injection An injection into a vein.

In vitro fertilization (IVF) A type of assisted conception where fertilization occurs outside of the womb and embryos are transferred back into the womb.

Kangaroo care A technique, adopted especially with premature babies, where baby and parent have prolonged skin-to-skin contact. This is thought to provide warmth, stimulation, and to encourage breastfeeding.

Lanugo The fine soft hair that grows on the body of the fetus..

Lateral position The term used to describe the position of the baby's head in the birth canal when it is looking sideways, a common position in early labour.

Lie The position in which the baby is lying within the uterus.

Linea nigra A line of dark skin that appears down the centre of the abdomen over the rectus muscle in some women during pregnancy.

Lochia Postnatal vaginal discharge.

Longitudinal lie The position of the fetus in the uterus in which the spines of the fetus and the mother are parallel.

Low-birthweight baby A baby who weighs below 2.5kg (5lb) at birth.

Meconium The first contents of the bowel, present in the fetus before birth and passed during the first few days after birth. The presence of meconium in the amniotic fluid before delivery is usually taken as a sign of fetal distress.

Monozygotic See *Twins*.

Morula A stage in the development of the fertilized egg, 3–4 days after fertilization, when it has grown into 16–32 cells.

Nucleus The central part or core of a cell, containing genetic information.

Occipital anterior The position of the baby in the uterus when the back of its head (the crown or occiput) is towards the mother's front (anterior).

Occipital posterior The position of the baby in the uterus when the back of its head (the crown or occiput) is towards the mother's back (posterior).

Oedema Fluid retention, which causes the body tissues to be puffed out.

Oestrogen A hormone produced by the ovary and, in pregnancy, by the placenta.

Opioids (Narcotics) Painkilling drugs that induce drowsiness and stupor.

Palpation Feeling the parts of the baby through the mother's abdominal wall.

Pelvic floor The springy muscular structure set within the pelvis that supports the bladder and the uterus, and through which the baby descends during labour.

Perinatal The period from the 24th week of gestation to one week following delivery.

Perineum The area of soft tissues surrounding the vagina and between the vagina and the rectum.

Posterior See *Occipito posterior*.

Postnatal After the birth.

Postpartum After delivery.

Premature A baby born before the 37th week of pregnancy.

Presentation A term that describes the part of the fetus nearest the cervix before and during labour.

Preterm See *Premature*.

Primigravida A woman in her first pregnancy.

Progesterone A hormone produced by the corpus luteum and then by the placenta.

Prostaglandins Natural substances that stimulate the onset of labour contractions. Prostaglandin gel may be used to soften the cervix and induce labour.

Rhesus factor A distinguishing characteristic of the red blood corpuscles. All human beings have either rhesus positive or rhesus negative blood. If the mother is rhesus negative and the fetus rhesus positive, rhesus disease (the destruction of the red corpuscles by antibodies) may occur, unless prevented by an injection of anti-D gamma globulin.

Rooting The baby's instinctive searching for the breast.

Show A vaginal discharge of bloodstained mucus occurring before labour, resulting from the onset of cervical dilatation. A sign that labour is starting.

Stillbirth The delivery of a dead baby after the 24th week of pregnancy.

Surfactant A creamy fluid that reduces the surface tension of the lungs so that they do not stick together when deflated. Premature babies may have breathing difficulties if surfactant has not developed sufficiently.

Transcutaneous electronic nerve stimulation (TENS) A method of pain relief that uses electrical impulses to block pain messages to the brain.

Transducer An instrument that translates echoes of high-frequency sound waves, bounced off the developing fetus in the uterus, to build up an ultrasound image on a monitor. See also *Ultrasound scan*.

Transition A phase between the first and second stages of labour when the cervix is dilating to between 7 and 10cm.

Trial of labour A situation in which, although a Caesarean section may be necessary, the mother labours in order to see if a vaginal delivery is possible.

Twins The simultaneous development of two babies in the uterus. If two eggs are fertilized independently by two sperm, dizygotic or fraternal twins result; more rarely, one fertilized egg subsequently divides to produce monozygotic or identical twins.

Ultrasound scan A way of building up a picture of an object by bouncing high-frequency soundwaves off it. Ultrasound scans are used during pregnancy to show the development of the fetus in the uterus. See also *Transducer*.

Vernix A creamy substance that covers the fetus in the uterus.

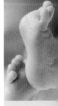

Resources

Fertility

www.gettingpregnant.co.uk
Fertility advice website

www.hfea.gov.uk
020 7291 8200
Human Fertilisation and Embryology
Authority

www.surrogacy.org.uk
01549 402777 or 0844 4140181
COTS (Childlessness Overcome Through
Surrogacy)

www.infertilitynetworkuk.com
0121 323 5025 or 0800 008 7464

www.fertilityuk.org
National fertility awareness and natural
family planning service

www.foresight-preconception.org.uk
01243 868001
Advice on preconceptual health

www.ivf-infertility.com

www.ivf.net

Pregnancy

www.arc-uk.org
0845 077 2290 or, via mobile, 0207 713 7486
Antenatal Results and Choices:
information and support for parents
throughout the antenatal testing process

www.bpas.org
0845 730 4030
British Pregnancy Advisory Service

www.babycentre.co.uk
Online information and advice for
expectant and new parents

www.fpa.org.uk
Helpline 0845 122 8690
Family Planning Association

www.maternityaction.org.uk
0845 600 8533
Advice for pregnant women and new parents

www.midwivesonline.com
Information on pregnancy, birth, and
new families

www.rcog.org.uk
020 7772 6200
Royal College of Obstetricians and
Gynaecologists
Information on pregnancy complications

Labour and birth

www.activebirthcentre.com
020 7281 6760

www.aims.org.uk
Helpline 0300 365 0663
Association for Improvements in the
Maternity Services

www.birthchoiceuk.com
Information on choosing where to
have a baby

www.birthtraumaassociation.org.uk

www.caesarean.org.uk

www.doula.org.uk
0871 433 3103
Support for women during labour and birth

www.homebirth.org.uk

www.hypnobirthing.co.uk
Self hypnosis for childbirth and labour

www.independentmidwives.org.uk
0845 4600 105

www.midwivesonline.com

www.nct.org.uk
Pregnancy and birth helpline 0300 330 0700
National Childbirth Trust

www.rcm.org.uk
The Royal College of Midwives

Breastfeeding

www.abm.me.uk
Helpline 0300 330 5453
Association of Breastfeeding Mothers

www.babyfriendly.org.uk
0207 375 6052
The Baby Friendly Initiative by Unicef
promoting breastfeeding

www.breastfeedingnetwork.org.uk
0300 100 0210 or 0300 100 0212

www.laleche.org.uk
Breastfeeding helpline 0845 120 2918

www.midwivesonline.com
Breastfeeding advice

www.nct.org.uk
Breastfeeding helpline 0300 330 0700
National Childbirth Trust

Support groups

www.apec.org.uk
Helpline 0208 427 4217
Action on Pre-Eclampsia

www.apni.org
020 7386 0868
Association for Postnatal Illness

www.asthma.org.uk
0800 121 6255

www.bliss.org.uk
Helpline 0500 618140
Support for families of premature and
special care babies

www.clapa.com
020 7833 4883
Cleft Lip and Palate Association

www.cafamily.org.uk
Helpline 0808 808 3555
Contact A Family: advice and support for
parents whose children have special needs

www.cry-sis.org.uk
Helpline 08451 228669
Advice for parents dealing with excessive
crying and sleep problems

www.diabetes.org.uk
Careline 0845 120 2960
Diabetes UK

www.diabetes.co.uk
0247 671 2201

www.downs-syndrome.org.uk
Helpline 0333 1212 300

www.eczema.org
Helpline 0800 089 1122

www.endo.org.uk
Helpline 0808 808 2227
The National Endometriosis Society

www.epilepsy.org.uk
Helpline 0808 800 5050

www.hyperemesis.org
Advice and information on hyperemesis
gravidarum

www.lupus.org.uk
St Thomas' lupus trust

www.miscarriageassociation.org.uk
Helpline 01924 200799

www.ocsupport.org.uk
The Obstetric Cholestasis Support website

www.pni.org.uk
Information and advice on postnatal
depression

www.scope.org.uk
Helpline 0808 800 3333
Information and advice on cerebral palsy

www.steps-charity.org.uk
Helpline 01925 750271
Information and advice on talipes
(club foot)

www.pre-eclampsia.co.uk

www.uk-sands.org
020 7436 5881
Stillbirth And Neonatal Death Society

Parent Groups

www.bestbear.co.uk
08707 201277
Information and advice on finding
childcare

www.dad.info
Information and guidance for expectant
and new dads

www.fatherhoodinstitute.org
0845 634 1328
Support for fathers

www.gingerbread.org.uk
0800 018 4518
Advice and information for single-parent
families

www.multiplebirths.org.uk
020 3313 3519
The Multiple Births Foundation

www.pacey.org.uk
0845 880 0044
Professional Association for Childcare
and Early Years

www.parentlineplus.org.uk
Helpline 0808 800 2222
Support and advice for parents

www.relate.org.uk
0300 100 1234
Relationship counselling

www.tamba.org.uk
Twinline 0800 138 0509
Twins & Multiple Births Association
(TAMBA)

www.twinsuk.co.uk
01670 458624

www.sitters.co.uk
0844 736 7367
Babysitting website

Rights and benefits

www.citizensadvice.org.uk

www.gov.uk
Employment and benefits

www.dwp.gov.uk
Department for Work and Pensions

www.hse.gov.uk
0845 345 0055
Health and Safety Executive

www.maternityaction.org.uk
Maternity rights and benefits

www.workingfamilies.org.uk
020 7253 7243
Advice and support for working parents

www.worksmart.org.uk
Information on maternity rights

General

www.bcma.co.uk
0845 345 5977
The British Complementary Medicine
Association

www.drinkaware.co.uk
020 7766 9900
Advice on drinking alcohol

www.eatwell.gov.uk
Advice on healthy eating

www.food.gov.uk
020 7276 8829
Food Standards Agency

www.smokefree.nhs.uk
0800 022 4332
NHS helpline for quitting smoking

www.homeopathy-soh.org
01604 817890

www.iaim.org.uk
020 8989 9597
International Association of Infant
Massage

www.nhs.uk
NHS choices: Health advice
and information

www.nhs.uk/nhsdirect/symptoms
Online symptom checkers

www.nhs.uk/111
Helpline 111
If you need medical help fast, but it's
not a 999 emergency

www.nimh.org.uk
01392 426022
The National Institute of Medical
Herbalists

www.nutrition.org.uk
020 7557 7930
Promoting nutritional wellbeing

www.quit.org.uk
Quitline 0800 002200
Helping smokers to stop

www.reflexology-uk.net
International Institute of Reflexology

www.talktofrank.com
Helpline 0800 776600
Information and support for drugs and
alcohol addiction

www.trusthomeopathy.org
01582 408675
British Homeopathic Association

www.vegsoc.org
0161 925 2000
Information on vegetarian diets during
pregnancy and for infants

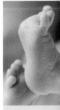

Index

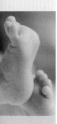

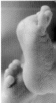

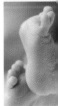

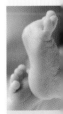

luteinizing hormone (LH) 38, 43, 47, 49
lying positions
    getting up safely 340
    in labour 421, 425

M

malaria 28–9
manganese 44
manicures 191
marijuana 24
"mask of pregnancy" 170, 190, 467
massage
    baby massage 458
    for back pain 296
    bump 175
    for constipation 171
    in labour 383
    pain relief 400
    perineal 336
    in second trimester 224, 257
    in third trimester 300
    see also reflexology
mastitis 475
maternity allowance (MA) 348, 349
maternity benefits 267
maternity bras 121
maternity leave 267
    arranging 140, 255
    beginning 361
    finances 291
    making the most of 366
    planning 281
    rights 348
    twins 237
maternity pay 255, 291, 337, 348–9
maternity stockings 225
maternity towels 443
mattresses, cot 269
MCADD (medium chain acyl-codehydrogenase deficiency) 454
measles 110
measurements
    baby's head 132
    bump 233
    crown-rump length (CRL) 131, 132, 139, 141, 185
    dating scan 139
    fundal height 279, 284
    growth charts 284
    newborn baby 463
    in second trimester 214
    small for dates 255
    ultrasound scans 159, 284–5
meat 14
    cravings 191
    fat content 204
    food safety 17, 101
    pork 164

"mechanisms of labour" 423
meconium 234, 328, 429
    fetal distress 474
medical history 122, 129
medical interventions, labour 415
medication
    after conception 60
    free prescriptions 349
    pain relief 402–7
    for pre-existing conditions 20–1
    safety in pregnancy 23
    speeding up slow labour 415
Mediterranean diet 104
melanin
    eye colour 354
    "mask of pregnancy" 190
    newborn baby 207
melon 127
membranes 304
    delivery of 428
    manual rupture 415, 417, 432
    membrane sweep 380, 393, 401, 432
    premature delivery 431
    waters breaking 304, 411
memory
    development of 240
    memories of labour 369
    memory problems 229, 271, 321
menstrual cycle 34–8
    after conception 56
    irregular cycles 65
menstruation see periods
mental problems, after birth 475
mercury pollution, in seafood 17, 96, 169
metabolism 77, 282
midwives 103, 146
    antenatal care 91, 102
    antenatal classes 265
    booking-in appointment 122, 129
    community midwives 445
    home birth 413
    independent midwives 91, 102
    midwifery-led units 103
    and post-birth trauma 459
    postnatal checks 446, 450, 457, 461
    role of 129
    shared care 102
    shortages of 387
    talking to 175
migraine 117
milia ("milk spots") 458, 477
milk see breast milk
milk teeth 110, 216
mineralocorticoids 266
minerals 15, 16
    baby's needs 340
miscarriage 144, 472
    after diagnostic tests 153
    causes 94

    conception after 47, 94
    exercise and 96
    late miscarriage 94
    twins 59
    types of 87, 94
    ultrasound scans 79
    in very early pregnancy 67
missed miscarriage 87, 94
mittelschmerz 43
mobile epidurals 404
mobile phones 25
moles 140, 170
Mongolian blue spots 476
monitoring 418–19, 426
    fetal heartbeat 188, 285, 381, 418–19
    multiple pregnancies 434
    twin births 435
monitors, baby 309, 329
monoamniotic twins 434
Montgomery's tubercles 309
mood swings 84, 101
morning sickness see nausea and vomiting
morning-after pill 73
morula 50, 57, 58
Moses baskets 269
mother's helps 332
mouth (baby's)
    cleft lip and palate 21, 476
    development of 118,136
    newborn baby 443
    rooting reflex 444
mouth (mother's), excess saliva 92
movements 218, 221, 233, 246
    active fetus 285
    changes in 257
    discomfort 277
    kick counts 273, 285
    in second trimester 178, 193, 206, 213, 219, 246
    in third trimester 273, 279, 304, 322, 380
    twins 222
MRSA superbug 389
mucus
    cervical 38, 43, 45
    in fetal lungs 182
    "show" 372, 391, 410, 411
multi-cultural society 82
multiple births see triplets; twins
mumps 110
muscles
    abdominal 89, 249, 313, 250, 278, 462
    baby's 89, 166, 322
    carb loading 366
    exercise in third trimester 356
    leg cramp 246, 470
    post-delivery exercises 456
    strengthening and toning exercises 90

music
    during labour 377
    music therapy 93
    playing to unborn baby 174, 252, 319
muslins 347
myths
    owls 374
    sex of baby 375

N

naevi
    spider 134, 140
    strawberry 476
nails (baby's)
    development of 222, 249, 330
    newborn baby 443, 457
nails (mother's)
    changes in pregnancy 26–7
    manicures 191
    varnish 27
nalaxone 403
names
    choosing 230, 231, 392
    Hawaiian 231
    for twins 231
nannies 332
nappies 238
    changing 445, 451
    contents 455
    crying baby and 454
    for twins 294
    types of 269, 291
nappy rash 451
naps
    in late pregnancy 379
    newborn baby 457
narcotic drugs 403
nasal congestion 165
National Childbirth Trust (NCT)
    antenatal classes 199, 265
    second-hand sales 301
natural birth 311
natural pain relief 398–41
nausea and vomiting 81, 111, 145, 467–8
    acupressure wristbands 111
    and food aversion 109
    hyperemesis gravidarum 111, 472
    ginger and 81
    medication for 23
    natural remedies 81
    in second trimester 159
    snacks and 80
    twin pregnancies 132
navel, protruding 319, 327
neck, development of 120, 128, 135, 168
neonatal intensive care units (NICU) 245, 452–3
neonatal nurses 453
neonatologists 103

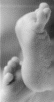

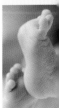

support belts (belly bands) 179, 278, 325, 329
support networks
    after birth 371
    single mothers 287
support pants 179
Sure Start Maternity Grant 349
surfactant 252, 356, 431
surgery, Caesarean section 406–7, 438–9
sutures, skull 386
swallowing
    amniotic fluid 146, 182, 220, 239
    baby's reflexes 282
swearing, in labour 378
sweat glands, development of 207
sweating 248, 270
sweeping the membranes 380, 393, 401, 432
swimming
    in late pregnancy 379
    safety of chlorine 25
    swimwear 213
    in second trimester 187
    in third trimester 268, 329, 350, 353
swollen feet and ankles 306, 353, 466–7
symphysis pubis dysfunction (SPD) 286
syndactyly 476
syntocinon/Syntometrine 428, 432, 439, 442
syphilis 123
systemic lupus erythematosus 21

T

"tail", embryo 78, 101
talipes (club foot) 476
talking to your baby 157
tanning beds 27
tanning lotions 27, 172
taste, sense of 135, 186, 328
tea
    green tea and fertility 46
    herbal teas 21, 134
    raspberry leaf tea 391
team midwifery care 102
tears, perineal 427
    assisted birth 436
    and baby's position 415
    perineal massage and 336
    problems 475
    stitches 442
teeth
    dental care 27, 133, 349
    development of 110, 193, 216
television 174
tendons, stretching 197, 208
TENS (Transcutaneous Electrical Nerve Stimulation) 399

terminal hair 364
testes (testicles)
    development of 128, 130, 226
    hydrocele 276
    undescended 276, 476
testosterone 266
    and fertility problems 56
    and ovulation 47
    and sex of baby 200
tests
    blood tests 122–3
    diagnostic tests 120, 129, 143, 152–3
    glucose tolerance test 305
    Guthrie test 454
    ovulation 43, 56
    pregnancy tests 63, 71
    screening tests 120, 123, 129, 142–3
    in second trimester 151, 179
    special care babies 453
    urine tests 123, 299
tetanus vaccination 105
tetracyclines 23, 107
thalassaemia 123
third stage of labour 397, 428–9
threatened miscarriage 87, 94
3D ultrasound scans 178, 209, 240, 258
throat infections 107
thrush 22, 133, 226, 471
thumb-sucking, in uterus 174, 176, 190, 219, 234, 242, 258, 315
thyroid gland
    development of 170
    problems 21
thyroxine 294
tiredness 466
    after birth 463
    in first trimester 84, 145
    in late pregnancy 379
    in second trimester 217
    in third trimester 279, 307, 337
toddlers see children
toenails see nails
toes
    development in first trimester 97, 108, 118, 125
    development in second trimester 155, 179, 213
    syndactyly 476
tokophobia 319
tongue, development of 110
toning exercises 90
tooth buds 193
topping and tailing 446
toxoplasmosis 56
    avoiding 17, 86, 101
    symptoms 25, 101
    testing for 123
trains, travelling on 344
trans fats 15, 204
transition stage 397, 416

transverse lie 336, 415
    twins 312
trauma, post-birth 459
travel 28–9
    deep vein thrombosis (DVT) 186
    in first trimester 131
    holidays 106
    on public transport 339, 344
    in second trimester 185
    to hospital 413
    vaccinations 105, 131
    see also cars
travel cots 269
tretinoin 27
triple test 142, 143, 151, 179
triplets
    antenatal care 162
    birth weight 335, 435
    conception 51
    labour 435
    length of pregnancy 312
    occurrence 155
    weight gain 141
trisomy 13 and 18, 142, 143, 152
trousers 151, 179
tryptophan 172, 177, 292, 379
turning a breech baby 364, 433
20-week scan (anomaly scan) 200, 208, 214–15
twins 59, 312
    amniotic fluid 316
    antenatal care 221
    antenatal classes 199
    birth weight 312, 335, 435
    bonding with 312, 355
    bonding with each other 177, 222
    breastfeeding 351, 448
    Caesarean section 307
    choosing names for 231
    clothes 294, 320
    conception 44, 49, 51
    coping strategies 450
    cots 288, 335
    delivery 434, 435
    diet in pregnancy 14
    exercise and 306
    in first trimester 132
    growth 294
    growth differences 190
    home birth 434
    incidence of 155
    induction of labour 432
    labour 435
    length of pregnancy 312
    lie in uterus 312
    maternity leave 237
    monitoring during pregnancy 434
    monoamniotic twins 434
    movements 222
    placenta 130

    premature labour 335
    risk factors 155
    screening tests 120
    in second trimester 186
    signs of 124
    in third trimester 274
    twin-to-twin transfusion syndrome (TTTS) 130, 434
    ultrasound scans 124
    weight gain 99, 141
    see also identical twins

U

ulcerative colitis 21
ultrasound scans
    "combined" test 142
    dating scan 74, 137, 138–9
    Doppler scans 188, 224, 285, 324, 418
    4D scans 258
    early scans 79
    hearing and 248
    measuring baby 159, 284–5
    monitoring labour 418
    nuchal translucency scan 120, 132, 142, 143
    safety 144
    sex of baby 211, 215
    3D scans 178, 209, 240, 258
    20-week scan (anomaly scan) 200, 208, 214–15
    twins 124
ultraviolet rays 29
umbilical cord 113, 126, 129, 136, 166, 247, 292
    blood vessels 98, 157
    coils 132, 205
    collection of stem cells 302
    "cord blood" 310
    cutting 428, 442
    delivery of placenta 428–9
    development of 68, 78, 84, 118, 134
    lotus birth 363
    monoamniotic twins 434
    prolapse 474
    round baby's neck 426
    stump 446
    in third trimester 390
    20-week scan 214
    twin births 435
    water birth 307
underweight
    body mass index 17
    and conception problems 40
    risks of 77
    weight gain 99, 195
unsaturated fats 14, 204
upright positions, in labour 424
upright row exercise 196
urethra 125
urge incontinence 475

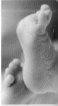

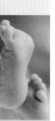

Index

Acknowledgments

Maggie Blott's acknowledgments

I would like to thank the Pregnancy and Childcare team at Dorling Kindersley for their help, guidance, and expert knowledge. In particular I would like to thank Andrea Bagg for her patience and support. I would also like to thank my children Polly, Jess, and Eddie for their love and for putting up with me and my preoccupation during this project.

Publisher's acknowledgments

Indexer Hilary Bird
Proofreader Angela Baynham
Additional Editorial Assistance Suhel Ahmed, Ann Baggaley, Terry Moore, Helen Murray, Diana Vowles
Additional Design Assistance Isabel de Cordova, Charlotte Seymour
New Photography Ruth Jenkinson
Art Direction for Photography Emma Forge
Illustration Assistance Amanda Williams
Additional illustrations Philip Wilson
Picture Librarian Romaine Werblow
Additional Picture Research Jenny Baskaya
Hair & Make-up Stylist for Photography Alli Williams
Photographer's Assistants Sarah Bailey and Carly Churchill
Assistant to Art Director for Photography Susie Sanford
Location Agency www.1st-Option.com

Dorling Kindersley would like to thank all the authors and illustrators for their expertise and dedication. We are grateful to the following individuals and organizations for their help:
Dr Mary Steen RGN, RM, BHSc PGCRM, PGDipHE, MCGI, PhD for consultancy work and editorial assistance.
Catharine Parker-Littler SRN, RSCN, SCM, DPSM (Advanced midwifery), BscMid (Hons) for permission to reuse text from *Ask a Midwife*.
Dr Paul Moran MD, MRCOG for consultation and expert advice on all embryonic and fetal images. His invaluable contribution provided not only the fetal text and all fetal captions, but he also sourced, scanned, and supplied images when all other image sources had been exhausted. Paul would like to thank the women who helped him to provide the images for this book and Maggie Blott for the opportunity to work on such a fascinating title.
Dr Pranav Pandya BSc, MRCOG, MD for advice on embryonic and fetal images.
The women at the Royal Victoria Infirmary who gave permission for their scans to be used in this book.
Nicola, Joe and Leo Hayward and **Reuben Marcus** for allowing us to use photographs of themselves.

A special thank you to:
University College Hospital London for permission to photograph in the new Elizabeth Garrett Anderson (EGA) Wing. Many thanks also to the midwives, who helped and advised during photography and who also in some cases modelled for us.

The new University College Hospital Elizabeth Garrett Anderson (EGA) Wing opened its doors to women and their babies in the first week of November 2008. The £70 million wing includes three floors dedicated to the care of mothers and babies and has been specially designed to ensure all women have ready access to the integrated care they and their babies may require. Maternity care is provided by midwifery, obstetric, neonatal and anaesthetic consultants with their teams and core midwifery staff working together to deliver up to 6,000 babies a year.

Mothers will receive care from the same team of midwives throughout their pregnancy. All women who are anticipated to have low risk pregnancies and deliveries will be offered the facilities of the Bloomsbury Birthing Centre – providing a home-from-home philosophy.

The Elizabeth Garrett Anderson (EGA) Wing houses antenatal and post-natal beds, high-dependency maternity unit beds, birthing rooms, birthing pools, special care cots, and neonatal intensive care cots. As well as providing care for women with normal pregnancies, the staff also care for women with very complicated, high risk pregnancies and treat some of the sickest and most vulnerable babies in the UK with the most modern equipment and up-to-date and highly trained medical, midwifery, and nursing teams.

Picture credits

Most of the scans and photographs of the developing baby in this book are of the embryo and fetus live in utero, pictured using endoscopic and ultrasound technology. When this has not been possible, images have been taken by reputable medical professionals as part of research or to promote educational awareness.

Dorling Kindersley would like to thank the following for their kind permission to reproduce their photographs:
(Key: a-above; b-below/bottom; c-centre; f-far; l-left; r-right; t-top)
Alamy Images: 322tl; Angela Hampton Picture Library 266bc; Avatra Images 33cra, 84br; Marie-Louise Avery 135cl; Peter Banos 58cr; Bubbles Photolibrary 10tr, 20br, 148br, 185cr, 233bc, 242br, 317br, 328br; Adam Burton 125br; Camera Press Ltd 255bc, 268bc; Form Advertising 338br; David J. Green 76bc; Jennie Hart 47bl; Juergen Hasenkopf 95br; Janine Wiedel Photolibrary 405bl, 438br; Martin Hughes-Jones 154cr; Medical-on-Line 381cl; Picture Partners 235c, 369br, 380c; Pregnancy Maternity And Motherhood/Mark Sykes 365bl; Profimedia International s.r.o. 3fcla; Chris Rout 119bc, 148bc, 193c, 232cr; **babyarchive.com:** MJ Kim 42cl; **Babybond® www.babybond.com:** 2clb, 146tl, 149bc, 149bl, 149fbl, 173tl, 183tl, 199tl, 206bc, 206bl, 206br, 218tl, 256bc, 257tl, 258tl, 262fcl, 262ftl, 262tl, 263bc, 281tl, 282tl, 283tl, 286tl, 287tl, 288tl, 289tl, 292tl, 294tl, 306tl, 310tl, 311tl, 320tl, 323br, 327tl, 328tl, 329tl, 330tl, 332tl, 333tl, 336tl, 337tl, 338tl, 339tl, 340tl, 353tl; **BSIP:** 166tl, 235tl, 253tl; Ramare 174tl, 240bc, 343tl, 350tl, 351tl; SGO 131tl, 270tl, 271tl, 296tl; **Bubbles:** Moose Azim 333bl; **Corbis:** Heide Benser / zefa 180br; Brooke Fasani 341bc, 382bl; Rolf Bruderer 198c; Cameron 426c; Kevin Dodge 77bl; Annie Engel / zefa 200bl, 335bc, 375bc; Wolfgang Flamisch / zefa 387c; Owen Franken (sidebar); Rick Gomez 3fcrb, 10tc, 32cra, 158bc, 177c; Ole Graf/zefa 32bc; Rune Hellestad 389bc, 438bl; A. Inden / zefa 171cl; JLP/Sylvia Torres 2fcla; Michael A. Keller 60cr, 64bc; Jutta Klee

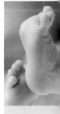

140c; Mika / zefa 80bl, 101bc; Markus Moellenberg/zefa 2crb, 31tc; Moodboard 273cl; Kevin R Morris 314br; Peter Pfander / zefa 351bc; Shift Foto / zefa 261bc; Ariel Skelley 6fbl, 464cl; Tom Stewart 245cr; Larry Williams 6fcr, 205br, 289br, 297cr, 395cr; **Custom Medical Stock Photo:** 127tl; **Dreamstime.com:** Monkey Business Images 37br, 57cl, 65cr, 292bc; Pliene 159tl; Shahar 204br; Shipov 180tl; Starush 256bl; Studio1one 162tl; **fotolia:** Liv friis-larsen 134cl; Nyul 75cr; **Getty Images:** 83bc, 311cr, 374c; Altrendo 412bc; Altrendo Images 356bl; B2M Productions 54l; Blend Images 73cr; Blend Images/Jose Luis Pelaez Inc 6cra, 30tr; Blend Images/PBNJ Productions 33bl; Leland Bobbe 313cr; Daniel Bosler 287br; Noah Clayton 164bc; Taxi / Colorstock 157br; Donna Day 270bc; DK Stock 63br; DK Stock / Michael Rowe 172br; Dorling Kindersley / Sian Irvine 173br; Gazimal 117bl; George Doyle 339bc; Vladimir Godnik 309bc; Sammy Hart 354c; Frank Herholdt 263br; Dorling Kindersley / Ian Hooton 209br; Ian Hooton 295br; Iconica 45c; Iconica / Andersen Ross 241br; Image Bank/Tracy Frankel 263bl; Image Source 149cra; Blend Images / Jose Luis Pelaez Inc 251br; Ruth Jenkinson 306cr; Christina Kennedy 223br; Jutta Klee 169cr; The Image Bank / Bernhard Lang 115cr; Lecorre Productions 145cr; StockFood Creative / Louise Lister 114br; LWA 462c; LWA/The Image Bank 367c; Laurence Monneret 385br; Nacivet 371br, 373br; Peter Nicholson 131br; Sarma Ozols 357cr; Barbara Peacock 262bc; Iconica / Jose Luis Pelaez 110c; Photonica 97bc; Louie Psihoyos 453tl; Riser 44cr, 116bc; Riser/ Frank Herholdt 3crb; Riser/Laurence Monneret 263cr; Stockbyte 86c, 263ftl, 327br; Stockbyte/George Doyle 2cla; StockFood Creative 33ca; Stone 39c, 105br; Stone / James Baigrie 207br; Stone/Jerome Tisne 148; Jonathan Storey 246bc; Studio MPM 283c; Taxi 66br; Taxi / Bernd Opitz 252tl; Taxi / DreamPictures 106br; Jerome Tisne 151br; Titus 275bc; Tobias Titz 127cl; Paul Venning 379cr; Simon Wilkinson 139br; ZenShui / Laurence Mouton 316cr; **iStockphoto.com:** Alex Bramwell 104br; Dirk Richter 259c; **Prof. J.E. Jirasek MD, DSc.:** 3cra, 11tl, 32br, 33tc, 33tl, 68tl, 69tl, 71tl, 72tl, 73tl, 75tl, 76bl, 83tl, 87tl, 96cr, 96tl, 101tl, 104tl, 107tl, 110tl, 114tl, 115tl, 149tl, 149tr, 232tl, 242tl, 249tl; **jupiterimages:** Pixland 91cl; **Lennart Nilsson Image Bank:** 33ftl, 65tl, 87cr, 91tl, 93cr, 93tl, 99tl, 100tl, 107cr, 126cr, 156cr, 219tl, 231c; **Life Issues Institute:** 125tl, 181tl, 200tr, 260tl; **LOGIQlibrary:** 113br, 138c; **Masterfile:** 191cl, 237bc; Jerzyworks 224c, 304cr; Michael A. Keller 180bc; **Mediscan:** 120tl, 211tl, 237tl; **Mother & Baby Picture Library:** 262br, 282bc, 426cl, 435cr; Dave J. Anthony 238bc; Moose Azim 307br, 427bc, 427br; Ian Hooton 6bl, 6cla, 6fcl, 6tr, 12tr, 26br, 28br, 30tc, 33br, 103bc, 122bc, 122cb, 138b, 142l, 146cl, 199c, 229bc, 230c, 243cr, 262tr, 263tl, 267cr, 278br, 279br, 286bc, 299c, 300br, 302br, 321bc, 348, 383bc, 393c, 394cl, 397c, 402cr, 411tr, 465cl; Ruth Jenkinson 3fcra, 6cl, 6crb, 11tc, 13tr, 239cr, 288br, 319cr, 331cr, 394c, 399tl, 407cr, 409bl, 416br, 432bc, 441tc; Eddie Lawrence 6cr, 395cl, 399b; Paul Mitchell 8-9, 31tl, 149cl, 203cr, 320br; James Thomson 13tc, 19; **Dept of Fetal Medicine, Royal Victoria Infirmary, Newcastle upon Tyne:** 97tl, 111, 140tl, 161tl, 165tl, 167tl, 170tl, 187tl, 188tl, 274tl, 275tl, 276tl, 277tl, 278tl, 279tl, 297tl, 299tl, 300tl, 304tl, 305tl, 314tl, 316tl, 317tl, 325tl, 370tl, 374tl, 375tl, 377tl, 378tl, 379tl, 380tl, 381tl, 382tl, 383tl, 385tl, 386tl, 388tl,

389tl, 392tl; **Dr Pranav P Pandya:** 143c, 143cr, 285c, 285cr; **Photolibrary:** Banana Stock 2fclb, 103cl, 429b, 464c; Pierre Bourrier 133cr; Brand X Pictures 167bc; Neil Bromhall 226bl; OSF / Derek Bromhall 190tl; OSF / Neil Bromhall 221tl, 223tl, 229tl, 233tl, 255tl; OSF / Densey Clyne 193tl, 194br, 194tl, 203tl; Fresh Food Images/Robert Lawson 32tl; Henry Horenstein 366tl; Robert Lawson 322c; Graham Monro 430; Andersen Ross 323bc; Joy Skipper 332cr; **Phototake:** Dr Benoit/Mona Lisa 365tl; Sovereign 355tl; **PunchStock:** 442; **Reflexstock:** Agencja Free / Rafal Strzechowski 221br; **Rex Features:** 309tl; Prof Stuart Campbell 105tl, 106tl, 151tl, 154tl, 172tl, 189tl, 198tl, 209tl, 216tl, 217tl, 225tl, 226tl, 245tl, 252, 261tl, 269tl, 293tl, 295tl, 307tl, 321tl, 345tl, 361tl, 363tl, 387tl; **Science Photo Library:** 21tl, 77tl, 120bc, 169tl, 207tl, 240tl, 262c, 284tl; AJ Photo 335tl; Anatomical Travelogue 49tl, 63tl, 64tl, 67cl, 79tl, 81tl, 84tl, 86tl, 89tl, 92tl, 117tl, 129tl, 133tl, 145tl, 158tl, 174c, 197tl, 291tl, 344tl, 362tl, 364tl, 371tl; Samuel Ashfield 343br, 364c; Bernard Benoit / Kretz Technik 341tl; Thierry Berrod, Mona Lisa Production 354tl; Biophoto Associates 36tl; Neil Borden 215tc, 215tl; Neil Bromhall 230tl, 241tl, 243tl; Neil Bromhall / Genesis Films 227tl; BSIP Estiot 57tl; BSIP VEM 40tl; BSIP, ASTIER 395c, 434bl; BSIP, ATL 324tl; BSIP, Cavallini James 124bl; BSIP, Laurent 418br; John Burbridge 47tl; CIMN, ISM 266tl, 273cr; Clouds Hill Imaging Ltd 10tl; Clouds Hill Imaging Ltd. 53cr; CNRI 428c; Kevin Curtis 378bl; Dopamine 135tl, 163tl, 175tl, 178tl, 179tl; Dr Keith Wheeler 43tl; Du Cane Medical Imaging Ltd 367tl, 386c; Edelmann 41c, 72cr, 100c, 109tl, 119tl, 124tl, 132tl, 134tl, 144tl, 148ftr, 148tr, 155tl, 157tl, 166bl, 171tl, 182br, 185tl, 213tl, 222tl, 234tl, 238tl, 239tl, 256tl, 347tl, 369tl; Simon Fraser 141tl, 370br; GE Medical Systems 372tl, 373tl; Steve Gschmeissner 37tl, 41tl, 46tl, 48tl; Ian Hooton 1c, 2cra, 2fcrb, 3cla, 4-5c, 6fbr, 14, 24bc, 46br, 103bl, 129c, 149cb, 149ftl, 188cl, 214bc, 263c, 398br, 455c, 464cr, 465cr; Dr Isabelle Cartier, ISM 45tl; Jean-Claude Revy-A. Goujeon, ISM 66tl; K.H. Kjeldsen 60tl; Mehau Kulyk 186tl, 246tl, 251tl; Dr Najeeb Layyous 95tl, 116tl, 121tl, 126tl, 130tl, 137tl, 156tl, 182tl, 186bc, 204tl, 208tl, 212tl, 222bl, 231tl, 267bc, 268tl, 274br, 313tl, 357tl, 358tl, 359tl; Living Art Enterprises, Llc 215c, 215cl; Cecilia Magill 6fcra, 31tr; Manfred Kage 39tl; Matt Meadows 346tl, 391tl; Hank Morgan 206tl; Dr Yorgos Nikas 50bl, 50br, 50fbr; Dr Yorgos Nikos 59bc, 59tl; Susumu Nishinaga 44tl; Lea Paterson 20bc; D. Phillips 50fbl, 53tl; Photo Researchers, Inc / Nestle / Petit Format 205tl; Alain Pol, ISM 248tl; Prof. P. Motta / Dept. of Anatomy / University 56tl; Prof. P. Motta / Dept. of Anatomy / University "LA SAPIENZA", Rome 49bc; Professors P.m. Motta & J. Van Blerkom 32tr; Professors P.M. Motta & S. Makabe 35tr; R. Bick, B. Poindexter, UT Medical School 67tl; P. Saada / Eurelios 138tc; Sovereign, ISM 139tl, 177tl, 178cr; James Stevenson 259tl; BSIP, Kretz Technik 319tl; Tek Image 310br; Alexander Tsiaras 132cr, 162cr; Zephyr 38tl, 331tl; **University College London Hospitals:** 271cr; **Wellcome Library, London:** 80tl, 164tl, 190br, 191tl, 195tl, 224tl, 265tl; Yorgos Nikas 61tl; Anthea Sieveking 429tr; **Wikipedia, The Free Encyclopedia:** Acaparadora 43bl

All other images © Dorling Kindersley
For further information see: www.dkimages.com